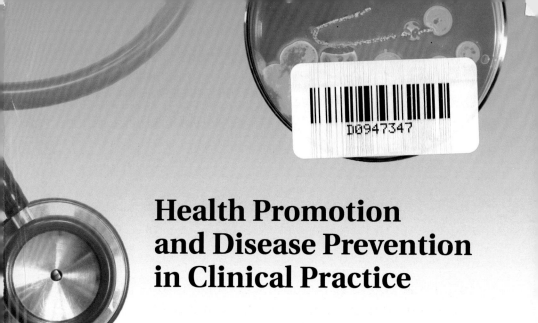

Health Promotion
and Disease Prevention
in Clinical Practice

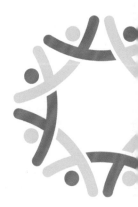

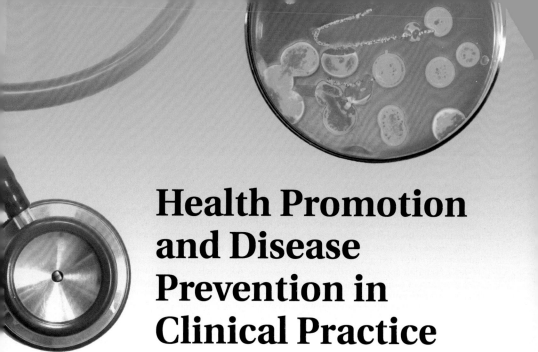

Health Promotion and Disease Prevention in Clinical Practice

THIRD EDITION

Jessica Coviello, DNP, APRN, ANP-BC
Associate Professor of Nursing
Yale School of Nursing
Orange, Connecticut

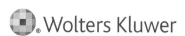. Wolters Kluwer

Philadelphia • Baltimore • New York • London
Buenos Aires • Hong Kong • Sydney • Tokyo

Executive Editor: Rebecca Gaertner
Development Editors: Ashley Fischer, Eric McDermott
Editorial Coordinator: Annette Ferran
Marketing Manager: Rachel Mante Leung
Senior Production Project Manager: Alicia Jackson
Senior Designer: Joan Wendt
Senior Manufacturing Coordinator: Beth Welsh
Prepress Vendor: TNQ Technologies

Printed in China

Library of Congress Cataloging-in-Publication Data

Names: Coviello, Jessica Shank, editor.
Title: Health promotion and disease prevention in clinical practice / [edited by] Jessica Coviello.
Description: Third edition. | Philadelphia : Wolters Kluwer, [2020] | Includes bibliographical references and index.
Identifiers: LCCN 2018059851 | ISBN 9781496399960
Subjects: | MESH: Preventive Health Services | Health Promotion | Preventive   Medicine | United States
Classification: LCC RA427.8 | NLM WA 108 | DDC 613–dc23
LC record available at https://lccn.loc.gov/2018059851

shop.LWW.com

The author wishes to acknowledge all previous and current contributors who have dedicated their lives to health promotion and disease prevention with the hope that we will all come to see a healthier America.

Foreword

"Treatment without prevention is simply unsustainable."
—Bill Gates

Up until this century, the biggest threats to our humanity have been famine, plague, and war, which wreaked unspeakable suffering and early death. These three hazards were solely responsible for wiping out entire families and large swaths of the global population in short periods of time. For the first time in humankind, famine, plague, and war have been replaced by overeating and suicide as the leading cause of premature death and disability. Consider the following facts:
In 2012,[1] 56 million people died across the globe.

- 6,200,000 to human violence
  - 120,000 to war
  - 50,000 to crime
  - 800,000 committed suicide
- 1.5 million died of diabetes

More people die from eating too much than from eating too little; we are dying of old age rather than infectious disease. More of the world's population dies prematurely due to their own hand in suicide rather than terrorism, war, or crime *combined*. There is more disability and premature death from eating highly palatable, low-nutrient food than from famine, drought, Ebola, or ISIS attacks combined. We are experiencing high rates of addiction, loneliness, lack of belonging, disconnection, and untreated mental illness. These social factors are all precursors to suicide or other less permanent self-destructive behaviors, such as binge eating, gambling, or Internet addiction. The World Health Organization[2] has identified 4 health habits that are most responsible for disability and early death across the globe and that are entirely preventable:

1. Insufficient exercise
2. Unhealthy food
3. Alcohol abuse
4. Tobacco

---

[1] Harari YN. *Homo deus: A brief history of tomorrow*. Harper Collins Publishers; 2016.
[2] The World Health Organization Global Observatory Data (2015–2017). *Non-communicable diseases*. Retrieved from World Health Organization: http://www.who.int/gho/ncd/en/index.html.

These alarming data present a cosmic shift that requires health care providers to look up and out at the environment we are all living in, toward a new way of helping people and society prevent disease and promote health. This requires a shift in mindset that looks at risk clear-eyed. It often requires a herculean emotional and physical effort to overcome a lifestyle that allows people to "host" a chronic preventable illness. The challenges in promoting health and preventing disease are enormous and cannot be left to a single profession or scientific body of knowledge. This is an adaptive problem; it will require the interdisciplinary cooperation of multiple areas of expertise, laid out in this book.

COMPLEXITY

We are all promoting health and preventing disease in a highly complex world, one with far more moving parts and layers than previous generations experienced. This VUCA world, one which is Violative, Uncertain, Complex, and Ambiguous, creates a health care habitat that requires a different approach to the patients that present to us. We are confronted with the demand to do more with less and a public that has access to unlimited (and uncurated) information that does not necessarily draw from an evidence base or translate to wisdom. Three examples that make promoting health and preventing disease especially demanding for clinicians are the "anti-vaxxer" movement, the weight loss industry, and novel devices that deliver the known carcinogen, tobacco.

- **The anti-vaxxer movement** whose insistence that vaccines are toxic have led to resurgence of measles, mumps, pertussis and whooping cough across the country. This group is especially impervious to scientific fact. The opposition to vaccines stems largely from a deep distrust of science than for religious reasons. This distrust of science can extend to health care providers who do not support homeopathic remedies lacking an evidence base for deadly diseases, making disease prevention for this population uniquely difficult.
- **The $7 billion weight loss industry** is largely unregulated and for the most part lacks any evidence whatsoever. An Internet search on "weight loss" finds commercial products claiming $40 vegan skinny oil, B12 patches, cleanses, detox powders, and thousands of supplements and bars. It is not easy to find a place to learn how to relate to real food in a healthy way. We have food desserts where impoverished communities have no access to unprocessed food. We have a food industry that does not concern itself with health and a health system that does not concern itself with food. Getting sound solution to the obesity epidemic is no simple matter.
- **New ways of using known carcinogens.** There is growing alarm that tobacco delivery systems are attracting adolescent users at high rates

in the form of vaping, e-cigarettes, and Juuls. Some of these systems deliver tobacco in smoke-free "microdoses" with added sweetener. Thus, they are creating the illusion that the known carcinogen is "nontoxic" and "not addictive." They are being marketed as mood enhancers, and the delivery system resembles a USB flash drive, creating a novel and alluring approach to getting young people addicted.

"What cruel mistakes are sometimes made by benevolent men and women in matters of business about which they can know nothing and think they know a great deal."
—Florence Nightingale, Notes on Nursing, 1859

We are seeing shockingly low levels of the population receiving even the minimal recommended preventive measures and continue to face challenges with patients making scheduled preventive visits. The chapters contained in this book are a "how-to" for clinicians to address these multifaceted challenges. The remedy for complexity is to move away from the one-on-one approach and develop high-functioning teams and systems to move prevention to the center stage. This book directly focuses on the complex environment in which preventive services are delivered with the remedies of sharing decision making with patients by interdisciplinary teams. It asks the provider to consider how to design office systems to make health promotion and disease prevention the default and to automate these services and integrate them into the workflow and "sick visits."

THE FUTURE

As we look to the future in health promotion and disease prevention, we can expect to see more integration of wearable devices with electronic medical record (EMR), liquid biopsies, more population-based "scalable" interventions, and more customized health risk profiles using DNA. There are successful trials deploying home health robots to keep shut-in elders in their homes as companions, to provide basic care services, and to communicate remotely with the health care team. This will require skills in which the clinician is more innovative with integration of technology and expertise in the science of how people initiate and sustain intentional change described in this book. We may see more employers making health promotion the default such as what some exemplars are doing by pricing their cafeteria food, deeply discounting healthy whole food and up charging processed food. Or having standing desks, walking meetings, and requiring tobacco users to contribute more for their health insurance coverage.

We have known for centuries that social determinants of health have the largest impact on health status. Risk factors often clump together, and patients can be encased in an environment that goes directly against the pursuit of wellness. There are many forces working against health promotion and disease prevention, and this important book, by a wide range of experts, outlines the best practices and skills necessary for modern clinicians. The editors and authors of *Health Promotion and Disease Prevention in Clinical Practice 3rd Edition* have described the enormous challenges by providing a blueprint for individual clinicians to improve the health of the nation.

Eileen T. O'Grady, PhD, RN, NP
Certified Nurse Practitioner and Wellness Coach
Founder, The School of Wellness

Preface

"Be the change you wish to see in the world."
—Mahatma Gandhi

This book was originally published in 1996 as a how-to guide for delivering preventative health care services. Its contents extended beyond presenting the evidence to providing the details associated with the actual delivery of the care, such as performing a pap smear or a rectal examination or counseling a patient in lifestyle change.

The second edition, published in 2008, continued in this tradition by providing updated guideline evidence, supporting data, and resources. This book was meant for a wide audience of providers, and contributors were physician experts in the field of preventative care.

The purpose of the this third edition is to provide updated evidence in support of preventative care as seen through the lens of population health and told by an interdisciplinary team of expert providers. Patient-centered, interdisciplinary approaches add value to the primary health care team by increasing access to diagnostic and therapeutic services and represent the trend in care delivery. Contributors include a wide range of disciplines, including registered dietitians, exercise physiologists, nurse practitioners, physician assistants, psychologists, public health experts, and physicians. The focus of this book remains risk factor identification and reduction rather than a specific symptom complex or problem. It does not discuss the detailed treatment for existing disease. The emphasis is on health promotion, a plan for health maintenance, and strategies for assisting patients in adopting a healthy lifestyle. It is a practical guide to health promotion and disease prevention, and although clinical practice guidelines are used to validate approaches to care, absent is original research or systematic review that can be accessed using the online resources as seen in Online Appendix A ⊕. Contents of the book take into consideration the changes in health care policy, reimbursement, technology, resources, and data since 2008. One of the most important policy changes in the delivery of health promotion services in the United States was the enactment of the Patient Protection and Affordable Care Act (ACA) of 2010. The ACA removes barriers to the delivery of preventive services by mandating that nearly all private health plans with plan-years beginning on or after September 23, 2010, cover these services without cost to the patient. Leading scientific and medical authorities, with federal support, have provided evidence documenting cost-effectiveness of evidence-based preventive services, ultimately resulting in the mandate for all private health plans to provide evidence-based screening, counseling, routine immunizations, and preventive services for children, youth, and women. Although coverage has been in flux with the recent change in the political environment, preventative services remain a focus in care.

Another major change since the last edition is the change seen in technology, in EMR programs, and in applications that address office management of preventative services. Resources in this area are now extensive with experts in their operation weighing the advantages of a specific platform based on the size and extent of the office practice. Please visit the eBook to view Online Appendix A 🌐 for resources.

The text aims to answer several questions related to risk development and identifies factors associated with health risk both in the individual and the community. (1) What is population health and why does it matter? (2) How does population health work, particularly in health care systems? (3) What are some best practices of population health management in health care delivery systems? (4) How do we assess for individual risk? (5) How do we help patients lead a healthy lifestyle? (6) What are desired outcomes? How do best practices guide us? What are EMR methods in following individual and population-based outcomes?

The text opens with a new chapter to this edition, a presentation of population health. This term is increasingly used in health care delivery systems, public health, academia, research, advocacy, and policy-making arenas as a key to improving health outcomes for all people. The continuous increase in population, migration, longevity, lack of access to health care, and unsustainable growth of health care costs and disparities in health and outcomes has forced the United States to embrace the population health approach as a viable way for improving our health status and health care delivery systems.

In Chapters 2–5, we take the reader from population risk to the process of individual risk assessment. The finer points of the history and physical examination as a guide to identifying health behaviors, health decision making, and preclinical disease are presented. Chapter 5 identifies standard laboratory screening tests and their meaning and documentation.

Principles of health behavior change and health promotion strategies are presented in Chapters 6–17. These chapters provide expert advice to translate the evidence into meaningful information addressing a patient's health risk, social determinants, ways of knowing, and decision making. Tools found in these chapters help the provider engage the patient in education to modify recognized risk, establish a health maintenance program, and structure decisions related to follow-up, treatment, and immunizations. Recommendations are validated with specific evidence-based practice guidelines that can be found and accessed online and through applications that can be downloaded to iPad, iPhone, or android. A list of these applications can be found in Online Appendix A 🌐 accessible through the eBook bundled with this text.

The practice environment has changed since 2008. The use of technology as a quick, up-to-date resource to information that guides decision making in the patient care environment is wide spread even in the most rural areas in the United States. In keeping with this change, Online Appendix A 🌐 provides the reader with a list of resources that can be downloaded to iPhone, iPad, or android. Resources cover practice guidelines, patient educational resources, and general guides to practice. This list of resources has been thoughtfully created by our contributors who are providers and academicians active in providing direct care, the policy arena, health care systems management, and academia. It is a ready list that will evolve as the practice guidelines change ensuring access to the most recent data.

Immediately before the publication of the last edition, the Centers for Medicare and Medicaid Services proposed pay for performance (P4P) as a solution to the sustainable growth problem in Medicare. Since that time, health care has been transforming to a value-based system characterized by the move from fee for service to alternative payment models and from sole practices and freestanding hospitals to medical homes, accountable care organizations, large hospital systems, and organized clinics, such as Kaiser Permanente, for example. The purpose of this move was to reward clinicians and health care organizations that are capable of achieving high performance quality measures. Data show outcomes shifts, however, are yet to be actualized.

Along the lines of reimbursement, the 10th revision of the International Statistical Classification of Diseases and Related Health problems, a medical classification of the World Health Organization, also known as the ICD-10 code, was revised in October 2015. The ICD-10 is a globally recognized international system for recording diagnoses that follows an international standard making certain the diagnosis is interpreted the same way by every profession. The new coding system increased diagnostic codes from approximately 14,000 to more than 68,000 and procedure codes from 4,000 to 87,000 with the promise to improve quality reporting and outcomes measurement as well as streamline reimbursement processes. Clinical resources and coder education helped make the transition in the United States possible by ensuring that clinicians met the level of coding specificity needed to obtain reimbursement, comply with regulatory requirements, and accurately reflect patient care. Efforts to enhance coding accuracy through training between clinicians and coders ensured that documentation accurately reflected the quality of care provided. Better documentation provides for better reimbursement. The Current Procedure Terminology (CPT) codes were revised in October 2017 and are used to identify services provided and are used by insurance companies to determine how much a provider will be paid for services. Resources for both ICD-10 and CPT coding, specific to preventative services, can be found in Online Appendix A 🌐.

We end the book with a glance into the future of health promotion and disease prevention with a sense of optimism and adventure. Several ideas are presented and provide opportunity for readers to discuss and debate how this vision for health promotion and disease prevention in primary care can be realized. Future and current health care providers are challenged to consider the chapter's content, assess the current state of health promotion and disease prevention policy, discuss possible goals and measurable outcomes, and develop strategies for potential change. The reader is challenged to become an agent of change and is asked to consider the complex issues of policy development, funding, implementation, and evaluation so that health care for all people can be actualized.

Jessica Coviello, DNP, APRN, ANP-BC
Associate Professor of Nursing
Yale School of Nursing
Orange, Connecticut

Contributors

Nancy C. Banasiak, DNP, PPCNP-BC, APRN
Associate Professor
Yale University School of Nursing
Department of Nursing
Orange, Connecticut

Babette Biesecker, FNP-BC, PhD
Clinical Assistant Professor and
  Program Director of FNP and Holistic
  Sequence
NYU Rory Meyers College of Nursing
Department of Graduate Nursing, FNP
New York, New York

David Brissette, MMSc, PA-C
Assistant Professor
Yale University School of Medicine
  Physician Associate Program
Department of Internal Medicine
New Haven, Connecticut

Carolynn Spera Bruno, FNP-C, PhD
Clinical Assistant Professor
New York University Rory Meyers
  College of Nursing
Department of Nursing
New York, New York

Alison Moriarty Daley, PhD
Associate Professor
Yale University School of Nursing
Master's Program
Orange, Connecticut

Mary Dietmann, EdD
Clinical Associate Professor
Sacred Heart University College of
  Nursing
College of Nursing
Fairfield, Connecticut

Lisa M. Fucito, PhD
Associate Professor
Yale University School of Medicine
Department of Psychiatry
New Haven, Connecticut

Linda T. Gottlieb, MA
Research Associate III
Yale University School of Public Health
MEPH School of Public Health
New Haven, Connecticut

Janelle Guirguis-Blake, MD
Clinical Professor
University of Washington
Department of Family Medicine
Tacoma, Washington

Russell Harris, MD, MPH
Emeritus Professor
University of North Carolina at Chapel
  Hill
Department of Medicine
Chapel Hill, North Carolina

Kelly F. Holtz, EdD
Certified Health Education Specialist,
  Educator
Wilton High School
Department of Health
Wilton, Connecticut

Lisa Kimmel, MS, RD, CDN
Director of Wellness and Health
  Education
Yale University
Department of Wellness
Milford, Connecticut

Leslie Ann Kole, PA-C, MS
Physician Assistant
Mobile Medical Care
Heart Clinic
Bethesda, Maryland

Geraldine F. Marrocco, EdD
Associate Professor
Yale University School of Nursing
Department of Nursing
West Haven, Connecticut

Martha Okafor, PhD
Lecturer
Yale University
Yale School of Nursing
Orange, Connecticut

Susanne J. Phillips, DNP
Associate Dean of Clinical Affairs
University of California Irvine
Sue & Bill Gross School of Nursing
Irvine, California

Elizabeth Roessler, MMSc, PA-C
Assistant Professor
Yale University School of Medicine
Department of Internal Medicine
New Haven, Connecticut

Mary Savoye, RDN, CDE
Clinical and Research Dietitian &
    Associate Director, Pediatric Obesity
Yale University School of Medicine
Department of Pediatric & Adult
    Endocrinology
New Haven, Connecticut

Erica S. Spatz, MD, MHS
Assistant Professor
Yale University School of Medicine
Department of Cardiovascular
    Medicine
New Haven, Connecticut

Linda Trinh, DNP, FNP-C, PMHNP-BC, MPH
Doctor of Nursing Practice, Family NP,
    Psychiatric Mental Health NP
Optihealth
Psychiatric Mental Health
Irvine, California

Robert M. Weinrieb, MD
Physician
University of Pennsylvania Perelman
    School of Medicine
Department of Psychiatry
Philadelphia, Pennsylvania

Contents

🌐 Indicates material is available online through the eBook bundled with this text. Please
see the inside front cover for eBook access instructions.

Acknowledgments

The editor and authors of the third edition would like to thank those who contributed to the previous editions of this text.

First edition

Henrietta N. Barnes, David H. Bor, Willard Cates, Jr., Bruce V. Davis, Paul S. Frame, Dorian Lizabeth Ravenese, Alan R. Greene, John C. Greene, David A. Grimes, Tee L. Guidotti, Hilliard Jason, Mark B. Johnson, Steven Jonas, William J. Kassler, John M. Last, Robert S. Lawrence, Perrianne Lurie, Marc Manley, Thom A. Mayer, Marion Nestle, Julian Orenstein, Michael D. Parkinson, Thomas H. Payne, Michael E. Stuart, Stephen H. Taplin, Robert S. Thompson, Edward H. Wagner, Judith N. Wasserheit, Jane Westberg, Steven H. Woolf

Second edition

Randall T. Brown, Karen T. Feisullin, Laura E. Ferguson, Michael F. Fleming, Daniel E. Ford, Paul S. Frame, Russell E. Glasgow, Michael G. Goldstein, Russell Harris, John M. Hickner, Steven Jonas, Evonne Kaplan-Liss, Linda S. Kinsinger, Charles M. Kodner, Alex H. Krist, Robert S. Lawrence, Terence McCormally, J. Michael McGinnis, Virginia A. Moyer, Heidi D. Nelson, Betsy Nicoletti, J. Marc Overhage, Kevin Patrick, Michael Pignone, Stephen F. Rothemich, Kavitha Bhat Schelbert, Roger A. Shewmake, Leif I. Solberg, Carolyn L., Westhoff, Robert M. Wolfe, Steven H. Woolf

Introduction

JESSICA SHANK COVIELLO

Many of you will be starting your academic journey in health care. You represent the next generation of health care providers. You will carry on the mission that many of us started with the anticipation that the next 25 years will further advance our understanding of how lifestyle influences health and wellness. Our current knowledge makes it clear that one's health is affected by everything that goes on in and around a person's environment in meeting the challenges of lifestyle, stressors, and societal demands. As our understanding of this relationship grows, the ability to reduce overall health risk through health promotion takes center stage. Health promotion and disease prevention[1] have an inherent logic: it has always seemed more sensible to prevent the occurrence of diseases, or to stop them early in their natural history, than to delay treatment until the process of pathogenesis has resulted in irreversible damage to body tissues, organ systems, and physiologic processes. Clinicians know too well how ineffective medical and surgical interventions can become at this late stage in the process, when controlling symptoms and forestalling progression, rather than curing the disease itself, are often all that can be offered to patients.

Yet 92.1 million Americans are living with some form of cardiovascular disease (CVD), be it heart failure or stroke. The cost of these CVDs is estimated to total more than 329.7 billion, accounting for both health expenditures and lost productivity.[3] In 2017, new cases of cancer were projected to be 1,688,780 with over 600,000 deaths in the United States.[4]

---

[1]*Health promotion* is defined as "any combination of educational, organizational, economic, and environmental supports for behavior and conditions of living conducive to health."[1] Modifying personal health behaviors to reduce the risk of disease and injury is often described as health promotion. *Disease prevention* encompasses primary, secondary, and tertiary prevention. "*Primary preventive* measures are those provided to individuals to prevent the onset of a target condition (e.g., routine immunization of healthy children), whereas *secondary preventive* measures identify and treat asymptomatic persons who have already developed risk factors or preclinical disease but in whom the disease itself has not become clinically apparent. Obtaining a Pap smear to detect cervical dysplasia before the development of cancer and screening for high blood pressure are forms of secondary prevention. Preventive measures that are part of the treatment and management of persons with clinical illnesses ... are usually considered *tertiary prevention*."[2]

Obesity is one of the biggest drivers of preventable chronic disease, such as heart disease, cancer, renal failure, stroke, and diabetes. In 2013-2014, 2 of every 3 adults were considered overweight with 1 in 6 children considered obese.[5] Obesity is expected to overtake smoking as the leading cause of death and to give today's children a shorter life expectancy than their parents,[6] not to mention its psychosocial consequences. The estimated annual health care costs of obesity-related illness are nearly 21% of the annual medical spending in the United States.[5] If current obesity trends continue, it is estimated that obesity will increase future Medicare beneficiary spending by 34%.[5,6]

Tobacco, alcohol, and drug abuse add to this disease burden, forcing the health care system to invest heavily in caring for complications from these conditions, rather than in preventing the disease processes that caused them. In comparison with the cost of chronic disease–related end-stage disease, only 3% of the total health care spending goes toward prevention.[7] As providers in today's health care system, we see our intensive care units, emergency rooms, and long-term care facilities dedicated to the care of and sophisticated technologies used to support those with preventable chronic disease.

Important trends make it likely that the prevalence and costs of chronic diseases will worsen over the coming years. The "baby boom" generation began to reach 60 years of age in 2006. The number of seniors in the United States is expected to be 72 million in 2030,[8,9] with the prevalence of chronic diseases increasing as advances in medical care improve life expectancies and lengthen life spans. Currently, almost half of Americans have one or more chronic illnesses, and the number is expected to grow to 171 million in 2030,[10] with the costs of medical care for those chronic diseases climbing rapidly.[11] It is a safe prediction that the convergence of these trends will result in a higher prevalence of chronic diseases and that health care costs to treat the complications of those diseases will climb. Economic pressures from rising costs are already substantial for major employers, and the trends just mentioned portend a growing threat to corporate America and to the solvency of the Medicare program.

Chronic diseases, such as heart disease, cancer, and diabetes, are responsible for 7 of every 10 deaths among Americans each year and account for 75% of the national health spending.[12] With the surge in disease anticipated with the aging of America, prevention offers individuals, the health care community, and society at large a more rational strategy for dealing with disease and promoting health than the current model of deferring treatment until illness develops, often with little success. The logic behind prevention is obvious. It is more rational to screen for and treat asymptomatic persons than for years later to treat their end-stage disease. Benjamin Franklin understood this principle well when he popularized the maxim: "An ounce of prevention is worth a pound of cure."[13]

THE HISTORY OF THE HEALTH PROMOTION MOVEMENT

Despite this logic, the critical role of health promotion and disease prevention was not well recognized as a priority area of national health policy until the early 1970s. At that time, a seminal Canadian document, the Lalonde Report, presented a new model that raised awareness about the importance of an integrated health promotion policy for improving the health status of the population as a whole.[14] The Lalonde Report signaled the transformation of health promotion from the preceding "wellness" movement, a succession of vitamin and stress-reduction fads with little supporting scientific evidence, to a well-recognized epidemiologic and clinical science linking behavioral risk factors to specific disease outcomes. The incorporation of these principles into national health policy was formalized in the United States in 1979-1980, when the federal government published *Healthy People: The Surgeon General's Report on Health Promotion and Disease Prevention*[15] and *Promoting Health/Preventing Disease: Objectives for the Nation*,[16] setting specific goals to be achieved by 1990. By the time that new objectives for the year 2010 (*Healthy People 2010*) were released in 2000,[17] health promotion and disease prevention had become a well-accepted component of national health policy. The 2020 objectives, launched in December 2010, represented 30 years Healthy People had been committed to improving the quality of the nation's health by producing a framework for public health prevention priorities and actions. In just the last decade, preliminary analyses indicate that the country has either progressed toward or met 71% of its Healthy People targets. Health promotion policy has now diffused to the regional and local level, where initiatives to promote wellness and preventive care are common priorities of local governments, health care institutions, insurance plans, employers, and retailers.[18]

AFFORDABLE CARE ACT COMPREHENSIVE HEALTH CARE REFORM

In March 2010, the Affordable Care Act (ACA) was signed by President Obama. The law has 3 primary goals:

- Make affordable health insurance available to more people. The law provides consumers with subsidies ("premium tax credits") that lower costs for households with incomes between 100% and 400% of the federal poverty level.
- Expand the Medicaid program to cover all adults with income below 138% of the federal poverty level. (Not all states have expanded their Medicaid programs.)
- Support innovative medical care delivery methods designed to lower the costs of health care generally.[19]

The ACA addressed public health goals in 3 ways: it expanded public health capacity by establishing new programs and structures that focused on public health objectives and enhanced funding for existing programs, it increased access to clinical preventive services, and it provided new incentives for prevention and wellness programs in the private sector.[19] By the third quarter of 2016, the percentage of Americans lacking health coverage was at the lowest level ever recorded, and measures of access to care had improved substantially.[20–23] Many saw health reform as an opportunity to address the social determinants of health well beyond medical care. There were calls for more community-based prevention and to increase the proportion of health spending going to population health[24] and chronic disease prevention.[24,25] There was a call to bolster enrollment outreach for existing insurance programs that had prevention components, such as Medicaid and the Children's Health Insurance Program (CHIP).[26] The focus of the law was in eliminating health disparities and improving health across communities.

The final bill, signed into law by President Barack Obama on March 23, 2010, included a prevention or public health component, Title IV, Prevention of Chronic Diseases and Improving Public Health.

The law created both the National Prevention, Health Promotion, and Public Health Council. A total of $15 billion was set aside for the Prevention and Public Health Fund; together, these represented the first time that a comprehensive public health strategy, with dedicated funding, was articulated in federal law.

The final prong of the ACA's public health initiatives consisted of various incentives to states, providers, patients, and employers to improve health. To create healthier workplaces, the law lifted the ceiling on workplace wellness incentives from 20% of health care costs to 30%. It allowed employers to increase premiums up to 50% for participation in smoking cessation programs.[27]

In addition, grant funds were made available for small businesses to create workplace wellness programs. The ACA's wellness incentives allow employers to reward employees with a discount of up to 30% of their insurance premium for undertaking wellness activities. The ACA differed from most prior US health care reform legislation in putting prevention squarely into the coverage and cost containment mix. The Act bolstered financing for building public health and prevention capacity, improved access to preventive services, and encouraged private employers and insurers to incorporate prevention and wellness into workplaces and coverage policies. The ACA generated substantial benefits for Americans, greatly expanding insurance coverage, spurring delivery system reforms, and protecting the financial security of American families. It also generated great progress in the prevention of ill-health among Americans through increases in capacity, coverage, and incentives. The law has been the center of political discourse since its signing in 2010. At this writing, Congress continues to work to improve and change the law as we move into the next election cycle.

Society can practice health promotion and disease prevention through several channels: (1) controlling communicable diseases, (2) protecting the environment, (3) modifying personal behaviors that affect health, and (4) preventing, or reducing the severity of, noncommunicable and chronic disabling conditions.[28] The last century has witnessed achievements in health promotion and disease prevention in each of these areas. Through improved public sanitation, housing, immunization programs, and nutrition, infectious diseases that were the leading causes of death and disability in the United States at the beginning of the 20th century have now become uncommon. Government and industry have worked to improve the cleanliness of air, water, and soil and to increase the safety of products and transportation services, thereby reducing the incidence of infectious diseases, environmental and occupational illnesses, and injuries. Recent outbreaks of both Zika and Ebola, however, act to remind us of the importance of continued vigilance and efforts in both prevention and disease containment.

Personal health consciousness has been integrated into daily American life. Joggers and power walkers became common sights on residential streets in the 1970s. Concerns about nutrition and the importance of lifestyle in preventing infection with human immunodeficiency virus grew in the 1980s. Now, other examples of health promotion have become evident in society: print and television advertisements feature messages about healthy, low-fat products and physical fitness; motorists routinely fasten their seat belts; children are protected by car safety seats and bicycle helmets; no-smoking policies have been adopted by local and state governments, employers, airlines, restaurants, and other public facilities; and celebrities, advertisers, and public service announcements encourage cancer screening, safe sex, and avoiding drug and alcohol abuse and drunk driving. The personal health behaviors of Americans have changed and provided improvements in cancer and cardiovascular deaths. Behavioral risk factor modification accounts for a large proportion of these reductions. Reduced stroke mortality is believed to be due to early detection and treatment of hypertension. Age-adjusted mortality for lung cancer has been decreasing since 1991 due largely to decreased tobacco use.[29]

These achievements aside, far too many Americans continue to suffer from diseases and injuries that are largely preventable. The health status of the population is far lower than it should be, primarily because the full benefits of health promotion and disease prevention have yet to be realized. Heart disease remains the leading cause of death in the United States, killing almost 800,000 Americans annually.[30] More than 90 million Americans carry a diagnosis of CVD. Among non-Hispanic (NH) blacks 20 years and older, 46.0% of males and 47.7% of females live with CVD in the United States. Stroke accounts for 1 of 20 deaths in the United States. Approximately every 40 seconds, someone experiences a stroke in the United States. Death rates due to stroke have declined. As adults with stroke survive, stroke has become the leading cause of long-term disability in the

United States. NH blacks have a risk of first ever stroke that is almost twice that of whites.[30] The estimated yearly stroke incidence of new and recurrent attacks is 45,000 for NH black men and 60,000 for NH black women. NH blacks between the ages of 45 and 64 years are at 2 to 3 times the risk of stroke as whites.[30] About 40% of the excess stroke risk in NH blacks is due to traditional stroke risk factors, with levels of systolic blood pressure (SBP) accounting for approximately one-half of this impact.[30] For each 10-mm Hg increase in SBP, the increased stroke risk in whites is ≈8%; however, a similar 10-mm Hg increase in SBP in NH blacks is associated with a 24% increase in stroke risk, an impact 3 times greater than in whites.[30] An estimated 85.7 million Americans (34% of the population) have high blood pressure. An estimated 45% of Americans with hypertension do not have controlled blood pressure.[30] Today, over 100 million Americans are living with diabetes or prediabetes. In 2015, an estimated 1.5 million new cases of diabetes were diagnosed among people 18 years and older. Nearly 1 in 4 adults living with diabetes—7.2 million Americans—did not know they had the condition. Only 11.6% of adults with prediabetes knew they had it.[31] Worldwide, the prevalence of diabetes is expected to increase to 7.7% in the year 2030. Approximately one-third of such deaths are potentially preventable, caused by a short list of modifiable risk factors (tobacco use, unhealthy diet, physical inactivity, and problem drinking).[29] Mortality from motor vehicle injuries (approximately 40,000 deaths each year) could be reduced in half if seat belt use was maximized and drinking and driving were curtailed.[29] A total of 38,658 deaths in 2016 were caused by firearms[29], a situation that prudent handgun policies could remedy.

Of great importance is that the inequities in health outcomes in the United States continue to grow. The incidence, morbidity, and mortality of certain diseases are disproportionately higher among disadvantaged and minority populations. These health disparities are disproportionately experienced by groups of people, in different socioeconomic classes and geographic locations and at various times as Dr. Martha Okafor's chapter in this book so clearly outlines.

The reasons for the inadequacies in the availability and use of health promotion and disease prevention services are multifactorial. Strategies available to society for preventing diseases are limited by logistic, political, financial, religious, and philosophic obstacles. Regulations to protect the safety of the environment place economic and administrative burdens on private industry and governmental agencies. Vaccines and screening services are costly to society and often unavailable to persons with limited access to health care. The biologic efficacy of vaccines and antibiotics to control infectious diseases is threatened by the emergence of new organisms, antibiotic-resistant strains, and vaccine failure. Perhaps the most effective means of promoting health, convincing individuals to change personal behaviors, cannot succeed if individuals lack the motivation or resources to change behavior. To change behavior voluntarily is difficult because unhealthy behaviors are often enjoyable or deeply ingrained in lifestyle and culture. Unhealthy foods, tobacco, and alcohol products are actively promoted by advertisers. Forcing changes in behavior, such as requiring motorcyclists to wear helmets, poses philosophic, ethical, political, and legal problems and generally conflicts with American preferences for individual freedom.

PRACTICE

It is in this context of societal efforts that this book explores the role of clinicians in promoting health and preventing disease. Clinicians play a vital role in promoting health. The limitations of this effort, however, are as immediately apparent as their capabilities. We cannot ensure the cleanliness of water and food supplies, cannot redesign motor vehicles to improve safety, cannot redesign the built environment to facilitate outdoor physical activity. We can guide, educate, and encourage our patients but cannot control their behavior.

Nonetheless, our potential capabilities in promoting health are substantial. Clinicians, perhaps better than anyone, know the consequences of allowing conditions to progress to their final stages and the futility of offering treatments late in the natural history of disease. We are therefore among the most persuasive advocates of health promotion. Clinicians also have special access to the population. In 2016, 84.6% of Americans had contact with a clinician each year, averaging more than 3 office visits per year.[29] Patients value our advice. Studies suggest that patients' decisions to stop smoking, undergo a mammogram, or have their child immunized are often traceable to clinician encouragement. The clinician is essential to the delivery of many preventive services (e.g., Pap smears, screening colonoscopy, and prescription medication to help with smoking cessation).

Clinicians have therefore always tried to emphasize preventive services in clinical practice. For decades we have prioritized health promotion and disease prevention issues during well-baby and well-child visits. We have emphasized nutrition, exercise, and other aspects of wellness. Much of the prenatal care is dominated by prevention topics. We devote much of our time to encouraging patients to modify cardiac risk factors, screen for colorectal cancer, encourage the prevention and early detection of skin cancer, screen for glaucoma, and so on.

Most clinicians, however, do fall short in providing the preventive services that are recommended for their patients. Results from a 2015 study survey show that only 8% of Americans 35 years and older reported having received all of the appropriate, high-priority clinical preventive services recommended for them and nearly 5% reported having received none of them. The results also show that comprehensive preventive care is achievable: more than 20% of adults reported receiving more than 75% of the services.[32]

BARRIERS TO THE DELIVERY OF CLINICAL PREVENTIVE SERVICES

The most pressing reason for inadequate attention to preventive services in the clinical setting has been related to the time constraints in a patient visit. In recent years, this has been resolving with the advent of a more interdisciplinary practice model and the use of the electronic medical record where preventative prompts and digital educational materials are readily available. Yet, many patients see their clinicians only when sick, which calls to mind the need to "seize the moment" when the opportunity presents itself. With new models in interdisciplinary education, this need to seize the moment has been recently emphasized as part of practice. The ACA has had prevention as its main focus, and we see this as an important outcomes measure in regard to reimbursement for services.

A second disincentive to providing clinical preventive services is skepticism about their effectiveness. Uncertainty about the ability of screening tests, counseling, and immunizations to reduce morbidity and mortality has been a long standing obstacle to preventive care for many years. It was this skepticism that prompted the U.S. Public Health Service to establish the U.S. Preventive Services Task Force (USPSTF) in 1984. The USPSTF, modeling its approach after that of the Canadian Task Force on the Periodic Health Examination (now the Canadian Task Force on Preventative Health Care),[33] carefully examined the evidence for more than 200 clinical preventive services. Although it found that many preventive services lacked sufficient evidence to reach conclusions about their effectiveness or ineffectiveness, it was able to identify a core package of clinical preventive services for which there was compelling evidence of significant health benefits.[2] The USPSTF findings have been regularly updated over 3 decades and have been reinforced by other expert panels and medical groups. Together, the findings of these groups provide a strong scientific argument for emphasizing these measures in daily patient care.

Which specific clinical preventive services should be provided? The recommended clinical preventive services for patients in specific age and risk groups have been specified by the USPSTF and other groups. Specific downloadable websites and application of these groups can be found in Online Appendix A.

The details of *how* to perform the recommended clinical preventive services are the principal focus of this book and include how to collect risk factor information during the history, physical, and laboratory examination. In addition, the ways and means of using that information to help patients modify risk factors and to determine appropriate follow-up tests, treatments, immunizations, and counseling are included.

Health insurers, employers, and the Medicare program have widened coverage of clinical preventive services as part of their efforts to control the rising costs of health care. Preventative services are popular with consumers, and many plans compete for patient enrollment by advertising their respective preventive services packages. The performance review criteria used by organizations that evaluate the quality of health care (e.g., the National Committee for Quality Assurance, quality improvement organizations for Medicare, and the National Quality Foundation) emphasize preventive services delivery as a cornerstone for judging the quality of care provided to patients. Secondary prevention is also a driver with readmission rates a main concern for health care organizations. Since the ACA in 2010, clinicians and health care organizations reimbursement has been dependent on the achievement of high performance on quality indicators.[34]

The emphasis on the clinical setting as a venue for preventive care has been accompanied by the growing recognition of the importance of population-based efforts and community programs in health promotion and disease prevention. A counterpart to the USPSTF—the Task Force on Community Preventive Services—has been working since the 1990s to identify evidence-based strategies outside the clinical setting that are effective and actionable.[35] The greatest promise lies in leveraging the power of both venues through partnerships between clinicians and such community programs. For example, more effective smoking cessation counseling can occur when primary care clinicians augment efforts in the office by referring smokers to proactive telephone counseling provided by quit lines. Success in addressing obesity requires the collective efforts of families, retailers, and school systems to facilitate behavior change and collaborations between clinicians and community resources (e.g., commercial weight loss programs) to deliver intensive weight loss counseling.

THE IMPORTANCE OF PATIENT EDUCATION AND COUNSELING IN PREVENTIVE MEDICINE

The clinical preventive services that clinicians should provide are classified by the USPSTF as (1) counseling interventions, (2) screening tests, (3) immunizations, and (4) chemoprophylaxis. *Counseling interventions* refer to efforts to educate patients about the consequences of personal health behaviors (e.g., smoking, diet, physical inactivity, substance abuse, sexual practices, and injury prevention) and to work in a collaborative manner on strategies for risk factor modification. *Screening tests* are special tests or standardized examination procedures for the early detection of preclinical conditions (e.g., cervical dysplasia) or risk factors (e.g., elevated serum cholesterol) in asymptomatic persons. *Immunizations* include the use of vaccines and immunoglobulins to prevent infectious diseases.

Chemoprophylaxis refers to the use of drugs, nutritional and mineral supplements, or other natural substances by asymptomatic persons to prevent future disease.

This book gives special emphasis to counseling patients about risk factors. Modifying personal health behaviors is probably the most effective way for patients to prevent disease. According to one analysis, a 45-year-old female smoker is 23 times more likely to avoid a premature death by stopping smoking than by getting a screening mammogram.[36] Despite the relative superiority of health behavior change over testing as a strategy to prevent disease, the former is more challenging and a typical patient is more likely to see the latter emphasized in clinical practice. As in other areas of health care, preventive care is dominated by procedures and testing. In the past, patients seeking preventive care were more likely to undergo a rectal examination or cholesterol test than to be asked whether they smoke, what they eat, or whether they exercise. With renewed focus on preventative value-based care, the use of electronic medical records, and the interdisciplinary model of education, we are seeing this change.

Modifying behaviors early in the natural history can prevent (or, in some cases, reverse[37,38]) progression of the disease many years before it would be detectable by physical examination or screening tests. The general ineffectiveness of screening tests stands to reason. If one considers the time line of the natural history of disease, it becomes apparent that screening tests cannot detect a disorder until the disease process has produced a measurable pathophysiologic abnormality, even if it is asymptomatic. Treatment interventions at this stage are often of limited effectiveness because the pathophysiologic process has often advanced to the point of producing irreversible disease. Personal health behaviors that cause disease, on the other hand, play a key etiologic role much earlier on the time line. Attention to these causes of disease and injury can accomplish real prevention, whereas the inherent nature of screening requires one to wait for the disease process to begin.

PRINCIPLES OF EXCELLENCE AND QUALITY IN PREVENTIVE HEALTH CARE

Basic to the practice of good preventive care is taking a thorough history. The clinician cannot determine which preventive services are indicated for a particular patient without first considering the patient's risk factors. It is self-evident that the clinician cannot recognize the need to advise a patient to stop smoking without first inquiring whether he or she smokes. The need to advise an adolescent about sexual practices will not become apparent until the clinician determines whether the teen is sexually active. The need to begin colorectal screening at an earlier age because of hereditary polyposis will not become apparent unless the clinician inquires about the family history. A diagnostic approach to risk factors is of as much importance in designing a plan for prevention as is a diagnostic approach in determining how to treat symptomatic patients. Proposing a uniform ("one size fits all") health maintenance plan for all patients is as inappropriate as suggesting a single treatment plan for all patients with chest pain. The history, physical, and laboratory examination must be used to construct an individual risk profile. Only then can one determine which preventive services are indicated and which deserve priority.

The risk factors identified in the evaluation should be treated as real problems, recorded on the patient's "problem list" along with diseases, physical findings, and symptoms. Unhealthy personal behaviors, inadequate screening, and overdue immunizations represent problems that require as clear and as determined a follow-up plan as atrial fibrillation, rectal bleeding, a palpable spleen, or a new systolic murmur. Indeed, the fact that a patient does not exercise, has multiple sexual partners, consumes a high-fat diet, drinks and drives, or has not had a mammogram in 5 years may represent a more serious threat to the patient's health than most conditions that appear on conventional problem lists. Certainly, they require as much attention if the patient is to reduce the risk of adding new diseases to the problem list in future years. The bulk of this book is devoted to advising the clinician on how to address risk factors once they are identified.

This book is targeted at primary care clinicians, who are most knowledgeable about the patient's complete medical history, have the skills to diagnose and manage the broad array of clinical problems that arise in health promotion and disease prevention, and have a relationship with the patient that facilitates continuity in the health maintenance program. The primary care clinician is best suited to coordinate the patient's referrals to specialists, ensuring that patients receive necessary expert care in categorical areas without allowing other problems to "fall through the cracks." They are the captain of the health care ship.

Discussions in this book about patient education and counseling emphasize a shared decision-making model and a respectful style of discourse between clinicians and patients. This approach differs from the old-fashioned paternalistic counseling style in which the doctor "tells the patient what to do." The philosophy espoused in this book is that patients are entitled to make informed decisions about how they live their lives and about their health care. Clinicians have a professional responsibility to ensure that patients' decisions are based on complete and accurate health information but do not have a right to force the outcome of decisions. Once they have given the patient the necessary information about benefits and harms, they must respect the patient's preferences, even if the patient decides against doing what the clinician recommends. An authoritarian approach to promoting personal behavior change is rarely effective and does not contribute to establishing a trusting relationship. Instead, this book encourages a collaborative model for decision making, which permits the clinician and patient to work together to determine the best choice for that individual. The book speaks of choices, not "orders"; patient initiative, not "compliance"; and partnership, not "prescription."

Although this trend in patient empowerment in decision making is occurring throughout health care, it is especially appropriate in the practice of preventive health care. In health promotion, the "locus of control" lies more with the patient than with the clinician. In curative medicine, the clinician can often perform a procedure to solve the patient's problem (e.g., by placing a cast, removing an infected gallbladder, or suturing a laceration). In health promotion, only the patient can solve the problem. Stopping smoking, changing eating habits, increasing physical activity, and other changes in lifestyle are under the control of the patient and occur outside of the clinician's office or clinic. The clinician can, and should, provide information about the health risks associated with the behavior, encourage change, and suggest strategies for doing so, but the ultimate determinant of whether change occurs is the patient and not the clinician. The patient's feelings and attitudes about these health issues therefore require the full attention and respect of the clinician. The clinician can also act as community advocate and collaborate with public health colleagues to support changes in environmental factors, such as advertising for unhealthy foods, which interfere with even the most highly motivated patient's ability to practice health-promoting behaviors. In this way, the clinician promotes not only individual risk factor reduction but also the risk factor reduction of a community.

This book's emphasis on standards of care and patient education is reflected in Online Appendix A 🌐 where practice guidelines as well as other websites and resources are available to download into your phone or tablet. Characteristic of the current "information age" and the growth of medical consumerism, the scope of health information available to patients and the technologies for obtaining it are expanding rapidly. This information can supplement and reinforce the counseling provided by the clinician and can help the patient frame new questions, as well as identify the resources for answering them. It is the clinician's responsibility to ensure that patients are aware of these information resources and how to obtain them. Of all the services that clinicians can provide in the practice of health promotion and disease prevention, information is certainly the most valuable.

Finally, excellence in the practice of health promotion requires a holistic approach to understanding "health." Clearly, health is more than the absence of disease and comprises more than the discrete biophysical entities that we are currently capable of measuring. Our understanding of the interconnections between the mind and body continues to grow. Health is influenced by the social determinants of health that influence biophysical factors. One's health is affected by emotional and spiritual life, family dynamics and relationships, work satisfaction, income, food security, educational status, personal achievements, and social support.

Failure to consider the broader context of health can limit or undermine the clinician's efforts to help patients. A clinician who is preoccupied with a patient's "noncompliance" in getting a mammogram, without considering her personal life and the barriers she faces, may never discover that depression over her husband's death has diminished her interest in living longer. An overweight inner-city youth concerned about basic survival and gang-related shootings will be helped little by a clinician preoccupied with weight management as a singular focus. Clinicians need to consider these issues. By learning more about their patients' lives, clinicians can enjoy satisfying relationships with their patients and their families. Their suggested strategies for behavior change are more likely to be relevant to their patients' living conditions and, accordingly, are more likely to achieve results. Defining health objectives more broadly gives clinicians the gratification of knowing that their efforts are directed toward goals that are meaningful to their patients and that relate directly to the overall quality of their lives.

ACKNOWLEDGMENTS

The author wishes to acknowledge the original contributions of this introduction by Steven H. Woolf, Robert S. Lawrence, and Evonne Kaplan-Liss.

REFERENCES

1. Green LW. Prevention and health education. In: Last JM, Wallace RB, eds. *Maxcy-Rosenau-Last. Public health and preventive medicine*, 13th ed. Norwalk: Appleton & Lange, 1992:787–802.
2. U.S. Preventive Services Task Force. *Guide to clinical preventive services*, 2nd ed. Baltimore: Williams & Wilkins, 1996.
3. Benjamin EJ, Virani SS, Callaway CW, et al. on behalf of the American Heart Association Council on Epidemiology and Prevention Statistics Committee and Stroke Statistics Subcommittee. Heart disease and stroke statistics 2018 update: a report from the American Heart Association [published online ahead of print January 31, 2018]. *Circulation*. DOI: 10.1161/CIR.000000000000055)
4. Siegel RL, Miller KD, Ahmedin J. *Ca: Cancer A Journal for Clinicians* Cancer statistics, First published: 05 January 2017. https://doi.org/10.3322/caac.21387 2017.
5. Cawley J, Meyerhoefer C. The medical care costs of obesity: an instrumental variables approach. *J Health Econ*. 2012;31(1):219–230. https://www.niddk.nih.gov/health-information/health-statistics/overweight-obesity
6. Grover SA, Kaouache M, Rempel P, et al. Years of life lost and healthy life-years lost from diabetes and cardiovascular disease in overweight and obese people: a modelling study. *The Lancet Diabetes Endo*, 2014: doi:10.1026/S2213-8587(14)70229-3
7. The Prevention and Public Health Fund: *A critical investment in our nation's physical and fiscal health*. American Public Health Association Center for Public Health Policy, Issue Brief, June 2012. https://www.apha.org/~/media/files/pdf/factsheets/apha_prevfundbrief_june2012ashx
8. He W, Sengupta M, Velkoff VA, et al. U.S. Census Bureau. *Current population reports, P23-209, 65+ in the United States: 2005*. Washington, DC: U.S. Government Printing Office, 2005.

9. Horvath J. *Chronic conditions in the U.S.: implications for service delivery and financing.* Rockville: Agency for Healthcare Research and Quality, http://www.ahrq.gov/news/ulp/hicosttele/sess2/horvathstxt.htm. Accessed 2007.

10. Eyre H, Kahn R, Robertson RM. ACS/ADA/AHA Collaborative Writing Committee. Preventing cancer, cardiovascular disease, and diabetes: a common agenda for the American Cancer Society, the American Diabetes Association, and the American Heart Association. *CA Cancer J Clin.* 2004;54:190–207.

11. Benjamin EJ, Virani SS, Calloway CW et al. on behalf og the American Heart Association Council on Epidemiology and Prevention Statistics Committee and Stroke Statistics Subcommittee. Heart disease and stroke statistics 2018 update: a report from the American Heart Association [published online ahead of print January 31, 2018]. *Circulation* doi: 10.1161/CIR.000000000000055

12. *Agency for Health Care Research and Quality-Medical Expenditure Panel Survey.* https://www.HHS.org.

13. Independence Hall Association. *The quotable Franklin.* Philadelphia: Independence Hall Association, at http://www.ushistory.org/Franklin/quotable/quote67.htm. Accessed 2007.

14. Lalonde M. *A new perspective on the health of Canadians.* Ottawa: Information Canada, 1974.

15. U.S. Department of Health, Education, and Welfare. *Healthy people: The Surgeon General's report on health promotion and disease prevention.* HEW Publication No. 79–55071. Washington, DC: U.S. Department of Health, Education, and Welfare, 1979.

16. U.S Department of Health and Human Services. *Promoting health/preventing disease: objectives for the nation.* Washington, DC: U.S. Department of Health and Human Services, 1990.

17. U.S. Department of Health and Human Services. *Healthy People 2010: Understanding and Improving Health.* 2nd ed. Washington, DC: U.S. Government Printing Office, November 2000.

18. U.S. Department of Health and Human Services: *Healthy People 2020.* Washington, DC: US Department of Health and Human Services. https://www.healthypeople.gov/sites/defaulty/files/DefaultPressRelease_1.pdf.

19. Chait N, Glied S. Promoting prevention under the Affordable Care Act. *Ann Rev Pub Health*, 2018; 39: 507–24.

20. Altman D. *The Affordable Care Act's little-noticed success: cutting the unin-sured rate.* October 12, 2016. Kaiser Family Foundation, Menlo Park, Ca: https://www.Kff.org/uninsured/perspective/the-affordable-care-acts-littl-noticed-success-cutting-the-uninsured-rate/

21. Avery K, Fiengold K, Whitman A. *Affordable Care Act has led to historic sidespread increase in health insurance coverage.* Issue brief, September 29. https://www.aspe.hhs.gov/system/files/pdf/207946/ACAHistoricIncreaseCoverage.pdf, Assist, Secr. Plan.Eval., Washington, D.C.

22. Shartzer A, Long SK, Anderson N, et al. Access to care and affordability have improved following Affordable Care Act implementation: problems remain. *Health Affair* 2015: 35: 161–68.

23. Skopec L, Waidmann TA, Sung J, et al. *Access to health care improved during early ACA market place implementation.* Brief http://www.aarp.org/content/dam/aarp/ppi/2015/access-to-health-care—improved-during-early-aca-%20marketplace-implementation.pdf, January 2015, AARP Public Policy Inst., Washington, DC.

24. Bassett MT. Bold steps for the health of Americans: yes we can. *Am.. J. Public Health* 2009; 99: 587.

25. Farley TA. Reforming health care or reforming health. *Am. J. Public Health* 2009; 99: 588–90.

26. Skopec L, Sommers BD. *Seventy-one million additional Americans are receiving preventative services coverage without cost sharing under the Affordable Care Act.* Issue Brief https://www.aspe.hhs.gov/sytem/files/pdf/76626/ib_prevention.pdf, March 18, 2013, Assist.Secr.Plan.Eval., Washington, DC.

27. Madison K, Schmidt H, Volpp KG. Smoking, obesity, health insurance, and health incentives in the Affordable Care Act. *JAMA*, 2013; 310: 143–44.

28. Last JM, Wallace RB, eds, *Maxcy-Rosenau-Last public health and preventative medicine*, 13th ed. Norwalk: Appleton & Lange, 1992.

29. Heron M. *National Vital Statistics Reports*, 2018; 67:6.

30. Benjamin EJ, Blaha MN, Chiuve SE. et al. Heart Disease and Stroke Statistics- 2017 Update: A report from the American Heart Association. *Circulation*, 2017; 135: 1. https://www.ahajournals.org/doi/full/10.1161/CIR. (13)05485.

31. Centers for Disease Control. *New CDC report: More than 100 million Americans have diabetes or pre-diabetes*, July 18, 2017. https: www.cdc.gov/media/releases/2017/p0718-diabetes-report.html.

32. Borsky A, Zhan C, Miller T. et al. few Americans receive all high-priority, appropriate clinical preventative service. *Health Affair*, 2018:37:6. https://www.healthaffairs.org/doi/10.1377/hlthaff.2017.1248.

33. Canadian Task Force on the Periodic Health Examination. *The Canadian guide to the clinical preventative health care.* Ottawa: Canada Communication Group, 1994.

34. Burns LR, Pauley MV. Transformation of the health care industry: Curb your enthusiasm? *Milbank Quarterly.* 96;1: 57–109. https://www.milbank.org/quarterly/.../transformation-health-care-industry-curb-enthus.

35. Zaza S, Briss PA, Harris KW, eds. *The guide to community preventive services: what works to promote health? Task Force on Community Preventive Services.* Oxford University Press, 2005.

36. Woolf SH. The need for perspective in evidence-based medicine. *JAMA* 1999;282: 2358–2365.

37. Ornish D, Scherwitz LW, Billings JH, et al. Intensive lifestyle changes for reversal of coronary heart disease. *JAMA*, 1998;280:2001–2007.

38. Franklin BA, Brinks J, Friedman H. Foundational factors for cardiovascular disease: Behavior change as a first-line preventative strategy. Professional Heart Daily Resources for Cardiovascular and Stroke Clinicians and Scientists.

PART ONE

Gathering Information

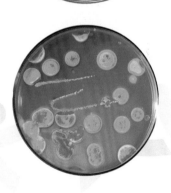

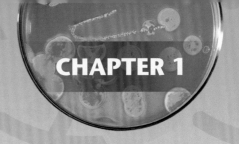

CHAPTER 1

Population Health

MARTHA OKAFOR

BACKGROUND

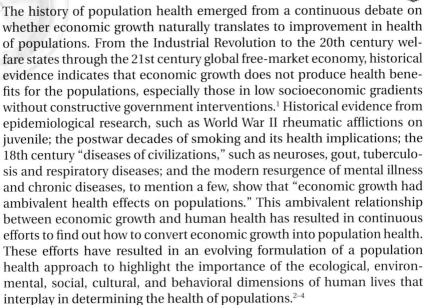

The history of population health emerged from a continuous debate on whether economic growth naturally translates to improvement in health of populations. From the Industrial Revolution to the 20th century welfare states through the 21st century global free-market economy, historical evidence indicates that economic growth does not produce health benefits for the populations, especially those in low socioeconomic gradients without constructive government interventions.[1] Historical evidence from epidemiological research, such as World War II rheumatic afflictions on juvenile; the postwar decades of smoking and its health implications; the 18th century "diseases of civilizations," such as neuroses, gout, tuberculosis and respiratory diseases; and the modern resurgence of mental illness and chronic diseases, to mention a few, show that "economic growth had ambivalent health effects on populations." This ambivalent relationship between economic growth and human health has resulted in continuous efforts to find out how to convert economic growth into population health. These efforts have resulted in an evolving formulation of a population health approach to highlight the importance of the ecological, environmental, social, cultural, and behavioral dimensions of human lives that interplay in determining the health of populations.[2–4]

Thus, there is no one definition of population health. The phrase "population health" is defined in various ways based on the context and lens of the entity defining this term, although all definitions aim at improving health outcomes of a population. The use of this term has shifted the focus on people, as a group, to understand who is healthy and who is sick, and why those people? It also seeks to understand under what circumstances do people experience health and illness? What causes and contribute to their condition? When and where do these occur? These questions must be addressed to improve health and achieve health equity. Put simply, population health is the health of a population and the conditions that optimize equitable health outcomes. This term is increasingly used in health care delivery systems, public health, academia, research, advocacy, and policy-making arenas as a key promising approach to improve health outcomes for all people. The continuous increase in population, migration, longevity, lack of access to health care, and unsustainable growth of health care costs and disparities in health and outcomes have forced the United States to embrace the population health approach as a viable way for improving our health status and health care delivery systems. This chapter explores the following: (1) What is population health and why does it matter? (2) How does population health work, particularly in health care systems? and (3) What are some best practices of population health management (PHM) in health care delivery systems?

WHAT IS POPULATION HEALTH AND WHY DOES IT MATTER?

Introduction

We have lived our lives with the assumption that how well our health care delivery systems are funded determines how well our health status and outcomes shall be. We have been wrong. We have extensively funded the health care delivery systems in the United States but have one of the lowest health status and worse outcomes when compared with other high-income nations.[5,6] In addition to the high cost and fewer outcomes, we have widespread disparities in health outcomes. These health disparities are disproportionately experienced by groups of people, in different socioeconomic classes and geographic locations and at various times. The inequities in health outcomes in the United States continue to grow with the increase in funding and cost of our health care. It is evident that we must change our assumption based on this paradoxical situation, if we want to improve the health status in the United States and ensure that the improved health outcomes are equitably experienced by all populations. This imperative to optimize health care delivery systems and improve equitable health outcomes has resulted in different actions aimed at improving population health in the United States.

Definitions: What Is Population Health?

Despite the differences in the fields of thoughts and lenses from which many entities have defined population health over decades ago, there are certain commonalities in their definitions and espousals as outlined in the following context:

Dunn and Hayes (1999) described population health as "The health of a population as measured by health status indicators and as influenced by social, economic and physical environments, personal health practices, individual capacity and coping skills, human biology, early childhood development, and health services." To them, the health status of a population must take into account the factors outside the health care delivery systems that influence the overall health status.

Also, Kindig and Stoddart (2003) defined population health as "the health outcomes of a group of individuals, including the distribution of such outcomes within the group." They pointed out in their definition the need to identify who shares what health outcomes with whom within a group of people and the determinants of those health outcomes ranging from wellness to disease prevention and disease control. Their definition plays a significant role in advancing population health.

Meanwhile, Young (2005) defined population health as a "conceptual framework for thinking about why some populations are healthier than others," as well as the policy development, research agenda, and resource allocation that flow from it. One can say that Young's thought about population health extends beyond Kindig and Stoddart's definition by including the need to take necessary actions to appropriately address "why" people share those health outcomes.

Berwick, Nolan, and Wittington (2008) heightened the essence of population health when they made it one of the three fundamental elements of the Institute for Healthcare Improvement's (IHI) Triple Aim for "improving the health systems and health of populations while reducing cost." The IHI Triple Aim presented a new framework for organizing and optimizing health systems through (1) improving individual patient experience of care, (2) reducing per capita cost of care, and (3) improving population health.

In 2009, the U.S. Department of Health and Human Services (HHS) through the Centers for Medicare and Medicaid Services (CMS) enacted the Health Information Technology for Economic and Clinical Health (HITECH) Act as part of the American Recovery and Reinvestment Act. The HITECH Act of 2009 facilitated a major "shift" of health care delivery systems toward population health. This legislation authorizes up to $27 billion in federal subsidies to eligible health professionals, doctors, and hospitals for the adoption and "meaningful use" of electronic health records (EHRs) aimed at: (1) improving quality, safety, and efficiency; (2) engaging patients in their care; (3) increasing coordination of care; (4) improving the health status of populations; and (5) ensuring privacy and security.[7]

The U.S. federal government in 2010 also initiated the Patient Protection and Affordable Care Act that encourages health care providers to provide patient-centered medical homes and take more responsibility for the cost, quality of care, and health outcomes of their patients. This provision of the law authorizes demonstration of alternative payment from fee-for-service to bundled payment based on value of care as measured through quality care, efficiency, and healthful population outcomes.

In 2012, the CMS established a shared-savings program for Accountable Care Organizations (ACOs).[8] The ACOs are groups of doctors, hospitals, and other health care clinicians who come together to form a robust network of providers committed to working together to provide highly coordinated quality care with reduced cost and improved outcomes for their patients, particularly those in Medicare. In this provision of the law, the providers are the ones to join the ACOs and not the patients, which is a shift from the prior practice of having the beneficiaries or patients join the Health Maintenance Organizations. The law also allows CMS to apply a portion of the reimbursement for hospitals as base incentives to promote quality care and penalize hospitals for avoidable readmissions as part of their performance measures. The goal is to make clinicians more accountable for the delivery of health care, including the cost, quality, and outcomes.

Meanwhile, Bostic (2012) espoused how the use of "health in all policies" approach could advance population health in the United States. This approach encourages both health and nontraditional health agencies of the U.S. government to see how their work has the potential to affect health and health equity, for example, food, housing, transportation, education, finance, employment, welfare, environment, trade, and commerce. The aim of "health in all policies" approach is to galvanize these agencies to work together, across sectors, in formulating, implementing, and evaluating their policies to measure how they help or hinder health conditions for the populations.

Summary Application

It is clear from the highlighted definitions that population health is beyond the auspices of public health traditional responsibility. It requires significant participation and more responsibility from health care delivery systems and shared accountability from entities whose action can cause and/or contribute to health conditions or outcomes. The broad array of determinants of health that are interconnected in population health warrant a robust integration of multiple factors to improve health outcomes. I would ask you to quickly review the highlighted definitions and identify the following:

1. Which of the definitions stood out to you, and why did you choose this particular definition?
2. Choose up to additional two definitions from the above-mentioned list that share specific common elements with your selected definition in question #1?
3. Identify and write up to five key components to be covered in a population health approach?

In summary, looking at Figure 1.1, how many of the listed factors did you identify in your response to question #3? Use the figure to add more components to your list, and notice the level of coordination, collaboration, and partnerships needed to successfully improve population health.

Why Does It Matter?

There is an increasing recognition that health care delivery systems cannot be isolated from the rest of other causal and contributing factors that influence health outcomes in the society. Health of an individual, family, or population is determined within the social, economic, and demographic context.

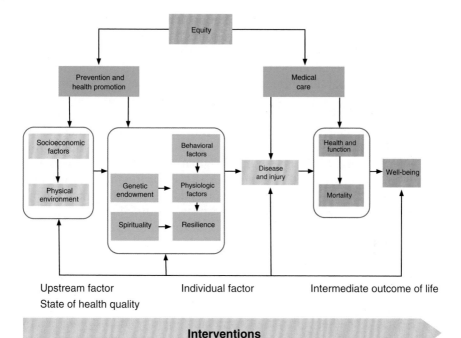

Figure 1.1 IHI population health composite model. This figure depicts the synergistic effect of multiple factors operating along the health spectrum to improve population health. Adapted from Stiefel M, Nolan KA. *Guide to Measuring the Triple Aim: Population Health, Experience of Care, and Per Capita Cost. IHI Innovation Series white paper.* Cambridge, Massachusetts: Institute for Healthcare Improvement; 2012. Available on www.IHI.org.

Population health matters because health status in the United States with higher per capita cost lags behind most of other comparable developed countries.[9] In addition, the U.S. health outcomes are not equitably experienced by all populations. The growing disparities in health are disproportionately shared among racial and ethnic groups, people in low socioeconomic conditions, those living in disadvantaged zip codes, and those with minority orientations and demographics, to mention just a few.

Population health matters because the HHS-CMS, which is the federal agency that administers the Medicare program and oversees the state government administration of Medicaid and the Children's Health Insurance Program (CHIP), and other government sponsored health insurance programs have integrated key elements of population health as part of their mission statement and priorities. It emphasizes key elements of: (1) patient empowerment and partnership in the care delivery, (2) improved quality and accessible and affordable care, and (3) improving the health of populations they serve. The implementation of medical homes, ACOs, and value-based reimbursement systems requires physicians and eligible clinicians to shift from traditional fee-for-service practice to a PHM approach.

Similarly, other nongovernment health insurance entities (private insurance) have parallel efforts supporting the federal government CMS direction and are moving toward a PHM practice to cut cost and improve quality care and health outcomes. As a result, physicians and eligible health care clinicians are being held accountable for health outcomes of the population they serve, as members of the ACOs. To accomplish this level of accountability, doctors and eligible providers are expected to address the upstream factors in Figure 1.1 (such as food insecurities and access to healthy food, safe neighborhoods and access to parks, walking trails or in-house exercise for active lifestyles, health education and prevention strategy for addressing obesity, and care coordination of medical visits) to improve health outcomes of all their populations.

The enactment of the Affordable Care Act (ACA) advances the population health approach. The expanded coverage of people who were uninsured is aligned with the CMS mission to increase access to care for U.S. populations. The patient-centered medical home practice requires clinicians to work together with patients and meaningfully address their health needs to improve their health outcomes. This law also motivates providers through incentives to encourage prevention of diseases and health promotion. The establishment of the National Strategy for Quality Improvement, CMS Center for Medicare and Medicaid Innovations, and Patient-Centered Outcomes Research Institute serves as resources to support the successful transition of the health care delivery systems.

Likewise, the National Prevention, Health Promotion and Public Health Council was established to develop standards and strategies for advancing prevention in the communities and primary care settings. Community transformation grants are made available to support this effort. In addition, incentives in the form of grants are made available to small businesses to advance workplace wellness programs and insurance discounts for employees participating in wellness plans. All these actions and more provisions[10] not mentioned in this chapter, including workforce development and training for health professionals, are put in place to build the necessary capacity and help clinicians transition from being accountable for their individual patients to being accountable for health of populations.

For hospitals, the ACA requires them to conduct community health needs assessment (CHNA) once every 3 years to address the spectrum of health, in Figure 1.1, particularly upstream and individual factors to facilitate healthier communities. The CHNA allows hospitals to engage members of their communities, the public health agency, and other stakeholders to identify their needs and strengths/assets, prioritize community needs, and identify solutions to meet the diverse needs of their unique populations.

It enables hospitals to influence broader determinants of health. This law also introduced a new Internal Revenue Service requirement with reporting and imposition of excise tax for hospitals that fail to meet the CHNA requirements aimed at creating healthier communities.[11]

Population health matters to public health since improving health of the public is the mission of public health agencies. The advancement of population health presents the public health agencies with a broader framework and tools to actively address the social determinants of health (SDH)[12] by engaging broader stakeholders operating in the SDH (Fig. 1.2) below to assure that: (1) conditions in which people are born, grow, live, work, and age are healthy, and (2) health equity is experienced by all populations in the United States. In addition, it allows public health to support health care delivery systems with epidemiological reports and surveillance services to address health inequities and leverage opportunities to improve health outcomes for all the populations they serve.

Population health acknowledges the importance of access to medical care and recognizes that without addressing the SDH factors that arise mostly as upstream factors, we cannot positively influence population health and eliminate health disparities, particularly health inequities. Health "inequities" are not the same as "inequalities" because inequalities are differences, whereas inequities are unfair. Health inequities are differences in health that are unnecessary, avoidable, unfair, and unjust.[13] They are often revealed and fostered through unfair and systematic patterns of access or outcomes across populations with differential levels of underlying social advantage or disadvantage[14] expressed by race, wealth, power, prestige, gender, sex, or other markers of social stratification.[15]

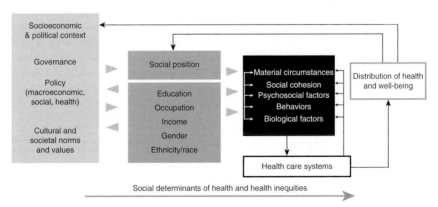

Figure 1.2 World Health Organization Commission on Social Determinants of Health, a conceptual framework linking social determinants of health and distribution of health. Adapted from *World Health Organization's Commission on Social Determinants on Health (CSDH) Framework Last version*, 48. Available on www.who.int.

A population health approach recognizes that these differential advantages and disadvantages stemming from health inequities are translated into differences in access to health promotion, preventive, curative, or palliative health services resulting in differences in outcomes, such as health, disability, morbidity, and mortality. It also acknowledges that, to advance equity in health of populations, we must address inequities, and to address inequities, we have to influence the SDH.

According to World Health Organization Commission on Social Determinants of Health framework:

> The social and economic context (e.g., employment conditions, national taxation schemes, and global trade agreements) gives rise to a set of unequal socioeconomic positions. Social position reflects the unequal distribution of materials and other resources in every society, which can be portrayed as a system of social stratification or a social hierarchy, including educational achievement, income level, occupational status, and gender, often captured by markers of discrimination (e.g., race/ethnicity). These social positions are characterized by differential exposure to health-damaging conditions and differential vulnerability, in terms of health conditions and material resource availability. Social stratification likewise determines differential consequences of ill health for more and less advantaged groups. The framework also highlights a collection of intermediary factors covering differential exposures, vulnerabilities, and consequences as playing an important part in the explanation of health inequities, which include the health system itself. The outcomes that emerge at the end of the social "production chain" of health inequities are the measurable impacts of social factors on comparative health status and outcomes among different population groups (i.e., health equity).[2,16]

The Commission on Social Determinants of Health presents the dynamics between the SDH and the distribution of health as well as how the absence of prohealth conditions determines ill health conditions and possible ways to close the health inequity gaps.

The causes of inequalities in health are dynamic with complex multiple determinants.[17] Yet, a major element of population health aims at achieving health equity in populations. To accomplish this aim, there should be a diffuse accountability whereby communities must establish and facilitate effective partnerships of public health agencies, health care delivery systems, and key SDH stakeholders to be responsible and share accountability as vital contributors to population health outcomes (IOM 1997, 2010, 2012). With the IHI Triple Aim identification of population health as one of its goals, it calls for similar engagement of a broad network of stakeholders to cooperate to improve population health outcomes since no single sector can accomplish this goal alone without being an integrator that leverages collective strengths of others.

How Does Population Health Work, Particularly in Health Care Systems?

Introduction

In this section, we attempt to answer the question of "how population health works, particularly in health care systems" by elucidating principles that underpin population health and discussing how these principles apply to a PHM in health care systems. As illustrated in the first section, population health approach has been in existence for decades. We would now focus mostly on "how to" manage population health and what makes it work to improve the outcomes for all groups of people we serve, particularly in the health care systems. Our focus on health care delivery systems is crucial because of the recent implementation of the ACA, the IHI Triple Aim for organizing effective health care systems, and the changing health care reimbursement for hospitals, clinician groups, health centers, and other eligible providers. The overarching goal of these recent changes is to achieve quality care, cost containment, and equitable health outcomes by shifting the paradigm of health systems: (1) from volume to value, (2) from being a sick care to a health care, (3) for health care organizations to provide patient-centered care and not clinician-centered care, (4) to be cost-effective with appropriate prevention and quality care delivered in collaboration with other stakeholders, and (5) contribute to health outcomes of their patients.

How Does Population Health Work in Health Care Systems and What Guides This Approach?

In brief, one can say that a population health approach promotes conditions of health for all populations to improve health outcomes of groups of individuals, including distribution of such outcomes within each group, to reduce health inequities. Promotion of the conditions of health will require addressing many determinants of these conditions, which fall outside the health care systems and include factors such as: housing, transportation, education, culture, gender, language, literacy, income, social status, poverty, race/ethnicity, occupation, age, and environment.

To improve health outcomes, population health has shifted the health care delivery systems to focus on promoting health conditions to prevent illness, providing early and continuous interventions with quality care to treat illnesses and cure diseases, and maintaining health and wellness, including self-management support, in appropriate settings, for all populations. Based on literature review, Figure 1.3 depicts seven principles of population health that guide how this approach works:

1. Defining and planning for population health

    Population in health care systems could be defined in many ways. It can be a group of people in a community or a defined place or with specific

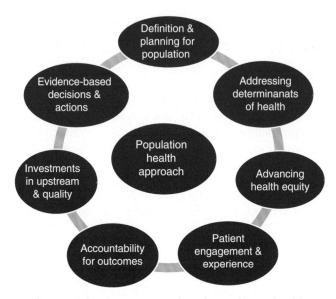

Figure 1.3   Seven principles of population health.

characteristics or markers, or shared experiences or other traits. A doctor and a nurse practitioner would see their patients as their population. Public health practitioners would see the community or the public they serve as their population. What drives a clinician to apply a population health approach in his or her practice is the willingness to improve the health outcomes of people he or she serves or a personal health experience or when the clinician is aware of avoidable negative health outcomes of others. It is normal to focus inward first by asking some question such as who shares what conditions in your practice, and why those people? Do people who have the same diagnosis have the same health outcomes? If yes, what determines their shared health outcomes? If no, what determines their differential health outcomes? Who influences those determinants of health outcomes, and why? What do you want as expected health outcomes? Where do you start (define the group, why and what)?

According to the American Academy of Pediatrics,[18] a possible way of defining and planning for population health in a pediatric health care delivery system includes but is not limited to the following:

  i. Determine which patients are behind on preventive care visits or immunizations, and send reminder emails/texts.
  ii. Identify children with asthma in the practice, and identify those children in need of flu shots, those with excessive rescue treatments, or those who might benefit from group educational visits. Examine managed care patient lists and reach out to those who have not established care to date.

iii. Understand the chronic disease incidence in the practice, or health risks that patients and families face, and develop targeted educational interventions and identify relevant community resources. Consider budgeting and contracting based on any newly discovered factors.

Planning for population health in health care systems involves understanding the interactions between the patients and social determinants of their health in order to improve their health outcomes. Population health planning activities consist of: (1) identifying and defining the specific group of people whose health outcomes you want to improve, as outlined earlier, (2) determining indicators for measuring the health status of the population, (3) assessing the internal context, such as practice and clinic process, and the external context, such as patient lifestyles and conditions, (4) determining the benefits to the population and how the organization will benefit, (5) identifying a champion (engage the senior clinician) and forming a committed team, (6) planning for adequate resources and securing leadership support, (7) outlining action steps with measures and who is responsible and when, and (8) proactively engaging patients and staff in planning.

2. Addressing the determinants of health and their implications

Engaging partners early in planning for population health helps with building alliance in addressing the determinants of health. This early engagement of stakeholders that cause or contribute to health outcomes for your defined population should include forming a consensus on visible results and specific objectives the alliance agrees to work on, shared leadership, accountability, and benefits to the partners. Your proposal has to answer the question of what's in it for the partners? One of the goals for addressing these SDH is the recognition that other factors beyond what happens in the health care delivery settings determine who is sick, who is healthy, and what can help or hinder health.

There is a growing evidence linking SDH with health outcomes, for example, lead ingestion by children, particularly those aged 0 to 6 years living in substandard housing, have low cognitive function and stunted physical development[19,20]; pollution and allergens, which are disproportionately high in disadvantaged neighborhoods, are associated with high asthma rate[21,22]; the availability of alcohol in disadvantaged neighborhoods is associated with an increase in alcohol use among youth, affecting rates of alcohol-related traumatic injury[23]; disproportionate concentration of convenience stores is associated with tobacco use, even after adjusting for individual-level characteristics, such as educational attainment and household income[24]; and food desert with lower availability of fresh produce and concentrated fast-food outlets with few recreational opportunities are linked to poor nutrition and a less active lifestyle.[25,26]

Thus, a population health approach "measures, analyzes and addresses the full spectrum of factors and their interactions known to influence and contribute to health."[27] Addressing the determinants of health also requires the assessment of policies in the SDH agencies to measure the extent to which existing policies affect health conditions and outcomes of the population. For the partnership to become effective, the team has to identify the necessary actions to be taken, who will take what action, who will lead what subgroup, and role and policy change. For example, to reduce disparities in children with elevated blood lead level and asthma diagnoses, the team would first identify the children with the highest burden of this disparity and where they live (let us assume they cluster in public housing units), determine an intervention such as implementing healthy homes policy with no lead and asthma triggers for families with children 0 to 6 years who live in public housing as a solution, and then describe what results/outcomes are expected, what happens to the affected children if the proposed solution is not implemented, what the objectives are, how they are measured, how (action steps) to lead to expected results, who is responsible for each action, and so on. Addressing the SDH is very crucial because they are drivers of health considering that medical care accounts for an estimated 15% of preventable mortality in the United States.[17,28]

3.   Making decisions and taking actions based on reliable evidence

PHM is the platform for addressing key required changes in ACA, IHI Triple Aim, and other quality care measures. This requires the use of evidence-based tools and protocols for assessing, diagnosing, and treating patients in a consistent and efficient manner. The seven underlying principles of a population health approach are dependent on the use of best evidence available in practice, policy, program, and technology to appropriately assess, identify, stratify, plan, implement, measure, collect, use, and analyze data with automation needed to reduce cost and increase quality and outcomes. With the shift from volume to value, there is almost an accelerated need for use of health information and effective technology to automate appropriate tasks; optimize processes; and store, manage, and analyze data to continually inform decision, action, research, policy, and outcomes. Some of the tasks required in health care systems to advance population health are routine and standardized tasks that do not need to be done by human beings and can be automated for efficiency and accuracy. In addition, "automation also allows healthcare delivery organizations to better assess population needs and stratify populations based on geography, health status, resource utilization, and demographics."[29]

Most health care delivery organizations use EHRs to collect patients' health data and have care managers to coordinate care of patients grouped into categories by disease condition. This has been the traditional approach of disease management programs. Population health has shifted this approach from traditional disease management to an improved process of care management stratification of patients who are well and need preventive care; patients who are sick enough to require mild early intervention to become well with support from a care manager; patients who are sick diagnosed with less serious chronic conditions to require medical treatment and interventions to prevent them from getting worse; and patients who are chronically sick to require serious medical treatment and intensive care management. Reports using linked EHR information, claims data, financial data, patients' self-reports, and other patients' registries should be available to activate and support responsibilities of providers and management to advance population health. Such intelligent information presents the needed evidence on best practices that are working and sheds light on what is not working and where to change to improve quality, measure cost and patients' experience of care, and improve health equity in support of the IHI Triple Aim goals. A key to success of this principle is to assure that the data are clean, accurate, complete, and validated for reporting of performance.

4. Investing in upstream, integrative, and quality interventions

Studies have shown that shifting the balance of care from curative to preventive or primary care is not only cost-effective but also quality care. Likewise shifting the investment in upstream interventions that address what causes people to be sick in the first place instead of mainly in the downstream where people are sick and getting treated in the hospitals or experiencing avoidable deaths is encouraged by population health.[30] It is established that medical care, although important, accounts for about 15% of health outcomes, whereas a wide spectrum of social factors apart from medical care significantly affect health outcomes.[16,31,32] To optimize the impact of health care delivery systems, we have to integrate upstream prevention with primary care, hospital, and home care in a patient- and family-centered approach.

As a result, an assessment of population health should include a vast range of interventions based on thorough assessment and problem definition of the holistic needs for the patients' panel or population. At the individual level, the use of evidence-based assessment tools is highly recommended to determine the health problems and identify strengths that could be protective to inform authentic solutions. In addition, a cost-benefit analysis to help determine priorities for investment must be conducted. This process of priority setting should leverage investments in other sectors with viable potentials to positively influence health. Furthermore, there should be stratification of risks and assets pertaining to both the clinicians (health care and social) and the patients. Also, determination of opportunities for improvements based on evidence is needed to demonstrate possible return on investment of the interventions across the spectrum of health continuum. The existence of reliable assessments and use of big data, such as the public health vital records, hospitals' CHNA, patients'

EHR, claims payment data, hospital discharge data, and motor vehicles crash data, could inform and evaluate appropriateness of investment to be made by the partners in achieving the health outcomes. Remember the main question for the chief financial officer and the Board, where applicable, is whether your proposed intervention(s) for investment by the organization is cost-effective. Therefore, cost-benefit analysis and best evidence of practice, including investment from other sectors, are crucial in securing investment for upstream interventions as well as immediate, short-term, and long-term results.

A similar process is applicable to secure investment for integrative and quality interventions within the health care settings. In addition to demonstrating how the absence of requested investment to support the proposed intervention will affect the organization (e.g., by resulting in fragmented, high cost, less quality care, and undesirable outcomes) you should align your "ask" with agency or leadership priorities. Also, there is a need to identify interventions to divest or discontinue to improve health outcomes. In addition, to improve health outcomes of the population being served by a health care center, a primary care clinic, or a hospital, the clinician must participate, if possible lead, this effort with the patients and other clinical staff and administrative staff. Everybody must be involved and understand the mission, population goals, and priorities. The strategy for integrating and coordinating care to meet patients' needs should be clearly understood as part of standard practice. To effectively integrate care and respond adequately to the health needs of the population, automation of data sources to reliably deploy relevant health information is necessary. An example is Bon Secours Medical Group, Richmond, Virginia; Robert Fortini, the Vice President, said that they "use a service that maintains a registry of our patient population. By applying clinical protocols to the registry data, this service generates automated messages to patients who need to be seen. Last year, the system made 78,000 telephone calls; as a result, patients scheduled 17,000 appointments with their clinicians. Our organization doesn't have the manpower to do that kind of outreach manually."[33] Likewise, a hospital call center that performs a traditional role of answering and helping patients who call them can send automated messaging to all discharged patients reminding them to see their clinicians, fill their prescriptions, and call the hospital if they have any questions about their care plan. This could provide much needed time for care managers to address more complex needs such as calling only patients with history of noncompliance. Likewise, automated health promotion messages could be sent to patients with chronic disease, such as type 2 diabetes.

5. Advancing health equity by reducing disparities in health

The U.S. Healthy People 2020 recognizes that "Health disparities adversely affect groups of people who have systematically experienced greater obstacles to health based on their racial or ethnic group; religion;

socioeconomic status; gender; age; mental health; cognitive, sensory, or physical disability; sexual orientation or gender identity; geographic location; or other characteristics historically linked to discrimination or exclusion."[34] The release of the landmark report by the Institute of Medicine Unequal Treatment: Confronting Racial and Ethnic Disparities in Health shows significant pervasive evidence of issues concerning access to care, quality of care received, and improvement in health outcomes among different groups, with minority groups receiving unequal treatment and health outcomes.[35] David Satcher et al. stated "that using 2002 data, an estimated 83,570 excess deaths each year could be prevented in the U.S. if the black-white mortality gap could be eliminated."[1] Population health requires health care providers to address health disparities to advance health equity. It expects health care providers to know the population they serve and have a better understanding of their health needs presented at the clinical settings as well as their social needs that affect their health outcomes. This means that health care delivery systems are to be involved in the community in which patients reside to know the factors that might worsen their vulnerability, increase their risks, or be protective and build their resilience. Measuring and demonstrating advancement in health equity and reduction of disparities in health is complex based on social determinants and social gradient in health. Michael Marmot (2017) suggested five actions health professionals could take to improve the social conditions that constrain health: (1) education and training, (2) seeing the patient in a broader perspective, (3) the health service as an employer, (4) working in partnership, and (5) advocacy.[9] Conditions in which people are born, live, work, play, grow, and age shape and determine health outcomes of a population, to a large extent. Some researchers have argued that synergy surrounding race, ethnicity, and gender make them to be the fundamental causes of health status.[13] Adding equity protocols to health registries, clinical information, and claims data will help health professionals perform the five actions, as well as produce standard reporting to track levels of inequities and advance equity.

For health care systems to apply this requirement, they should always ask: (1) who is vulnerable (non-breast-feeding mothers by choice), (2) who is underserved (has no car or public transportation), or excluded (missing medical appointment with no annual visit), and (3) under which circumstances, and how the vulnerability or exclusion materializes into health risks or disease status of one group versus another group within a patient panel or population served by the same medical home or hospital is crucial. For instance, breast-feeding provides lasting health benefits to both mothers and their babies, and rates of breastfeeding initiation, intention, and duration in the United States differ by race, ethnicity, income, and nativity.[36] Some people have linked the disproportionate low intention, initiation, and duration of breast-feeding among African Americans to the historical use of black mothers as "wet nurses" for the white mothers during slavery in the United States. The suggested intersection between this historical experience and the present disparity in breast-feeding among this population requires further studies. Intersectionality suggests that larger structures of oppression and privilege converge on individuals and groups of individuals to pattern advantage and disadvantage.[37] To apply equity lens to a noncommunicable disease goal of obesity reduction by 10% in 1 year as a goal, one has to first identify who has this disease and why. Who contributes, to what proportion, to this burden of disease in the clinic, and why those people? The next steps include determining what SDH is associated with the patients' condition, including stress, sleep, and occupation factors, such as sedentary work, job stress, and working long hours with no time to engage in activities that mitigate these negative effects. It is important to be mindful that health disparities have existed for more than a century in the United States with the racial and ethnic health disparity gap growing wider.[3]

The use of health data and evidence are crucial in assessing, determining, and defining the problem to solve, strategies to use, scope of actions to take as potential solutions or interventions, and results to target and where (multiple settings). Also, public interest, measures of success to track, and coordinating mechanism for accountability should be addressed. The question to continually ask is whether health needs of every individual, group of people, or all populations are met, and how the health outcomes are distributed among the groups. Camara Jones states that "racial health disparities are produced on at least three levels: differential care within health care system; differential access to health care; and differences in exposures and life opportunities that create different levels of health and disease."[13] It is imperative for health care providers to continually evaluate the health outcomes of populations they serve at different settings to ensure that appropriate, adequate, and equitable interventions are provided in response to their needs to demonstrate measurable reduction in health disparities in targeted areas for all populations. Leaderships across sectors internal to the organization and external partners are to be engaged based on the SDH framework to address the social context that affects inequities.

6.   Proactively engaging patients across the continuum of care

The patient-centered medical home (PCMH) of ACA requires primary care clinicians to engage patients and families in patient care to adequately and appropriately improve their health outcomes.[38] PCMH goals include incenting primary care practices with payment to effectively coordinate services and be responsive to patients' unique needs, culture, values, preferences, including language and after hour offices, self-care support, engaging patients as partners in their care, and involved in quality, practice, and policy improvements.[38] Based on the spectrum of care continuum in population health as depicted in Figure 1.1, a PCMH practice has to engage the patients before the medical visit or encounter, during the encounter, after the encounter, and in between encounters through a coordinated team of providers.

One of the commonly shared challenges of the health care system is "how do we recruit the patients?" The Institute for Family-Centered Care recommended the following tips for recruiting patients and their families in health care systems seeking to proactively engage patients:

i. Ask patients and families who are already involved if they have a friend who might be interested in participating.
ii. Ask providers to identify patients and families.
iii. Contact family networks, support groups, or advocacy organizations (in the community you serve).
iv. Post notices in appropriate languages on bulletin boards in waiting areas in clinics and in hospital emergency rooms.
v. Post notices in appropriate languages on bulletin boards at educational, recreational, and social service programs and clinics serving patients and families.
vi. Include information about opportunities for patients and families to participate as advisors in the program's or hospital's consumer satisfaction surveys.
vii. Ask patients and families who participate in neonatal intensive care unit and postpartum reunion gatherings.
viii. Ask individuals and families who participate in cancer survivor meetings.
ix. Create a Web page for the Patient and Family Advisory Council and include recruitment information on the site. Link with other relevant websites in the community and encourage them to link with the Council site.
x. Develop radio and television public service announcements in the language of the communities you are trying to reach.
xi. Place a story in community newspapers.
xii. Use "key informants"—people in the community who are knowledgeable about patients' and families' needs and are a link to other patient and family groups.
xiii. Ask community and church leaders (also ask barbers and beauty shop owners).
xiv. Send notices to social and cultural clubs in the community.
xv. Place posters in community locations—at large employers, churches, housing projects, clinics, gas stations, social service agencies, and kindergarten registration (also place posters in local grocery stores and laundromats).
xvi. Send a letter home with school children.[39]

Patients' engagement adds a unique quality to the coordination of care connecting interventions to address the social and medical needs of the patients to influence their health outcomes. The complexities of care required to meet health needs of patients through provision of culturally appropriate and responsive services is not to be underestimated. Some of the questions to guide health care practitioners in engaging their patients include but are not limited to: (1) who are the patients with less optimal outcomes or exacerbated health conditions to be improved, (2) what are their care gaps, (3) where do they live, (4) how do we proactively partner with patients to improve their health, (5) what interventions should be provided and when, where, and by whom, (6) how could the conditions of health for a group of patients be positively influenced, and (7) who could help address these health conditions to improve population health outcomes? Patients must be engaged in their care planning, be involved in codesigning their interventions to increase potentials of their effectiveness, and participate in quality improvements. Applying effective strategies to improve patients' experience of and satisfaction with care is vital to improving their health outcomes. The main activator of patient engagement is the primary care clinician or provider (PCP), and the level of quality relationship between the PCP and patients determines the level of motivation, engagement, and satisfaction of the patients. Also, leveraging upstream interventions and information technology could help achieve PCMH goals.

7. Demonstrating accountability for health outcomes

Implementation of population health requires formation of partnerships internally and externally with networks of providers and the patients plus their families, where applicable, to be successful. The health care systems to demonstrate accountability of health outcomes have to establish an accountability culture in their organizations. This will require a clearly developed and actionable results-based accountability framework that is underpinned with principles of execution and continuous quality improvement. Using existing requirements by payers (such as ACA, PCMH, EHR, CMS' Physician Quality Reporting Initiative) and applying notable organization tools and metrics (e.g., IHI Triple Aim) could help galvanize and facilitate the organization culture to become more accountable for population health outcomes. This shift requires a clinician to change his or her practice and become an integrator working in a team-based practice to coordinate and deliver appropriate care. Accountability demands identification of where patient's health status is at the point of encounter to establish baseline measures and set targets for health improvement.[27] Data collection, analysis, and application are crucial parts of population health approach beginning from needs assessment to diagnosis to direct care services and interventions addressing associated SDH factors to measuring outcomes and tracking progress toward equitable health status across all populations. The shift from a traditional approach to health care delivery to a population health approach depends on business intelligence applications to conduct essential standardized tasks, such as automation of messaging health information and alerts to patients for medical visit reminders, post–medical visit reminders on care plan compliance actions, hospital discharge messages on next steps, and pharmacy prescription drug pick-up reminders. The same intelligence application of data analytics could help with stratification of patients' risks and assets, morbidity, mortality, health status, disease management, wellness, and patient experience. To facilitate accountability, targeted goals must have associated clear objectives with measures and indicators of success. This accountability culture needs a coordinated mechanism for data sharing, reporting progress, celebrating success, and continuously improving health outcomes of the populations. There should be a shared accountability with other factors including "public health interventions, aspects of the social environment (income, education, employment, social support, and culture) and of the physical environment (urban design, clean air and water), genetics, and individual behavior"[40] affecting population health.

Most designed business intelligence applications are developed to measure mortality, health status, morbidity, and patient experience. Linking and integrating financial information, clinical information, patients' registries, and other practice data into the business intelligence application is highly encouraged to provide population-wide reports needed to measure input, output, process, and outcome indicators of improvements being made toward quality and equitable population health. With the help of big data and standardized reporting, one can show information on partners' progress and identify trends, gaps, and opportunities for improvement of population health outcomes.

Table 1.1 has examples of population health outcome metrics to be considered.

Keep your mind focused on patient's experience, choose one population health outcome from the list in Table 1.1, and write out associated strategy, measures, and resources needed to implement it.

WHAT ARE SOME BEST PRACTICES OF POPULATION HEALTH MANAGEMENT IN HEALTH CARE DELIVERY SYSTEMS?

Introduction

This section discusses PHM and uses best practices to explicate how a population health approach works in health care delivery systems. The HHS Agency for Healthcare Research and Quality introduced a concept called "practice-based population health," which is defined as "an approach to care that uses information on a group of patients within a primary care practice or group of practices to improve the care and clinical outcomes of patients within that practice."[41] As illustrated in prior sections of this chapter, population health shifts the focus of the health care delivery clinician from taking care of patients on an individual basis to taking care of group of individuals or the patient panel with the goal of improving equitable health outcomes. Based on countless research, the definition and

TABLE 1.1   Examples of Population Health Outcome Metrics to be Considered

Mortality	Morbidity	Inequities	Primary/Preventive
Neonatal (<28 d)	<Ventilator-acquired pneumonia	Stratified by race, ethnicity, income, sex, education level, social class, wealth, or zip code	Satisfactory patient experience and timely access to treatment
Infant (<1 yr)	Reduced Infection	Same as above	Completeness of vaccines and periodic preventive visits
Disease specific	Reduced type 2 diabetes incidence	Same as above	Active lifestyle and healthy eating
Injury specific	Reduced fall (>55 yr)	Same as above	Hospital admission or readmission
Disability related	Reduced depression	Same as above	Stress management, adequate sleep, and self-care support
Smoking related	Improved cardiac care	Same as above	Education and cessation treatment
Occupation linked	>Medication safety, e.g., pain	Same as above	Safe work place

principles of population health, it is established that medical care is one of the factors amid other SDH. Evidence shows that, although medical care plays an important role when people are already sick, it plays a very limited role in determining who becomes sick or injured in the first place.[15,42,43] With the population health approach, the health care delivery systems are now influencing health conditions outside the clinical settings through partnership and investing on upstream interventions.

The similarity between population health and PHM is their common goal to improve health outcomes of group of individuals or a population, including to advance equitable distribution of such outcomes within the group or population. The difference between population health and PHM is that the former is a broader perspective and can take place anywhere by health organization entity (e.g., public health), whereas the latter takes place in health care settings, such as health care centers, health clinics, and hospitals. The goal of PHM is to improve health outcomes of the patient population by keeping "a patient population as healthy as possible, minimizing the need for expensive interventions such as emergency department visits, hospitalizations, imaging tests, and procedures"[6] and it systematically addresses the preventive and chronic care needs of every patient.[29] This approach recognizes that individuals' ability to change is socially contextualized. The changing social circumstances lead to changes in individuals' vulnerability and the distribution of health risks. Therefore, population management seeks to continuously assess, track, and modify these factors that make people sick or exacerbate their illnesses, while improving health outcomes. No single health care organization is capable of addressing all of these factors without collaborating with community resources, such as transportation, public health agencies, social service agencies, schools, chamber of commerce, city planning, and other associated local entities, to improve the overall health of their populations.

Sample Best Practices on Population Health Management

There are growing demonstrations of best practices on PHM especially since the enactment of the Health Information Technology for Economic and Clinical Health Act of 2009 and the subsequent ACA of 2010 in the United States. PHM is fundamental to the transformation of the health care delivery system as already described in this chapter. The Care Continuum Alliance defined population health as an improvement model that highlights three components: (1) the central care delivery and leadership roles of the primary care physician, (2) the critical importance of patient activation, involvement, and personal responsibility, and (3) the patient focus and capacity expansion of care coordination provided through wellness and disease and chronic care management programs.[44] Based on the seven principles that underpin population health approach, let us look at some examples of best practices on some of these principles.

Example #1

PHM requires a practice shift in health care delivery systems from clinician management of patients to management of a patient population's health outcomes. Clinicians will have to become accustomed to thinking in terms of caring for an entire population and not just for the individual patients who actively seek care. This is a significant change in the way of thinking and the practice patterns of clinicians and requires appropriate training and development of new skills to successfully operationalize this new approach. One of the fundamental strategies to support the clinician accountability for population health is to integrate the care continuum linking preventive with primary to curative and palliative care. There are many ways of redesigning care to be integrative, and the following is just one example.

Sample Best Practice on Integrative Care

At Kaiser Permanente, we put a lot of effort into customizing our EHR as part of the implementation process, which took several years. One reason for this was that the EHR they had purchased lacked many of the features needed for PHM. For example, "we had to develop registries and automation tools to identify care gaps, do patient outreach, and stratify populations into subgroups such as people with chronic illnesses and people at the end of life." Health care organizations that are trying to do PHM must also, like Kaiser, find a way to integrate their EHR across inpatient, ambulatory, and continuing care settings. This approach helps to improve the coordination of care and also provides other opportunities for proactive care management. For instance, Kaiser has been leveraging its EHR in a unique approach to proactively care for patients so that when they come in for acute health problems, they also receive care for their chronic conditions. To illustrate how they have leveraged their systems integration, for instance, if patients come in for a laboratory test and it is discovered that they have not refilled their medications for a chronic condition, the laboratory will arrange that. And if members are in the pharmacy and it is found they are in need of a mammogram, the pharmacist will ask their clinician to order one. This has been a fundamental shift for Kaiser and has had a dramatic impact on filling those care gaps and improving their performance on quality measures. Kaiser also regards patient engagement as a crucial part of PHM. Their patient portal allows members to schedule appointments, review medications, see laboratory results, e-mail clinicians with questions, and receive health information materials. Their patients can also view their medical information in a personal health record. All of this involves the patient partnership more in their own care, while allowing families to participate more fully with the patient's permission. This example supports meaningful use of data and health information exchange to improve population health outcomes. It also fosters team work, care coordination, and a culture of shared responsibility.

Source: Adapted from the Institute for Health Technology Transformation (iHT2) Guide to Population Health by: Alide Chase, Senior Vice President, Quality and Service Matt Stiefel, Senior Director, Care and Service Quality Kaiser.[4,27]

Example #2

Patient and family engagement or patient experience of care is one common measure, element, principle of not only population health but also ACA, AQHR, IHI Triple Aim, and quality improvement metrics. A focus on the patient who is the ultimate customer of health care service as a key driver of health outcomes makes sense in light of the recognition of other social determinant factors that can help or hinder patient's health. To create the right culture and environment for accomplishing this vital part of PHM improvement, one should first assess the extent to which any given health care organization (e.g., primary care office, hospital, health center, or clinic) operates as a patient- and family-centered care entity. The following presents an assessment to guide the health care delivery organization in knowing where they are in their culture and operations and identifying opportunities for their improvement.

Sample Best Practice on How to Assess Organizational Culture of Patient- and Family-Centered Care

Initial Assessment of Organizational Culture and Philosophy of Care

- Do the organization's vision, mission, and philosophy of care statements reflect the principles of patient- and family-centered care and promote partnerships with the patients and families it serves?
- Has the organization defined quality health care, and does this definition include how patients and families will experience care?
- Has the definition of quality and philosophy of care been communicated clearly throughout the health care organization, to patients and families and others in the community?
- Do the organization's leaders model collaboration with patients and families?
- Are the organization's policies, programs, and staff practices consistent with the view that families are allies for patient health, safety, and well-being?

Patient and Family Participation in Organizational Advisory Roles

- Is there an organizational patient and family advisory council?
- If there is a patient and family advisory council, is patient safety a regular agenda item?
- Do patients and families serve on committees and work groups involved in
  - Patient safety?
  - Quality improvement?
  - Facility design?
  - Patient/family education?
  - Service excellence?
  - Discharge/transition planning?
  - Staff orientation and education?
  - Ethics?

Architecture and Design

- Does the health care organization's architecture and design
  - Create welcoming impressions throughout the facility for patients and families?
  - Reflect the diversity of patients and families served?
  - Provide for the privacy and comfort of patients and families?
  - Support the presence and participation of families?
  - Facilitate patient and family access to information?
  - Support the collaboration of staff across disciplines and with patients and families?

Patient and Family Access to Information

- Are patients and families viewed as essential members of the health care team? For example, are they encouraged and supported to participate in care planning and decision-making?
- Are there systems in place to ensure that patients and families have access to complete, unbiased, and useful information?
- Are patients and families encouraged to be present and to participate in rounds and nurse change of shift?
- Are patients and families encouraged to review their medical records and work with staff and physicians to correct inaccuracies?
- Are patients and families provided with practical information on how to best assure safety in health care?

Education and Training Programs

- Do orientation and education programs prepare staff, physicians, students, and trainees for patient- and family-centered practice and collaboration with patients, families, and other disciplines?
- Are patients and families involved as faculty in orientation and educational programs?

Research

- In research programs, do patients and families participate in
  - Shaping the agenda?
  - Conducting the research?
  - Analyzing the data?
  - Disseminating the results?

Human Resources Policies

- Does the organization's human resources system support and encourage the practice of patient- and family-centered care?
- Are there policies in place to ensure that
  - Individuals with patient- and family-centered skills and attitudes are hired?
  - There are explicit expectations that all employees respect and collaborate with patients, families, and staff across disciplines and departments?

Source: Adapted from Hospitals & Health Networks, on the MCG Health System in Augusta, Georgia 23; 3.[47]

Example #3

The PHM is centered on primary care and the critical role of PCPs. This requires a continuous supply of primary care physicians to ensure that patients receive appropriate preventive and long-term care in the primary care settings.[45] The shortage of PCPs and an increase in population and longevity, among other factors, have led to increased unmet expectation of PCPs. The expanded role of nurse practitioners as PCPs in most areas aims at addressing this provider demand and unmet health needs of U.S. populations. The shift of health care practice from individual patient care to population health can be achieved only through a care team of providers led by physicians or nurse practitioners, or other eligible clinicians in partnership with the patients and families plus other relevant professionals. These care teams are increasingly including mid-level practitioners, such as medical assistants, dietitians, physical therapists, nurses, care managers, and health coaches.[32] The use of care teams has also resulted in a practice redesign with different work flow, and in some places, enhanced automation of care is added. The next example describes one best practice of a care team.

Sample Best Practice on Evidence-Based Care Management

One of the evidence-based practices is the use of Standing Orders and Core Responsibilities of Care Team Medical Assistant (CTMA). The U.S. Preventive Services Task Force levels A and B evidence have put in effect through standing orders what the CTMA can execute. This evidence defines the roles and responsibilities of the CTMA by standing orders to support the CTMA in focusing on the activities of prevention, referrals, and patient follow-up as part of PHM.[46] Preventive care standing orders covered reviewing the need for a number of cancer screenings and immunizations, such as breast cancer, cervical cancer, and shingles. Standing orders were also created for chronic disease management and for routine referrals by CTMAs to other members of the care team. For example, standing orders covered referrals to care management, pharmacy, social work, and nutritionists.

Using the Penobscot health care organization experience, assigning these tasks to medical assistants was a major departure from standard practices at Penobscot. Traditionally, clinicians at Penobscot had made referrals on their own, including routine referrals to pharmacists, licensed clinical social workers, care managers, and physical therapists. To further support clinicians, the CTMA role was expanded beyond population health and previsit planning to include clinicians' desktop management. This responsibility included tasks such as prioritizing abnormal laboratory results in providers' inboxes for their review. With a focus on prevention and population health, the CTMA:

- Uses a registry to identify patients' overdue for chronic disease care and preventive care.
- Orders overdue care for patients based on applicable standing orders.
- Calls patients who are overdue on preventive screenings and uses motivational interviewing techniques to encourage patients to come in.

For advance previsit planning (1–2 weeks ahead of patient's scheduled visit), the CTMA

- Updates and resolves medications such as antibiotics for acute or short-term conditions identified in the medical record.
- Follows up on previous orders and consults with providers outside Penobscot.
- Documents data from new patient records and specialist reports.
- Orders overdue or upcoming care, using motivational interviewing to discuss services due with patients.

For clinician desktop management, the CTMA

- Prioritizes laboratory tests and test results.
- Updates previous medical, social, and surgical history from consults, emergency department, and hospital reports.
- Enters data in discrete and appropriate fields.
- Ensures follow-up if appropriate.
- Orders additional testing per standing orders.
- Helps clinicians organize and prioritize messages on their desktops by using flags so that clinicians can respond to messages more efficiently.

Based on the aforementioned examples of three sample best practices:

1. Determine and assign the seven principles of population health to the three examples as you deem appropriate.
2. Why did you choose the principles, and what made you to match them with the examples?
3. Identify one practice you would like to implement in your organization, and why?

SUGGESTED RESOURCES AND MATERIALS

Affordable Care Act. New Requirements for 501(c)3 Hospitals Under the Affordable Care Act.
https://www.irs.ov/charities-non-profits.
https://www.aap.org/en-us/professional-resources/practice-transformation/Implementation-Guide/Pages/Population-Health.aspx.
https//www.hhs.gov/healthcare/about the Affordable Care Act.
www.ipfcc.org/resources/Patient-Safety-Toolkit-04.pdf.
www.who.int/social_determinants/sdh.
www.who.int/social_determinants/en/.

REFERENCES

1. Satcher D, Fryer GE, McCann J, Troutman A, Woolf SH, Rust G. What if we were equal? A comparison of the black–white mortality gap in 1960 and 2000. *Health Affairs*. 2005;24(2). doi:10.1377/hlthaff.24.2.459.
2. Solar O, Irwin A. *A Conceptual Framework for Action on the Social Determinants of Health. Discussion Paper for the Commission on Social Determinants of Health.* Geneva: World Health Organization; 2007. Available at http://www.who.int/social_determinants/resources/csdh_framework_action_05_07.pdf [cited 2013 JulA 8].

3. Srinivasan S, Williams SD. Transitioning from health disparities to a health equity research agenda: the time is now. *Public Health Rep.* 2014;129(suppl 2):71-76.

4. Stiefel M, Nolan KA. *Guide to Measuring the Triple Aim: Population Health, Experience of Care, and Per Capita Cost. IHI Innovation Series White Paper.* Cambridge, Massachusetts: Institute for Healthcare Improvement; 2012. Available at www.IHI.org.

5. Szreter S. The GRO and the public health movement 1837-1914. *Soc His Med.* 1991;4:435-463.

6. Mahon M. *U.S. Spends More on Health Care Than Other High-Income Nations But Lower Life Expectancy, Worse Health.* The Commonwealth Fund. Accessed at http://www.commonwealthfund.org/publications/issue-briefs/2015/0ct/us-health-care-from-aglobal-perspective.

7. Blumenthal D, Tavenner M. The "meaningful use" regulation for electronic health records. *N Engl J Med.* 2010;363:501-504.

8. Center for Medicare and Medicaid Innovation. http://innovations.cms.gov/.

9. Marmot M. The health gap: doctors and the social determinants of health. *Scand J Public Health.* 2017;45(7):686-693. doi:10.1177/1403494817717448.

10. https//www.hhs.gov/healthcare/about the Affordable Care Act.

11. https://www.irs.ov/charities-non-profits – New Requirements for 501(c)3 Hospitals Under the Affordable Care Act.

12. www.who.int/social_determinants/sdh.

13. Jones CP. Levels of racism: a theoretical framework and a gardener's tale. *Am J Public Health.* 2000;90(8):1212-1215.

14. Szreter S. Rethinking McKeown: the relationship between public health and social change. *Am J Public Health.* 2002;92:722-725.

15. Jones CP. *Confronting Institutionalized Racism.* National Center for Chronic Disease Prevention and Health Promotion, Center of Disease Control and Prevention; 2000. https//www.unnaturalcauses.org.

16. World Health Organization. *Closing the gap in a Generation: Health Equity Through Action on the Social Determinants of Health. Final Report of the Commission on Social Determinants of Health.* Geneva: WHO; 2008. Available at http://www.who.int/social_determinants/thecommission/finalreport/en/index.html.

17. McGuinnis JM, Williams-Russo P, Knickman JR. The case for more active policy attention to health promotion. *Health Aff (Millwood).* 2002;21:78-93.

18. https://www.aap.org/en-us/professional-resources/practice-transformation/Implementation-Guide/Pages/Population-Health.aspx.

19. Lidsky T, Schneider JS. Lead neurotoxicity in children: basic mechanisms and clinical correlates. *Brain.* 2003;126(1):5-19. doi:10.1093/brain/awg014.

20. Afeiche M, Peterson KE, Sanchez BN, et al. Windows of lead exposure sensitivity, attained height, and body mass index at 48 months. *J Pediatric.* 2012;160:1044-1049.

21. Race PB. Class and environmental health: a review and systematization of the literature. *Environ Res.* 1995;69:15-30.

22. Lanphear BP, Kahn RS, Berger O, Auinger P, Bortnick SM, Nahhas RW. Contribution of residential exposures to asthma in U.S. children and adolescents. *Pediatrics.* 2001;107:E98.

23. Pollack CE, Cubbin C, Ahn D, Winkleby M. Neighborhood deprivation and alcohol consumption: does the availability of alcohol play a role? *Int J Epidemiol.* 2005;34:772-780.

24. Chuang YC, Ubbin C, Ahn D, Winkleby MA. Effects of neighborhood socio-economic status and convenience store concentration on individual level smoking. *J Epidemiol Community Health.* 2005;59:568-573.

25. Cummins S, Mcintyre S. Food environment and obesity-neighborhood or nation? *Int J Epidemiol.* 2006;35:100-104.
26. Gordon-Larsen P, Nelson MC, Page P, Popkin BM. Inequality in the built environment underlies key health disparities in physical activity and obesity. *Pediatrics.* 2006;117:417-424.
27. https://www.hse.ie/eng/about/who/population-health/population-health-approach/population-health-strategy-july-2008.pdf.
28. Braveman P, Gotlieb L. It's time to consider the causes of causes. *Public Health Rep.* 2014;129(suppl 2):19-31. doi:10.1177/00333549141291S206.
29. Hodach R. The promise of population health management: New Technologies are required to automate expanded physician workflow. *Phytel White Paper.* 2013.
30. Rose G, Marmot MG. Social class and coronary heart diseases. *Br Heart J.* 1981;45:13-19.
31. Marmot M, Bell R. Fair society, healthy lives. *Public Health.* 2012;126(suppl 1):S4-S10.
32. Kindig DA, Stoddart G. What is population health? *Am J Public Health.* 2003; 93:3669.
33. Institute for Health Technology Transformation – www.exerciseismedicine.org/population health management.
34. U.S. Department of Health and Human Services Office of Health Promotion and Disease Prevention [US-HHS]. *Health People 2020.* Washington, DC: US Department of Health and Human Services; 2010.
35. Institute of Medicine (IOM). *Unequal Treatment: Confronting Racial and Ethnic Disparities in Health Care.* Washington, DC: The National Academies Press; 2003. doi:10.17226/10260.
36. Bowleg L. The problem with the phrase women and minorities: intersectionality—an important theoretical framework for public health. *Am J Public Health.* 2012;102(7):1267-1273.
37. Fabiyi C, Peacock N, Hebert-Beirne J, Handler A. A qualitative study to understand nativity differences in breastfeeding behaviors among middle-class African American and African-born women. *Maternal Child Health J.* 2016;20(10):2100-2111.
38. Strategies to Put Patients at the Center of Primary Care – PCM – AHRQ: http://www.pcmh.ahrq.gov.
39. Jeppson E, Thomas J. *Essential Allies: Families as Advisors.* Bethesda, MD: Institute for Family Centered Care.
40. World Health Organization. *Social Determinants of Health: The Solid Facts*; 2013. Number 18000264. ISBN:9789289014014.
41. Cusack CM, Knudsen AD, Kronstadt JL, Singer RF, Brown AL. Practice-based population health: information technology to support transformation to proactive primary care. *AHRQ.* 2010;4. Publication No. 10-0092-EF.
42. Alder NE, Marmot M, McEwen BS, Stewart J, eds. *Socioeconomic Status and Health in Industrial Nations: Social, Psychological, and Biological Pathways.* New York: New York Academy of Sciences; 1999.
43. Braveman P, Egerter S, Williams DR. The social determinants of health: coming of age. *Annu Rev Public Health.* 2011;32:381-398.
44. Care Continuum Alliance. Advancing the Population Health Improvement Model. http://www.fiercehealthit.com/story/hennepin-health-project-looksbuild-countywide-ehr-program-national-implica/2012-01-10.
45. Chen EH, Bodenheimer T. Improving population health through team-based panel management. *Arch Intern Med.* 2011;171:17.

46. Grantham S. Redesigning Health Care Teams for Population Health and Quality. https://www.ahrq.gov/systems.
47. American Hospital Association and the Institute for Family-Centered Care. *Strategies for Leadership—Patient and Family-centered Care Toolkit.* Washington, DC; 2004. Available at http://www.aha.org/aha/issues/Quality-and-Patient-Safety/strategiespatientcentered.html.

Please see Online Appendix: Apps and Digital Resources for additional information.

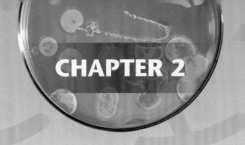

CHAPTER 2

Principles of Risk Assessment

ELIZABETH ROESSLER

INTRODUCTION

Case 1: *A 21-year-old male college student was brought to the emergency department following a motor vehicle accident. He was the unbelted driver of an automobile involved in a high-speed collision. The patient was ejected from the vehicle on impact and thrown 50 yd, sustaining fatal head injuries. The deceased patient's blood alcohol concentration was 0.24%. Past medical history revealed that he had been seen for acute gastritis at the student health center on three occasions in the last year. The records revealed no discussion of his alcohol use, which had been a problem since high school, or his regular practice of driving without using a seat belt.*

    Case 2: *A 52-year-old woman presented to a gastroenterologist with a 3-month history of progressive left lower quadrant abdominal pain, weight loss, and fatigue. In the last few days she had noted bloody stool. A colonoscopic examination with biopsy revealed an obstructing adenocarcinoma of the sigmoid colon. The patient underwent a partial colectomy and colostomy placement. Past medical history was noteworthy for ulcerative colitis, which was diagnosed when the patient was 24 years old but which had not required extensive medical care. The patient's previous clinical encounters had been limited to preventive visits to her gynecologist, who had never discussed her ulcerative colitis and had not recommended periodic colonoscopy or sigmoidoscopy.*

    Case 3: *A 49-year-old corporate executive was brought to the emergency department 45 minutes after clutching his chest and collapsing during a business meeting. The electrocardiogram revealed 3-mm ST-segment depression in the anterior leads. Shortly thereafter the patient developed ventricular fibrillation and could not be resuscitated. Postmortem examination revealed a blood cholesterol level of 356 mg/dL and large stenotic plaques in the left main and anterior descending coronary arteries. Family members indicated that the patient had been gaining weight and smoking more heavily in recent years but was otherwise healthy. His siblings were also considered to be healthy, but two sisters were being treated for elevated* *serum lipid levels. The patient's father and uncle had also died at a young age from unanticipated heart attacks. The patient visited a clinician only three times as an adult, primarily for treatment of joint injuries received during unsuccessful attempts at jogging. The provider's notes addressed the joint injuries but did not discuss the patient's tobacco use, family history, eating habits, or physical inactivity. No prior record of the patient's lipid levels could be found in the chart.*

Case 4: *A 20-month-old girl was admitted to the hospital with a 1-day history of fever, headache, and increasing lethargy. Physical examination was suggestive of meningitis, and culture of the cerebrospinal fluid demonstrated the presence of* Haemophilus influenza type b. *After completion of intravenous antibiotic therapy, the patient was discharged from the hospital but was noted to have permanent hearing impairment. Review of the family provider's records revealed that the patient had received appropriate immunizations until 9 months of age, but subsequent appointments for well-child examinations were canceled by the parents for unexplained reasons and therefore the* Haemophilus *vaccination series was never completed. The patient's mother did see the family provider on two occasions for treatment of facial lacerations, but the child's immunization status and the conditions at home were not discussed. Six months later, a telephone call from a neighbor prompted an evaluation by the local child protective services agency, which revealed that both the child and mother were regular victims of beatings by the father.*

What these unfortunate cases have in common is clear to the reader: each patient suffered from or died of conditions that were potentially preventable earlier in life. Diseases (e.g., coronary artery disease, colon cancer), injuries (e.g., motor vehicle accidents, physical abuse), and infections (e.g., meningitis) were preceded months, years, and decades earlier by the presence of risk factors or preclinical disease states that were amenable to prevention but that escaped detection and intervention.

Unfortunately, prevention failures of this magnitude are neither exceptional nor uncommon in the United States. Each day, many thousands of Americans undergo treatment for conditions that could have been prevented earlier in their lives if the underlying causal risk factors had been identified. The failure to detect and treat those risk factors while patients are otherwise healthy often culminates years later in the need for aggressive medical interventions (e.g., chemotherapy, surgery, dialysis) and in chronic impairment (pain, paralysis, mental illness, disability, death). Such personally, socially, and financially costly consequences can be prevented through relatively simple interventions, such as modifying harmful health behaviors (e.g., smoking), immunizations, and screening for early detection of disease before it becomes clinically apparent. The reality that so many Americans do not take these steps, despite being under the care of a clinician, has created a growing concern among both professionals and the public.

Americans receive only half of recommended clinical preventive services.[1] Preventive care in the United States is inadequate for many reasons, including limited access to health services, patient noncompliance, and cost. In many cases, however, the failure to receive preventive care is attributable to the failure of clinicians to include risk assessment in their routine care of asymptomatic and healthy patients. The purpose of this chapter is to review the importance of clinical risk assessment and the theoretic principles that underlie the related activities discussed in this book. See Chapters 3–5 for details on how to perform risk assessment as part of the history, physical examination, and laboratory testing.

THE PLACE OF PREVENTION IN ILLNESS VISITS

In this book, the terms *asymptomatic* and *healthy* are not meant to describe patients without complaints; relatively few patients visit their doctor without complaints for the sole purpose of obtaining preventive checkups. Rather, the terms refer to the absence of signs or symptoms of *target conditions*. For example, the executive who was seen on three occasions for joint injuries was "symptomatic" in the usual sense of the term—he had acute joint pain—but he was asymptomatic with respect to the target condition of coronary artery disease.

This, in fact, is the usual context of preventive care: the detection of risk factors in patients who are asymptomatic with respect to target conditions often occurs during clinical encounters that have been scheduled by the patient to address other, more immediate problems. For example, a patient schedules an appointment to address sinusitis but is found to be physically inactive and returns home with *both* an exercise and antibiotic prescription. A patient presents with a vaginal yeast infection but is noted not to have had a Papanicolaou smear for 5 years. A preschool boy with inadequate well-child care is rushed to the emergency department for treatment of acute otitis media and receives his second measles-mumps-rubella vaccination before being discharged.

See Chapter 21 for further discussion of the advantages and disadvantages of delivering preventive care opportunistically during such illness visits, as opposed to during well-person examinations dedicated to prevention.

WHAT IS RISK ASSESSMENT?

Risk assessment in the clinical setting refers to the collection of information about risk factors during the history, physical, and laboratory examination.[a] *Risk factors* are personal characteristics, physiologic parameters,

---

[a]Population-based risk assessment, such as the measurement of environmental and other health risks facing society (e.g., pandemics, bioterrorism), is not discussed here.

symptoms, or preclinical disease states that increase the likelihood that an individual has or will develop a particular disease. Examples of personal characteristics that can increase risk are personal health behaviors (e.g., smoking), family history, genotype, environmental exposures, and occupation. Examples of physiologic risk factors, which can be determined by measurement, include laboratory test results (e.g., serum lipid levels), anthropomorphic measurements (e.g., body mass index), and other laboratory information (e.g., audiometry results). Similarly, symptoms and past or present disease states may also increase a patient's likelihood of developing a related disease.

Chapters 3–5 discuss how to perform risk assessment during the history, physical, and laboratory examination, respectively. Part II of this book discusses what to do with the findings.

Risk assessment should not be regarded as a unique clinical activity, separate from routine patient care. It is, after all, a well-established component of the thorough history, physical, and laboratory examination taught throughout clinical training. Personal characteristics that increase health risk, such as smoking and family history, are commonly addressed in the social and family history sections of the history. Preclinical disease states are sought in a careful physical examination. Physiologic risk factors are often detected in conventional laboratory tests. Yet many clinicians perform incomplete risk assessments when evaluating healthy patients for preventive care.

THE IMPORTANCE OF RISK ASSESSMENT

Why do not clinicians conduct complete risk assessments? Why, for example, did the businessman's clinician not investigate his family history and cardiac risk factors? In some cases, the oversights are due to *lack of knowledge* and the clinician's unfamiliarity with current guidelines. The gynecologist may not have remembered that ulcerative colitis is a risk factor for colon cancer and that periodic endoscopic surveillance may be necessary. In other instances, the oversight is due to *lack of time*. The provider in a busy student health center may have lacked the time to ask about the patient's drinking habits or seat belt use. In some cases, the oversight is due to *distraction* by the patient's current complaints. The family provider's concentration on suturing the mother's facial lacerations may have made him less attentive to the source of her injuries or her daughter's missed appointments. Sometimes the oversight is *attitudinal*, due to a lack of appreciation of the clinical importance of prevention. Problem drinking, seat belt use, unsuccessful attempts at regular exercise, unhealthy eating habits, and missed appointments may all have seemed unimportant at the time, and the serious consequences of overlooking them may have been unapparent. Finally, *inadequate reimbursement* by insurers lessens the enthusiasm of some clinicians to devote large portions of office visits to preventive care.

An important reason for incomplete risk assessments is the unwillingness of clinicians to believe that preventive interventions are worthwhile. Many do not appreciate the linkage between the quality of preventive care provided and the thoroughness of risk assessment, despite its obviously logical basis—clinicians cannot provide patients with rational advice on health maintenance or intervene with early-stage disease without first identifying the risk factors and disease states that most deserve their attention. A standardized "prevention package" for all patients is rarely appropriate, effective, or well received. The prevention priorities for a 55-year-old smoker with a family history of premature heart disease obviously differ from those of the health-conscious young athlete, the drug-using, depressed adolescent who talks of suicide, or the elderly nursing home patient. If the clinician is to have a meaningful and effective impact on the patient's risk of future disease, the prevention message must be tailored to the risk profile of that individual.

Risk assessment is also necessary for the rational ordering of screening tests. For many years, clinicians administered a standard battery of laboratory tests as part of annual checkups, such as screening blood counts and chemistries, urinalyses, chest radiographs, and electrocardiograms. Many clinicians continue this practice now. One problem with this approach, aside from its enormous cost, is that it generates large numbers of false-positive results (see Chapters 5 and 20). This, in turn, leads to a so-called screening cascade of what in fact are unnecessary diagnostic workups and treatment interventions.

Because these adverse effects are less likely when screening is targeted to patients with specific risk factors (in whom the pretest probability and positive predictive value are increased), expert panels, such as the U.S. Preventive Services Task Force (USPSTF),[2] have recommended that clinicians avoid routine test batteries and instead order selected screening tests based on the patient's individual risk profile. This recommendation obviously requires the clinician to first identify the patient's risk factors. It also reinforces the need for clinicians to return to the time-honored traditions of careful history taking and physical examination to limit the currently common overreliance on laboratory testing.

THE BASIS OF INCOMPLETE RISK ASSESSMENT BY CLINICIANS: THE ILLNESS-BASED VERSUS THE RISK FACTOR–BASED THOUGHT PROCESSES

The tendency of clinicians to perform incomplete risk assessments may result from using the wrong thought process when evaluating patients. The commonly used clinical thought process when evaluating symptomatic patients identifies the chief complaint(s) as the primary problem(s) and has as its objective the clarification of the diagnosis and treatment plan. This *illness-based thought process* is, appropriately, oriented to the present and not the future. In such patients, risk assessment—the collection of risk factor information in the history, physical, and laboratory examination—is performed to explain the patient's *current* symptoms and signs. In this context, assessment of *future* risk plays a relatively minor role. Experienced clinicians know that the history of present illness and physical examination findings are usually all that are needed to make the diagnosis. Although risk factor information can occasionally enhance diagnostic accuracy, most clinicians discover over time that their diagnostic accuracy is rarely compromised by an incomplete social, family, or occupational history. Clinicians accustomed to caring for symptomatic patients are therefore not driven to thorough questioning about risk factors.

In preventive medicine, risk assessment has a different purpose, because the patient has not yet developed clinical evidence of the target conditions. Therefore, a different *risk factor–oriented thought process* is necessary. The patients' risk factors, not their current complaints, come to be viewed as the primary problem. In contrast to their relatively minor role in evaluating current symptoms, risk factors constitute the primary problem in preventive care. Therefore, risk assessment becomes the essential starting point for addressing the scope of the problem. What should follow in the thought process is a problem-oriented examination of how to evaluate and modify the identified risks.

A patient with the risk factors of tobacco use, prior exposure to tuberculosis, and susceptibility to influenza requires a special program of smoking cessation counseling, tuberculin skin testing, and influenza vaccination. A patient with the risk factors of multiple sexual partners, injection drug use, and a history of dysplastic nevi requires a special program of sexual practices and substance abuse counseling, screening for sexually transmitted infections and malignant melanoma, and vaccination against hepatitis B. These interventions will not be carried out if the clinician does not first establish the risk factor "problem list" through risk assessment.

Clinicians are more accustomed to the thought process used for symptomatic patients than to the thought process used for preventive care. Their tendency to use the customary illness-based thought process in preventive care probably accounts for the frequency of incomplete risk assessments. To further illustrate the consequences of this mismatch, let us return to the example of a provider accustomed to the illness-based thought process who enters the examination room of the previously mentioned patient with sinusitis. Because the illness-based thought process defines current complaints as the primary problem, the clinician immediately identifies purulent rhinorrhea and maxillary tenderness as the primary matter at hand. With additional physical examination findings to confirm the diagnosis, there is little reason to pursue risk assessment. For a patient with obvious sinusitis, why should the clinician obtain a social, family, or occupational history? The only risk factors to which the illness-based thought process might direct the clinician are those related to sinusitis. The patient would be sent home with an antibiotic prescription but without a discussion of the need to engage in regular exercise.

High-quality preventive care requires the clinician to adopt a risk factor–oriented thought process that is independent of the evaluation of current complaints. Once the current complaints have been addressed, the next step is to switch to a risk factor–oriented thought process, which begins a comprehensive search for unrecognized risk factors. In a systematic process that takes less than a few minutes to complete, the clinician supplements the sinusitis history with information about the risk factors discussed in Chapter 3 and checks whether the patient is up to date on the recommended physical examination and laboratory screening procedures discussed in Chapters 4 and 5. In this example, questions drawn from Chapter 2 would call attention to the patient's physical inactivity and would prompt a discussion of regular exercise or arrangements for a return visit devoted to this topic.

The risk factors identified through this process vary among patients. Each patient's risk factor "problem list" constitutes an *individual risk profile*. It provides global information on the patient's overall risk for developing future disease, as well as a framework for tailoring the health maintenance plan to the patient's particular needs. For example, consider a patient who makes an appointment with a clinician to obtain a bone density measurement. Rather than simplistically responding to this request, the provider performs a brief but thorough risk assessment to review the individual's risk profile. This reveals that the patient has multiple risk factors for other diseases, including a family history of premature coronary artery disease and a personal history of smoking, hypertension, overweight, and hypercholesterolemia. This "big picture" perspective enables the clinician and patient to review the complete list of risk factors and to work together to "triage" the priorities. They first agree that the cardiac risk factors pose a greater threat to future health than does osteoporosis, defer the bone density measurement, and use the remaining time to devise a plan for cardiac risk factor modification. It is rarely appropriate or possible to address all risk factors at once. Health maintenance planning involves collaborative work with the patient: setting priorities by determining which problems the patient is willing and able to address first and agreeing on a follow-up plan for addressing other risk factors. See Chapter 6 for further details about this process.

SETTING REASONABLE LIMITS AND PRIORITIES IN RISK ASSESSMENT

There are at least hundreds of personal characteristics, physiologic parameters, environmental exposures, symptoms, and preclinical disease states that can increase an individual's risk for future disease. Practical and scientific reasons make it implausible for clinicians to screen for all risk factors during risk assessments. The most important practical constraint is lack of time; a typical office visit can accommodate a discussion of no more than two or three risk factors. Moreover, for many risk factors, there is insufficient scientific evidence that they pose *significant* risks or that attempts to modify them are effective in improving health. At its best, devoting time to these unproved measures may be useless. At its worst, this practice can divert the clinician and patient away from more important risk factors that deserve their attention. Up to half of all premature (or early) deaths in the United States are due to behavioral and other preventable factors, including modifiable habits such as tobacco use, poor diet, and lack of exercise.[3]

How, then, should the clinician select the factors to address in risk assessment? These are the key questions to ask: (1) How serious is the target condition? (2) How common is the risk factor? (3) What is the magnitude of risk associated with the risk factor? (4) How accurately can the risk factor be detected? (5) What is the evidence that potential interventions improve health outcomes? (6) How does this information compare with other health priorities? Similar questions are pertinent in setting reasonable limits for almost every topic in this book.

How Serious Is the Target Condition?

Risk factors for a trivial health problem may not deserve attention. The burden of suffering from the target condition is best judged by its frequency and severity. Frequency is typically measured in terms of incidence or prevalence. *Incidence* is the proportion of the population that acquires the condition in a given period of time. *Prevalence* is the proportion of the population that has the condition at any given time. A variety of outcome measures are used to estimate the severity of a health condition. Traditional measures include morbidity, mortality, and survival rates, but health services research has encouraged the use of more meaningful measures of quality of life, functional status, and overall well-being. In terms of mortality, a convenient ranking of the importance of diseases is the leading causes of death, which can be determined for the general population (see Table 2.1) or stratified by specific risk groups. Table 2.2 lists the leading causes of death for specific age groups.

How Common Is the Risk Factor?

A risk factor that is extremely uncommon may not be worthy of routine screening, and some risk factors that are extremely common may be weak predictors of future disease. Like target conditions, the frequency of the presence of a risk factor in the population is generally measured by prevalence and incidence rates and may vary considerably in different segments of the population.

TABLE 2.1   Leading Causes of Death in the United States

Rank	Cause of Death	Number of Deaths, 2015	Age-Adjusted Death Rate (per 100,000)	Percentage of Total Deaths
1	Heart disease	633,842	168.5	23.4
2	Malignant neoplasms	595,930	158.5	22.0
3	Chronic lower respiratory diseases	155,041	41.6	5.7
4	Unintentional injuries	146,571	43.2	5.4
5	Cerebrovascular diseases	140,323	37.6	5.2
6	Diabetes mellitus	79,535	21.3	2.9
7	Influenza and pneumonia	57,062	15.2	2.1

Adapted from National Center for Health Statistics. *Health, United States, 2016: With Chartbook on Long-term Trends in Health.* Hyattsville, MD; 2017. http://www.cdc.gov/nchs/data/hus/hus16.pdf#listtables.

WHAT IS THE MAGNITUDE OF RISK ASSOCIATED WITH THE RISK FACTOR?

The magnitude of risk conferred by a risk factor can be defined in terms of relative or absolute risk. *Relative risk* is the ratio between the risk of disease among persons with the risk factor and the risk among those without the risk factor. A relative risk of 2.0 suggests that persons with the risk factor are twice as likely to develop the disease as persons without the risk factor. Such ratios, which are often used in both the medical literature and lay media to emphasize (and sensationalize) the magnitude of risk, can be misleading if not accompanied by information about the *absolute risk,* the actual proportion of persons with the risk factor who will develop the disease.

To clarify the distinction, consider hypothetical risk factors A and B. Risk factor A is a risk factor for disease A, risk factor B is a risk factor for disease B, and both diseases are fatal. The relative risk of risk factors A and B are 2.0 and 1.1, respectively. Readers of the medical literature and lay media are likely to conclude at first glance that risk factor A is almost twice as dangerous as risk factor B. The missing information is the absolute risk.

TABLE 2.2   Leading Causes of Death, United States, by Age Group, 2015

1–4 yr	5–14 yr
Unintentional injuries	Unintentional injuries
Congenital malformations/deformations/chromosomal abnormalities	Malignant neoplasms
Homicide	Suicide
Malignant neoplasms	Congenital malformations/deformations/chromosomal abnormalities
Diseases of the heart	Homicide
Influenza and pneumonia	Diseases of the heart
Septicemia	Chronic lower respiratory diseases
Conditions originating in the perinatal period	Cerebrovascular diseases
Cerebral vascular diseases	Influenza and pneumonia
Chronic lower respiratory diseases	In situ neoplasms/benign neoplasms/neoplasms of uncertain/unknown behavior
15–24 yr	**25–44 yr**
Unintentional injuries	Unintentional injuries
Suicide	Malignant neoplasms
Homicide	Diseases of the heart
Malignant neoplasms	Suicide
Diseases of the heart	Homicide
Congenital malformations/deformations/chromosomal abnormalities	Chronic liver disease and cirrhosis
Chronic lower respiratory diseases	Diabetes mellitus
Diabetes mellitus	Cerebrovascular diseases
Influenza and pneumonia	Human immunodeficiency virus disease
Cerebrovascular diseases	Septicemia
45–64 yr	**65 yr and Older**
Malignant neoplasms	Diseases of the heart
Diseases of the heart	Malignant neoplasms
Unintentional injures	Chronic lower respiratory diseases

(Continued)

TABLE 2.2 Leading Causes of Death, United States, by Age Group, 2015   (Continued)

Chronic liver disease and cirrhosis	Cerebrovascular diseases
Chronic lower respiratory diseases	Alzheimer disease
Diabetes mellitus	Diabetes mellitus
Cerebrovascular diseases	Unintentional injuries
Suicide	Influenza and pneumonia
Septicemia	Nephritis, nephrotic syndrome, nephrosis
Nephritis, nephrotic syndrome, nephrosis	Septicemia

Adapted from National Center for Health Statistics. *Health, United States, 2016: With Chartbook on Long-term Trends in Health.* Hyattsville, MD; 2017. http://www.cdc.gov/nchs/data/hus/hus16.pdf#listtables.

Suppose the absolute risk for persons with risk factor A is 1:50,000, whereas the risk is 1:100,000 for persons without risk factor A. Therefore, although it is true that the relative risk is 2.0 (1:50,000 is twice the risk of 1:100,000), the patient's absolute risk of developing disease A is increased by only 0.001% (1:100,000 subtracted from 1:50,000) by having risk factor A. Put differently, 99.998% of persons with risk factor A will not develop the disease.

Next consider the situation for risk factor B, which has a lower relative risk (1.1) than risk factor A (2.0). Suppose, however, that the absolute risk for disease B is 1:10 (0.1) among persons with this risk factor and 1:11 (0.0909) for persons without this risk factor. Therefore, although it is true that the relative risk associated with risk factor B is 1.1 (0.1/0.0909), it increases the absolute risk for disease B by 0.9% (0.1–0.0909). Recall that the absolute risk for disease A was increased 0.001% by risk factor A. Therefore, although the relative risk of risk factor B (1.1) is approximately half that of risk factor A (2.0), the absolute risk data tell us that persons with risk factor B are 900 times (0.9/0.001) more likely to develop disease B than are persons with risk factor A to develop disease A. (Note that, even with this higher risk, 90% of persons with risk factor B will not develop the disease.)

Absolute risk helps to clarify the distinction between risk factors and real disease, a common source of confusion among both clinicians and the public. Once the relation between a risk factor and a disease is established and public education campaigns are launched to raise awareness of the risk factor, there is a tendency for both clinicians and patients to feel that a disease has been discovered when they detect a risk factor. Both patients and clinicians often need reminders and reassurance that heightened risk, whether from an increase in high-density lipoproteins, C-reactive peptide, prediabetes, or prehypertension, warrants attention but is not tantamount to disease.

Unfortunately, it is all too common for the public, policymakers, and clinicians to overlook these details when they make arguments for or against health-promoting interventions. For example, based on the information given in the earlier example, is it appropriate for a newspaper headline to claim that risk factor A or B is a more serious problem? The answer is that neither relative nor absolute risk data provide sufficient information to answer the question. The analysis is incomplete without considering the *population-attributable risk*, the proportion of the population affected. Suppose that 1 million Americans have risk factor A, but only 1000 have risk factor B. Reducing the absolute risk of disease A by 0.001% will save 1000 (1 million × 0.001%) lives, whereas reducing the absolute risk of disease B by 0.9% will save only 9 (1000 × 0.9%) lives. Therefore, whether in the government or clinic, the importance of a risk factor requires consideration of relative, absolute, and population-attributable risk.

How Accurately Can the Risk Factor Be Detected?

Even if the target condition and risk factor are serious, efforts to detect risk factors may be ineffective or harmful if the screening test is inaccurate. Inaccurate screening tests can produce *false-positive* results, which suggest incorrectly the presence of the risk factor, or *false-negative* results, which suggest incorrectly the absence of the risk factor. False-positive results can generate unnecessary anxiety, follow-up testing, and treatment. False-negative results can lead to delays in the detection and treatment of the risk factor. The accuracy of a screening test is measured in terms of *sensitivity, specificity,* and *predictive value*. In general, a screening test is more likely to produce false-positive results if the risk factor is uncommon in the population. See Chapter 5 for definitions of these terms and for further discussion of these concepts.

What Is the Evidence That Potential Interventions Improve Health Outcomes?

Even if the risk factor and target condition are important and the available screening tests are accurate, there is little point in screening if there is inadequate evidence that available interventions improve outcomes. The best evidence to this effect are intervention studies demonstrating that patients who undergo risk factor modification achieve better health outcomes than those without the intervention. More often, however, all that is available is epidemiologic evidence suggesting that the presence of the risk factor is causally associated with the disease. In such cases, proponents of risk factor modification may use this evidence of causality to infer that modifying the risk factor will be effective in reducing the incidence of the disease.

Unfortunately, such assumptions are not always valid. For example, there is considerable evidence of an association between dietary fat and cancer, but prospective trials have not convincingly demonstrated that lowering dietary fat intake reduces the incidence of cancer. In exceptional cases, the effectiveness of risk factor modification can be inferred from the strength and consistency of the evidence. For example, there has never been a controlled intervention study demonstrating that smoking cessation reduces the incidence of cancer. The performance of such a study is highly unlikely for both ethical and legal reasons. The enormous strength and consistency of the causal evidence and the lower rates of disease in persons who stop smoking are considered adequate evidence, even without a controlled trial, to infer that such measures are effective.

How Does This Information Compare With Other Health Priorities?

Individual risk factors and diseases do not exist in a vacuum. In deciding whether to devote limited time and energy to a particular risk factor or health problem, the conscientious clinician must also consider its relative importance in relation to the other risk factors and health problems that also require attention. Advising patients about dietary fiber intake may be important, but is it more important than using the same time to discuss dietary fat consumption, tobacco use, the need for breast cancer screening, or blood pressure monitoring? Advocates of prostate cancer screening may emphasize that almost 30,000 Americans die each year from this disease, but, by examining the data in Table 2.1, the clinician can put these numbers in perspective as they relate to other serious diseases the patient and clinician must consider.

SETTING PRIORITIES

Fortunately for the clinician, the risk factors and screening tests that most often deserve attention in the clinical encounter have already been identified by several expert panels, which have devoted years of research to examining the aforementioned issues. The USPSTF[2] is an independent panel established by the federal government in 1984 to develop evidence-based recommendations on which preventive services to include in the periodic health examination. The USPSTF recommendations can be accessed at https://www.uspreventativeservicestaskforce.org. Some clinicians prioritize the services to which the Task Force gives an "A" or "B" recommendation, indicating strong evidence of net health benefit. Comprehensive preventive care recommendations have also been issued by medical specialty societies, and more specific recommendations on screening tests, immunizations, and health behaviors have been issued by government agencies, medical groups, and private organizations.[4] These recommendations form the basis for the risk factor evaluations and screening tests discussed in Chapters 3–5.

Tools have been developed for clinicians to quickly determine which preventive services are recommended for an individual patient. For example, the Agency for Healthcare Research and Quality (AHRQ) has created both research tools and an app (ARHQ ePSS) that can be used online or downloaded to a handheld device, which uses clinical information input by the clinician to identify the services recommended by the USPSTF for an individual with that history (see http://epss.ahrq.gov/PDA/index.jsp).

For most primary care practices, however, the complete list of preventive services recommended by these programs is too extensive to offer in a single office visit or even a routine health maintenance examination. A widely cited estimate is that it would take 7.8 hr/d for most clinicians to deliver all of the preventive services recommended by the USPSTF.[5] Choices must be made. As discussed further in Chapter 21, practices must often focus on ensuring the delivery of a subset of the preventive services that they consider most important.

Assistance in deciding which preventive services are most important is provided in the 2006 report of the National Commission on Prevention Priorities,[6] which ranked preventive services based on their relative clinical effectiveness and cost-effectiveness (see Table 2.3). Clinicians should consult these rankings when setting priorities and establishing protocols for their own practices, considering the local contextual issues discussed in Chapter 21 (e.g., patient population needs, agreement from colleagues). Moreover, as discussed earlier, the most important preventive services for individual patients are likely to differ based on personal risk profiles.

TOOLS TO HELP INDIVIDUALIZE RISK ASSESSMENT

A variety of tools are available to help clinicians compile and analyze information about patients' risk factors. For generations it has been customary for patients to provide such information on forms completed when they register at practices and, less consistently, for this database to be updated over time. Health risk appraisals, introduced in the 1970s to collect risk data from patients and generate epidemiologically based, personalized risk projections, are still in use by some practices. See Chapter 3 for further discussion of the role of questionnaires about risk factors and health history.

The emergence of electronic health records has introduced a more systematic means for organizing and maintaining information about individual risk factors. Interoperable electronic databases also enable risk factor data to be shared between practices, hospitals, and other institutions and to be updated as changes occur.

Beginning with the use of handheld mini records and health passports in the 1980s, patients have assumed an active role in keeping track of their personal health information and, increasingly, are using interactive websites and software for self-management of their health. They use their

TABLE 2.3 Rankings of Clinical Preventive Services by National Commission on Prevention Priorities

Preventive Service	Clinically Preventable Burden	Cost-Effectiveness
Childhood immunization series	5	5
Tobacco use screening and brief intervention, youth	5	5
Tobacco use screening and brief counseling, adults	5	5
Alcohol misuse screening and brief counseling	3	5
Aspirin chemoprophylaxis	3	5
Cervical cancer screening	4	4
Colorectal cancer screening	4	4
Chlamydia and gonorrhea screening	3	4
Cholesterol screening	4	3
Hypertension screening	4	3
AAA screening	2	4
Healthy diet and physical activity counseling for those at higher risk of CVD	5	1
HIV screening	2	4
HPV screening	3	3
Influenza immunization	4	2
Obesity screening, adults	5	1
Syphilis screening	1	5
Vision screening, children	2	4
Breast cancer screening	3	2
Depression screening, adolescents	2	3
Depression screening, adults	3	2
Obesity screening, children and adolescents	4	1
Pneumococcal immunization	2	3
Herpes zoster immunization	1	3
Osteoporosis screening	2	2

TABLE 2.3 Rankings of Clinical Preventive Services by National Commission on Prevention Priorities (Continued)

Preventive Service	Clinically Preventable Burden	Cost-Effectiveness
Folic acid chemoprevention	1	2
Meningococcal immunization	1	1
Tdap/Td booster	1	1

How to Interpret the Scores

Score	Clinically Preventable Burden (QALYs Saved)	Cost-Effectiveness (Dollars/QALY Gained)
5	>700,000	Cost saving
4	190,000–700,000	0–3,500
3	70,000–190,000	33,500–50,000
2	18,000–70,000	50,000–75,000
1	<18,000	>75,000

Adapted from Maciosek MV, LaFrance AB, Dehmer SP, et al. Updated priorities among effective clinical preventive services. *Ann Fam Med.* 2017;15(1):14-22.

Services that produce the most health benefits received the highest clinically preventable burden (CPB) score of 5. Services that are most cost-effective received the highest cost-effectiveness (CE) score of 5.

AAA, abdominal aortic aneurysm; CVD, cardiovascular disease; HIV, human immunodeficiency virus; HPV, human papillomavirus; QALY, quality-adjusted life year.

computers and handheld devices, including smartphones, to obtain health information from websites and to maintain personal health records—the consumer counterpart to the electronic health record maintained by clinicians. Interactive websites and software products on which patients store past medical history and risk factor data can be programmed to advise patients about unhealthy behaviors (e.g., physical inactivity, smoking) and preventive services recommended for individuals with their risk profile. They can print out summaries and prompts for patients to bring to their doctor, and some systems can, with the patient's permission, interface directly with electronic health records to transfer patient-entered data directly into the practice database and to review results of laboratory tests.

Finally, clinicians must often rely on specific risk calculation tools to determine whether some preventive services are indicated. For example, body mass index calculators, which can be accessed at websites or stored on smartphones help clinicians quickly determine whether patients are overweight or obese and require counseling about weight management (see Chapters 8, 9 and Appendix A). Decisions about the chemoprevention of coronary artery disease and treatment of elevated serum lipids are often guided by the Framingham risk equation (see Chapters 16 and 19), which can be calculated for individual patients using the guide in Figure 2.1 or by using handheld or online software tools. Similarly, the appropriateness of medications to prevent breast cancer, such as tamoxifen and raloxifene, are influenced by the 5-year risk of breast cancer, which can be calculated using the Gail model (see Chapter 16). Online calculation tools are listed at the end of this chapter, and further details about their application in decisions about chemoprevention are provided in Chapter 16.

APPLYING THE PRINCIPLES OF RISK ASSESSMENT IN PRACTICE

Applying the principles of risk assessment requires more than implementing guidelines and using risk assessment tools, although these are helpful. Each day, clinicians have the opportunity to incorporate the principles discussed in this chapter when counseling patients and when setting policy in their practice. When counseling patients about the meaning of risk factors, the conscientious clinician will provide information about both relative and absolute risk, allowing the patient to make a more informed decision about the importance or unimportance of the risk factor and limiting unnecessary anxiety. For example, providing only relative risk information to patients with risk factor A—telling them that they are twice as likely to develop a fatal disease than persons without the risk factor—is more likely to generate anxiety than if the absolute risk is also described. Patients who realize that their absolute risk of disease is only 0.002% will put this information in proper perspective and will be less likely to abandon more important health concerns to address this risk factor. Also, the realization that 99.998% of persons with risk factor A will not develop disease will also help them avoid the pitfall of confusing risk factors with disease.

The principles of risk assessment can also be applied when developing policy for one's practice. Although national guidelines are available to define important health priorities, local practice conditions or the emergence of new information following publication of the guidelines may prompt the need to supplement or modify recommendations for local practice. For example, organizations disagree about the appropriateness of routine screening for diabetes in the general population. However, clinicians caring for Native Americans, in whom the prevalence of diabetes is high among certain tribes, might need to examine whether a different policy is indicated in their practice. Local news reports may heighten a community's concern over a particular risk factor (e.g., exposure to hazardous emissions), a health problem (e.g., avian influenza), or a bioterrorist incident, which may exert pressure on clinicians to screen for this condition. Finally, the medical literature may provide new information about the importance of a risk factor or the availability of a new screening test before national expert panels have had an opportunity to publish recommendations.

To calculate 10 year risk of CHD

Age	Points	
	M	F
20–34	–9	–7
35–39	–4	–3
40–44	0	0
45–49	3	3
50–54	6	6
55–59	8	8
60–64	10	10
65–69	11	12
70–74	12	14
75–79	13	16
Points		

Total Cholesterol	Age 20–39		Age 40–49		Age 50–59		Age 60–69		Age 70–79	
	M	F	M	F	M	F	M	F	M	F
<160	0	0	0	0	0	0	0	0	0	0
160–199	4	4	3	3	2	2	1	1	0	1
200–239	7	8	5	6	3	4	1	2	0	1
240–279	9	11	6	8	4	5	2	3	1	2
>280	11	13	8	10	5	7	3	4	1	2
Points										

HDL	Points
>60	–1
50–59	0
40–49	1
<40	2
Points	

Systolic BP	If untreated		If treated	
	M	F	M	F
<120	0	0	0	0
120–129	0	1	1	3
130–139	1	2	2	4
140–159	1	3	2	5
>160	2	4	3	6
Points				

Smoking	Age 20–39		Age 40–49		Age 50–59		Age 60–69		Age 70–79	
	M	F	M	F	M	F	M	F	M	F
Non smoker	0	0	0	0	0	0	0	0	0	0
Smoker	8	9	5	7	3	4	1	2	1	1
Points										

Points: Age ___ + Total Cholesterol ___ +HDL___ + Systemic BP___ + Smoking___ =

Men 10 year risk of coronary heart disease in the next 10 years																			
Points	<0	0	1	2	3	4	5	6	7	8	9	10	11	12	13	14	15	16	17
Risk %	<1%	1	1	1	1	1	2	2	3	4	5	6	8	10	12	16	20	25	>30%

Women 10 year risk of coronary heart disease in the next 10 years																		
Points	<9	9	10	11	12	13	14	15	16	17	18	19	20	21	22	23	24	>24
Risk %	<1%	1	1	1	2	2	3	4	5	6	8	11	14	17	22	27	>30%		

Figure 2.1 Calculation of a patient's Framingham risk score. Risk factors included in the Framingham-based calculation of 10-year coronary artery disease risk are age, total cholesterol, high-density lipoprotein (HDL) cholesterol, systolic blood pressure, treatment for hypertension, and smoking status. Points are assigned for each risk factor according to the tables, and the sum of points is used in the gender-specific tables to determine the 10-year risk to develop coronary heart disease. The cholesterol and HDL cholesterol values should be the average of at least two measurements. The systolic blood pressure should be the current blood pressure, but the need for antihypertensive therapy is an additional risk factor. *BP*, blood pressure; *CHD*, coronary heart disease. Adapted from National Cholesterol Education Program. *Detection, Evaluation, and Treatment of High Blood Cholesterol in Adults (Adult Treatment Panel III).* Available at https://www.nhlbi.nih.gov/health-topics/management-blood-cholesterol-in-adults. Last updated in 2013.

In each of these cases, the clinician should use the principles discussed in this chapter to determine the relative importance of the risk factor and its relation to other established health priorities. How serious is the target condition? How common is the risk factor? What is the magnitude of risk associated with the risk factor? How accurately can the risk factor be detected? What is the evidence that potential interventions improve health outcomes? How does this information compare with other health priorities?

Clinicians should also examine the source of articles advocating increased clinical attention to a particular risk factor. As noted in the preceding text, such recommendations often originate from individuals, medical organizations, or government agencies that have a specialized interest in the topic. If an individual's research or an organization's mission is devoted to the eradication of a particular disease or risk factor, it may advocate full attention to this problem without first considering the effect of its recommendations on other serious health problems outside its focus of concern. Clinicians, who have the responsibility to address all of the patient's health needs, must be careful to use independent judgment before adding such topics to their risk assessment protocol. See Chapter 7 for a helpful list of questions to consider in making such choices.

CONCLUSION

What follows in Chapters 3–5 are the details of how to perform risk assessment during the history, physical, and laboratory examination. Part II of this book contains chapters devoted to the risk factors that clinicians are most likely to encounter during risk assessments. These chapters are designed to provide the clinician with detailed information about what to do when a particular risk factor is discovered, including further questions for completing the risk assessment, screening tests for related disorders, counseling, and treatment. These efforts are paramount if the clinician is to have a meaningful impact on helping patients to reduce their risk of developing diseases in later life.

SUGGESTED RESOURCES AND MATERIALS

Alvin J. Siteman Cancer Center at Washington University School of Medicine
Your Disease Risk
https://siteman.wustl.edu/prevention/ydr/?ScreenControl=YDRGeneral&
   ScreenName=YDRWhat%20Does%20My%20Risk%20Mean

National Cancer Institute. Cancer Risk
Understanding the Puzzle
http://understandingrisk.cancer.gov/

AHRQ Electronic Preventive Services Selector. http://epss.ahrq.gov/PDA/index.jsp

Online Risk Calculation Tools

BODY MASS INDEX

National Heart, Lung, and Blood Institute
Calculate Your Body Mass Index
https://www.nhlbi.nih.gov/health/educational/lose_wt/BMI/bmicalc.
  htm(downloadable format iPhone and Android devices)

CORONARY ARTERY DISEASE (FRAMINGHAM RISK) CALCULATOR

The Framingham Risk Equation is often used to estimate the patient's
  10-year risk of cardiovascular events, using an appropriate risk calculator. The estimate for a specific patient can be obtained from Figure
  2.1 or can be calculated automatically using online tools. See National
  Heart, Lung, and Blood Institute. *Risk Assessment Tool for Estimating
  10-year Risk of Developing Hard CHD (Myocardial Infarction and
  Coronary Death)*. Available at https://www.framinghamheartstudy.org/
  risk-functions/cardiovascular-disease/10-year-risk.php

BREAST CANCER RISK CALCULATOR

The Gail model is an assessment tool that calculates a woman's risk of
  developing breast cancer over the next 5 years and over her lifetime. See
  National Cancer Institute *Breast Cancer Risk Assessment Tool*. Available
  at http://www.cancer.gov/bcrisktool/

REFERENCES

1. McGlynn EA, Asch SM, Adams J, et al. The quality of health care delivered to adults in the United States. *N Engl J Med.* 2003;348:2635-2645.
2. U.S. Preventive Services Task Force. *Guide to Clinical Preventive Services*; 2014. Available at http://www.ahrq.gov/sites/default/files/publications/files/cpsguide. pdf.
3. U.S. Burden of Disease Collaborators. The state of US health, 1990-2010: burden of diseases, injuries, and risk factors. *JAMA.* 2013;310:591-606.
4. *American Academy of Family Physicians Summary of Recommendations for Clinical Preventive Services*; 2017. Available at https://www.aafp.org/dam/AAFP/documents/patient_care/clinical_recommendations/cps-recommendations. pdf.
5. Yarnall KS, Pollak KI, Ostbye T, Krause KM, Michener JL. Primary care: is there enough time for prevention? *Am J Pub Health.* 2003;9(3):635-641.
6. Maciosek MV, Coffield AB, Edwards NM, Flottemesch TJ, Goodman MJ, Solberg LI. Priorities among effective clinical preventive services: results of a systematic review and analysis. *Am J Prev Med.* 2006;31:52-61.

Please see Online Appendix: Apps and Digital Resources for additional
  information.

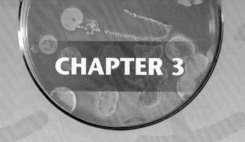

CHAPTER 3

The History: What to Ask About

ELIZABETH ROESSLER

INTRODUCTION

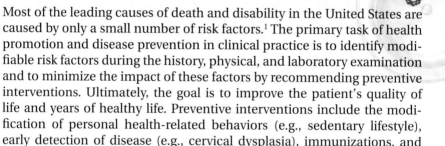

Most of the leading causes of death and disability in the United States are caused by only a small number of risk factors.[1] The primary task of health promotion and disease prevention in clinical practice is to identify modifiable risk factors during the history, physical, and laboratory examination and to minimize the impact of these factors by recommending preventive interventions. Ultimately, the goal is to improve the patient's quality of life and years of healthy life. Preventive interventions include the modification of personal health-related behaviors (e.g., sedentary lifestyle), early detection of disease (e.g., cervical dysplasia), immunizations, and chemoprophylaxis.

This chapter discusses how clinicians should approach collecting risk factor information while obtaining a history from their patients. Two types of questions are used to collect a preventive history. *Primary screening questions* are those that determine whether more detailed, *exploratory questions* are necessary. The chapter assumes that the patient is asymptomatic, i.e., lacking signs or symptoms of the target condition. Patients who have already developed the target condition will often require different risk assessment questions. An example of a primary screening question is, *"Do you smoke?"* More detailed questions such as *"At what age did you start smoking"* or *"How many packs do you smoke each day?"* are examples of exploratory questions and will be addressed in the chapters in Part II.

This chapter offers examples of potential *primary screening* questions that should be asked during history taking. Chapters 4 and 5 discuss how to obtain further evidence of risk factor exposure during the physical and laboratory examination, respectively. The chapters in Part II of this book address specific risk factors and the appropriate exploratory questions and techniques that should be used for learning more about these risk factors. Part II also addresses the interventions that should be recommended once a risk factor is identified.

A prevention history is not the same as a conventional medical history. The conventional history that is taken when evaluating symptomatic patients includes questions about chief complaints, history of present illness, past medical and surgical history, current medications, drug allergies, and a review of systems, all of which relate to the *current* situation. This chapter focuses on how to question patients about *past and present* risk factors for *future* disease or injury, with the hopes of intervening and preventing their occurrence or minimizing their impact. As noted in Chapter 2, in the evaluation of current complaints the questions that relate to future risks are generally not stressed. Clinicians often consider this information to be less relevant than establishing a diagnosis for a current complaint. Instead, many clinicians reserve detailed questions about modifiable risk factors for special visits, separate from acute care or disease management visits, such as when they first meet a patient or when a patient presents for a periodic health examination (PHE) (i.e., annual physical, preventive checkup) (see Chapter 21 for further discussion of this topic).

General Approach to the Prevention History

Clinicians can use a wide range of information sources to collect a prevention history, including the patient, family, friends, caregivers, outpatient records, and hospital records, as well as prior laboratory, radiographic, and procedure results. Before entering the room, preferably, the clinician should briefly review the patient's medical record to determine which risk factors have been discussed at previous visits, to recall the patient's previous successful or unsuccessful attempts at risk factor modification, and to determine which risk factors and clinical preventive services deserve attention at the current visit. A preventive care "problem list" or reminder notes, displayed prominently in paper-based or electronic medical records, will obviously facilitate performing such a review. In fact, having to comb through a multipaged medical record to compile a current risk factor list diminishes the likelihood that such a task will be undertaken. If the patient has already successfully modified a risk factor (e.g., smoking cessation), the clinician will want to offer positive reinforcement during the current visit and to verify that the patient has not relapsed. Other risk factors and outstanding preventive services that have not been addressed should then be identified, and, working with the patient, the clinician should determine which deserve attention in the current interview.

Patients may be psychologically unprepared for a detailed discussion of their lifestyle, especially at a visit other than a scheduled preventive checkup. When risk assessment questions are introduced, patients (or parents of young patients) may be surprised by the sudden change of subject or may be uneasy or offended by the personal nature of the questions. Transition statements serve an important function in laying the groundwork for such questions:

"Well, Mrs. Jones, I'm glad you've agreed to see Dr. Smith for an opinion on having gallbladder surgery. It will be good to get that resolved. You know, sometimes we can get so preoccupied with a specific medical problem—such as your gallbladder—that we lose sight of other important health matters. I'd like to run through a short list of questions to make sure we aren't overlooking something important that also needs our attention. Is that alright with you?"

"So, Mr. White, I anticipate that your back pain will ease up if you follow the plan that we discussed, but I want you to let me know next week if it still bothers you. By the way, there are some personal health matters we haven't discussed in the past that, although they have nothing to do with your back, might someday affect your health in other ways. I'd hate for something important to fall through the cracks. For example, you once mentioned that you had been dating several people. As you know, there can be important health implications to sexual activity. I wonder if you might be willing to discuss how many sexual partners you have had in the last year."

"Mrs. Jackson, I think your daughter's ear infection will respond well to the antibiotic I'm prescribing today. I'd like to see her again in a few weeks to reexamine her ear. Before you leave, though, I want to ask you a few questions about Tracy, double-check her shot record, and go over some conditions at home that might affect her risk of future illness or injuries. Is that all right?"

During both the introductory statement and the question period, the clinician should monitor the patient's emotional reactions. The patient's comments, vocal quality (tone, pitch, tempo), and nonverbal communication may signal discomfort, impatience, or a reluctance to discuss certain lifestyle issues. Recognizing these reactions and sharing the observations with the patient through reflection (e.g., "*You seem uncomfortable talking about this.*") are important for several reasons. First, if patients do not bring these emotions to the surface, they may suppress them or develop feelings of resentment or anger toward the clinician. Second, open discussion of the emotions and their validation by the clinician can often reduce patient anxiety. Third, although some patients use their discomfort or impatience as an excuse for changing the subject, the clinician's open acknowledgment of their feelings gives many patients the strength to return to the topic in greater detail. Often these patients will "open up" with disclosures that would not have been mentioned if the clinician were less empathic.

The clinician should also monitor the patient's choice of words, which may disclose important information about risk factors. Clues are often deeply imbedded in dialogue about other problems. The clinician may obtain more information by carefully listening to these subtle comments than from the patient's answers to routine screening questions:

"The chest pains seem to occur after meals, although lately I've wondered whether it's because of the way my life is going. Anyway, I tried antacids..."

"Doctor, you know it's got to be bad for me to come in—I haven't been to a doctor in years—I hate all those tests—but I just can't stand this shoulder pain anymore."

"I didn't start the baby on the medicine yet because I needed John to pick it up for me. He's been on a short string lately and I'm afraid to push him, with the way he gets. Now the baby has a fever and pulls on her ears..."

"No, my stomach pain isn't any worse after fatty meals. Lately, with my schedule, I've been getting a daily dose of French fries and greasy food, but that has never brought on the pain. It's only when I don't eat..."

"I doubt the headaches are due to the birth control pills. I stopped taking those things two months ago. My boyfriend thinks I've got migraines, which do run in our family..."

TECHNIQUES FOR TAKING THE PREVENTION HISTORY

Collecting a prevention-focused history requires a unique set of history-taking skills that includes the *integration* of a range of topics into an encounter, *prioritization* of essential topics for discussion, and an *appropriately timed and systematic* approach.

Integration

Sick visits comprise most patient encounters at the office, clinic, emergency department, hospital, or nursing home. Therefore, if risk assessments and preventive interventions are omitted from sick visits and offered only during well visits, then only a small percentage of patients will benefit from preventive care. As Chapter 21 discusses further, many clinicians therefore attempt to incorporate preventive medicine into routine illness visits. Acute care and disease management visits often pose a greater challenge for integrating a prevention history, however, because patients and clinicians frequently have a predefined problem-focused agenda. The most appropriate means for integrating a prevention history into a clinical encounter will vary from clinician to clinician, patient to patient, and encounter to encounter. Primary screening questions can be an effective and simple means for a clinician to introduce a prevention topic during a sick visit. By systematically administering health risk assessments before the encounter, practices can set the tone that prevention will routinely be addressed. In addition, patients themselves frequently give cues to potential prevention needs through their chief complaint or history.

Aside from sick visits, visits by new patients and PHEs provide additional and often more conducive opportunities to address prevention. Visits by new patients represent a unique opportunity to get to know a patient. History taking commonly extends beyond the presenting problem and naturally includes topics such as the patient's occupation and social or health behaviors. The PHE is, by design, centered on prevention. Therefore, the issue is not how to integrate the taking of a prevention history into the visit, but rather how to ensure that all appropriate topics are addressed when such a history is obtained.

Prioritization

It is obviously unrealistic for clinicians to address all risk factors during a short patient visit. Prioritization is essential (see Chapter 2 for general information about how to prioritize risk factors and other preventive services, and see Chapter 21 for guidance on how priorities should be tailored by individual practices). The average primary care office visit lasts 16 minutes,[2] and most of that time must be devoted to the patient's chief complaints. Investing more than a few minutes in risk assessment is rarely feasible. These minutes do provide enough time, however, to ask a few primary screening questions. A clinician can leverage small amounts of time for maximum health benefit by selecting questions about risk factors that could potentially yield the greatest health benefit for a patient or that a patient is mostly likely to act upon. Given that tobacco use is the leading cause of preventable death in the United States,[1] clinicians who have time for only one question should probably ask the most valuable primary screening question: "*Do you smoke?*" The same question should be asked of parents regarding their children or adolescents (refer to Chapters 9 and 18 for further details).

Timing

- **Identifying risk factors.** When is the right time during a sick visit to ask questions about risk factors? Inserting the questions into the history obtained for the presenting problem is one approach. Another is to first address the presenting problem and, at the conclusion of the visit, to bring up the matter of the patient's risk factors. Both models are illustrated in the subsequent text for a hypothetical patient who has visited the clinician for a chief complaint of flu-like symptoms.

During the History

Clinician: "… So, to summarize, you've had a fever since Friday, and for the past two days you've had muscle aches, a sore throat, and fatigue. I want to examine you but, before I do, let me ask you a question that also relates to your health. Do you smoke?"

At the End of the Clinical Encounter

Clinician: "… and remember to drink plenty of fluids. Call me if you feel that you are getting worse or if you notice new symptoms. Before you leave, I want to address an unrelated issue that also affects your health. How much exercise do you get?"

- **Giving advice and counseling.** Another timing issue is when during the encounter to advice and counsel a patient. Clinicians may be tempted to counsel a patient about an unhealthy behavior during the questioning period, when the patient first mentions it. Compared with waiting until the end of the encounter, this has the advantage of limiting the possibility of forgetting to address the health behavior later and being faced with the challenge of delivering multiple counseling messages on a range of topics. It is a potential pitfall, however, to provide counseling before collecting the entire history. It can diminish the impact of the counseling message if patients feel that the clinician has not heard their entire story. Furthermore, the clinician may neglect other important information, obtained later in the encounter that would alter advice or could be used as further motivation when counseling the patient.

This book includes separate chapters on the history, physical examination, and screening tests. However, during an encounter these tasks will often be appropriately undertaken together. Specific findings on physical examination should prompt further risk assessment questions (such as asking about alcohol consumption in much greater depth if a patient is found to have hepatomegaly). In addition, many elements of the physical examination do not require silence, allowing an opportunity to ask primary screening questions during inspection and palpation. Caution is warranted in determining which questions are appropriate during portions of the examination. Some questions might make patients uncomfortable, and clinicians should monitor nonverbal cues as they perform the physical examination.

- **Using windows of opportunity.** During a problem-focused visit, whether for a new problem or chronic disease management, opportunities may arise in which clinicians can address prevention. These opportunities can serve as tools for both prioritizing and integrating the prevention history into the encounter. They allow for natural transitions in conversation from the presenting problem to a prevention topic and can create a "teachable moment." Teachable moments will often occur when a patient's problem is caused or exacerbated by a modifiable risk factor. Through improved health behaviors, a patient may not only be able to significantly ameliorate the presenting problem but may also secure a better health future. One example of a teachable moment is a smoker who presents with a community-acquired pneumonia. By asking about smoking status and then providing brief counseling, the patient may recognize how his behaviors have contributed to his illness, increasing his receptivity to smoking cessation and providing him with further reasons to quit.

- **Longitudinal history taking.** Clinicians should not view the prevention history as an isolated event. Not only do risk factors and health behaviors change over time but also clinicians lack the time to effectively address all of the questions listed in this chapter during a single visit. Patients lack the capacity to act on all potential interventions. Taking advantage of a longitudinal relationship between a clinician and patient can allow for the more effective delivery of preventive care across a patient's lifespan. Establishing a system to track which preventive questions have been asked, which primary screening questions deserve follow-up, and which modifiable risk factors need to be addressed is necessary to allow for longitudinal preventive care. Coupling such tracking systems with reminders can assist clinicians in remembering to address timely prevention topics and to reinforce past discussions at future encounters. Clinicians should schedule a return visit dedicated to addressing those risk factors that cannot be covered in the current visit. The latter may be the best option for patients who visit the clinician sporadically only for illness visits.

Systematic Approach

Despite the best intentions, many clinicians overlook important risk factors, even when they are attempting to be complete. A systematic approach to asking about risk factors can help ensure a complete prevention history. Many such strategies exist and can be used alone or in conjunction with one another. Some examples of systematic approaches include health risk assessments, regular questionnaires such as intake forms, flow sheets, checklists, electronic medical record prompts, team-based delivery of care, and information collection performed as part of the "vital sign" process performed by nursing staff.

Another option is for clinicians to regularly use an organized verbal script to collect a prevention history. This is more time consuming for clinicians and may result in missing some questions. However, the approach allows for patient-specific individualization of the history taking as seen in the Patient-Centered Medical Home (PCMH). The PCMH with its successful team approach to whole patient care, which utilizes several members of the medical team to collect elements of the prevention history at designated stages of the intake and discharge process (see "vital sign" procedure on page 59), initiates the delivery of counseling interventions and referrals. This patient-centered and team approach has been shown to take the burden off of the individual clinician, allows for duplication of history collection (increasing the likelihood of completeness), increases office and medical staff satisfaction, and ultimately improves patients' health status by improving receipt of preventive services.[4]

WHAT TO ASK ABOUT

This section provides sample language for screening questions, but the clinician, who can identify the optimal communication strategy for his or her patient, best determines the wording in clinical practice. Moreover, for most risk factors, research has not yet determined the "correct" wording for such questions nor tested their sensitivity and specificity. (see discussion of "Screening Questionnaires.") The wording that clinicians use when asking risk factor questions should reflect their practice style and their relationship with the patient. The questions also need to be sensitive to the patient's age, educational background, primary language, culture, and health belief model. Because questions about risk factors often address sensitive aspects of personal behavior, the clinician should avoid judgmental or directive questions or those that will put most patients on the defensive. Patients who are asked *"You aren't homosexual, are you?"* or *"I assume that you don't drink and drive"* may be reluctant to answer honestly. Similarly, facial expressions (e.g., raised eyebrows) and other nonverbal communications that suggest the clinician's disapproval are inappropriate.

Table 3.1 gives examples of the type of primary screening questions that clinicians should employ on a routine basis to begin constructing an individual's risk profile. In the subsequent text we discuss the major topics in some detail. These questions address a fundamental set of risk factors: health behaviors (tobacco use, physical activity, dietary intake, sexual practices, alcohol and other drug use, injury prevention, exposure to ultraviolet light, dental hygiene); mental health and functional status; risk factors from past medical and family history; occupational and environmental exposures; travel history; and the status of recommended screening tests, immunizations, and chemoprophylaxis. Questions for pediatric patients need to be tailored to the patient's age to determine the content of the question and whether the patient or parents should be asked. General principles are discussed here; see Chapter 18 for details about the pediatric and adolescent examinations.

Health Behaviors

Tobacco Use

Sample primary screening question: *"Do you smoke cigarettes or use other types of tobacco?"*

TABLE 3.1   Sample Primary Screening Questions About Key Risk Factors

---

Note: **See text for complete wording of questions. Different questions are indicated for patients in specific age or risk groups and for parents of infants and small children.**

Do you smoke cigarettes or use other types of tobacco?

How much exercise do you get?

What foods have you eaten in the last 24 hr?

Do you have sex with men, women, or both? How many partners do you have now, and how many were there in the past? Do you regularly use condoms? Are you interested in getting pregnant, or are you using some form of birth control?

Do you drink alcohol? Have you ever used cocaine or other drugs? Have you ever injected any drugs?

Do you always fasten your seat belt when you are in a car? Do you ever drive after drinking or ride with a driver who has been drinking?

Do you protect yourself from the sun when you are outdoors?

How often do you brush your teeth and how often do you floss? When did you last visit the dentist?

How are your spirits these days?

Have you ever been told that you had heart trouble, cancer, diabetes or a serious infectious disease?

Is there a family history of heart trouble, cancer, or diabetes?

What sort of work do (did) you do?

Have you ever been in other countries, or are you planning a trip to one?

When was your last _____?

    (recommended screening test)

When was your last _____?

    (recommended immunization)

Are you taking daily aspirin?

Exploratory Questions and Follow-Up

If there is only one risk factor that a clinician can address in a clinical encounter, it should be tobacco use. One means to ensure that smoking status is assessed at every clinical encounter is to include smoking status as a "vital sign" routinely collected at the same time as other vital signs (see Chapter 10). Tobacco use accounts for 480,000 deaths each year in the United States.[3] All adults, adolescents, and, occasionally, older children should be asked whether they smoke or use smokeless tobacco. If they do not currently use tobacco, the clinician should inquire whether they used tobacco previously and, if so, when they quit. Exposure to environmental smoke (at home or at work), i.e., "second hand smoke" should also be addressed. Because patients who stop smoking often relapse, tobacco use should be readdressed periodically throughout the clinician's relationship with the patient. The topic also needs to be revisited regularly with children and adolescents, who are always at risk of starting to smoke or use smokeless tobacco for the first time.

Physical Activity

Sample primary screening question: *"How much exercise do you get?"*

Exploratory Questions and Follow-Up

Physical inactivity, an important risk factor for coronary artery disease, hypertension, obesity, and other chronic conditions, should be addressed with adults (including the elderly) as well as with children and adolescents (see Chapter 7). Depending upon their age such questions may need to be directed to the parents. Both the clinician and patient should have a clear understanding of what they mean by the term *exercise*. *"Well, doc, what I mean by 'exercise' is that I have to take several walks through the factory each day to inspect production lines. I also have a flight of stairs at my apartment."* At a minimum, further questions should explore the intensity, frequency, and duration of physical activity.

Dietary Intake

Sample primary screening questions: *"Tell me about your typical diet. How many servings of fruits and vegetables do you eat in a typical day? Do you typically try to avoid fatty foods?"*

Exploratory Questions and Follow-Up

The range of nutritional issues that can be addressed by the clinician is broad, including dietary intake of calories, saturated fat, *trans* fats, cholesterol, carbohydrates, fruits and vegetables, sodium, iron, calcium, and vitamins (see Chapter 8). Clinicians cannot offer meaningful counseling about these nutrients without first performing a dietary assessment of the foods that the patient typically eats. It is difficult to ask a single primary screening question that identifies all patients in need of counseling, and a *complete* dietary assessment for each food category is usually beyond the scope of a single visit (and may well be beyond the competency of the given clinician). However, of all the nutrients and foods in the patient's diet, those that most affect the patient's future health are total calories, fat, and fruits and vegetables (see Chapter 8). At a minimum, clinicians with limited time should consider exploring these topics. Further questions can explore consumption of meat, fried food, and fast foods as well as the general frequency of food consumption, meal skipping habits, and portion sizes. In patients with poor dietary habits, exploring their barriers for eating healthier foods and reviewing improvement strategies that they have tried in the past can help to guide clinicians with the counseling that follows.

Infants and Children

Nutritional questions are essential during well-baby and well-child examinations. However, primary screening questions about nutrition should also be considered during other visits, especially if compliance with recommendations made during well-child examinations is not anticipated or poor feeding practices are suspected. The most important nutritional priorities during childhood are to ensure that the diet is appropriate for healthful growth and development and that intake of dietary fats and sweets is limited. Chapter 8 provides further details on nutritional guidelines for infants and children.

Older Adults

Older adults, in addition to the nutritional issues that confront them, face the added risks of nutritional deficiencies and malnutrition. They can also experience potentially harmful interactions between their dietary practices and their medical conditions and medications. Clinicians should assess whether the patient suffers from impaired functional status and whether this impairment may be caused by nutritional deficiencies. Impaired functional status can further exacerbate poor dietary intake by creating barriers to obtaining and preparing healthy foods. One specific nutritional deficiency to recognize in older adults is inadequate calcium intake, which results in an increased risk for osteoporosis and subsequent fractures (see Chapter 8).

Sexual Practices

Sample primary screening questions: *"Do you have sex with men, women, or both? How many partners do you have now, and how many did you have in the past? Are you interested in getting pregnant, or are you using some form of birth control? How do you protect yourself against sexually transmitted infections? Do you use condoms?"*

Exploratory Questions and Follow-Up

The U.S. Preventive Services Task Force (USPSTF) recommends screening for several sexually transmitted infections in populations at risk for acquiring the infection, such as human immunodeficiency virus (HIV), hepatitis C, syphilis, gonorrhea, and Chlamydia (see Chapters 12 and 13). This requires clinicians to take an appropriate sexual history on all adolescent and adult patients to ascertain each patient's risk. Clinicians must, of course, be exceedingly careful and sensitive in asking such questions and may want to develop their own approaches and preferred language. The information is important, however, for identifying high-risk individuals who could benefit from further laboratory screening or specific counseling. Owing to the sensitive nature of this topic, clinicians often need to introduce questions about sexual behavior by explaining its relevance to their health; see Chapter 13 for suggested language. This introduction is especially important if the patient is being seen for an unrelated health problem. Clinicians also frequently need to overcome their own discomfort with discussing sexual behavior. Even in practices that see high-risk patients, universal practices were not common: risk assessment (56%), prevention counseling (60%), STD tests (30%), and HIV tests (19%).[5]

Depending on the patient's answers to screening questions about sexual practices, further questions are often necessary regarding the use of condoms, birth control methods, duration of current sexual relationships, current or prior sexual practices (e.g., anal or oral sex, association between alcohol or drug use and sexual activity, prostitution), and sexual contact with partners who used injection drugs, had multiple partners, or had known sexually transmitted infections. The sexual history may reveal evidence of dysfunctional relationships (e.g., *"I don't need birth control because we hardly make love anymore," "Don't tell my wife, but I've been with other women in the past year"*). Such findings deserve further exploration for psychosocial reasons.

Adolescents

The Centers for Disease Control and Prevention (CDC) suggest that 41% of students in grades 9 to 12 report having had sexual intercourse, 43% did not use a condom the last time they had sex, and 21% had drunk alcohol or used drugs before the last sexual encoounter.[6] This helps inform the usual discomfort that patients experience when asked about sexual behavior is magnified further for adolescents, who are often reluctant to admit to sexual activity or are afraid that the information they provide to the clinician will not be kept confidential. A commonly used approach is to begin by normalizing and depersonalizing the practice (e.g., *"A lot of high school students are having sex these days"*) and assuring the patient of confidentiality before asking the first question about sexual habits, such as *"Have you ever had sex?"* Some clinicians ease into the subject by first inquiring about peers (*"How about your friends?"*) and showing a nonjudgmental demeanor as the patient describes the sexual activity of his or her friends. Many adolescents then become comfortable enough to discuss their own sexual histories. See Chapter 18 for further details.

Lesbian, Gay, Bisexual, and Transgender Individuals

It known that lesbian, gay, bisexual, and transgender (LGBT) individuals face health disparities linked to social stigma, discrimination, and denial of their civil and human rights. According to Healthy People 2020,[7] LGBT persons face discrimination that has been associated with high rates of psychiatric disorders, substance abuse, and suicide. Unfortunately, experiences of violence and victimization are frequent for LGBT individuals and continue to have long-lasting effects on the individual and the community. Given the desire to avoid potential discrimination, LGBT individuals are reluctant to disclose to their providers. Given potential risks of smoking, alcohol/drug use, intimate partner violence, and suicide it is imperative to develop sensitive but direct primary screening questions. Establishing an inclusive and welcoming environment can help lessen these challenges. There are many recommendations for a brief self-administered multiple-choice survey that can be given before the clinician enters the room and the use of open-ended questions, mirroring the terms and pronouns that the patients use to describe themselves. It must be remembered that sometimes establishing a trusting relationship with LGBT patients may take a while and that is okay.

Alcohol and Other Drug Use

Sample primary screening questions: *"Do you drink alcohol? Have you ever used any drugs such as marijuana or cocaine?"*

Exploratory Questions and Follow-Up

The USPSTF, National Academy of Medicine, American Academy of Pediatrics, and other groups recommend screening all adult and adolescent patients for evidence of alcohol dependence, problem drinking, or excessive alcohol consumption (see Chapter 11). Patients who report drinking alcohol should be asked about the quantity and frequency of their consumption as well as whether drinking has resulted in any adverse effects on their life (such as causing trouble with work or relationships). However, patients' self-reports of their alcohol use may not provide accurate information to identify problem drinking. The reported sensitivity of historic inquiry about alcohol use is only 10% to 50%. Similarly, patients with a current or past history of illicit drug use may be even more reluctant to discuss the subject because of its legal implications. Clinicians must often rely on clues in the patient's responses and to other aspects of the medical history and lifestyle to detect a problem. For example, the answer *"I just drink socially"* requires further exploration.

Commonly used alcohol abuse questionnaires, such as the CAGE and Alcohol Use Disorders Identification Test (AUDIT) instruments or the Michigan Alcoholism Screening Test (MAST) (see Chapter 11 for further details), can provide a nonthreatening approach for patients to honestly report alcohol habits. Long-term continuity relationships between primary clinicians and patients can also foster trust over time by creating a safe environment for patients to accurately describe their alcohol and drug use. Patients with a history of drug use or sexually transmitted infections should be asked specifically about past or present injection drug use. Patients who use either alcohol or other drugs should be asked about driving while intoxicated and about binge drinking.

Adolescents

As with sexual behavior, adolescents may be reluctant to admit to alcohol or other drug use for fear of disapproval or disclosure to parents, teachers, or the legal authorities. Nonetheless, because, for example, intoxication accounts for approximately half of adolescent deaths in motor vehicle crashes, and because substance abuse often begins at this age, broaching this subject with teens is especially important. Again, it is often useful to first depersonalize the practice (e.g., *"A lot of high school students drink or use drugs these days"*), assure confidentiality, inquire about peers (*"How about your friends?"*), and then ask about the patient's habits (*"Have you ever used drugs?"*). See the discussion of respecting confidentiality with adolescents under "Patient Privacy."

Injury Prevention Practices

Sample primary screening questions: *"Do you always fasten your seat belt when you are in a car? Do you ever drive after drinking, or ride with a driver who has been drinking?"*

> *For parents of infants and small children:* "Is your child always secured in a safety seat when you or others transport him (her) in the car?"
> *For parents of older children:* "Does your child fasten his (her) seat belt whenever he (she) is transported in a car?"

Exploratory Questions and Follow-Up

Many clinicians believe that a patient's driving habits are not a clinical concern, and yet motor vehicle accidents account for approximately 50,000 deaths and 5 million injuries each year in the United States. They are the leading cause of injury-related deaths among persons younger than 45 years.[8] Clinician inquiry can further validate and support safe driving practices.

Older Adults

Falls are a common cause of injury in older adults, especially among those older than 75 years, in whom falls are the leading cause of injury-related deaths (due largely to the complications of hip fractures and head trauma). The clinician should ask the patient, family members, or caregivers whether the home has been inspected for fall hazards. A sample screening question is, *"Have you gone through the house to look for bad lighting; things that could cause you to trip or slip on the floor, steps, rugs, or bathtub; or sharp corners or hard floors that could hurt you if you fell?"* The clinician should also review the patient's medications, which may increase the risk of falls.

Exposure to Ultraviolet Light

Sample primary screening question: *"Do you protect yourself (your child) from the sun when you are outdoors?"*

Exploratory Questions and Follow-Up

Further questions could explore a patient's cumulative sun exposure, history of severe or frequent sunburns, activities (e.g., occupation, weekend hobbies, or visiting tanning salons) associated with increased sun exposure, methods used to avoid sun exposure (avoidance of midday sun or use of protective clothing), and use of sunscreen.

Excess exposure to the ultraviolet radiation of sunlight carries a significantly increased risk of all types of skin cancer. Reducing exposure to ultraviolet rays through avoidance of midday sun or the use of protective clothing can help to prevent skin cancer. In addition, use of sunscreen can prevent the development of squamous and basal cell skin cancers. Whether sunscreen prevents melanoma is less clear. If individuals who use sunscreen are more likely to increase the time they spend in the sun, melanoma risks could be increased, unless other preventive measures (e.g., sitting in the shade, protective clothing) are observed. Avoidance of ultraviolet radiation can decrease the risk of skin cancer, whereas there is insufficient evidence to demonstrate that clinician counseling changes patients' skin exposure behaviors.[6]

Dental Hygiene Practices

Sample primary screening questions: *"How often do you brush your teeth? How often do you floss? When did you last visit the dentist?"*

> *For parents:* "How often does your child brush his (her) teeth? When was he (she) last taken to the dentist? Does your child drink adequately fluoridated water? If not, is your child receiving fluoride supplements to prevent tooth decay?"

Exploratory Questions and Follow-Up

Further exploratory questions could include "Are you having any problems with your mouth, throat, or teeth? Do your gums bleed when you brush or floss? Do you have trouble chewing your food? Do you have any questions about your oral health?"

In general, patients should be encouraged to see their dentist at least once every 12 months. Patients may need prompt referral for inflamed or bleeding gums, decayed or loose teeth, or lesions suggestive of oral cancer. Patients should also be encouraged to avoid the risk factors for poor oral health, which include smoking, chewing tobacco, and consuming refined sugars (e.g., sodas), and to minimize the risks of dental injuries. Parents of infants should be asked about baby bottle-feeding practices, and clinicians should inquire about fluoride intake to determine if supplementation is necessary (see Chapter 18). The USPSTF endorses fluoride supplementation for those children 6 months of age and older whose primary water source is inadequately fluoridated and that primary care clinicians apply fluoride varnish to primary teeth of all infants and children starting at the age of primary tooth eruptions but found insufficient evidence for primary care clinicians to conduct routine pediatric screening for dental disease. The USPSTF has not recently reviewed evidence for adult dental care.[9]

Mental Health and Functional Status

Sample primary screening question (mental health): *"How are your spirits these days?"*

Sample primary screening question (functional status and development):

> *For parents:* "What has your child learned to do recently?"
> *For older adults:* "Are you having any trouble taking care of things at home, such as getting your meals or cleaning?"

Exploratory Questions and Follow-Up

See Chapters 15 and 18.

Mental Health

The scope of potential problems and complications that fall under this category is broad, ranging from poor self-esteem, depression, and abuse (as victim or perpetrator) to violence and suicidal behavior. A single primary screening question is often inadequate to detect these problems. Therefore, to detect a problem, the clinician must be alert to clues in the patient's behavior, affect, family dynamics, and physical examination findings, not only during the risk assessment visit but also throughout the relationship with the patient. Patients who have recently experienced an important loss (e.g., death, divorce, loss of job) are at increased risk of depression. If there is evidence of depression, the patient should be asked whether he or she has had suicidal or homicidal ideation (e.g., *"Have you ever thought of hurting yourself or others?"*). Commonly used screening instruments for depression include the Zung Self-Rating Depression Scale, Center for Epidemiological Studies Depression Scale, the Beck Depression Inventory, and the Patient Health Questionnaire (see Chapter 14).

The clinician must also remain alert for signs of interpersonal conflict, domestic violence, or other risk factors for intentional injuries (e.g., child abuse, spouse abuse, sexual violence, homicide). Because patients and family members often display their "best behavior" during clinical encounters, the clinician must be able to see past this presentation to unmask signs of escalating tensions in a relationship, an individual's inability to resolve conflicts nonviolently, or the physical findings of abuse or neglect. A patient or family member's grimace, shrug, or hesitation in answering a screening question, such as *"How are things at home?,"* or their responses to open-ended questions, such as *"What are the good things and bad things about your relationship?,"* are often the clinician's best clues in detecting an important problem at home. In responding to such questions, patients may give clues to their possible misuse of alcohol or other drugs or to the presence of other codependent behaviors. Although unproved, acting on these findings by arranging for psychotherapy, marital counseling, substance abuse treatment, or social services may improve family dynamics and the emotional well-being of its members. In more advanced cases, these interventions may prevent physical illnesses and injuries, emotional morbidity from abuse or neglect, unwanted pregnancies, family dysfunction, unintentional firearm injuries, and even homicide. We should always be cognizant that LGBTQ individuals are more likely than others to experience mental health issues, such as major depression or generalized anxiety disorder. The reluctance of coming out and potential of being discriminated against for sexual orientation or gender identities can lead to depression, posttraumatic stress disorder, thoughts of suicide, and substance abuse. Clinicians should be mindful of the risks of mental health disorders in this population and alert for any sign or symptoms the patient may display that is indicative of underlying mental health concerns.

Functional Status

Functional status refers broadly to an individual's ability to perform age-appropriate tasks of self-care and self-fulfillment. In childhood, this is often affected by abnormal physical or mental growth and development. Childhood development is covered in Chapter 18 and is therefore not discussed further in this chapter. In old age, functional status can be impaired by both physical and mental illness. The consequences affect other health-related behaviors, such as nutrition patterns and injury avoidance.

When examining older adults, clinicians should remain alert for evidence of difficulty in performing the activities of daily living. Screening for cognitive impairment is more difficult, because undertaking a lengthy mental status examination is often impractical in the brief clinical encounter and may lack accuracy or effectiveness as a screening test. The clinician must often seek readily obtainable clues in the patient's speech, ability to understand medical instructions, behavior in the office, and statements made about home or living conditions. In addition, if the clinician thinks that a patient may be cognitively impaired, the patient can be asked to complete the Mini-Mental State Examination, a screening instrument that provides a general measure of basic cognitive functions (see Chapter 14).

Obtaining the Presence of Risk Factors From the Past Medical History

Sample primary screening question: *"Have you ever been told that you had heart trouble, cancer, diabetes, or a serious infectious disease?"*

Exploratory Questions and Follow-Up

Beginning with an open-ended question and progressing to questions about specific conditions can be an effective means to elicit a comprehensive prevention-focused past medical history. However, there are other sources for obtaining such information. Prior health records may be more efficient and effective than direct questioning to acquire an understanding of a patient's past medical history. Whether obtained from direct questioning or the medical record, the past medical history can provide critical information for determining whether patients fall within risk groups requiring special screening tests, immunizations, or other preventive services (see Chapters 4, 5, 17, and 19 for details). The medical history form that patients usually complete before their first interview will often be very helpful in focusing the discussion.

Learning About Risk Factors from the Family History

Sample primary screening question: *"Do you have a family history of heart trouble, cancer, or diabetes?"*

Exploratory Questions and Follow-Up

A thorough conventional family history can cover a wide range of topics and conditions. However, from a prevention standpoint coronary artery disease, cerebrovascular accidents, cancers (colorectal, breast, ovarian, prostate, and skin), and diabetes represent potentially inherited conditions that place patients in risk groups requiring screening tests specified for high-risk populations or at an earlier age than routinely recommended for the general population (see Chapters 4 and 5). In particular, clinicians should inquire whether these conditions occurred in first-degree relatives, or in multiple family members, or if family members with the condition had an early age of disease onset. Although time consuming to complete, the family history can provide a comprehensive look at the patient's entire medical pedigree. A family history questionnaire (such as https://family-history.hhs.gov/) that a patient completes before the encounter can facilitate this process.

Occupational and Environmental Exposures

Sample primary screening questions: *"What sort of work do (did) you do? Does (did) your job or other activities expose you to loud noise, the sun, harmful chemicals, radiation, or other hazardous materials?"*

> *For parents:* "Where do you live, how old is your home, and what is the source of your drinking water?"
>
> *For older adults:* "Where do you live? Who do you live with? Who is available to assist you if needed?"

Exploratory Questions and Follow-Up

A thorough occupational or environmental history requires more detailed questions about risks of occupational illnesses and injuries than can be addressed in this book. The earlier questions are intended to screen for selected exposures that place patients in risk groups requiring routine screening tests and immunizations (see Chapters 4, 5, and 17). For example, skin and hearing screening may be warranted for patients with occupational or recreational exposure to excessive sunlight or noise, respectively. Health care workers are at increased risk of being exposed to or transmitting tuberculosis, hepatitis B, HIV, and other harmful organisms (e.g., rubella). Questions for determining a worker's need for occupational screening tests (e.g., air sampling, pulmonary function testing), however, are addressed in standard occupational medicine and environmental health texts.

Questions about living conditions can also provide important environmental risk information for tailoring the patient's health maintenance plan. Crowded or unsanitary living conditions, for example, increase the risk of tuberculosis, influenza, and other pathogens. Determining that a patient lives in a homeless shelter, correctional institution, nursing home, or migrant worker camp suggests the need for tuberculosis screening (see Chapter 5). A number of environmental factors are potentially relevant to children, some of which have already been addressed (e.g., passive exposure to environmental tobacco smoke). Characteristics of the home, such as its age (dwellings constructed before 1960 often contain lead-based paint) and the presence or absence of fluoride in the water supply, have special relevance to a child's risk of developing disease. The CDC was authorized by the 1988 Lead Contamination Control Act to initiate program efforts to eliminate childhood lead poisoning in the United States. In 2012, the CDC updated its recommendations on children's blood lead levels and shifted its focus to primary prevention of lead exposure, including reducing or eliminating dangerous lead sources in the child's environment before they are exposed.[10] For older adults, clinicians should determine the patient's living environment (e.g., private home, assisted living facility, or nursing home) and what support systems exist to help patients with their needs.

Travel History

Sample primary screening question: *"Have you (or your child) ever been in other countries, or are you planning a trip to one?"*

Exploratory Questions and Follow-Up

The risk of certain target conditions (e.g., hemoglobinopathies) or of exposure to infectious diseases (e.g., tuberculosis, hepatitis, HIV infection) is increased for immigrants from certain countries in Asia, the Pacific Islands, Africa, Central and South America, and the Mediterranean (see Chapters 4, 5, and 17). Patients traveling to developing countries or other regions in which malaria and other preventable infectious diseases are endemic require certain immunizations and chemoprophylaxis before their departure (see Chapter 17).

Clinical Preventive Services

The clinician should ask patients (or the parents of infants and children) whether they have received appropriate clinical preventive services—screening tests, immunizations, and chemoprevention regimens—that are recommended for their age and risk profile. Clarifying the risk group requires not only determining when the patient last received the service but also understanding the patient's risk for disease and the results of prior screening tests. Medical records, and flow sheets or screen prompts that summarize pertinent data, may be particularly helpful in gathering this information. Appendix A of this book lists the key screening tests that are indicated for average-risk adults. See Chapters 4, 5, 16, and 17 for further details on when screening tests, immunizations, and chemoprevention regimens are indicated for particular patients.

SPECIAL CONSIDERATIONS

Infants, Children, and Adolescents

See Chapter 18.

Older Adults

Obtaining accurate risk factor information from some older adults can be difficult for both organic and attitudinal reasons. Organic barriers in the elderly include the patient's difficulty in understanding questions or providing coherent answers, due to hearing loss, cognitive impairment, or other medical factors. Clinicians often need to accommodate these limitations through special measures, such as speaking more slowly in a loud, low voice; clearly writing the questions on paper; or obtaining the information from caregivers. Attitudinal barriers include the patient's hesitation to identify a risk factor as a problem because of a belief that it is a natural consequence of aging (e.g., hearing loss), it is something that should not be complained about (e.g., depression), it is too late in life to benefit from risk factor modification (e.g., smoking cessation after decades of tobacco use), or it will result in the loss of freedoms (e.g., the ability to drive or live independently). Clinicians often need to spend time with the patient to correct misconceptions, educate them about healthy aging, encourage open discussion, and foster a trusting and collaborative relationship.

Patient Privacy

Asking about risk factors with other individuals in the room is generally inappropriate for several reasons. First, taking a history under these conditions violates patient confidentiality. Second, the presence of other individuals often makes patients uncomfortable and reluctant to discuss personal behaviors. The patient may give inaccurate or incomplete information, such as denying or minimizing their involvement with behaviors that might be judged negatively by others (e.g., the adolescent who denies sexual activity or substance abuse when the parents are present). Third, if the visit includes a physical examination, the visitors must leave the room anyway to respect the patient's privacy.

On the other hand, family members, caregivers, or friends who accompany patients can often provide important information about risk factors that may not be volunteered by the patient. For example, a teenage patient denies tobacco use, but the mother tells the clinician that she routinely sees a cigarette package in his shirt pocket. A wife complains about her husband's drinking problem, although he denies such behavior. The children of an older adult, who denies problems at home, inform the clinician that they have witnessed frequent episodes of disorientation and memory loss. It is therefore useful, in the appropriate setting, to ask individuals who have accompanied a patient whether they have any health concerns that they would like to discuss. They should then be asked to leave the room.

Most individuals accompanying patients, once given an opportunity to express their concerns, are quite agreeable to leaving the examination room. Some parents of adolescents or older children may be surprised by or resistant to the request, in part because this practice was unnecessary when their children were younger, but a brief explanation will usually suffice to ease their anxieties. Some sample language may include, "*I always make sure to give my teenage patients a chance to ask questions.*" Or "*I routinely ask parents to step out of the room for a few minutes so that we can talk.*" Each clinician will develop and each patient encounter will dictate an individualized approach to interviewing patients and caretakers. A commonly used sequence is to interview everyone present, then interview the patient alone, conduct an examination, review the assessment and plan with only the patient, and summarize the encounter with everyone present, of course taking care to omit from that discussion any matters that any of the participants asked to be kept confidential. This can allow an opportunity for everyone to contribute to the history and the plan of action while maintaining patient privacy and providing the patient an opportunity to limit what will be shared with others. The adamant refusal of family members to leave the examination room or a tendency to dominate the interview should raise the clinician's index of suspicion that there are issues of abuse, neglect, or other problems that they do not want disclosed.

Interview Problems and Strategies

Silence, which frequently makes both clinicians and patients uncomfortable, is nevertheless often helpful in collecting risk factor information. Patients may introduce silence themselves, pausing after mentioning a risk factor to collect their thoughts or to marshal the courage to bring up a difficult topic. Rather than breaking the silence with another question, clinicians who wait for the patient to break the silence are often rewarded with additional information. *"No, I don't use any drugs, and I hardly touch alcohol ...* (silence introduced by patient) ... *Did I ever tell you, doctor, that I was once in a rehab program? I was using crack and heroin back then...."* Even if the patient does not introduce silence, the clinician may intentionally pause to see how the patient fills the silence. *"Things at home are fine, I guess...* (silence introduced by clinician) ... *I do wish things were better between my husband and the kids, though...."*

Resistance is often manifested by a patient's hesitation in answering questions, vagueness, or an abrupt change of subject. Only a few patients express anger or hostility when asked questions about lifestyle. As noted earlier, the clinician's reflection and validation of the patient's feelings will often overcome this resistance. It is, however, the patient's right to terminate discussion of difficult topics. The clinician should respect those preferences and move on to other subjects.

Communication barriers can include hearing loss, language and literacy barriers, cognitive limitations, and cultural differences. Information about risk factors can be obtained from deaf patients by relying on lip reading, written questionnaires, handwritten notes, or sign language. Clinicians who cannot speak the patient's language may require the aid of a translator to ask questions. If patients have partial command of the clinician's language, it is easy to mistakenly assume that the patient understands questions or instructions. A patient may nod in response to a yes/no question without truly understanding what was asked. For example, a Vietnamese-speaking patient who says "no" when asked whether she has ever had "hepatitis B" might answer "yes" if the disease was named in her language. Patients with cognitive limitations, due either to inadequate education or limited intelligence, may have difficulty in understanding complex words or sentences. The clinician should be careful to avoid sophisticated terminology (e.g., *saturated fats, hypertension, and monogamous relationships*) and should verify that the patient truly understands the questions. Even the most highly educated patients can get confused when presented with complex medical jargon.

Even if they have complete command of the clinician's language, patients with different *cultural background* may assign different meanings and weights to given risk factors or they may be offended by certain questions. It is therefore important for the clinician to be culturally competent: familiar with and sensitive to the attitudes and health belief model of the patient's culture. For example, the very concept of prevention may not be meaningful if patients believe that diseases develop from sinful behavior, rather than medical risk factors, or that suffering from disease leads to spiritual growth. Patients from certain ethnic or minority communities may be confused by the clinician's choice of words. For example, they may view a *"negative* test result" as unfavorable news. They may deny a history of "diabetes" or "hypertension" but admit to having "sugar" or "high blood."

Screening Questionnaires

Many practices ask patients to complete a medical history form at their first visit. If they ask questions about relevant risk factors, these forms can provide the clinician with useful risk assessment information and save time during the interview by identifying which topics require further investigation. They can also stimulate the patient's thinking, prompting the patient to bring up certain issues with the clinician that would otherwise be forgotten.

One limitation of such forms is that patients may not answer the questions honestly or may leave the questions unanswered. More comprehensive screening forms will take longer for patients to complete, increasing the likelihood of a patient not completing the questionnaire. The forms may not be understandable, especially if the patient speaks a different language or has difficulty reading. Finally, patients may become frustrated with the redundancy of completing multiple questionnaires over time, yet reserving such forms solely for new encounters may miss changes in a patient's modifiable risks. Therefore, clinicians must be careful to supplement and update risk factor information obtained from medical history forms.

As noted earlier, screening questionnaires, standardized instruments that have been validated as screening tools for specific conditions, have been developed for the detection of depression, alcohol abuse, cognitive impairment, and other health problems. These instruments have been designed out of concern that routine questions by clinicians have poor sensitivity and specificity in detecting these conditions. Unfortunately, most screening questionnaires also have limited sensitivity and specificity. That is, a patient with an abnormal score may not have the condition (false positive) and a patient with a normal score may have the condition (false negative). For example, in a recent study to assess the accuracy of the Mini-Mental State Examination, it was reported that 85% of people with dementia were be correctly identified using this screening questionnaire, whereas 15% would be wrongly classified as not having dementia, and 90% of those tested would be correctly identified as not having dementia, whereas 10% would be false positives and might be referred for further testing.[11] An expert panel judging the accuracy of 19 screening questionnaires for childhood developmental delay gave its highest rating to instruments with a sensitivity and specificity approaching 80% and 90%, respectively.[12] This means that the best performance of such instruments (assuming a sensitivity and specificity of 80% and 90%, respectively, and a 5% pretest probability of a developmental disorder) would be to falsely label two children as developmentally delayed for every true case detected; if the pretest probability is 1%, 12 children would be mislabeled for every true case detected.

In addition to the poor predictive value of questionnaires, completion of questionnaires is often too time consuming to be done during the clinical interview. Common solutions are to ask patients who are at risk for the problem to complete the questionnaires before meeting with the clinician, either in the waiting room or before the appointment. If the need for using the questionnaire first becomes apparent during the clinical interview, the patient can be asked to complete the form while the clinician moves on to another patient or, if necessary, with the help of someone from the medical team. The clinician can then return to the patient's room to discuss the results. Another solution is to send the patient home with the questionnaire with instructions to mail it to the clinician when completed or to provide the patient with the means to complete the survey electronically.

With technological advances, innovative new tools are emerging that link screening questionnaires with individualized risk factor profiles, personal guidelines on recommended services, patient information resources, and self-management tools. A unique aspect of these tools is that their use not only results in the collection of historic information but also initiates the delivery of care and empowers patients to assume active roles. The content of the screening questionnaires can range from the identification of a single target condition, as described in the preceding text, to more global assessments of preventive care needs. Frequently, these tools are electronic, rather than paper based, allowing for automated risk assessment calculations and automated delivery of information to the patient and/or clinician; the delivery systems can include websites, portable laptops, electronic mobile devices, and computer kiosks, all of which can be accessed in the clinician's office, elsewhere in the community, or at the patient's home. Examples of these innovative tools include www.HowsYourHealth.org and www.MyPreventiveCare.net (see Fig. 3.1). Linking this technology with electronic health records maintained by the practice and personal health records maintained by the patient can further enhance the efficient collection of information and foster patient-clinician communication. The information and advice generated by these tools can be powerful motivators for patients attempting lifestyle change. The clinician and patient can together review the information these systems generate as part of their discussion of health maintenance.

CONCLUDING THE RISK ASSESSMENT INTERVIEW

As noted earlier, the clinician can continue to collect elements of the history during the physical examination. This may be particularly useful if the clinician finds any abnormalities on examination that prompt further questions. Regardless, the focused encounter period for discussions about risk factors should be concluded with the courtesies that are extended at the end of any clinical interview. Patients should be asked whether they have any additional concerns that they would like to discuss. They should be provided a transition to the next stage of the encounter by being told what to expect. If the interview is to be followed by a physical or laboratory examination, a helpful statement may be: *"I want to talk with you further about the health issues that we have discussed. But before we do that, I'd like*

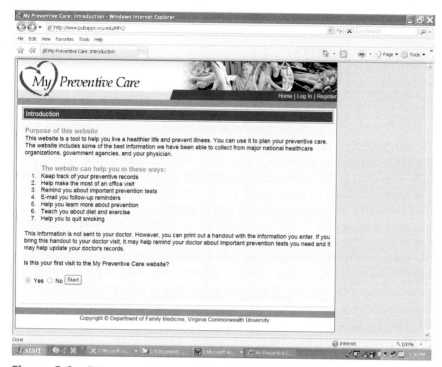

Figure 3.1 "My preventive care" is a Web-based personal health record used to collect the patient's prevention-related history and to offer individualized recommendations.

to examine you and perform a few tests so that we will have a complete picture of your risk factors. I'll step out for a few minutes so that you can change into this gown. Is that ok?"

Risk factors and preclinical disease states to anticipate in the physical examination are discussed in the next chapter.

OFFICE AND CLINIC ORGANIZATION

At a minimum, the clinician should document which risk factors were discussed in the notes for the visit. Clinicians should maintain a risk factor "problem list" for each patient. Entries on the problem list should indicate the dates when the risk factor information was obtained, previous attempts at risk factor modification, and the current status of the risk factor. Risk factors about which no information has been obtained should be flagged for attention at future visits.

SUGGESTED RESOURCES AND MATERIALS

Barker LR. The practitioner-patient relationship and communication during clinical encounters. In: Barker LR, Burton JR, Zieve PD, eds. *Principles of Ambulatory Medicine.* 7th ed. Philadelphia: Lippincott Williams & Wilkins; 2007:25-37.

Bickley LS, Szilagi PG. *Bates' Guide to Physical Examination and History Taking.* 12th ed. Wolters Kluwer; 2017.

Coulehan JL, Block MR. *The Medical Interview: Mastering Skills for Clinical Practice.* 5th ed. Philadelphia: F. A. Davis Company; 2006.

National Institute on Aging. *Talking With Your Older Patient.* Bethesda: National Institute on Aging; 2017. Available from https://www.nia.nih.gov/health/doctor-patient-communication/talking-with-your-older-patient.

Stewart M, Brown JB, Weston WW, et al. *Patient-Centered Medicine: Transforming the Clinical Method.* London: Radcliffe Publishing; 2014.

REFERENCES

1. Mokdad AH, Marks JS, Stroup DF, Gerberding JL. Actual causes of death in the United States, 2000. *JAMA.* 2004;291:1238-1245.

2. Tai-Seale M, McGuire TG, Zhang W. Time allocation in primary care office visits. *Health Serv Res.* 2007;42(5):1871-1894.

3. U.S. Department of Health and Human Services. *The Health Consequences of Smoking—50 Years of Progress: A Report of the Surgeon General.* Atlanta, GA: U.S. Department of Health and Human Services, Centers for Disease Control and Prevention, National Center for Chronic Disease Prevention and Health Promotion, Office on Smoking and Health; 2014.

4. Ferrante JM, Balasubramanian BA, Hudson SA, Crabtree BF. Principles of the patient-centered medical home and preventive services delivery. *Ann Fam Med.* 2010;8(2):108-116.

5. Montaño DE, Phillips WR, Kasprzyk D, Greek A. STD/HIV prevention practices among primary care clinicians: risk assessment, prevention counseling, and testing. *Sex Transm Dis.* 2008;35(2):154-166.

6. Centers for Disease Control and Prevention. Sexual identity, sex of sexual contacts, and health-related behaviors among students in grades 9-12—United States and selected sites, 2015. *MMWR.* 2015;65(SS-9).

7. US Department of Health and Human Services. *Healthy People 2020. Lesbian, Gay, Bisexual and Transgender Health.* Available from https://www.healthypeople.gov/2020/topics-objectives/topic/lesbian-gay-bisexual-and-transgender-health.

8. Adapted from National Center for Health Statistics. Health, United States, 2016: With Chartbook on Long-Term Trends in Health. Hyattsville, MD; 2017. http://www.cdc.gov/nchs/data/hus/hus16.pdf#listtables.

9. U.S. Preventive Services Task Force. *Guide to Clinical Preventive Services*; 2014. Available from http://www.ahrq.gov/sites/default/files/publications/files/cps-guide.pdf.

10. Centers for Disease Control and Prevention. Childhood Lead Poisoning Prevention Programs. Available from https://www.cdc.gov/nceh/lead/default.htm.

11. Noel-Storr AH, Trevelyan CM, Hampton T, et al. Mini-Mental State Examination (MMSE) for the detection of dementia in clinically unevaluated people aged 65 and over in community and primary care populations. *Cochrane Database Syst Rev.* 2016;(1).

12. American Academy of Pediatrics Committee on Children with Disabilities. Developmental surveillance and screening in infants and young children. *Pediatrics.* 2001;108:192-196.

⊕ Please see Online Appendix: Apps and Digital Resources for additional information

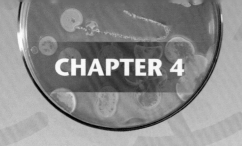

CHAPTER 4

The Physical Examination: Where to Look for Preclinical Disease

DAVID BRISSETTE

BACKGROUND

The physical examination is an important part of the delivery of preventive care to all patients. There are limitations to its direct value, as discussed in the subsequent text. It can be very beneficial, however, if performed in a skillful manner, integrated with other essential elements of the encounter, and used to support counseling and motivate patients to improve health behaviors. In the context of this chapter, the physical examination refers to the direct inspection, palpation, percussion, and auscultation of the patient's body. Other elements of an encounter, for example, obtaining the history (see Chapter 3), performing laboratory tests (see Chapter 5), and counseling the patient (see Section II), may occur during the physical examination but are discussed separately in other chapters.

This chapter focuses on physical examination procedures to screen for asymptomatic disease or risk factors rather than on the physical diagnosis of patients with symptomatic disease. Patients who present with complaints or abnormal physical findings require careful, focused examination techniques to make the correct diagnosis. Physical examination procedures that qualify as preventive interventions (as opposed to a diagnostic workup) are those that detect abnormalities in the absence of symptoms.

When seeing a clinician for preventive care, most patients expect to have their clinician perform a physical examination. It is an opportunity to detect abnormalities that the patient may not recognize, that the clinician may not have suspected based on historical information, or that may not be revealed by laboratory screening tests. Examination can potentially detect concerning signs of unhealthy behaviors (e.g., wheezing in a smoker suggesting early airway disease) or asymptomatic disease (e.g., xanthelasma in a patient with familial hypercholesterolemia). Findings

78

from an examination may also be necessary to properly interpret abnormal laboratory values; obtaining this information before the laboratory results may help to prevent unnecessary patient or clinician anxiety. For example, a slightly elevated prostate-specific antigen (PSA) test may be less concerning if the patient has a uniformly enlarged prostate consistent with benign prostatic hypertrophy.

Although virtually any component of the physical examination (Table 4.1) can detect early-stage disease in the absence of symptoms, there is little scientific evidence that healthy persons experience better outcomes because of head-to-toe physical examinations. Conducting studies to definitively evaluate the effectiveness of physical examination procedures is difficult because of the required size, logistics, expenses, and possibly, ethical considerations associated with such studies. Even for physical examination elements for which there is evidence of health benefits, the likelihood that an individual patient will have an abnormality during a specific examination is low (e.g., there is a low probability that a woman aged 50–55 yr will have a palpable breast mass on physical examination).

TABLE 4.1 The Comprehensive Physical Examination

Includes Examination of the Following:
Skin
Head, scalp, face, nares
Pupils, sclera, conjunctiva, retina, extraocular muscles
Buccal mucosa, teeth, gums, tongue, pharynx
Ear, tympanic membranes
Neck, cervical lymph nodes, jugular veins, carotid arteries
Thoracic and lumbar spine
Posterior lung fields
Breasts, axillae
Precordial impulse, heart sounds
Shoulders, upper arms, elbows, forearms, hands, fingernails
Abdominal viscera
Genitalia, rectum, inguinal canal, femoral pulses
Hips, thighs, knees, lower legs, ankles, feet, toenails
Peripheral pulses
Mental status and central nervous system
Cranial and peripheral nervous system

The time required for a thorough physical examination is an important opportunity cost. Busy clinicians often have limited time to spend with each patient. Leveraging that time for counseling or other preventive interventions has a much greater likelihood of improving the patient's health than spending that same time doing a head-to-toe examination. As a result of time constraints, some physical examinations may be more focused and cursory. Little may be gained by performing examination procedures in such a cursory manner (e.g., examining only a small portion of the patient's skin, briefly palpating for breast masses), which is often ineffective and therefore makes poor use of limited time.

An appropriate way to focus the routine physical examination, however, is to emphasize examination procedures that have demonstrated potential benefit as screening procedures in asymptomatic patients. Ensuring that these selected procedures are performed well helps to maximize the value of the prevention-focused physical examination. The history can help to guide the clinician in selecting additional examination procedures that may be indicated for a given patient based on individual risks. Because patients have come to expect clinicians to perform a comprehensive physical examination, the clinician may wish to explain the value of the focused physical examination and to highlight specific preventable conditions that merit attention.

Findings from the physical examination should be reviewed with the patient and used to inform and individually tailor counseling messages for patients. For example, the detection of wheezing in a smoker may prompt the clinician to say during their smoking cessation counseling, "*Mr. Smith, when I listen to your lungs, I can hear wheezing. This may be a sign that smoking is damaging your lungs. I would like to discuss with you what that means and how we can work together to improve your health.*"

This chapter focuses on the physical examination procedures for which there is at least some scientific evidence that routine screening may be beneficial. These include sphygmomanometry; routine measurement of height, weight, and head circumference; testing for abnormal hearing and visual acuity; oral cavity examination; clinical breast examination (CBE); digital rectal examination (DRE); and skin examination. See Chapter 18 for discussion of specific examination procedures for children (e.g., newborn examination for the pupillary light reflex). The reader should consult the suggested readings at the end of this chapter for information about other preventive examination procedures not discussed here (e.g., auscultation of the heart or carotid arteries, palpation for abdominal aortic aneurysms or thyroid nodules, testicular examination, or congenital hip dislocation). Other references should be consulted regarding examination procedures to screen for occupational illnesses and injuries.

The discussion of each examination procedure that follows includes a brief introduction describing the target condition and the rationale for the screening test, guidelines on how often screening should be performed and on which patients, a summary of official guidelines issued by major organizations and agencies, and suggestions on patient preparation and technique. (The sources of the recommendations in the "Official Guidelines" sections are listed under "Suggested Readings" later in this chapter.) The discussion of each examination procedure also includes sections on the potential adverse effects of screening, the accuracy of the examination procedure, and suggestions on how to organize the office or clinic and maintain medical records for optimal screening. Data cited in the "Accuracy and Reliability as Screening Test" sections of this chapter and Chapter 5 are drawn from a large body of evidence. The hundreds of studies on which these estimates are based are not cited explicitly in these chapters owing to space limitations. The reader interested in the source of the data is referred to other texts[1] that discuss the individual studies in more detail.

Because routine physical examination procedures usually detect no abnormalities, their most important value may lie in providing a setting for counseling patients about primary and secondary prevention of the target condition. Each section of this chapter therefore includes a "Standard Counseling" discussion of the reminders that clinicians should give all patients, even if no abnormality is detected, about how to prevent the target condition and when to return for additional screening. This section also refers readers to other relevant chapters in Section II of the book, which discuss in more detail how to counsel patients about specific health behaviors. This chapter does not discuss how to manage abnormal findings. For those instances the reader should refer to Chapter 19 for an overview of follow-up testing and treatment options.

SPHYGMOMANOMETRY

Introduction

Over the last four decades, substantial improvements have been made in the awareness and control of hypertension, a major risk factor for the development of cardiovascular disease. Approximately 75 million Americans are hypertensive, only 54% of whom have well-controlled blood pressure.[2] Studies have consistently shown that the early detection and treatment of hypertension can reduce all-cause mortality as well as the incidence of cardiac and cerebrovascular events.[3] Screening for hypertension is performed by periodic sphygmomanometry. In the typical office or clinic, this measurement is obtained when routine vital signs are taken before the clinician's examination.

Screening Guidelines. **All adults 18 years and older should undergo periodic screening for hypertension. The evidence is weaker for blood pressure screening of children and adolescents.**

Official Guidelines. The U.S. Preventive Services Task Force (USPSTF) recommends periodic measurement of blood pressure in adults 18 years and older. Adults aged 18 to 39 years with normal blood pressure (<130/85 mm Hg) who do not have other risk factors should be rescreened every 3 to 5 years. It recommends annual screening for adults aged 40 years or older and for those who are at increased risk for high blood pressure. Persons at increased risk include those who have high-normal blood pressure (130–139/85–89 mm Hg), those who are overweight or obese, and African Americans.

The American Academy of Family Physicians (AAFP) agrees with the recommendations of the USPSTF. On the basis of expert opinion and the potential to detect treatable causes of secondary hypertension (up to 28% of children with elevated blood pressure have secondary hypertension), the American Academy of Pediatrics (AAP), the National Heart, Lung, and Blood Institute, and the American Heart Association recommend that children over 3 years and under 18 years have annual screening and once during every health care episode. Children under 3 years should have their blood pressure measured in special circumstances such as a history of being very low birth weight, a history of recurrent urinary tract infections, and congenital heart disease. The Joint National Committee on Detection, Evaluation, and Treatment of High Blood Pressure recommends that screening be repeated in adults every 2 years if the previous reading was in a normotensive range (less than 120/80) and every year if the reading was in a prehypertensive range (120–139/80–89). Patients with stage 1 or 2 hypertension need more frequent monitoring. The American College of Obstetricians and Gynecologists (ACOG) recommends blood pressure screening as part of women's annual health care visits.

Patient Preparation

Accurate blood pressure measurement is essential in diagnosing hypertension. The patient should be seated for 5 minutes before blood pressure is measured. Relaxation should be encouraged. The arm should be at the level of the heart, comfortably supported on a firm surface, and slightly flexed. Clothing with constricting arm sleeves should be removed. The patient should not have exercised, smoked, or ingested caffeine for 30 minutes before measurement.

The examiner should select the proper cuff size to accommodate the size of the patient's arm (Table 4.2). A normal-sized adult cuff will produce falsely elevated pressures on an obese arm and falsely low pressures on a thin arm or on that of a child. Therefore, choose a cuff with a bladder width that is 20% wider than the diameter of the arm or 40% of the circumference of the arm. The length of the bladder should be approximately 80% of the circumference so that it does not completely encircle the limb. In children, the bladder width should not exceed two-thirds the length of the upper arm and the bladder length should not encircle more than three-fourths of the circumference of the arm.

TABLE 4.2 Proper Cuff Sizes for Accurate Blood Pressure Measurement

Patient	Recommended Cuff Size (cm)	Arm Circumference Range at Midpoint (cm)
Newborn	4 × 8	–
Infant	6 × 12	–
Child	9 × 18	–
Small adult	12 × 22	22–26
Adult	16 × 30	27–34
Adult	16 × 36	35–44
Adult	16 × 42	45–52

Adapted from Smith L. New recommendations for blood pressure measurement. *Am Fam Physician.* 2005;72(7):1391-1398.

Technique

The cuff should be placed snugly around the upper arm, with the lower edge approximately 1 in above the antecubital fossa, the bladder over the brachial artery, and the tubing over the medial aspect of the arm. For a manual measurement, both the palpable systolic pressure and the audible Korotkoff sounds should be determined. Electronic devices automate this process and do not require audible or manual assessment. At least two measurements should be made, and the average of the two should be recorded as the patient's blood pressure. If an abnormality is detected, the blood pressure can be compared in both arms in supine, sitting, and standing positions; in children, blood pressure can be measured in the lower extremities to rule out aortic coarctation. Differences of up to 10 mm Hg between arms are within the normal range.

For adults, blood pressure is considered *normal* if it is less than 120/80 mm Hg. The threshold for blood pressure that is *elevated* is 120 to 129 mm Hg systolic and less than 80 mm Hg diastolic. *Hypertension stage 1* is 130 to 139 mm Hg systolic or 80 to 89 mm Hg diastolic. *Hypertension stage 2* is ≥140 mm Hg systolic or ≥90 mm Hg diastolic. For children and adolescents, hypertension is based on normative distributions of blood pressure in healthy children on the basis of sex, age, and height. See Table 4.3 for the criteria for elevated blood pressure in children. Isolated blood pressure elevations can be due to anxiety and other factors (e.g., "white coat" hypertension), and the diagnosis of hypertension should therefore not be made until the patient has had two consecutive visits in which elevated blood pressure has been documented.

TABLE 4.3 Criteria for Elevated Blood Pressure (BP)	
For Children Aged 1–13 yr	**For Children Aged ≥13 yr**
Normal BP: <90th percentile	Normal BP: <120/<80 mm Hg
Elevated BP: ≥90th percentile to <95th percentile or 120/80 mm Hg to <95th percentile (whichever is lower)	Elevated BP: 120/<80 to 129/<80 mm Hg
Stage 1 hypertension (HTN): ≥95th percentile to <95th percentile + 12 mm Hg, or 130/80 to 139/89 mm Hg (whichever is lower)	Stage 1 HTN: 130/80 to 139/89 mm Hg
Stage 2 HTN: ≥95th percentile + 12 mm Hg, or ≥140/90 mm Hg (whichever is lower)	Stage 2 HTN: ≥140/90 mm Hg

Adapted from Clinical practice guideline for screening and management of high blood pressure in children and adolescents. *Pediatrics.* 2017;140(3):e20171904.

Standard Counseling

Patients should be reminded that regular physical activity (see Chapter 7), adoption of the DASH diet—Dietary Approaches to Stop Hypertension—(see Chapter 8), weight management (see Chapter 9), and alcohol moderation (see Chapter 11) will help control blood pressure and that their blood pressure should be measured again in the appropriate interval (see Table 4.4). Patients with an isolated blood pressure elevation should be informed that the elevation is not considered "high blood pressure" until repeat measurements are obtained, but the importance of returning for repeat measurements should be emphasized.

Potential Adverse Effects

There are no direct adverse effects from measuring blood pressure, but the results can be inaccurate, producing psychological, behavioral, and even financial consequences if the results affect insurance or employment eligibility or require repeat office visits to rule out hypertension. Although patients may experience anxiety over the possibility of having high blood pressure, studies have inconsistently demonstrated higher rates of work absenteeism among persons who receive the label of "hypertension."[1] Antihypertensive medications may produce side effects. Inaccurate sphygmomanometry can also produce false-negative results, allowing hypertensive persons to escape detection.

Accuracy and Reliability as Screening Test

Office sphygmomanometry is less accurate than invasive techniques (e.g., intra-arterial monitoring) for measuring blood pressure, but its exact sensitivity and specificity are uncertain. The type of instrument, the technique of the examiner, and the physiologic state of the patient affect the

TABLE 4.4 Recommended Follow-Up Interval Based on Initial Blood Pressure (BP) Level

Initial Blood Pressure	Follow-up Recommended
Normal (<120/80 mm Hg)	Evaluate yearly, encourage healthy lifestyle changes to maintain normal BP
Elevated (120–129/80–89 mm Hg)	Recommend healthy lifestyle changes, reassess in 3–6 mo
Hypertension stage 1: 130–139 mm Hg systolic or 80–89 mm Hg diastolic	Assess the 10-yr risk for heart disease and stroke: If risk less than 10%, start with lifestyle changes and reassess in 3–6 mo If risk is greater than 10% and the patient has known cardiovascular disease, diabetes mellitus, or chronic kidney disease, recommend lifestyle changes and treat with BP-lowering medication and reassess in 1 mo If goal is met after 1 mo, reassess in 3–6 mo If goal is not met after 1 mo, consider titration or different medication and monthly follow-up until control is achieved
Hypertension stage 2: ≥140 mm Hg systolic or ≥90 mm Hg diastolic	Recommend healthy lifestyle changes and BP-lowering medication If goal is met after 1 mo, reassess in 3–6 mo If goal is not met after 1 mo, consider different medications or titration and continue monthly follow-up until control is achieved

Adapted from Detailed Summary from the 2017 Guideline for the Prevention. Detection, evaluation and management of high blood pressure in adults. *Am Heart Assoc.* 2017.

accuracy and reliability of the test. Given that patients' blood pressure varies throughout the day, a single office-based measurement may not reflect a patient's average blood pressure over time. Some evidence suggests that continual ambulatory blood pressure monitoring, which provides an average blood pressure measured over 24 hours, more accurately predicts clinical cardiovascular outcomes. However, whether this information more effectively guides treatment decisions remains uncertain.

Office and Clinic Organization for Routine Screening

Intake procedures for obtaining vital signs should provide sufficient time to allow the patient to relax for several minutes before the blood pressure is measured. The office or clinic should be equipped with a variety of cuff sizes for adults and children. Sphygmomanometers become inaccurate over time and should be recalibrated periodically. Reminder systems should be in place to ensure that patients return for routine screening, obtain consecutive repeat measurements for elevated values, and obtain appropriate counseling and treatment if hypertension is diagnosed.

Medical Record Documentation

The blood pressure recorded in the medical record should be the average of two blood pressure readings obtained during the office visit. If the blood pressure is measured in both arms and the readings are significantly different, the arm and recorded values should be documented. Until elevated blood pressure has been confirmed on two consecutive visits, the finding should be described in the medical record as "elevated blood pressure" and not as "hypertension" or even "high blood pressure." The follow-up plan for elevated blood pressure readings should be documented.

HEIGHT, WEIGHT, AND HEAD CIRCUMFERENCE

Introduction

In the United States, 35% of adult men, 40% of adult women, and 17% of children and adolescents are obese or overweight.[4] By maintaining a healthy weight, patients can reduce their risks of developing hypertension, heart disease, other chronic diseases, and premature mortality.[5] Screening has been advocated as a means of detecting patients who are overweight and obese and of initiating exercise and nutritional interventions to prevent complications, which are discussed in Chapters 7–9. The principal screening tests are height, weight (used to calculate the body mass index [BMI]), and other anthropomorphic measurements. In infants and children, frequent height, weight, and head circumference measurements are used to screen for abnormal growth velocity (including both delayed growth and obesity) and to institute nutritional and social service interventions (see Chapter 18). Some screening tests for obesity (e.g., skinfold thickness and other measures of body fat, waist and limb circumference) are not reviewed here.

Screening Guidelines. **The height and weight of adults should be measured periodically and used to calculate the BMI, but there is no scientific evidence regarding the proper interval. The height, weight, and BMI (and head circumference of infants and small children) should be measured at every childhood visit (unless recent measurements have been obtained within the last few weeks) and should be plotted on an appropriate growth chart (see Chapter 18).**

Official Guidelines. The USPSTF and the AAFP recommend that clinicians screen all adult patients for obesity and offer intensive counseling and behavioral interventions to promote improvements in weight status for obese adults with a BMI of 30 kg/m². The American Heart Association recommends that adults have their BMI calculated at least once a year. The AAP recommends that infants undergo height, weight, and head circumference measurement at well child visits between the ages of 0 to 24 months and annually from ages 2 to 6 years; it also recommends annual BMI measurements for all children and adolescents.

Patient Preparation

Patients should remove heavy clothing and shoes.

Technique

Height and weight are generally measured with a standing platform scale and a height attachment. Electronic scales are common and do not require calibration, but platform scales should be calibrated to zero before the patient is weighed. When height is measured, patients should stand erect with their back against the scale or measuring wall and with their feet together. They should look straight ahead, with the outer canthus of the eye on the same horizontal plane as the external auditory canal.

Infants and small children should be weighed on an infant platform scale. The height of infants and small children is measured by placing the child in a recumbent position on a measuring board, holding the feet against a fixed foot piece, and moving the headpiece to touch the vertex. Head circumference should be measured by wrapping a measuring tape around the child's head at the level of the occipital protuberance and the supraorbital prominence. See Chapter 18 for more details on the examination of infants and children.

The height and weight determine the BMI (Table 4.5), which in turn classifies patients as overweight (BMI = 25–29.9 kg/m^2) or obese (BMI greater than or equal to 30 kg/m^2) (see Chapter 8). There are three classes of obesity: class I (BMI = 30–34.9 kg/m^2) is low risk, class II (BMI = 35–39.9 kg/m^2) is moderate risk, and class III (BMI = 40 kg/m^2 and above) is high risk. The BMI is calculated by dividing the patient's height in kilograms by the height in meters squared (kg/m^2). Many electronic health records, calculators on mobile device apps, and website tools (www.nhlbi.nih.gov/health/educational/lose_wt/BMI/bmicalc.htm) can make this calculation automatically.

For infants and young children, the height, weight, and head circumference are used to detect abnormal size and growth velocity by plotting the data on age- and gender-specific growth curves that reflect population norms. Since 2000, the growth charts from the Centers for Disease Control and Prevention have included a BMI-for-age growth chart to help better identify obese children and those at risk for obesity. These growth charts are discussed in further detail in Chapter 18.

Obtaining regular body weights is not always easy to do with older or frail patients. If weight loss is suspected, repeat weighing should be done. For the BMI, the patient's height before age 50 years should be used as the reference height. Clinically significant weight loss is considered to be weight loss exceeding 2% of baseline in 1 month, 5% in 3 months, or 10% in 6 months. The importance of the relationship of lean body mass and excess body fat should be taken into account. Less technical measurements such as BMI and waist circumference correlate well to total body fat but are not good indicators of visceral fat stores.

TABLE 4.5 Table of Body Mass Indices

Body weight (pounds)

	Normal						Overweight					Obese										Extreme Obesity														
BMI kg/m²	19	20	21	22	23	24	25	26	27	28	29	30	31	32	33	34	35	36	37	38	39	40	41	42	43	44	45	46	47	48	49	50	51	52	53	54
Height (inches)																																				
58	91	96	100	105	110	115	119	124	129	134	138	143	148	153	158	162	167	172	177	181	186	191	196	201	205	210	215	220	224	229	234	239	244	248	253	258
59	94	99	104	109	114	119	124	128	133	138	143	148	153	158	163	168	173	178	183	188	193	198	203	208	212	217	222	227	232	237	242	247	252	257	262	267
60	97	102	107	112	118	123	128	133	138	143	148	153	158	163	168	174	179	184	189	194	199	204	209	215	220	225	230	235	240	245	250	255	261	266	271	276
61	100	106	111	116	122	127	132	137	143	148	153	158	164	169	174	180	185	190	195	201	206	211	217	222	227	232	238	243	248	254	259	264	269	275	280	285
62	104	109	115	120	126	131	136	142	147	153	158	164	169	175	180	186	191	196	202	207	213	218	224	229	235	240	246	251	256	262	267	273	278	284	289	295
63	107	113	118	124	130	135	141	146	152	158	163	169	175	180	186	191	197	203	208	214	220	225	231	237	242	248	254	259	265	270	278	282	287	293	299	304
64	110	116	122	128	134	140	145	151	157	163	169	174	180	186	192	197	204	209	215	221	227	232	238	244	250	256	262	267	273	279	285	291	296	302	308	314
65	114	120	126	132	138	144	150	156	162	168	174	180	186	192	198	204	210	216	222	228	234	240	246	252	258	264	270	276	282	288	294	300	306	312	318	324
66	118	124	130	136	142	148	155	161	167	173	179	186	192	198	204	210	216	223	229	235	241	247	253	260	266	272	278	284	291	297	303	309	315	322	328	334
67	121	127	134	140	146	153	159	166	172	178	185	191	198	204	211	217	223	230	236	242	249	255	261	268	274	280	287	293	299	306	312	319	325	331	338	344
68	125	131	138	144	151	158	164	171	177	184	190	197	203	210	216	223	230	236	243	249	256	262	269	276	282	289	295	302	308	315	322	328	335	341	348	354
69	128	135	142	149	155	162	169	176	182	189	196	203	209	216	223	230	236	243	250	257	263	270	277	284	291	297	304	311	318	324	331	338	345	351	358	365
70	132	139	146	153	160	167	174	181	188	195	202	209	216	222	229	236	243	250	257	264	271	278	285	292	299	306	313	320	327	334	341	348	355	362	369	376
71	136	143	150	157	165	172	179	186	193	200	208	215	222	229	236	243	250	257	265	272	279	286	293	301	308	315	322	329	338	343	351	358	365	372	379	386
72	140	147	154	162	169	177	184	191	199	206	213	221	228	235	242	250	258	265	272	279	287	294	302	309	316	324	331	338	346	353	361	368	375	383	390	397
73	144	151	159	166	174	182	189	197	204	212	219	227	235	242	250	257	265	272	280	288	295	302	310	318	325	333	340	348	355	363	371	378	386	393	401	408
74	148	155	163	171	179	186	194	202	210	218	225	233	241	249	256	264	272	280	287	295	303	311	319	326	334	342	350	358	365	373	381	389	396	404	412	420
75	152	160	168	176	184	192	200	208	216	224	232	240	248	256	264	272	279	287	295	303	311	319	327	335	343	351	359	367	375	383	391	399	407	415	423	431
76	156	164	172	180	189	197	205	213	221	230	238	246	254	263	271	279	287	295	304	312	320	328	336	344	353	361	369	377	385	394	402	410	418	426	435	443

Adapted from Clinical Guidelines on the Identification. *Evaluation, and Treatment of Overweight and Obesity in Adults: The Evidence Report. NIH Publication No.98-4083.* Bethesda, MD: National Heart, Lung, and Blood Institute in cooperation with The National Institute of Diabetes and Digestive and Kidney Diseases; 1998.

Standard Counseling

Patients should be counseled about the healthful benefits of regular physical activity (see Chapter 7), dietary modifications (see Chapter 8), and weight management through lifestyle modifications (see Chapter 9).

Potential Adverse Effects

There are no direct adverse effects from measuring height and weight, but the results can produce psychological, behavioral, and even financial consequences if they affect insurance and employment eligibility and can incur inconvenience and costs to have the abnormality evaluated. Significant social stigma exists for patients with obesity, although it is unclear whether defining and medicalizing obesity by clinical measurement increases this stigma. Some aggressive treatments for obesity, such as medications, very-low-calorie diets, and bariatric surgery are associated with significant potential side effects and complications (e.g., 1%–2% postoperative mortality for weight reduction surgery). False-positive results in measurements of infants and small children can create unnecessary parental anxiety about the possibility of a growth disorder.

Accuracy and Reliability as Screening Test

Height, weight, and BMI are easy to measure and highly reliable. The body fat percentage calculated from BMI correlates with directly measured body fat with an estimation error of only 4%. In addition, the BMI has been linked with a wide range of health outcomes. The BMI does not account for body fat distribution or the relative weight of muscle versus fat, which are also independent predictors of health outcomes.

Office and Clinic Organization for Routine Screening

Offices and clinics should be equipped to measure height and weight for adults and to calculate BMIs easily with conveniently posted BMI conversion tables or automated BMI calculators (see page 88). Likewise, offices with pediatric patients should be equipped with infant platform scales, measuring boards, measuring tape, and a complete supply of pediatric growth charts for boys and girls of all ages. The office should have reminder systems in place to ensure that parents of children with abnormal growth velocity keep appointments for follow-up visits and that the children receive appropriate evaluation and treatment.

Medical Record Documentation

Height, weight, BMI, and other anthropometric data should be recorded in an area of the medical record that allows easy comparison with previous measurements and early detection of important trends. The appropriate age- and gender-specific growth chart should be prominently displayed in the medical record of pediatric patients and should be filled out at each visit. The follow-up plan for abnormal height and weight should be documented in the medical record.

HEARING TESTING

Introduction

Approximately 28 million Americans have chronic hearing impairment, more than 1 million of whom are younger than 18 years.[6] Approximately 5 million Americans cannot hear and understand normal speech, and approximately 10 million persons have noise-induced hearing loss. Screening for hearing impairment is performed because it has the potential to improve communication skills and functional status and because it may improve language development when detected in infants and young children. Screening tests to assess hearing can include simple physical examination techniques, which are discussed in this section, and laboratory tests (e.g., audiometry, auditory-evoked responses, otoacoustic emissions testing).

Screening Guidelines. **Clinicians should inquire periodically about difficulties with hearing in children and in the elderly. There is little evidence to support routine screening of adolescents and adults. Physical examination findings may further corroborate positive responses to inquiries about hearing difficulties.**

Official Guidelines. The AAFP recommends periodic inquiry about hearing difficulties in the elderly but does not make recommendations supporting objective measurements for any age group. The AAP recommends periodic historical inquiry about hearing during infancy and childhood and objective hearing testing by a "standard testing method" at ages 4, 5, 6, 8, 10, and 12 years, then once between ages 11 to 14, 15 to 17, and 18 to 21 years. Newborn hearing screening is discussed further in Chapter 18. In 1996 and 2001, the USPSTF found insufficient evidence to recommend for or against routine hearing screening of infants, children, and adults, but the recommendations are currently under reevaluation. Hearing screening is required by law in some states.

Patient Preparation

Hearing should be examined in a quiet area with minimal background noise.

Technique

Simple physical examination tests of hearing include the whispered voice and watch-tick tests. In the whispered voice test, the examiner softly whispers words from a distance of 2 ft while the patient blocks the opposite ear by placing a finger on the tragus; the patient should be able to repeat at least half the words correctly. To avoid the patient from reading lips, the examiner can conduct the test from 2 ft behind the patient. Alternatively, the examiner can ask patients to close their eyes if testing from the front of the patient. In the watch-tick test, the examiner checks high-frequency hearing by moving a ticking watch toward the patient's ear and noting the distance at which the sound is first heard. The patient's eyes should be closed for this test also.

The hearing of young children is tested qualitatively by observing their response to whispered voice or sounds and the progress of their developing speech skills (e.g., delayed vocalization). For example, the examiner can stand or crouch behind the child and whisper softly to determine whether the child turns to the sound or responds to a simple question. See Chapter 18 regarding otoacoustic emissions and audiometry screening of newborns and young children.

Standard Counseling

Parents should be encouraged to contact the clinician if they or teachers note that the child has poor hearing, speech, or language skills. All patients, especially adolescents and young adults, should be reminded that occupational or recreational exposure to loud noise (e.g., loud music through earbuds at unsafe volumes) increases the risk of hearing loss. Older adults should be counseled that, although loss of hearing is common with increasing age, it should not be accepted as "normal," can compromise their quality of life, and is often treatable with hearing aids.

Potential Adverse Effects

There are no known adverse effects from hearing testing, but inaccurate results may produce unnecessary anxiety, especially among the parents of young children; may affect insurance and employment eligibility; and may incur cost and inconvenience for appointments and testing to rule out a disorder. Inaccurate testing may produce false-negative results, allowing hearing impairment to escape detection.

Accuracy and Reliability as Screening Test

There are few data available regarding the sensitivity and specificity of physical examination techniques for hearing.

Office and Clinic Organization for Routine Screening

Examination rooms in which hearing screening is performed should be located away from loud working areas or noisy machines. The office or clinic should have referral and reminder systems in place to ensure that patients with abnormal screening tests receive appropriate diagnostic studies (e.g., audiometry, tympanometry) either on site or through a referred specialist and that patients found to have hearing disorders receive proper treatment. The patient education literature about hearing aids and the need to treat presbycusis can be helpful to older adults.

Medical Record Documentation

The results of hearing tests should be recorded for each ear. The data can include the proportion of correctly heard words (whisper test) or the distance to hear watch sounds (watch-tick test). The follow-up plan for abnormal hearing should be documented.

VISUAL ACUITY TESTING

Introduction

Approximately 1% to 4% of American children have amblyopia, and an estimated 5% to 7% of preschool children have refractive errors.[7] Screening for abnormal visual acuity is performed because the detection of amblyopia and amblyogenic risk factors can improve visual acuity through treatments such as surgery for cataracts or strabismus, use of glasses or refractive surgery treatments, and visual training to treat amblyopia (e.g., patching). Although 6% of adults have visual impairment, there is little evidence that early detection of visual impairment reduces morbidity for school-aged children, adolescents, and young adults. Detection of impairment in older adults, however, may prevent injuries and improve functional status. Testing for abnormal visual acuity can range from simple acuity testing by primary care clinicians to sophisticated refraction measurements by eye specialists. Chapter 18 provides further details on testing of visual acuity and screening tests for amblyopia and strabismus in young children.

Screening Guidelines. **Screening for amblyopia, strabismus, and defects in visual acuity is recommended for children aged 3 to 5 years. Periodic screening for impaired visual acuity is appropriate in older adults, but there is no scientific evidence regarding the optimal interval. Asymptomatic adolescents and young adults do not require routine visual acuity screening.**

Official Guidelines. The USPSTF recommends vision screening for all children at least once between the ages of 3 and 5 years, to detect the presence of amblyopia or its risk factors, but there is insufficient evidence to recommend vision screening for children <3 years of age. The USPSTF concludes that the current evidence is insufficient to assess the balance of benefits and harms of screening for impaired visual acuity in adults 65 and older. The AAFP is in agreement with the USPSTF recommendations. On the basis of expert opinion, the American Academy of Ophthalmology and the AAP recommend vision assessment in children aged 6 months to 3 years with physical examination (e.g., external inspection, the fixation and follow test, the red reflex test, and pupil examination). Instrument-based vision screening (with autorefractors or photoscreeners) may be used, when available, in children aged 1 to 3 years. Visual acuity screening may be attempted at age 3 years using HOTV or Lea Symbols charts; children aged 4 to 5 years should have visual acuity assessed using HOTV or Lea Symbols charts, the cover-uncover test, and the red reflex test. Vision screening of preschool and school children is also required by law in some states and in a number of federal programs. For adults, the American Academy of Ophthalmology recommends comprehensive eye examination that includes visual acuity testing and dilation every 1 to 2 years for all adults 65 years or older who do not have risk factors or more frequently if risk factors are present.

Patient Preparation

Individuals with a known refractive error and prescribed corrective lenses should wear their glasses or contact lenses for the examination.

Technique

To test visual acuity, the patient should sit or stand 20 ft from a standard Snellen eye chart (Fig. 4.1). With one eye covered, the patient should read the letters aloud, moving from top to bottom, and then the test should be repeated with the other eye covered. The last full row of letters that the patient can read correctly indicates the acuity level. If the upper row of large letters cannot be seen at 20 ft, the patient should step forward until they become visible; the distance should be recorded in the upper figure (at a distance of

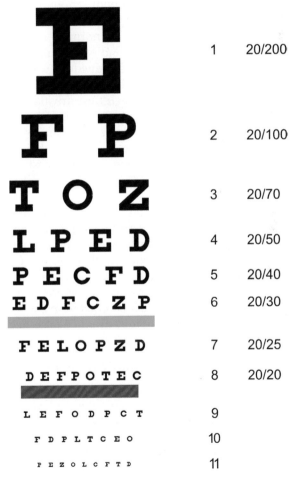

Figure 4.1   Snellen chart. Reprinted with permission from Ball JW, Dains JE, Flynn JA, et al. *Seidel's Guide to Physical Examination*. 8th ed. St. Louis: Elsevier Mosby; 2015:44.

5 ft, the notation would be "5/200"). An acuity of 20/30 or better is generally considered normal for adults. If a standard Snellen wall chart is unavailable, acuity can be tested with pocket eye charts (Rosenbaum or Jaeger charts) held at a distance of 14 in or, more approximately, by comparing the patient's ability to read printed material with that of the examiner. Illiterate and non-English speaking patients can be tested with the Snellen "E" chart by asking whether the letter faces up, down, to the left, or to the right.

Chapter 18 discusses the evaluation of visual acuity in children, screening techniques for amblyopia and strabismus, and other examination procedures (e.g., detection of red reflexes).

Standard Counseling

Parents should be encouraged to contact the clinician if they or teachers note that the child has difficulty seeing or has poor school performance. Older adults should be reminded that, although worsening vision is common with increasing age, it should not be accepted as "normal," can limit functional independence, increases the risk of falls and other unintentional injuries, and is often treatable with corrective lenses. Individuals with impaired vision may need to receive counseling about safe driving practices, ranging from modifying driving habits (e.g., reducing nighttime driving for older individuals with visual contrast impairment) to being advised to refrain from any future driving. Older adults at high risk for eye conditions, such as cataracts or glaucoma, or with early disease states (e.g., ocular hypertension) may also benefit from routine examinations by an eye specialist.

Potential Adverse Effects

There are no known adverse effects from visual acuity testing, but inaccurate results can produce unnecessary anxiety, especially among the parents of young children; may affect insurance and employment eligibility; and may incur costs and inconvenience for visits to eye care specialists to rule out a disorder. There is a potential for overly aggressive treatment of early disease or predisease, such as ocular hypertension, which may result in medication-related or surgical complications, with limited benefit. Conversely, inaccurate screening may produce false-negative results, allowing visual disorders to escape detection.

Accuracy and Reliability as Screening Test

Few studies have examined the sensitivity and specificity of visual acuity testing. In children, Snellen letters are estimated to have a sensitivity of 25% to 79% and a specificity of approximately 85%.

Office and Clinic Organization for Routine Screening

Offices and clinics should be equipped with a Snellen wall chart, a Snellen "E" chart, and eye covers. Visual acuity testing should not be performed in high-traffic areas, where the test is likely to be interrupted by the movement of staff or patients. A floor marker should identify the proper standing position.

Nurses and physician assistants can perform visual acuity testing before the clinician's examination. All staff performing the test should be trained in proper technique for performing the test and for recording the results. The office or clinic should have referral and reminder system in place to ensure that patients with abnormal visual acuity receive appropriate referrals to eye specialists and to verify that follow-up appointments are kept.

Medical Record Documentation

Visual acuity should be recorded for each eye. When the Snellen eye chart is used to determine the lowest row of letters that the patient can read correctly, indicate the number of letters from the next row that were read correctly (e.g., "20/25 + 2" means that the patient was able to read two letters from the 20/20 row). If strabismus is detected, indicate whether the eye is nasally deviated (esotropia) or temporally deviated (exotropia). The follow-up plan for abnormal visual acuity should be documented.

ORAL CAVITY EXAMINATION

Introduction

According to the Centers for Disease Control and Prevention in 2012, approximately 40,000 new cases of oral cancer were diagnosed in the United States, with about 9000 deaths attributed to cancers of the oral cavity and pharynx. Screening the oral cavity for cancer is advocated because of the potential to improve outcomes through the detection of early-stage disease and because there is little harm or cost associated with the examination. There is little direct evidence, however, that screening for oral cancer results in improved outcomes. Conversely, targeted counseling for modifiable risk factors, such as smoking cessation or alcohol moderation, may be a more effective use of a clinician's limited time. Human papilloma virus (HPV) has been linked to cancers of the oropharynx; however, more research is needed to determine if HPV itself can cause oral pharyngeal cancers or if smoking and alcohol use interact with the HPV to cause cancer. Nonetheless, this can be part of routine counseling on safe sexual practices for all patients and ensuring that adolescents and adults aged 26 years and younger are vaccinated against HPV, which may prevent some types of cancers of the oral cavity.[8]

Screening Guidelines. **Oral cavity screening of asymptomatic persons may be indicated in patients who use tobacco, drink excessive amounts of alcohol, or have found suspicious lesions on self-examination. There is little scientific evidence, however, regarding the effectiveness of or optimal interval for oral cavity screening.**

Official Guidelines. The USPSTF and the AAFP conclude that there is insufficient evidence to recommend for or against routine screening for oral cancer in asymptomatic adults. The American Cancer Society (ACS) recommends including an oral cavity examination in the general periodic health examination, which it recommends at regular intervals based on age group.

Technique

The oral cavity cancer examination begins with the lips, a potential site of both oral cavity and skin cancer. Dental appliances such as dentures should be removed. Using a tongue blade and a light source, the examiner should systematically inspect the buccal mucosa, gums, dorsum of the tongue, and hard palate. A nodule or growth on the palate, especially if it is not in the midline, should be evaluated further. The teeth should be inspected for plaque and carious lesions. The gums should be inspected for signs of inflammation, bleeding, or recession. The posterior pharynx should be inspected by depressing the tongue with a tongue blade and noting abnormalities in the tonsillar architecture. The hypopharynx can be viewed with a number 5 mirror (or pharyngoscope).

Ask the patient to touch the tongue tip to the hard palate and inspect the floor of the mouth and the ventral surface of the tongue. Using a gloved hand, wrap the tongue with gauze, pull it to each side to inspect the lateral borders, and palpate the tongue for masses or nodules. White or red material should be scraped to distinguish between food particles and leukoplakia, a precursor to oral neoplasms. An ulcer, nodule, or thickened white patch on the lateral or ventral surface of the tongue may represent a malignancy. Leukoplakia should be suspected if an immovable white lesion resembling white paint is detected on the buccal mucosa, lower lip, tongue, or floor of the mouth.

Standard Counseling

Patients who use tobacco should be advised to stop smoking or chewing tobacco (see Chapter 10), and those who drink excessive amounts of alcohol should receive appropriate counseling (see Chapter 11). All patients should be counseled regarding preventive dental care.

Potential Adverse Effects

The only direct adverse effect of the noninvasive oral cavity examination is the minor discomfort associated with the gag reflex and manipulation of the tongue. The detection of suspicious lesions can produce anxiety until a tissue diagnosis is obtained, however, and follow-up appointments with specialists may incur costs and inconvenience.

Accuracy and Reliability as Screening Test

Few studies have examined the sensitivity and specificity of the oral cavity examination, and the results have been variable, depending on the population, the skills of the examiner, and the study design: a sensitivity of 18% to 94%, specificity of 54% to 99%, and positive predictive value of 17% to 86% have been reported in studies on screening for oral cancer. More comprehensive examinations are likely more sensitive than the brief visual inspection of the oral cavity that is commonly performed by busy clinicians, but they also represent a greater opportunity cost because of the time required to perform the examination. No studies reported on harms from the screening test or from false-positive or false-negative results.[9]

Office and Clinic Organization for Routine Screening

The examination room should be equipped with a good light source, tongue blades, and cotton gauze. Referral and reminder systems should be in place to ensure that patients with abnormal findings receive appropriate referrals to otolaryngologists, dentists, and other appropriate specialists; that the appointments are kept; and that patients with documented disease receive appropriate counseling and treatment.

Medical Record Documentation

The examiner should document that an oral cavity examination was performed and should describe the location, size, and appearance of abnormal lesions. The follow-up plan for suspicious findings should be documented.

CLINICAL BREAST EXAMINATION

Introduction

In 2018, it is estimated that 268,670 new cases of breast cancer will be diagnosed in the United States.[10] It is the second leading cause of cancer death in women and is estimated to cause 40,920 deaths in 2018.[10] Although few studies have evaluated the effectiveness of CBE alone compared with no screening, the CBE is a component of most trials that evaluated mammography. Mammography is discussed in Chapter 5 and breast self-examination in Chapter 15.

Screening Guidelines. **CBE as an adjunct to mammography may be offered to all women aged 40 years or older for breast cancer screening.**

Official Guidelines. The USPSTF concludes that the current evidence is insufficient to assess the additional benefits and harms of CBE beyond screening mammography in women 40 years or older. The AAFP supports the Task Force's recommendation. The ACS states that research has not shown a clear benefit of regular clinical breast examination performed by a health care professional; however, it advises that patients should be familiar with how their breast look and feel normally and report any changes to their provider immediately. The ACOG recommends that CBE should be offered every 1 to 3 years for women aged 25 to 39 years and then annually for women 40 years and older.

Patient Preparation

The examination room should have adequate lighting. The patient should disrobe to the waist, remove her brassiere, and dress in a gown. A female chaperone may be advisable, especially if the examiner is a man.

Technique

The clinician should be sensitive to the anxiety of patients undergoing this examination, who often have been sensitized to the risks of breast cancer through lay media or the illnesses of family or friends. The clinician should inspect the breasts for size, symmetry, contour, skin color, and obvious lesions. Dimpling or retractions of the skin, edema resulting in *peau d'orange* texture (appearance of thick skin with large pores and accentuated markings), visible venous networks in one breast, or an abnormal nipple (e.g., bleeding, discharge, ulceration, inversion, retraction) may suggest carcinoma (see Fig. 4.2). Breast inspection is best performed in different positions: first with the patient seated and arms at the side, then with the arms over the head, with the hands pressed against the hips (or palms pushed against each other) to contract the pectoralis muscles, and, finally, with the patient leaning forward to place traction on the suspensory ligaments (see Fig. 4.3).

The breasts (including the nipples and subareolar tissue), axillae, and supraclavicular areas should be palpated in a systematic manner, feeling for lumps, nodules, or lymphadenopathy, with the patient in upright and supine positions. Currently, the vertical strip pattern approach to palpating the breast is the best validated technique in the detection of breast masses (see Fig. 4.4). The most important requirement is that each portion of the breast be fully examined in a systematic manner. Always palpate the tail of the breast, because 40% of malignancies occur in the upper-outer quadrant. The tail is made accessible to palpation by having the patient raise her arms over her head. The entire axilla and supraclavicular areas should be palpated for lymphadenopathy, including the lateral portion along the undersurface of the arm, the anterior wall along the pectoralis muscles, and the posterior portion along the scapular border. Supraclavicular nodes are best palpated by having the patient turn her head toward the side being examined while raising the shoulder and bending the head forward to relax the sternocleidomastoid muscle.

If a breast mass is palpated, the examiner should note its location, size, shape, consistency, tenderness, mobility, and borders. In premenopausal women, it is also important to note the stage of the patient's menstrual cycle. Breast carcinoma is more likely to be firm and nontender and to produce dimpling or edema of the skin. Breast enlargement, nodularity, and tenderness that occur in monthly cyclical patterns and in different locations of the breast are often related to fibrocystic disease. These patterns are not consistent, however, and malignancy generally cannot be ruled out without careful

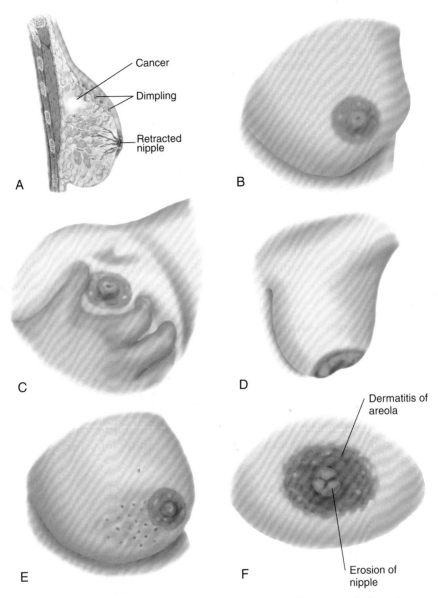

Figure 4.2   Visible signs of breast cancer. A, Retraction signs. As breast cancer advances, it causes fibrosis (scar tissue). Shortening of this tissue produces dimpling, changes in contour, and retraction or deviation of the nipple. Other causes of retraction include fat necrosis and mammary duct ectasia. B, Abnormal contours. Look for any variation in the normal convexity of each breast, and compare one side with the other. Special positioning may again be useful. Shown here is marked flattening of the lower outer quadrant of the left breast. C, Skin dimpling. Look for this sign with the patient's arm at rest, during special positioning, and on moving or compressing the breast,

(*Continued*)

as illustrated here. D, Nipple retraction and deviation. A retracted nipple is flattened or pulled inward, as illustrated here. It may also be broadened and feels thickened. When involvement is radially asymmetric, the nipple may deviate or point in a different direction from its normal counterpart, typically toward the underlying cancer. E, Edema of the skin. Edema of the skin is produced by lymphatic blockade. It appears as thickened skin with enlarged pores, the so-called *peau d'orange* (orange peel) sign. It is often seen first in the lower portion of the breast or areola. F, Paget disease of the nipple. This uncommon form of breast cancer usually starts as a scaly, eczema-like lesion on the nipple that may weep, crust, or erode. A breast mass may be present. Suspect Paget disease in any persisting dermatitis of the nipple and areola. Often (>60%) presents with an underlying in situ or invasive ductal or lobular carcinoma. Reprinted with permission from Bickley LS. *Bates' Guide to Physical Examination and History Taking.* 12th ed. Philadelphia: Wolters Kluwer; 2017.

documentation, repeat examinations, imaging studies, cyst aspiration, and/or tissue biopsy (see Chapter 18). Although small, 3 to 5 mm, mobile axillary lymph nodes are common in adults, the examiner should note the location, size, consistency, and degree of fixation of any palpable nodes.

Standard Counseling

Women aged 50 years and older should be advised about obtaining a biennial screening mammogram. The CBE may be repeated annually, but the clinician should ensure that the patient understands its limitations, risks, and potential benefits. Women should be advised to notify the clinician if suspicious masses or lesions are noted on self-examination. If women are performing breast self-examinations, they should be counseled on the appropriate technique. See Chapter 15 for further information about breast self-examination.

Potential Adverse Effects

The direct adverse effects of the CBE are embarrassment and discomfort during palpation. The detection of suspicious masses can produce significant anxiety until a tissue diagnosis is obtained and can lead to invasive and uncomfortable procedures such as needle aspiration and biopsy. Up to 80% of abnormal CBEs represent false positives. The costs and inconvenience associated with repeat office visits and appointments with specialists can be significant. Inaccurate or incomplete examinations can produce false-negative results, allowing premalignant and malignant lesions to escape detection.

Accuracy and Reliability as Screening Test

Comparing CBE alone with mammography and interval cancer development, CBE (without mammography) has a sensitivity of 40% to 69%, a specificity of 86% to 99%, and a positive predictive value of 4% to 50%. The

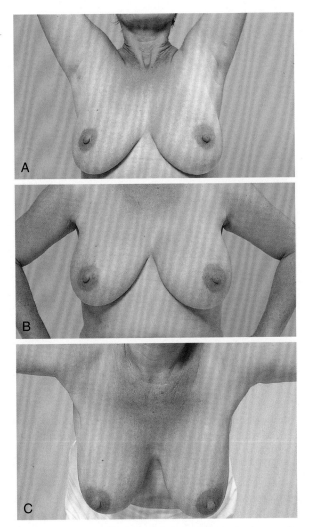

Figure 4.3 Patient positions for breast inspection. A, Arms extended over-head. B, Hands pressed against hips. C, Leaning forward to place traction on the suspensory ligaments. Reprinted with permission from Bickley, LS. *Bates' Guide to Physical Examination and History Taking.* 12th ed. Philadelphia: Wolters Kluwer; 2017.

accuracy and reliability of CBE are affected by the skills of the examiner and the age of the patient: as patients age, fatty tissue replaces fibrocystic tissue and the CBE becomes more accurate.

Office and Clinic Organization for Routine Screening

Examination rooms used for CBE should offer complete privacy, comfortable temperature, and good lighting. The CBE provides an important

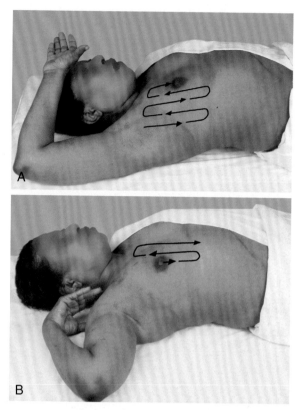

Figure 4.4 Vertical strip pattern for systematic palpation of the breasts. A, Lateral breast. B, Medial breast. Reprinted with permission from Bickley LS. *Bates' Guide to Physical Examination and History Taking*. 12th ed. Philadelphia: Wolters Kluwer; 2017.

opportunity for recommending mammography (see Chapter 5) and, if advocated by the clinician, for teaching breast self-examination (see Chapter 15). The office or clinic should therefore have systems in place to easily provide referrals for screening mammograms at the time of the breast examination and, if breast self-examination is recommended, to provide instructions and printed materials on proper technique. The office or clinic should have reliable referral and reminder systems in place to ensure that women return for their next breast examination within 1 to 2 years; that patients with abnormal findings on breast examination return for follow-up evaluations and, when indicated, receive referrals to surgeons or radiologists; that appointments with outside specialists are kept; and that women found to have breast disease receive appropriate counseling and treatment.

Medical Record Documentation

The examiner should document that a complete breast examination was performed. If a breast lesion is found on examination, the clinician should document the location by noting the quadrant, its diagonal relationship to the nipple ("3 o'clock, 3 cm from the nipple"), its size in centimeters, and the consistency, mobility, and tenderness of the mass. The presence or absence of skin, nipple, and lymph node findings should also be documented. A diagram of the breast, indicating the specific location of the mass, may be helpful for future reference and for describing the findings to other examiners. The follow-up plan for abnormal findings should be documented in the medical record.

PELVIC EXAMINATION

Introduction

The pelvic examination is part of the screening procedure for cervical cancer. It provides a means to visualize the cervix, which is necessary both to collect the Pap smear and to inspect for cervical lesions. The pelvic examination also allows for visualization of labial or vaginal lesions, such as squamous carcinomas, and palpation of masses that could be suggestive of uterine or ovarian pathology. In 2018, an estimated 13,240 cases of cervical cancer, 63,230 cases of uterine cancer, 22,240 cases of ovarian cancer, and 6190 cases of vulvar and 5170 cases of vaginal cancer will be diagnosed.[10] Aside from its role in cervical cancer screening, there is little evidence that the pelvic examination is beneficial in detecting other pathology. Vaginal cancers are uncommon and often present symptomatically at an early stage. The pelvic examination is an insensitive means to detect early-stage ovarian or uterine pathology. Chapter 5 reviews the Pap smear, whereas this chapter focuses on the pelvic examination itself.

Screening Guideline. **The recommendation for pelvic examination varies and is usually done in conjunction with the Pap smear to screen for cervical cancer. There is little evidence to support performing a pelvic examination without a Pap smear as a means to screen for cervical, ovarian, uterine, or vaginal cancers. Shared decision-making between patient and clinician may be a helpful tool in determining the need for pelvic examination (see Chapter 22).**

Official Guidelines. The AAFP and the USPSTF recommend against performing screening pelvic examinations in asymptomatic, nonpregnant adult women; however, the ACOG recommends performing pelvic examinations annually in all patients 21 years and older. The Well-Woman Task Force, convened by the ACOG in 2013, recommends that for women 21 years and older, external examination may be performed annually and that inclusion of speculum examination, bimanual examination, or both in otherwise healthy women should be a shared, informed decision between patient and clinician (see Chapter 22).

The ACOG and the ACS recommend periodic pelvic examination for women older than 19 or 20 years, respectively, or 3 years after the onset of sexual activity.

Patient Preparation

Patient preparation for the pelvic examination involves disrobing from the waist down and donning a gown or drape, lying supine on the examining table, and placing the legs in stirrups. A chaperone is recommended for this physical examination, especially if the examiner is a man.

Technique

A speculum of appropriate size and shape for the patient's vagina should be lubricated and warmed with warm water; jelly lubricants may interfere with cytologic studies for standard Pap smears. With two fingers placed at the introitus, the examiner should gently press down on the perineum and, with the other hand, slowly and gently introduce the closed speculum over the fingers (see Fig. 4.5). The discomfort of pressing on the urethra can be minimized by holding the blades of the speculum obliquely and advancing them along the posterior vaginal wall. Once the speculum enters the vagina, the fingers of the other hand should be removed from the introitus and the blades rotated to a horizontal position. When the speculum is fully advanced, the blades of the speculum should be opened, and the speculum should be maneuvered until the cervix comes into view.

The examiner should inspect the cervix and external os for ulcerations, nodules, masses, bleeding, leukoplakia, or discharge. The

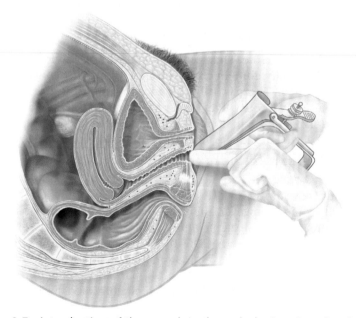

Figure 4.5 Introduction of the speculum through the introitus. Reprinted with permission from Bickley LS. *Bates' Guide to Physical Examination and History Taking.* 12th ed. Philadelphia: Wolters Kluwer; 2017.

squamocolumnar junction (or transformation zone), the region from which 90% to 95% of cervical cancers arise, should be visualized. The squamocolumnar junction is located on the ectocervix or in the endocervical canal. It often migrates inward with age, so that visualization in older women can be difficult. Any discharge obscuring the view of the cervix should be wiped away. See Chapter 5 for details on performing the Pap test at this stage of the examination.

After removing the speculum, the examiner can perform a bimanual examination. Lubricant should be placed on the index and middle fingers of the examiner's dominant hand, and the fingers should be inserted into the vagina until the tips touch the cervix. The examiner should place the nondominant hand on the patient's suprapubic region. The examiner should then palpate the cervix, uterus, and both adnexa between the two hands, feeling for consistency, mobility, tenderness, and masses.

Standard Counseling

The patient should be advised to return for repeat screening at the recommended interval and should be encouraged to reduce risks of unplanned pregnancy (see Chapter 12) and sexually transmitted infections (see Chapter 13), should these apply to the patient.

Potential Adverse Effects

The pelvic examination and Pap smear can be both embarrassing and uncomfortable. Falsely positive results can generate unnecessary anxiety and follow-up testing, including colposcopy, endocervical curettage, and other procedures. Women incur costs and inconvenience for follow-up cervical examinations. Falsely negative results may allow women with preventable cancers to escape detection.

Accuracy and Reliability as Screening Test

Chapter 4 discusses the accuracy and reliability of the Pap smear, in conjunction with the pelvic examination, in screening for cervical cancer. There is little evidence about the accuracy and reliability of the pelvic examination by itself. In general, however, the isolated pelvic examination is a poor means to identify cervical, ovarian, uterine, or vaginal cancers.

Office and Clinic Organization for Routine Screening

The routine performance of a pelvic examination for cervical cancer screening requires examination rooms with comfortable examination tables equipped with stirrups, good lighting, specula of varying sizes and shapes (including both Graves and Pedersen specula), gloves, lubricant, and gowns or other coverings. Reminder systems should be in place to ensure that patients return for repeat screening as necessary and that women with abnormal results receive appropriate follow-up and treatment.

Medical Record Documentation

The date and results of the pelvic examination should be placed in the medical record, preferably on a health maintenance flow sheet. The clinician should describe the appearance of the cervix and whether menstruation was noted. For future reference, it may be helpful to note in the medical record whether the uterus is retroverted and if a special speculum was required to visualize the cervix.

DIGITAL RECTAL EXAMINATION

Introduction

In 2018, it is projected that prostate and colorectal cancers together will account for more than 81,220 deaths and more than 313,520 new cases of malignancy in the United States.[10] Colorectal cancer is the second leading cause of cancer death among Americans, and prostate cancer is the second leading cause of cancer deaths among American men. DRE is among the oldest of the screening tests that have been recommended to detect these malignancies, but other tests discussed in Chapter 5 (e.g., PSA for prostate cancer and fecal occult blood testing and endoscopy for colorectal cancer) are far more sensitive. For example, only 3% of colorectal cancers are palpable on DRE. To date, no studies have demonstrated that performing a DRE leads to decreased mortality from prostate cancer or colorectal cancer or improved quality of life. Many clinicians are accustomed to performing the DRE for screening based on their training and their belief that it has benefits and few adverse effects. In addition, based on past experience, many patients expect a DRE as part of a comprehensive physical examination. The following explanation of how to perform the screening DRE does not necessarily imply an endorsement of the practice by the authors or editors.

Screening Guidelines. **It is reasonable for clinicians to defer a DRE, particularly after discussing its risks and benefits with the patient. Clinicians who do advocate routine DRE as a screening test recommend that the procedure be performed annually after age 50 years or after age 40 years for individuals at higher risk of developing prostate cancer.**

Official Guidelines. The AAFP, ACS, American Urological Association (AUA), and USPSTF do not recommend the DRE to screen for prostate cancer. The AUA does say that DRE in men with an elevated PSA may be a useful secondary test. Most organizations recommend that clinicians engage patients in a shared decision-making process before performing any prostate cancer screening examination or test. Further details about shared decision making are provided in Chapter 22. No organizations endorse DRE as a means to screen for colorectal cancer.

Patient Preparation

The examination can be performed in the Sim's (lying on left side with hips and knees flexed) or standing position. Explain to the patient why a DRE is indicated and acknowledge that it may be uncomfortable. The patient should be told that a cold-feeling lubricant will be used, that there may be a feeling of urgency for a bowel movement or to urinate, but that neither will occur. A chaperone may be advisable.

Technique

The gloved and lubricated examining finger is inserted through the anus and advanced along the anterior wall of the rectum to the prostate. The examiner should palpate the prostate gland and seminal vesicles across the anterior wall of the rectum. The finger may feel more of the prostate if the examiner's body is turned slightly away from the patient. The examiner should feel the median furrow and middle lobe of the prostate and then sweep the finger across the lateral lobes, noting whether the surface is smooth or nodular, as well as the consistency, shape, size, and mobility of the gland. The normal prostate gland is smooth, rubbery (consistency of a pencil eraser), and nontender, with well-defined borders. The normal size is approximately 3 to 4 cm in diameter (ordinarily twice the width of the examining finger), with less than 1 cm protrusion into the rectum; size generally increases with age. Prostatic carcinoma can present as one or more posterior nodules, which are often stony hard and painless. With more advanced disease, the entire gland may be stony hard and the median furrow may be obliterated. Once the examination is completed, the patient should be given tissues to remove the lubricant from the perianal area and should be invited to assume a more comfortable position.

As explained in Chapter 5, testing for occult blood after a DRE (as opposed to home testing) does not constitute adequate fecal occult blood testing for colorectal cancer screening and therefore should not be routinely employed. Doing so can increase the likelihood of false-positive results, originating from the trauma of examination, and has a much higher false-negative rate than utilizing three samples collected after normal bowel movements (see Chapter 5). The sensitivity of home occult blood testing on three samples is 23%, whereas that of a single post-DRE test is less than 5%.

Standard Counseling

Patients who receive a DRE should be advised that the examination can be repeated based on shared decision-making, which should occur before prostate examinations. Patients should be advised that the in-office DRE does not qualify as a screening test for colorectal cancer and should be encouraged to obtain the screening tests that are recommended in Chapter 5.

Potential Adverse Effects

The direct adverse effects of the DRE are embarrassment and discomfort (e.g., the sensation of having to defecate or urinate, mucosal irritation, anal sphincter spasm, pain from hemorrhoidal disease or anal fissures). If a suspicious prostate mass is detected, the patient may experience considerable anxiety until further testing is completed and may incur costs and inconvenience for follow-up office visits and procedures. Some follow-up tests, such as prostate needle biopsy, have more substantial adverse effects. Such testing may reveal nonaggressive (latent) prostate cancers that pose no risk to health but result in complications from treatments (see Chapters 5 and 20).

Accuracy and Reliability as Screening Test

The sensitivity of the DRE in detecting prostate cancer is limited because the examining finger can only palpate the posterior and lateral aspects of the gland and because stage A tumors, the stage for which screening is intended, are, by definition, nonpalpable. The reported sensitivity of the DRE in detecting prostate cancer in asymptomatic men is approximately 55% to 68%, but in some studies, it is as low as 18% to 22%. Moreover, interexaminer reliability, the consistency of findings between examiners, is poor. DRE does enhance the accuracy of the PSA test when performed together, increasing the yield of screening by 26%, but doing so also increases the rate of false-positive findings. Only 6% to 33% of men with suspicious findings on DRE have histologic evidence of prostate cancer on needle biopsy.[1] As already noted, only 3% of colorectal cancers are detectable by DRE.

Office and Clinic Organization for Routine Screening

Examination rooms used for routine screening should offer complete privacy and should be equipped with dressing gowns, gloves, and lubricant. The office or clinic should have reliable referral and reminder systems in place to ensure that the DRE is repeated at the interval recommended by the clinician, that patients with abnormal rectal examinations receive appropriate follow-up diagnostic studies and consultations with specialists, that appointments are kept, and that patients found to have documented disease receive appropriate counseling and treatment. Home stool testing kits and appropriate referral information for endoscopy should be available to help patients obtain colorectal cancer screening.

Medical Record Documentation

The examiner should document that a DRE was performed. Prostatic enlargement can be graded on the basis of diameter in finger breadths (e.g., 1+ = three fingerbreadths, 2+ = four fingerbreadths, 3+ = five fingerbreadths, 4+ occupies most of the anterior outlet with encroachment of the rectal wall) or of depth of protrusion into the rectum: grade I (1–2 cm), grade II (2–3 cm), grade III (3–4 cm), and grade IV (more than 4 cm). The follow-up plan for abnormal findings should be documented.

SKIN EXAMINATION

Introduction

Skin cancer, including malignant melanoma and squamous and basal cell carcinoma, is the most commonly diagnosed cancer in the United States. According to the American Academy of Dermatology, it is estimated that one in every five Americans will be diagnosed with skin cancer in their lifetime. Approximately 91,270 cases of malignant melanoma will be diagnosed in 2018, which will claim an estimated 9320 lives.[10] The outcome of malignant melanoma and other skin cancers can be improved significantly if detected early, for example, the mean thickness of melanomas is a predictor of survival, and comprehensive skin cancer screening examinations have therefore been recommended by some organizations. Direct evidence that such examinations reduce the morbidity or mortality of skin cancer is limited, however.

Screening Guidelines. **Although clinicians should remain alert for malignant skin changes in all patients, comprehensive screening examinations of the skin are recommended primarily for persons with a personal history of skin cancer, clinical evidence of precursor lesions (e.g., dysplastic nevi, actinic keratoses, certain congenital nevi), and those with increased occupational or recreational exposure to sunlight. There is no scientific evidence regarding the optimal interval for skin screening.**

Official Guidelines. The USPSTF and the AAFP found insufficient evidence to recommend for or against routine skin cancer screening by total-body skin examination. The ACS states that regular skin examinations are important for patients who are at increased risk for skin cancer.

Patient Preparation

Patients undergoing a comprehensive skin examination should be asked to remove street clothing. The patient should wear a gown during the examination, and skin surfaces should be covered after they are examined.

Technique

For patients undergoing a comprehensive skin examination, the entire skin surface should be examined in a systematic manner to ensure that all areas are inspected. Particular attention should be paid to sun-exposed areas (scalp, face, neck, shoulders, extensor surfaces of arms and hands) and to areas that are easily overlooked during routine self-examination (axillae, buttocks, perineum, backs of thighs, inner upper thighs, intertriginous surfaces). The skin cancer screening examination should search for evidence of basal cell carcinoma, squamous cell carcinoma, and malignant melanoma.

   Basal cell carcinoma can be nodular, pigmented, cystic, sclerosing, or superficial and usually occurs on the head (especially the face), neck, and back. It may have a translucent, smooth, "pearly" appearance with a central depression (see Fig. 4.6A) but can also be pigmented or hyperkeratotic. *Squamous cell carcinoma* often presents as a soft, mobile, elevated mass with a surface scale or a crusting nodule or plaque (Fig. 4.6B) but can also have other appearances (e.g., the red-brown lesion of squamous cell carcinoma in situ, Bowen disease). It usually occurs on sun-exposed areas such as the scalp, dorsal aspect of the hands, lower lip, and ear. *Malignant melanomas* include superficial spreading, nodular, lentigo, and acral-lentiginous forms. A pigmented lesion is more likely to be malignant if it is asymmetric, rapidly changes in size, or has irregular borders, variegated colors, or a diameter greater than 6 mm (see Fig. 4.7A–D). If suspicious

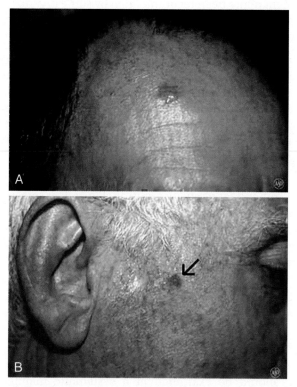

Figure 4.6 A, Basal cell carcinoma. This lesion does not metastasize but can extend below the skin to the bone. B, Squamous cell carcinoma. This lesion can increase in size, developing into large masses, and can metastasize. Reprinted with permission from the American Academy of Dermatology.

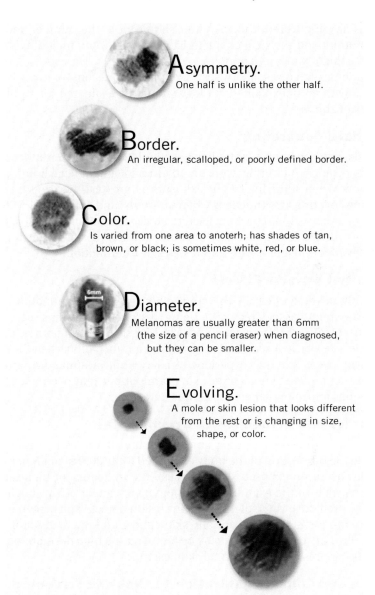

Asymmetry.
One half is unlike the other half.

Border.
An irregular, scalloped, or poorly defined border.

Color.
Is varied from one area to anoterh; has shades of tan,
brown, or black; is sometimes white, red, or blue.

Diameter.
Melanomas are usually greater than 6mm
(the size of a pencil eraser) when diagnosed,
but they can be smaller.

Evolving.
A mole or skin lesion that looks different
from the rest or is changing in size,
shape, or color.

Figure 4.7 The ABCDEs of melanoma: A, Asymmetry—one half unlike the
other half. B, Border—irregular, scalloped, or poorly circumscribed border.
C, Color—varied from one area to another: shades of tan and brown; black;
sometimes white, red, or blue. D, Diameter—larger than 6 mm, the diameter of a pencil eraser. E, Evolving—mole or lesion that looks different from
others or is changing in size, shape, or color. Reprinted with permission from
the American Academy of Dermatology.

lesions are discovered, the examiner should note the number, location, distribution, and physical characteristics of the lesion, including its size, shape, color, texture, and borders.

Patients with unusual bruises, lacerations, abrasions, or other signs of trauma with an unexplained etiology should be evaluated for a potential history of abuse.

Standard Counseling

Patients (and the parents of pediatric patients) should be reminded about the importance of limiting exposure to ultraviolet light (e.g., limiting time outdoors when ultraviolet light exposure is greatest, wearing hats and clothing covering arms and legs when outdoors, and applying SPF 50 sunblock). Patients should be counseled to advise the clinician if a skin lesion changes in size or appearance, becomes tender, or starts bleeding; see Chapter 15 for further details about skin self-examination.

Potential Adverse Effects

The only adverse effect of the comprehensive skin examination is the embarrassment associated with being disrobed. Screening can result in unnecessary treatments such as skin biopsies, which can be uncomfortable, may leave a scar, and may require a return office visit for suture removal. The patient may experience anxiety while awaiting the pathology report. Incomplete or inaccurate skin examinations may overlook important lesions and allow cancers to escape detection.

Accuracy and Reliability as Screening Test

Factors affecting the accuracy and reliability of the skin examination include the proportion of the body examined (only 20% of malignant melanomas occur on exposed skin surfaces), the frequency of the examination, the skills of the examiner, and the type of cancer being sought. The positive predictive value of a suspicious lesion detected on screening skin examination is 21% to 58% for any skin cancer and 6% to 19% for melanoma. Primary care clinicians may be less accurate than dermatologists in diagnosing preselected abnormal skin lesions.

Office and Clinic Organization for Routine Screening

Examination rooms used for routine skin cancer screening should offer complete privacy, dressing gowns, comfortable temperature, good lighting (preferably daylight or fluorescent lighting), and a magnifying lens or handheld light source to inspect lesions closely. Because the skin examination provides an important opportunity to counsel patients about avoiding ultraviolet light exposure, the patient education literature on this topic can be made available. In offices or clinics in which suspicious lesions are biopsied, equipment for performing biopsies and submitting pathology specimens should be easily accessible. Referral and reminder systems should be in place to ensure that patients return for repeat skin examinations at the interval recommended by the clinician, that patients with suspicious lesions obtain skin biopsies on site or receive referrals to a physician who performs them, that the results of skin biopsies are obtained from the pathologist and documented in the medical record, and that patients found to have skin disease receive appropriate counseling and treatment.

Medical Record Documentation

The examiner should document that a skin examination was performed and should describe which skin surfaces were inspected. The location, size, color, distribution pattern, and other physical characteristics of suspicious lesions should be described. Standard terms for skin lesions should be used (e.g., macule, patch, papule, nodule, tumor, plaque). A body diagram may be useful in mapping the exact location of lesions. Newer technologies allow clinicians to photograph lesions and incorporate them into the patient's medical record for more accurate longitudinal tracking. If a skin biopsy was performed, the clinician should describe the details of the procedure, including the size of the biopsy specimen (e.g., 3-mm punch), the section of the lesion that was taken (e.g., border, total excision), and the depth of the lesion that was excised (e.g., shave biopsy, full thickness). The follow-up plan for suspicious lesions should be documented.

CONCLUDING REMARKS

The prevention visit goes by many colloquialisms such as the "physical," "wellness examination," "health maintenance examination," or "checkup." These terms echo clinicians' and patients' frequent expectation that the key element of the visit will be a physical examination. Shared decision-making can also be an important part of navigating the screening physical examination and should not be overlooked (see Chapter 22). Although some elements of the examination are important, a thorough head-to-toe examination in asymptomatic individuals has low yield. The time it requires might be more effectively spent counseling patients about modifiable risk factors or arranging indicated screening tests and immunizations.[11] Conversely, performing validated examination elements in a hurried, cursory manner may leave important findings undetected. A beneficial prevention examination requires an appropriately systematized, deliberate, focused, and individually risk-based approach. Adopting such an approach is an essential skill set for clinicians who deliver preventive care.

SUGGESTED RESOURCES AND MATERIALS

Sphygmomanometry

National Heart, Lung, Blood Institute
The DASH Eating Plan
https://www.nhlbi.nih.gov/health-topics/dash-eating-plan.

American Heart Association
Changes You Can Make to Manage High Blood Pressure
http://www.heart.org/HEARTORG/Conditions/HighBloodPressure/Make
ChangesThatMatter/Changes-You-Can-Make-to-Manage-High-Blood-Pressure_
UCM_002054_Article.jsp#.WphyLkyZNBw.

Height, Weight, and Head Circumference

The National Institute of Diabetes and Digestive and Kidney Diseases
Talking With Patients About Weight Loss: Tips for Primary Care Providers
https://www.niddk.nih.gov/health-information/weight-management/
talking-adult-patients-tips-primary-care-clinicians.

National Heart, Lung, and Blood Institute
Aim for a Healthy Weight
https://www.nhlbi.nih.gov/health/educational/lose_wt/index.htm.

Hearing Testing

American-Speech-Language-Hearing Association
Speech and Language Development
http://www.asha.org/public/speech/development/.

National Institute on Aging
Hearing Loss: A Common Problem for Older Adults
https://www.nia.nih.gov/health/hearing-loss-common-problem-older-adults.

Visual Acuity Testing

American Academy of Family Physicians
Strabismus
http://www.aafp.org/afp/980901ap/980901a.html.

American Academy of Pediatrics
Eyes
https://www.healthychildren.org/English/health-issues/conditions/eyes/Pages/
default.aspx.

American Optometric Association
Eye Health
http://www.aoa.org/.

National Institute on Aging
Aging and Your Eyes
https://www.nia.nih.gov/health/aging-and-your-eyes.

Oral Cavity Examination

Oral Cancer Foundation
Oral Cancer Facts
http://www.oralcancerfoundation.org/facts/.

American Cancer Society
Learn About Oral Cavity and Oropharyngeal Cancer
https://www.cancer.org/cancer/oral-cavity-and-oropharyngeal-cancer.html.

Clinical Breast Examination

American Cancer Society
About Breast Cancer
https://www.cancer.org/cancer/breast-cancer/about.html.

National Cancer Institute
What You Need to Know About Breast Cancer
https://www.cancer.gov/publications/patient-education/wyntk-breast-cancer.

Digital Rectal Examination

American Cancer Society
Learn About Prostate Cancer
https://www.cancer.org/cancer/prostate-cancer.html.

Centers for Disease Control and Prevention
Screening for Prostate Cancer: A Decision for You and Your Doctor
https://www.cdc.gov/cancer/prostate/prostate-cancer-screening-fact-sheet.htm-
   National Cancer Institute.

Prostate Cancer Screening
https://www.cancer.gov/types/prostate/patient/prostate-screening-pdq.

Mayo Clinic
Prostate Cancer Screening: Should You Get a PSA Test?
https://www.mayoclinic.org/diseases-conditions/prostate-cancer/in-depth/
   prostate-cancer/art-20048087.

Skin Examination

American Academy of Family Physicians
Skin Cancer
https://familydoctor.org/condition/skin-cancer/.

American Cancer Society
Melanoma Skin Cancer
https://www.cancer.org/cancer/melanoma-skin-cancer.html.

American Cancer Society
Skin Cancer
https://www.cancer.org/cancer/skin-cancer.html.

SUGGESTED READINGS

American Academy of Family Physicians. *Clinical Preventive Services. American Academy of Family Physicians.* Available at https://www.aafp.org/patient-care/browse/type.tag-clinical-preventive-services-recommendations.html. Last updated July 2017.

American Academy of Pediatrics Committee on Practice and Ambulatory Medicine Section on Ophthalmology, American Association of Certified Orthoptists, American Association of Pediatric Ophthalmology and Strabismus, American Academy of Ophthalmology. Visual system assessment in infants, children, and young adults by pediatricians: Policy statement. Vision Screening Guidelines. *Pediatrics.* 2016;137(1):28-30.

American Cancer Society. *Guidelines for the Early Detection of Cancer.* Available at https://www.cancer.org/healthy/find-cancer-early/cancer-screening-guidelines/american-cancer-society-guidelines-for-the-early-detection-of-cancer.html. Accessed February, 2018.

American College of Obstetricians and Gynecologists. *Well Woman Recommendations.* Available at https://www.acog.org/About-ACOG/ACOG-Departments/Annual-Womens-Health-Care/Well-Woman-Recommendations. Accessed February, 2018.

American College of Physicians. *Current ACP Guidelines.* Available at http://www.acponline.org/clinical/guidelines/. Accessed February 2018.

Bickley LS. *Bates' Guide to Physical Examination and History Taking.* 12th ed. Philadelphia: Wolters Kluwer; 2017.

Canadian Task Force on the Periodic Health Examination. *CTFPHC Systematic Reviews and Recommendations*. Available at http://www.ctfphc.org/. Accessed January 2018.

LeBlond RF, Brown DD, Suneja M, Szot JF. *Dewogin's Diagnostic Examination*, 10th ed. New York, NY: McGraw-Hill; 2014.

Joint National Committee on Detection, Evaluation, and Treatment of High Blood Pressure. The Seventh Report of the Joint National Committee on Detection, Evaluation, and Treatment of High Blood Pressure (JNC VII). Available at http://www.nhlbi.nih.gov/guidelines/hypertension/jnc7full.htm. Accessed February 2018.

National Institutes of Health Consensus Development Conference. Diagnosis and treatment of early melanoma. *JAMA*. 1992;10:1-26.

Swartz MH. *Textbook of Physical Diagnosis: History and Examination*. 7th ed. Philadelphia: WB Saunders; 2014.

U.S. Preventive Services Task Force. *Agency for Healthcare Research and Quality*. Available at https://www.ahrq.gov/professionals/clinicians-providers/guide-lines-recommendations/uspstf/index.html. Accessed February 2018.

REFERENCES

1. U.S. Preventive Services Task Force. Agency for healthcare research and quality. Available at http://www.ahrq.gov/clinic/uspstfix.htm. Accessed February 2018.
2. Merai R, Siegel C, Rakotz M, et al. CDC grand rounds: a public health approach to detect and control hypertension. *MMWR Morb Mortal Wkly Rep*. 2016;65(45):1261-1264.
3. Joint National Committee on Detection, Evaluation, and Treatment of High Blood Pressure. The seventh report of the Joint National Committee on detection, evaluation, and treatment of high blood pressure. The JNCVII report. *JAMA*. 2003;289:2560-2572.
4. Flegal KM, Kruszon-Moran D, Carroll MD, Fryar CD, Ogden CL. Trends in obesity among adults in the United States, 2005 to 2014. *JAMA*. 2016;315(21):2284-2291.
5. *Healthy People 2020*. Washington, DC: U.S. Department of Health and Human Services, Office of Disease Prevention and Health Promotion. Available at https://www.healthypeople.gov/2020/topics-objectives/topic/nutrition-and-weight-status. Accessed 28 February 2018.
6. Caba AJ, Lee DJ, Gomez-Marin O, et al. Prevalence of concurrent hearing and visual impairment in US adults: the National Health Interview Survey, 1997-2002. *Am J Public Health*. 2005;95:1940-1942.
7. Kemper A, Harris R, Lieu T, et al. *Screening for Visual Impairment in Children 0 to 5 Years. Systematic Evidence Review No. 27 (Prepared by the Research Triangle Institute-University of North Carolina Evidence-based Practice Center under Contract No. 290-97-0011)*. Rockville, MD: Agency for Healthcare Research and Quality; May 2004. (Available on the AHRQ Web site at www.ahrq.gov/clinic/ser-files.htm).
8. Centers for Disease Control and Prevention. https://www.cdc.gov/cancer/head-neck/index.html. Accessed February 2018.
9. Olson CM, Burda BU, Beil T, Whitlock EP. *Screening for Oral Cancer: A Targeted Evidence Update for the U.S. Preventive Services Task Force*. Evidence Synthesis No. 102. AHRQ Publication No. 13-05186-EF-1. Rockville, MD: Agency for Healthcare Research and Quality; 2013.
10. Siegel RL, Miller KD, Jemal A. Cancer statistics. *CA Cancer J Clin*. 2018;68:7-30. doi:10.3322/caac.21442.
11. Stange KC, Zyzanski SJ, Jaen CR, et al. Illuminating the 'black box.' A description of 4454 patient visits to 138 family physicians. *J Fam Pract*. 1998;46(5):377-389.

Please see Online Appendix: Apps and Digital Resources for additional information.

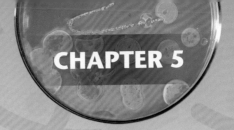

CHAPTER 5

Laboratory Screening Tests

DAVID BRISSETTE

BACKGROUND

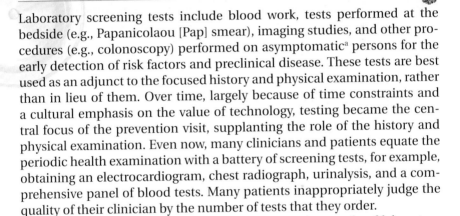

Laboratory screening tests include blood work, tests performed at the bedside (e.g., Papanicolaou [Pap] smear), imaging studies, and other procedures (e.g., colonoscopy) performed on asymptomatic[a] persons for the early detection of risk factors and preclinical disease. These tests are best used as an adjunct to the focused history and physical examination, rather than in lieu of them. Over time, largely because of time constraints and a cultural emphasis on the value of technology, testing became the central focus of the prevention visit, supplanting the role of the history and physical examination. Even now, many clinicians and patients equate the periodic health examination with a battery of screening tests, for example, obtaining an electrocardiogram, chest radiograph, urinalysis, and a comprehensive panel of blood tests. Many patients inappropriately judge the quality of their clinician by the number of tests that they order.

Several factors have contributed to the prominent role of laboratory screening in the periodic health examination. First, most patients and many clinicians believe that any noninvasive screening test can only be of benefit to a patient.[1] Issues about test accuracy (e.g., false positives or false negatives) and the downstream harms and costs of diagnostic workups should be considered when ordering what appears to be a "simple laboratory test" (see Chapter 20). For selected laboratory screening tests such as mammography and Pap smears, there is good evidence that periodic screening reduces morbidity and mortality. In many other cases, there is limited evidence about the benefits of the screening tests, but the voices of advocacy organizations and shared anecdotal experiences have led

---

[a]"Asymptomatic persons" refers to patients who lack signs or symptoms of the target condition, although they may be symptomatic for other reasons. Therefore, a woman with ulcerative colitis may be asymptomatic with respect to hyperlipidemia. "Asymptomatic" also excludes persons with a prior history of the target condition, such as a healthy woman with a prior history of breast cancer.

clinicians and patients to assume that screening is better than waiting for a disease to present clinically. Although they are often no more accurate than a careful history and physical examination, test results may be perceived as more reliable because they are generated by sophisticated technologies or because the results are quantitative. Numbers *seem* more accurate than subjective impressions, even if the numbers are inaccurate. Practical factors also promote overuse of screening tests. These include concerns about patient expectations, malpractice liability if tests are not ordered, local and state regulations for screening, and potential financial gain. Laboratory tests are convenient: it is often easier to simply order a battery of tests than to perform a methodical history and physical examination.

The potential harm of ordering laboratory screening tests extends beyond the financial and time costs to the patient and health care system. As discussed in detail in Chapter 20, laboratory screening tests can harm patients through direct physical complications, by generating inaccurate test results, and by setting off a cascade of follow-up tests and procedures that carry additional risks. These risks are influenced by the sensitivity, specificity, and positive predictive value (PPV) of the screening test.[b]

The PPV, the probability of true disease if a screening test is positive, depends on the prevalence, or pretest probability, of the disease. The PPV decreases, and the probability of producing falsely positive results increases, when patients at low risk of disease are tested, a common occurrence with screening. For example, if the pretest probability of disease is 1%, a test with a sensitivity and specificity of 90% has a PPV of 8.3%[c]; 11 patients will receive falsely positive results (and may require workups) for every true case of disease detected. If the probability is only 0.1%, the PPV falls to 0.9%; 111 patients will receive falsely positive results for every true case. For many blood tests, the "normal range" is defined on the basis of population statistics. These tests are usually flagged as "abnormal" on laboratory printouts if they fall outside the 95% confidence interval (i.e., if less than 5% of the normal population would have the result), not because the result is necessarily pathologic. Because "normal" is defined statistically, if the same test is repeated on 100 healthy persons, an abnormal result will occur an average of five times. For statistical reasons, the probability of such results increases when multiple tests are performed at once, as in blood chemistry panels that combine more than 20 tests at once. For example, when 20 independent variables are tested at once on a chemistry panel, there is a 64% probability of an "abnormal" result, even when no

---

[b]*Sensitivity* is the proportion of persons with disease who correctly test positive. *Specificity* is the proportion of persons without disease who correctly test negative.

[c]The disease would affect 1000 persons in a population of 100,000 (prevalence, 1%), meaning that 900 (1000 × 90%) persons with disease would correctly test positive, and 9900 (1 − [99,000 × 90%]) persons without disease would incorrectly test positive. Thus, only 8.3% (900/9900 + 900) of positive test results would reflect true disease.

abnormality exists. When such tests are ordered routinely on healthy persons receiving periodic health examinations, the probability of false-positive results is high and the clinician faces an ethical obligation to consider the potential adverse effects.

Given these concerns, what laboratory screening tests should clinicians perform routinely in the periodic health examination? With advances in medical technology, clinicians now have the ability to order hundreds of blood tests, imaging technologies, and other modalities that can detect diseases in asymptomatic persons. Since the late 1970s, authorities such as the Canadian Task Force on Preventive Health Care—CTF (previously known as the *Canadian Task Force on the Periodic Health Examination*), the U.S. Preventive Services Task Force (USPSTF), and the American Academy of Family Physicians (AAFP) have used formal criteria scientific evidence to weigh the benefits of such tests against their potential harms. In general, screening tests are not recommended unless there is scientific evidence (1) that the test can detect early-stage disease accurately (generating relatively few false-positive results) and (2) that early detection improves the clinical outcome. If the false-positive rate is unacceptably high for universal screening (i.e., because of low disease prevalence, test specificity, or PPV), *selective screening* may be recommended for specific high-risk groups rather than for all patients. Although restrictive recommendations for targeted screening are often viewed as a cost-control policy, their most important benefit often lies in protecting healthy patients from the psychological and physical morbidity associated with inaccurate test results and unnecessary workups. See Chapter 19 for more on the reasons to avoid certain preventive services, see Appendix A for a general list of preventive services recommended by the USPSTF.

SHARED DECISION MAKING

Shared decision making, also commonly referred to as *informed decision making*, or *evidence-informed patient choice*, is a patient-centered process in which both the patient and clinician exchange information with each other, jointly contribute to the decision-making process, and come to a conclusion about a plan of action.[2] Specifically, the USPSTF defines the goals of shared decision making as helping the patient to do the following:

1. Understand the risk related to or the seriousness of the illness or preclinical disease to be prevented.
2. Understand the preventive service, including the harms, benefits, alternative options, and uncertainties.
3. Weigh ones values regarding potential benefits and harms associated with the service.
4. Engage in the decision-making process at one's desired level of comfort.

It takes more time for a clinician to engage in shared decision making than to check boxes on a laboratory requisition form, accompanied by the parting words "you should get these tests." It is important, however, for clinicians to use a consistent, evidence-based approach to offering and informing patients about preventive screening tests. From a health perspective, evidence that shared decision making improves health outcomes is indirect and mixed; however, the ethical, practical, and educational reasons to engage in shared decision making are compelling. Some research on shared decision making suggest that patients have higher satisfaction and encounter less conflict in making decisions related to their medical care.[3] This approach may promote patient autonomy, foster trust in the patient-clinician relationship, increase adherence to care plans, and improve patient satisfaction. As Chapter 20 discusses in more detail, the scientific evidence for some preventive services is incomplete and the balance of benefits and harms is uncertain or "too close to call." In such situations, including patient values and preferences clarifies the balance of harms and benefits for the individual patient. Even for those preventive screenings grounded in good-quality evidence of benefit in population-level studies, the benefit to individual patients must incorporate their values about quality-of-life issues and their willingness and ability to comply with follow-up diagnostic and treatment interventions. Using the shared decision-making technique can help to foster a more realistic understanding about the harms and benefits of preventive care.

There are several barriers to shared decision making, including: patients' limited ability to understand complex medical topics, clinicians' uncertainty about the evidence for the benefit of a preventive service, limited time during clinical encounters, and lack of reimbursement for such discussions.[4] Concise decision aids (focused patient education materials) about specific choices in preventive care can help the patient to consider complex medical issues outside of the clinic visit setting and to return to the clinician in follow-up to ask informed questions and make decisions. Resources listed at the end of this chapter include decision aids on specific screening tests, as well as a useful website (the Cochrane Inventory of Patient Decision Aids) where many other decision aids can be located and evaluated.

Using evidence-based clinic protocols, nurses can follow a routine procedure to identify those tests for which a patient may benefit from shared decision making and give such patients appropriate decision aids for review while awaiting the clinician for the role of nurses and other staff in making these resources available systematically.

CONTENTS OF THIS CHAPTER

This chapter reviews the laboratory screening tests that are commonly recommended for asymptomatic persons (see Appendix A). Research has demonstrated that screening with these tests improves health outcomes (e.g., morbidity, mortality) or has other compelling scientific support. The chapter discusses tests that should be offered to all patients and tests that should be performed on a routine basis only in select subgroups of patients with risk factors, owing to low PPV in the general population or other concerns. These recommendations generally conform to the guidelines of evidence-based groups such as the USPSTF. The scientific evidence of the effectiveness of these tests and the arguments for why screening should be limited to selected populations or omitted completely are beyond the scope of this chapter. The reader should consult the references for more information about the scientific evidence for or against screening tests.[5] The information in this chapter about screening tests of unproven effectiveness is provided as a guide for those clinicians who choose to use them, but such tests are not necessarily advocated by the editors. The editors specifically discourage the routine use of the screening tests discussed in Chapter 20.

The discussion of each screening test includes a brief introduction describing the target condition and the rationale for the test, a summary of official guidelines issued by major organizations and agencies, and detailed instructions on patient preparation and technique. (The sources of the recommendations in the "Official Guidelines" sections of this chapter are listed under "Suggested Readings" later in this chapter.) Although routine screening rarely detects clinically significant abnormalities, it does provide a setting for counseling patients about primary and secondary prevention of the target condition. Each section of this chapter therefore includes a "Standard Counseling" discussion of the reminders that clinicians should give all patients, even if no abnormality is detected, about how to prevent the target condition and when to return for screening. This section also refers readers to relevant chapters in Section II of this book, which discuss in more detail how to counsel patients about specific health behaviors. Readers should consult Chapter 19 for guidance on proper follow-up of patients with abnormal results from the screening tests discussed in this chapter.

The discussion of each screening test also addresses the potential adverse effects of screening and the accuracy of the test, and suggestions on how to document screening in the medical record. Data cited in the "Potential Adverse Effects" and "Accuracy and Reliability as Screening Test" sections are drawn from a large body of evidence. The hundreds of studies on which these estimates are based are not cited explicitly in these chapters owing to space limitations. The reader interested in the source of these data is referred to other texts that discuss the individual studies in more detail, such as the USPSTF *Guide to Clinical Preventive Services*.[5]

To help address patients' questions or their anxiety about the risk of disease, clinicians may wish to provide educational materials such as those listed in the "Resources" section of this chapter, which can explain the meaning of a normal examination and encourage health behaviors for the primary prevention of the conditions for which the patients are being screened. Patient education materials for patients in whom screening tests are *abnormal* are listed in Chapter 19 and elsewhere in this book. The screening recommendations made in this chapter apply only to asymptomatic persons and therefore assume that the patient lacks clinical evidence of the target condition. Thus, for example, recommendations to limit chlamydia screening to persons with risk factors assume that the patient lacks signs or symptoms of infection. This chapter does not address laboratory tests performed in prenatal screening, occupational screening, pre-employment screening, or screening for admission to schools.

This chapter encourages clinicians to establish reminder systems in the office or clinic to ensure that patients receive recommended screening tests on time and return for repeat screening at the appropriate interval.

SCREENING BLOOD TESTS

Blood Glucose

Introduction

Within the chemistry panel, the glucose measurement is the only test for which there is even indirect evidence that screening improves health. Evidence indicates that early detection and treatment of diabetes when patients also have hyperlipidemia or hypertension may lead to improved health outcomes. In the general population, there is insufficient evidence that screening for diabetes is beneficial in averting either microvascular complications (e.g., nephropathy, retinopathy, neuropathy) or cardiovascular disease. See Chapter 20 for more details.

Screening Recommendations **Screening for diabetes in patients who are overweight or obese or have risk factors for the development of diabetes should be routinely offered as a part of periodic health screening. Screening those with risk factors for diabetes (e.g., obesity, family history of diabetes, certain racial/ethnic minorities) may be considered. There is limited evidence about the optimal frequency for screening; however, when testing is normal, intervals of every 3 years is acceptable.**

Official Guidelines Currently, the USPSTF recommends routine screening of all adults aged 40 to 70 years who are overweight or obese. Clinicians should consider earlier screening in patients who are at higher risk for developing diabetes, such as those with one of the following: family history of diabetes; members of certain racial and ethnic groups (i.e., blacks, American Indians or Alaska Natives, Asian Americans, Hispanics or Latinos, or Native Hawaiians or Pacific Islanders); personal history of gestational diabetes or polycystic ovary syndrome. The American Diabetes Association (ADA) notes that data from prospective studies are insufficient to determine the benefits of routine diabetes screening in the general population and recommends that the decision to test for diabetes should be based on clinical judgment and patient preference. On the basis of expert consensus and epidemiologic evidence that 50% of individuals diagnosed with diabetes have end-organ damage, the ADA recommends that clinicians consider screening for diabetes with the fasting plasma glucose (FPG) test beginning at age 45 years and at a younger age for individuals with risk factors, such as family history, overweight, and hypertension. If FPG testing is normal, it is reasonable to screen these patients every 3 years at minimum. The American College of Obstetricians and Gynecologists (ACOG) endorses the ADA recommendations.

Standard Counseling

Regardless of whether the clinician and patient decide to screen for diabetes, all patients should be counseled on exercise, eating a healthy diet, and maintaining a normal weight (body mass index of 20–25 kg/m^2) (see Chapters 7–9). More aggressive interventions to establish and maintain these behaviors should be considered for patients at increased risk for developing diabetes, especially those who are overweight or obese, have a family history of diabetes, or have a racial or ethnic background associated with an increased risk (e.g., Native Americans). Intensive dietary and physical activity programs should also be considered for patients who have impaired fasting glucose or impaired glucose tolerance, because good-quality evidence from large trials has demonstrated that these programs can reduce the incidence or even delay the development of diabetes in these patients.

Definition of Abnormal Result

Three tests have been used to screen for diabetes: FPG, 2-hour postload plasma glucose (2-hr PG), and hemoglobin A1c (HbA1c). As defined by the ADA, an abnormal FPG test suggests diabetes with a value greater than or equal to 126 mg/dL and impaired fasting glucose with a value of 100 to 125 mg/dL.[6] Guidelines advocate FPG for screening because it is easier to perform, more convenient for patients, and less expensive than other screening tests. It should be drawn in the morning after the patient has fasted for at least 8 hours overnight. The FPG is more reproducible than the 2-hour PG test, has less variation, and has similar predictive value for the development of microvascular complications. Compared with the FPG test, the 2-hour PG test may lead to more individuals being diagnosed with diabetes. HbA1c is less sensitive in detecting lower levels of hyperglycemia.

The random capillary blood glucose test has been shown to have reasonable sensitivity in detecting persons who have either an FPG level greater than or equal to 126 mg/dL or a 2-hour PG level greater than or equal to 200 mg/dL, provided the results are interpreted according to age and the length of time since the last meal. The random blood glucose test can be used for screening, but FPG is preferable.

The ADA recommends confirmation of a diagnosis of diabetes with a repeated FPG test on a separate day, especially for patients with borderline FPG results and patients with normal FPG levels for whom suspicion of diabetes is high.

Potential Adverse Effects

A diagnosis of diabetes could potentially cause "labeling" in asymptomatic individuals (e.g., anxiety, a negative change in self-perception, stigma) and could lead to social consequences (e.g., loss of insurability). Screening can produce false-positive results and subsequent psychological distress, especially in those with "borderline" abnormal results. Medications for diabetes and glucose intolerance can produce side effects (e.g., hypoglycemia, weight gain, gastrointestinal symptoms). For those identified as having impaired glucose tolerance, 30% to 50% of whom will become euglycemic and not develop diabetes, the side effects of medication could easily outweigh the benefits of pharmacologic treatment.

Accuracy and Reliability as Screening Tests

The sensitivity and specificity of the FPG, 2-hour PG, and HbA1c screening for detecting patients with retinopathy are approximately 75% to 80% at the following thresholds: FPG greater than or equal to 126 mg/dL, 2-hour PG greater than or equal to 200 mg/dL, or HbA1c greater than or equal to 6.5%.

Total Cholesterol and Lipid Profiles

Introduction

According to the Centers for Disease Control and Prevention (CDC), about 610,000 deaths per year in the United States can be attributed to heart disease of which coronary heart disease is the leading cause of morbidity and mortality, resulting in approximately 370,000 deaths each year. The risk for coronary heart disease increases with increasing levels of total cholesterol (TC) and low-density lipoprotein cholesterol (LDL-C) and declining levels of high-density lipoprotein cholesterol (HDL-C), in a continuous and graded manner with no clear threshold of risk. See Chapter 1 for Web-based tools to calculate a patient's 10-year risk of experiencing a coronary heart disease event, which influences the appropriateness of advising patients to consider aspirin prophylaxis (see Chapter 16).

Screening Guidelines All adults 20 years and older should have a fasting lipid profile to include total cholesterol, LDL-C, and HDL-C at least every 5 years as part of an assessment of CVD risk. Shorter intervals of screening may be necessary for those individuals who are close to warranting therapy based on CVD risk. Longer intervals may be acceptable in those who are not at increased CVD risk and have repeatedly normal levels.

Official Guidelines For adults aged 40 to 75 years, the USPSTF states that evidence on the role of statins in preventing CVD events across different populations has changed the focus from determining populations to be screened for dyslipidemia to populations who should be prescribed statin therapy based on CVD risk (history of CVD, CVD risk factors, and calculated 10-yr CVD event risk). Screening for elevated lipid levels is a necessary step in the overall assessment of CVD risk to help identify persons who may benefit from statin therapy. Periodic assessment of cardiovascular risk factors from ages 40 to 75 years, including measurement of total cholesterol, LDL-C, and HDL-C levels, is required to implement this recommendation. The optimal intervals for cardiovascular risk assessment are uncertain; however, measurement of lipid levels every 5 years is reasonable based on expert opinion and other guidelines. Shorter intervals may be necessary for patients whose risk levels are close to those warranting therapy, and longer intervals are appropriate for persons who are not at increased risk and have repeatedly normal levels. For adults aged 21 to 39 years the USPSTF recommends that clinicians use clinical judgement for screening patients in this group. The AAFP agrees with the recommendations of the USPSTF. The **National Cholesterol Education Program's Adult Treatment Panel III (ATP III), sponsored by the National Institutes of Health**, recommends a fasting lipoprotein profile (TC, LDL cholesterol, HDL-C, and triglyceride) in all adults older than 20 years once every 5 years.[7] This recommendation is similar to that of the American Heart Association, which recommends that all adults 20 years and older have a fasting lipid profile assessed every 4 to 6 years and work with their health care provider to determine their risk for CVD. The ACOG recommends screening women every 5 years beginning at the age of 45 years whereby screening for women aged 19 to 44 years is based on risk factors (see Chapter 18 for pediatric guidelines).

Standard Counseling

All patients, regardless of their lipid levels, should be advised regarding the health benefits of a diet low in saturated fat and high in fruits and vegetables, regular physical activity, avoiding tobacco use, and maintaining a normal weight (see Chapters 7–10).

Definition of Abnormal Results

TC and HDL-C can be measured on nonfasting or fasting samples. For nonfasting measurements, a TC greater than or equal to 200 mg/dL or HDL-C less than 40 mg/dL requires a follow-up lipoprotein profile to determine appropriate management. Optimal LDL, HDL-C, and TC as defined by ATP III are listed in Table 5.1.

Abnormal results should be confirmed by a repeated sample on a separate occasion, and the average of both results should be used for risk assessment.

TABLE 5.1   Adult Treatment Panel III (ATP III) Classification of Low-Density Lipoprotein (LDL), Total, and High-Density Lipoprotein (HDL) Cholesterol (mg/dL)

LDL Cholesterol
<100 Optimal
100–129 Near optimal/above optimal
130–159 Borderline high
160–189 High
>190 Very high
Total Cholesterol
<200 Desirable
200–239 Borderline high
>240 High
HDL Cholesterol
<40 Low
>60 High

Potential Adverse Effects

Screening for and identifying lipid disorders in adults do not appear to have important psychological sequelae or to produce important changes in indices of mental health, although labeling remains a potential harm. Screening low-risk individuals could lead to the costs and inconvenience of treatment with resultant small benefits. Statin therapy is associated with known adverse effects, including myalgias, rhabdomyolysis, increased liver transaminase levels, neuropathy, and other rare events.

Accuracy and Reliability as Screening Tests

The National Cholesterol Education Program has laboratory requirements for LDL-C testing to ensure precision (coefficient of variance less than 4%) and accuracy (bias less than 4%). Those laboratories meeting these requirements report highly accurate cholesterol values. At least two measurements are necessary to ensure that true values are within 10% of the mean of the measurements. Although most laboratories calculate LDL values, many offer direct LDL measurement, which is highly accurate and can be ordered on nonfasting samples.

Human Immunodeficiency Virus

Introduction

At the end of 2015, the CDC reports that there were 1.1 million persons living in the United States with human immunodeficiency virus (HIV-1) infection or acquired immunodeficiency syndrome. Fifteen percent of these individuals were unaware of their HIV status. Those at increased risk for HIV infection include men who have had sex with men after 1975; men and women having unprotected sex with multiple partners; past or present injection drug users; men and women who exchange sex for money or drugs or have sex partners who do; individuals whose past or present sex partners were HIV-infected, bisexual, or injection drug users; transgender women; persons being treated for sexually transmitted infections (STIs); and persons with a history of blood transfusion between 1978 and 1985. Individuals receiving care in certain high-risk settings are also at increased risk (e.g., STI clinics, correctional facilities, homeless shelters). Since the late 1990s, treatment with highly active antiretroviral therapy regimens has markedly reduced the morbidity and mortality associated with HIV. In pregnant women, early identification of maternal HIV seropositivity through universal screening and early antiretroviral treatment with multidrug regimens have been shown to significantly reduce maternal-infant transmission of HIV.

Screening Guidelines **All individuals at risk for HIV (see risk categories in preceding text) and those who receive medical care in high-risk settings should be offered HIV screening. Universal screening should be routinely offered to all pregnant women in the first trimester and rapid screening for those women who present in labor with unknown HIV status.**

Official Guidelines The USPSTF recommends HIV screening in adolescents and adults aged 15 to 65 years. Younger adults and older individuals who are at increased risk for HIV infection should also be screened. All pregnant women should be screened, including those who present in labor who are untested and whose HIV status is unknown. The AAFP, American College of Physicians, and ACOG recommend counseling and HIV testing of high-risk individuals. The CDC recommends universal HIV screening in patients in all health care settings after patient notification (opt-out screening) and that persons at high risk for HIV infection should be screened for HIV at least annually. The CDC recommends that separate written consent for HIV testing should not be required; general consent for medical care should be considered sufficient to encompass consent for HIV testing. The CDC also advises that clinicians should assess HIV-related risks for transgender patients based on current anatomy and sexual behaviors. Because of the diversity of transgender persons regarding surgical affirming procedures, hormone use, and patterns of sexual behavior, providers must remain aware of symptoms consistent with common sexually transmitted diseases (STDs) and screen for asymptomatic STDs on the basis of behavioral history and sexual practices, which applies to all STDs mentioned in this chapter. The American Academy of Pediatrics (AAP) recommends that all adolescents be counseled and offered HIV testing according to the USPSTF guidelines. Those adolescents at high risk should be tested and reassessed annually.

Standard Counseling

HIV testing should be accompanied by pretest and posttest counseling. Ideally, the clinician should disclose all HIV results in person, regardless of whether the test is positive or negative.

All sexually active individuals should be counseled regarding the importance of prevention of STIs; such preventive measures include counseling regarding abstinence, consistent condom and spermicide use, and maintenance of mutually monogamous relationships (see Chapter 13). All sexually active adolescents and adults should be made aware of the contribution of alcohol in risky sexual practices. Prevention of HIV transmission in individuals who use injection drugs includes referral to drug rehabilitation programs, use of clean needles and paraphernalia, and education regarding the dangers of impaired judgment leading to risky sexual activity while intoxicated. Clinicians who care for transgender women and men should have knowledge of their patients' current anatomy and patterns of sexual behavior before counseling them about HIV prevention.

Definition of Abnormal Results

The standard test for diagnosing HIV infection includes the repeatedly reactive enzyme immunoassay followed by confirmatory Western blot or immunofluorescent assay. A positive result on both the enzyme assay and confirmatory test identifies those individuals with HIV.

Potential Adverse Effects

Since false-positive test results are rare, harms associated with HIV screening are minimal. Potential harms of positive test results include increased anxiety, labeling, and effects on close relationships. Documented HIV infection can also influence insurance coverage and employment opportunities.

Accuracy of Screening Tests

Standard testing for HIV infection with the repeatedly reactive enzyme immunoassay followed by confirmatory Western blot or immunofluorescent assay has a sensitivity and specificity greater than 99%. False-positive test results are rare, even in low-risk settings. Compared with standard HIV testing, the reported sensitivities of rapid tests on blood specimens range from 96% to 100%, with specificities greater than 99.9%. Reported sensitivities and specificities of oral fluid HIV tests are also high (greater than 99%).

Syphilis

Introduction

In 2016, the CDC reported that the nationwide incidence rate of primary and secondary syphilis infection was 8.7 cases per 100,000 compared with 7.4 cases per 100,000 persons in 2015 (17.6% increase) and 5.0 cases per 100,000 persons in 2012 (74% increase). Syphilis, an infectious disease caused by the bacterium *Treponema pallidum*, causes a variety of symptoms depending on the stage of infection (primary, secondary, tertiary) and no symptoms during latent stages. Congenital syphilis results in fetal or perinatal death, as well as serious complications in surviving newborns. Populations at increased risk for syphilis infection include men who have sex with men (MSM) and engage in high-risk sexual behavior, commercial sex workers, persons who exchange sex for drugs, and those in adult correctional facilities. There is no evidence to support screening for syphilis among individuals currently or previously infected with another sexually transmitted organism.

Screening Guidelines **All high-risk adolescents and adults (see preceding discussion of high-risk groups) and all pregnant women should be offered syphilis screening.**

Official Guidelines The USPSTF strongly recommends screening asymptomatic, nonpregnant adults and adolescents who are at increased risk for syphilis infection and all pregnant women. Optimal screening intervals for individuals at increased risk for syphilis are not well established, but data suggest that, for MSM or persons living with HIV, detection may improve when screening occurs at 3-month intervals compared with annual screening. The AAFP clinical policy statement concurs with the USPSTF recommendations. The AAP and ACOG recommend prenatal screening for syphilis. The CDC recommends screening in all pregnant women at the first prenatal visit and repeat screening early in the third trimester and at delivery for all high-risk women (e.g., those who live in areas of excess syphilis morbidity, are previously untested, or have positive serology in the first trimester). The CDC also recommends screening in all sexually active MSM at least annually and every 3 to 6 months if at increased risk. Those individuals with HIV infection should be screened at the initial HIV evaluation and more frequently depending on individual risk behaviors and local epidemiology.

Standard Counseling

All sexually active individuals should be counseled regarding the importance of prevention of STIs; such preventive measures include counseling regarding abstinence, consistent condom and spermicide use, and maintenance of mutually monogamous relationships (see Chapter 13). Clinicians who care for transgender women and men should have knowledge of their patients' current anatomy and patterns of sexual behavior before counseling them about STI prevention.

Definition of Abnormal Results

Nontreponemal tests commonly used for initial screening are the venereal disease research laboratory or rapid plasma reagin tests, followed by a confirmatory fluorescent treponemal antibody absorption assay (FTA-ABS) or

Treponema pallidum particle agglutination (TP-PA) test. Positive results on the confirmatory FTA-ABS or TP-PA identify those individuals with *T. pallidum* infection. See Chapter 13 for proper follow-up and treatment of patients with abnormal results from screening.

Adverse Effects

Potential harms of screening may include opportunity costs to the clinician and patient (time, resources, and inconvenience). False-positive results may lead to stress, labeling, concerns about fidelity, and further testing. Harms of treatment include drug-related side effects, including penicillin allergy and the Jarisch-Herxheimer reaction (febrile reaction with headache, myalgia, and other symptoms), which may occur within the first 24 hours of any therapy for syphilis.

Accuracy of Screening Tests

The sensitivity of the rapid plasma reagin and venereal disease research laboratory tests is estimated to be 78% to 86% for detecting primary syphilis infection and 96% to 100% for later stages. Specificity ranges from 85% to 99% and may be reduced in individuals who have certain preexisting conditions (e.g., collagen vascular disease, pregnancy, injection drug use, advanced malignancy, tuberculosis, malaria, viral and rickettsial diseases). The confirmatory FTA-ABS test has a sensitivity of 84% and specificity of 97%. The PPV and number needed to screen (see Chapter 20) are highly dependent on the population prevalence of syphilis. For example, in a low-risk population, the NNS to detect a single case of syphilis is 24,000, whereas in a high-risk population of incarcerated women, the NNS would be only 10.

Prostate Cancer Screening With Prostate-Specific Antigen

Introduction

Prostate cancer is the second leading cause of cancer deaths in men. Incidence increases with age, and more than 75% of cases occur in men older than 65 years. Other risk factors include being African American and having a family history of a first-degree relative with prostate cancer. Although prostate cancer is a major cause of cancer death in men, many more men are diagnosed with the disease than die from it. Men in the United States have a 15% lifetime risk of being diagnosed with prostate cancer but only a 3% lifetime risk of dying from the disease. Prostate-specific antigen (PSA) and digital rectal examination (DRE) are the two predominant screening modalities for prostate cancer. Although it is certain that screening can detect prostate cancer in early stages, research has not proved whether screening reduces the death rate from prostate cancer. Given the known harms of the diagnostic workup that follows an abnormal PSA and the harms of treatment, the balance of the benefits and harms is uncertain.

Screening Guidelines Clinicians should not order the PSA test without first engaging the patient in a shared decision-making process (see "Shared Decision Making" Chapter 22). Based on the outcome of the shared decision-making process, the population who may benefit from screening is average-risk men between the ages of 50 and 70 years with at least a 10-year life expectancy and high-risk men (African Americans or men with a first-degree relative with prostate cancer) between the ages of 40 and 70 years.

Official Guidelines Since 2012, the USPSTF has recommended against PSA screening in all age groups, as evidence suggests that PSA screening results in the detection of many cases of asymptomatic prostate cancer. Furthermore, there is also convincing evidence that a substantial percentage of men who have asymptomatic cancer detected by PSA screening have a tumor that either will not progress or will progress so slowly that it would have remained asymptomatic for the man's lifetime. The AAFP concurs with this recommendation. The American Cancer Society (ACS) advises clinicians to discuss the potential harms and benefits with patients and to offer the test to all men 50 years and older who have at least a 10-year life expectancy and to younger men (approximately age 40 yr) at higher risk (African American men and men with a first-degree relative with prostate cancer). The American Urologic Association advises clinicians to use shared decision making for men aged 55 to 69 years, individualize screening decisions for higher-risk men 40 to 54 years of age, and to not screen men younger than 40 years, older than 70 years, or who have a life expectancy of less than 10 to 15 years.

Standard Counseling

Before ordering PSA testing, shared decision making should include the following: (1) discussion of the potential benefits and possible harms of PSA screening, including the false-negative and false-positive results, the downstream adverse effects of the diagnostic workup (pain, bleeding, infection following biopsy), and treatments (erectile dysfunction, urinary incontinence, bowel dysfunction following radical prostatectomy); (2) consideration of patient preferences with respect to the adverse effects of treatments; and (3) agreement as to whether or not to screen. Such counseling and the agreed-upon decision should be documented in the medical record.

Definition of Abnormal Results

A PSA value greater than or equal to 4.0 ng/mL is generally considered abnormal. PSA density (the PSA concentration divided by gland volume), percent free PSA (the proportion of PSA that is unbound), PSA velocity (the rate of increase in PSA per unit of time), and age-specific and race-specific normal references have been proposed to improve the sensitivity or specificity of total serum PSA measurement. It is uncertain whether these other measurements improve the detection of clinically significant disease and whether they reduce unnecessary biopsies from false-positive results.

Potential Adverse Effects

An abnormal screening test for prostate cancer often produces some anxiety. Less than 10% of men experience interference with daily activities as a result of prostate biopsy, a common feature of the diagnostic workup of an abnormal PSA. Fewer than 1% of patients undergoing biopsy have serious complications, including infections. Screening may lead to surgery, radiotherapy, or other treatments that carry a significant risk for complications, such as erectile, urinary, and bowel dysfunction. For indolent cancers, these adverse treatment effects occur without the benefit of a reduction in the risk of progressive prostate cancer.

Accuracy and Reliability

A PSA greater than or equal to 4.0 ng/mL has an estimated sensitivity of 72%, a specificity of approximately 93%, and a PPV of 25%.[8] Specificity decreases with increasing age and the presence of benign prostatic hyperplasia. The combination of DRE and PSA increases the sensitivity of screening, but it also increases the rate of false-positive results.

OTHER LABORATORY SCREENING TESTS

Pap Smears

Introduction

The Pap smear is performed routinely to detect cervical dysplasia, carcinoma in situ, and invasive carcinoma. In the United States, it is estimated that approximately 12,578 new cases of cervical cancer were diagnosed in 2014, and 4115 patients died from this disease. Women who have never been screened account for most invasive cervical cancers and cervical cancer–related mortality. Infection with human papillomavirus (HPV), a sexually transmitted organism, is a major risk factor for cervical cancer. HPV types 16 and 18 are known to be oncogenic. Other risk factors for cervical cancer include early onset of intercourse, a large number of sexual partners, and cigarette smoking.

Screening Guidelines **All adolescent and adult women aged 21 to 65 years with an intact cervix should be routinely offered Pap smear screening (regardless of HPV vaccination status). Those at low risk for cervical cancer can undergo screening every 2 to 3 years. For those aged 30 to 65 years who have HPV testing along with cytology may lengthen the interval for screening to every 5 years. Women at high risk for HPV and cervical dysplasia (e.g., documented HPV infection, history of abnormal**

Pap smears, early onset of intercourse, large number of sexual partners, and cigarette smoking) should undergo annual screening. Women who have had adequate screening with normal smears can discontinue Pap smear at age 65 years. Pap screening is unnecessary after a hysterectomy for a nonmalignant indication. There is no role for HPV testing as a screening test (it may be appropriate as part of *a diagnostic workup* for an abnormal Pap smear—see page 477). See Chapter 17 regarding HPV vaccination for the primary prevention of cervical cancer.

Official Guidelines The USPSTF recommends screening for cervical cancer in women who have a cervix regardless of sexual history aged 21 to 65 years with cytology (Pap smear) every 3 years or, for women aged 30 to 65 years who want to lengthen the screening interval, screening with a combination of cytology and HPV testing every 5 years. The USPSTF recommends against screening for cervical cancer in women younger than 21 years, women older than 65 years who have had adequate prior screening and are not otherwise at high risk for cervical cancer, and women who have had a hysterectomy with removal of the cervix and who do not have a history of a high-grade precancerous lesion (cervical intraepithelial neoplasia [CIN] grade 2 or 3) or cervical cancer. The USPSTF recommends against screening for cervical cancer with HPV testing, alone or in combination with cytology, in women younger than 30 years. The ACS/ASCCP/ASCP recommend that women aged 21 to 29 years be screened with cytology (cervical cytology testing or Pap testing) alone every 3 years. Women aged 30 to 65 years should be screened with cytology and HPV testing (co-testing) every 5 years or cytology alone every 3 years. The guidelines further state that no woman should be screened every year and that women aged 21 to 29 years should not be screened with HPV testing or combined cytology and HPV testing. The ACOG recommends that for average-risk women aged 30 to 65 years, co-testing with cervical cytology and high-risk HPV testing every 5 years is the preferred approach, with cervical cytology alone every 3 years as an acceptable screening strategy.

Patient Preparation

The Pap smear is usually obtained during the pelvic examination (see Chapter 3 for further discussion of the pelvic examination).

Technique

The selection and insertion of the speculum are discussed in Chapter 4. The examiner should inspect the cervix and external os for ulcerations, nodules, masses, bleeding, leukoplakia, or discharge. The clinician should visualize the squamocolumnar junction or transformation zone, located on the ectocervix or in the endocervical canal, where 90% to 95% of cervical cancers arise. Current evidence is equivocal as to whether the detection of cervical cancer is increased by sampling endocervical cells, but many laboratories consider smears inadequate if these cells are absent. The squamocolumnar junction often migrates inward with age, so that visualization in older women can be difficult. Any discharge obscuring the view of the cervix should be wiped away.

To maximize the likelihood of obtaining endocervical cells from the squamocolumnar junction, a complete Pap test requires the collection of specimens from the endocervical canal and the ectocervix. The two common collection techniques available at this time include (1) the wooden Ayre or extended-tip spatula and endocervical brush (see Fig. 5.1), and (2) the cervical broom (e.g., Cervex-Brush [see Fig. 5.2]). The adequacy of sampling is improved by using the cervical broom. In the first technique, the endocervical sample is obtained by inserting the endocervical brush into the canal and rotating it 180° between the fingers. The ectocervical specimen is typically obtained with a wooden Ayre spatula or an extended-tip spatula. (A plastic spatula is used with liquid-based technologies.) The longer end of the spatula is placed in the os, and the spatula is rotated in a circular manner so that a full scraping of the squamocolumnar junction is obtained. The second technique, in which the cervical broom is inserted and rotated five complete turns, allows simultaneous sampling of endocervical and ectocervical cells.

Conventional Pap smear techniques involve spreading specimens (obtained by either spatula/brush or broom) onto one or more glass microscope slides and immediately applying either 95% ether-alcohol or a spray fixative. When using liquid-based technologies, the samples are then placed into a vial containing an alcohol-based preservative.

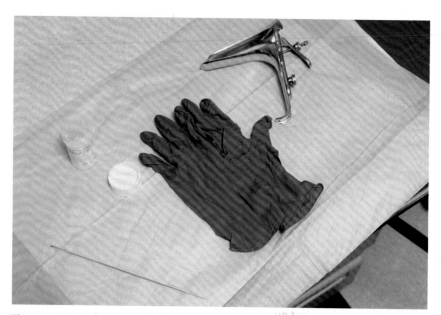

Figure 5.1   Equipment for Pap test. From Evans RJ, Yvonne M Brown YM, Evans MK. Canadian Maternity, Newborn & Women's Health Nursing. 2nd ed. Philadelphia, PA: Wolters Kluwer; 2014.

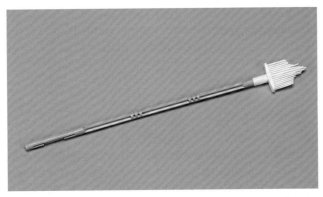

Figure 5.2 Cervical broom. From Weber JR, Kelley JH. *Health Assessment in Nursing*. 6th ed. Philadelphia, PA: Wolters Kluwer; 2017.

After plating the Pap smear and completing the examination, the patient should be told that the speculum will be removed; the speculum should be returned to the oblique angle before being gently withdrawn. Details about the patient's history (age, last menstrual period, type of contraception, previous cervical diagnoses or treatment) and relevant physical findings should be noted for the cytopathologist on the laboratory requisition form.

Standard Counseling

The patient should be advised to return for repeat screening at the recommended interval and should be encouraged to reduce risks of acquiring STIs (see Chapter 13).

Definition of Abnormal Results

The Pap smear may suggest the presence of cancer or its precursors if the laboratory reports squamous intraepithelial lesions, atypia including atypical squamous cells of unknown significance, dysplasia, CIN, squamous cell carcinoma, or adenocarcinoma. The presence of HPV is also abnormal, and many laboratories automatically perform HPV testing (commonly referred to as *reflex HPV testing*) when liquid-based Pap smears are abnormal. Cervical samples that are identified by the laboratory as inadequate (e.g., owing to absence of endocervical cells) may necessitate repeat testing, but there is little evidence regarding how many attempts should be made to obtain adequate specimens or whether the effort will result in improved cancer detection.

Potential Adverse Effects

The pelvic examination and Pap smear can be both embarrassing and uncomfortable. False-positive results can generate unnecessary anxiety and follow-up testing, including colposcopy with biopsy, endocervical curettage, and other procedures that carry associated risks (e.g., bleeding, infection, uterine perforation, cervical stenosis, or cervical incompetence). Women incur costs and inconvenience from follow-up cervical examinations. False-negative results may allow preventable cervical cancers to escape detection.

Accuracy and Reliability as Screening Test

Older studies reported that the Pap smear had a sensitivity of 47% (confidence interval, 30%–87%) and a specificity of 95% (confidence interval, 86%–100%) in detecting low-grade squamous intraepithelial lesions and CIN 2-3; this wide range in reported accuracy reflects limitations in study quality and heterogeneity in reference standards and disease prevalence rates. Recent trials comparing the Pap smear with liquid-based cytology suggest that sensitivity is similar, whereas the specificity of liquid-based cytology is lower for detecting CIN 2 or greater. Some studies performed outside the United States suggest that liquid-based cytology may yield superior specimens, but these conclusions may not be generalizable to the United States.

Medical Record Documentation

The date and results of the Pap smear should be documented in the medical record, preferably on a health maintenance flow sheet. The clinician should describe the appearance of the cervix and whether menstruation was noted. For future reference, it may be helpful to note in the medical record whether the uterus is retroverted and if a special speculum was required to visualize the cervix. When the Pap smear results are available, the presence of cellular atypia, dysplasia, or carcinoma on the smear should be carefully documented. The presence or absence of HPV should be noted as well when tested. Plans for follow-up and repeat testing should be clearly outlined.

Screening for Gonorrhea and Chlamydia

Introduction

Chlamydia trachomatis and *Neisseria gonorrhoeae* are the two most commonly reported notifiable diseases in the United States. Although chlamydia and gonorrhea are often considered similar STIs, chlamydia is far more common and underreported than gonorrhea. In 2016, the CDC reported a total of 468,514 cases of gonorrhea and 1,598,354 chlamydial infections were reported in the United States. Age is the strongest predictor of both chlamydial and gonorrheal infection: adolescent girls aged 15 to 19 years and men aged 20 to 24 years have the highest rates of chlamydia. Women and men aged 20 to 24 years have the highest risk of gonorrhea. Other risk factors include having multiple or new sexual partners, inconsistent use of barrier contraceptives, and a history of previous or concurrent STI. In women, chlamydial and gonorrheal infections cause urethritis, cervicitis, and pelvic inflammatory disease. In men, infection results in acute urethritis, epididymitis, or prostatitis and rarely chronic complications including chronic prostatitis and reactive arthritis. Treatment is highly effective.

Screening Recommendations **All sexually active women aged 24 years and younger, women at high risk (see preceding text for risk factors), and pregnant women should be offered screening for chlamydia and gonorrhea. Screening of nonpregnant women should be offered annually. Screening of pregnant women should be offered in the first trimester, followed by repeat screening in the third trimester for those at high risk. In areas with low prevalence of gonorrhea, clinicians may choose to screen only for chlamydia. Routine screening of men is not recommended except in adolescents and young adult males who have sex with males who engage in high-risk behaviors or who are in high-risk settings.**

Official Guidelines
Chlamydia. The USPSTF and AAFP recommend that clinicians routinely screen for chlamydia infection in all sexually active women younger than 25 years and all other asymptomatic women at increased risk. They also recommend screening all pregnant women younger than 25 years, as well as older pregnant women who are at increased risk. They conclude that there is insufficient evidence to recommend routine screening in men. The ACOG, AAFP, and AAP agree with these recommendations. The AAP also recommends routine annual screening for chlamydia in sexually active adolescent and young adult males who have sex with males if they engage in receptive anal or insertive intercourse; screening every 3 to 6 months for persons in this population if they are at high risk; and screening adolescents and young adults who have been exposed to chlamydia in the past 60 days from an infected partner. It also advises clinicians to consider annual screening for chlamydia in sexually active males in settings with high prevalence rates, such as jail or juvenile correction facilities. The CDC recommends annual chlamydia screening for sexually active women younger than 20 years and for older women who meet specific risk criteria. The CDC recommends that clinicians consider screening for chlamydia in sexually active young men in high-prevalence settings and annual screening for MSM, based on exposure history, with more frequent screening in populations at highest risk. Owing to the likelihood of reinfection, the CDC also recommends retesting of all patients diagnosed with chlamydia infections 3 months after treatment, regardless of whether or not sexual partners have been treated.

Gonorrhea. The USPSTF recommends that clinicians screen all sexually active women younger than 25 years and all other asymptomatic women at increased risk. Screening is also recommended for all pregnant women younger than 25 years, as well as older pregnant women who are at increased risk. The USPSTF recommends against routine screening for gonorrhea infection in men. The ACOG, AAFP, and AAP agree with these recommendations. The AAP also recommends routine annual screening for gonorrhea in sexually active adolescent and young adult males who have sex with males if they engage in receptive oral, anal, or insertive intercourse; screening every 3 to 6 months for persons in this population if they are at high risk; and screening adolescents and young adults who have been exposed to gonorrhea in the past 60 days from an infected partner. The CDC recommends that clinicians screen all sexually active MSM for genital gonorrhea at least annually. Screening for rectal and pharyngeal gonorrhea is also recommended if there is a risk of exposure. Owing to the likelihood of reinfection, the CDC also recommends retesting of all patients diagnosed with gonococcal infections 3 months after treatment, regardless of whether or not sexual partners have been treated. Complete treatment guidelines for chlamydia and gonorrheal infection are available from the CDC.[9] See Chapter 13 for more details.

Patient Preparation

In women, chlamydia and gonorrhea specimens are usually obtained during the pelvic examination. However, urine specimens can also be collected if a pelvic examination is not performed. For cervical collection, the patient must disrobe from the waist down, don a gown or drape, lie supine on the examining table, and place the legs in stirrups. Men must lower their trousers and briefs and should sit or lie supine to prevent falls from vasovagal reactions. The patient should be cautioned that the procedure may be uncomfortable. A chaperone may be advisable, especially if the patient is of the opposite sex of the examiner.

Technique

Screening can be accomplished using culture, nucleic acid amplification tests, and nucleic acid hybridization tests (nucleic acid probes). Culture isolates can be collected from endocervical swabs in women and urethral swabs in men. Chlamydia and gonorrhea screening are often performed with a single specimen collection. In many circumstances based on local epidemiology, clinicians may choose to screen for only one of these infections.

In women, the technique for cervical specimens (whether sent for culture, nucleic acid amplification tests, or nucleic hybridization tests) is similar: the specimen is obtained by inserting and rotating the swab or cytology brush in the endocervical canal; depending on the type of laboratory test, the duration that the swab should remain in the endocervical canal may vary. Instructions are available from swab manufacturers. Newer DNA amplification tests can be used with urine samples and cervical swabs. If urine is used, a midstream sample is sent to the laboratory for analysis; cervical swabs can be collected as described earlier.

In men, the urethral specimen is obtained by advancing the culture swab approximately 2 to 3 cm into the urethra. Just as in women, urine samples can be used for screening.

Based on patient sexual behaviors, samples may also be obtained by using culture swabs in the posterior nasopharynx and the tonsillar arches. For anal samples, a culture swab is inserted approximately 2 to 3 cm into the anal canal.

Standard Counseling

All sexually active patients should be counseled to maintain safe sexual practices and should receive instructions on the correct use of condoms and spermicides (see Chapter 13). Women at increased risk should receive information about the early signs and symptoms of pelvic inflammatory disease. Adolescents should be advised that abstinence from sexual intercourse is the most effective preventive strategy. Clinicians who care for transgender women and men should have knowledge of their patients' current anatomy and patterns of sexual behavior before counseling them about STI prevention.

Potential Adverse Effects

Specimen collection can be uncomfortable, in both men and women. This is especially so when specimens are obtained from the urethra of men, who can experience vasovagal reactions. False-positive results can cause unnecessary anxiety, concerns about infidelity, and unnecessary treatment. False-negative results can result in treatment delays and inadvertent transmission to other sexual contacts.

Accuracy and Reliability as Screening Test

Chlamydia screening tests that utilize amplified DNA assays (such as polymerase chain reaction and ligase chain reaction) have demonstrated sensitivity ranging from 86% to 100% and specificity ranging from 96% to 100% when compared with endocervical culture. For gonorrhea, sensitivity for nucleic acid amplification tests ranges from 90% to 100%, with specificity ranging from 97% to 100%. Nucleic acid amplification tests may be used with urine specimens in addition to endocervical and urethral swabs, and single specimens can be used to test for chlamydia as well as gonorrhea.

Medical Record Documentation

The date and results of the tests should be documented in the medical record. If the results are positive, notification of the patient and the treatment plan in addition to partner treatment and public health department notification (see Chapter 13) should be arranged and documented in the medical record.

Colorectal Cancer Screening

Introduction

Colorectal cancer (CRC) is the third most common cancer in the United States and is the second leading cause of cancer deaths, claiming 51,651 lives in 2014. Incidence is low until 45 years of age after which the incidence increases with each year of life. A 50-year-old person has a 5% chance of being diagnosed with CRC and a 2.5% chance of dying from this disease. Risk factors for CRC include age (older than 50 yr), first-degree relative with a history of CRC, a family history of hereditary nonpolyposis CRC or familial adenomatous polyposis, and a personal history of ulcerative colitis. However, most cases occur in persons of average risk with age older than 50 years as the sole risk factor. Studies demonstrate that screening reduces the incidence of and mortality from CRC. Screening facilitates the removal of premalignant adenomatous polyps and the detection of early-stage disease, which is more amenable to treatment. Although most polyps will not progress to CRC, the benefits of removing larger adenomatous polyps outweigh the risks of doing so.

Screening Guidelines **All adults 50 to 75 years of age should be offered screening for CRC. Acceptable screening tests include any of the following five options: (1) home fecal occult blood test (FOBT) every year, (2) flexible sigmoidoscopy every 5 years, (3) the combination of home FOBT every year and flexible sigmoidoscopy every 5 years, (4) colonoscopy every 10 years, or (5) double-contrast barium enema every 5 years. Barium enema is rarely used for screening, however. Colonoscopy should be offered earlier and more frequently for high-risk individuals (e.g., those with a first-degree family history of CRC or hereditary polyposis syndromes).**

Official Guidelines The USPSTF recommends screening for CRC in adults from 50 to 75 years of age using FOBT, sigmoidoscopy, or colonoscopy. It recommends against routine screening for CRC in adults 76 to 85 years of age; however, there may be considerations for screening in an individual patient. Screening is not recommended in adults older than 85 years. The ACS recommends screening average-risk adults beginning at age 50 years with flexible sigmoidoscopy every 5 years, a double-contrast barium enema every 5 years, CT colonography (virtual colonoscopy) every 5 years, or a colonoscopy every 10 years. A fecal immunochemical test (FIT), stool FOBT can be done yearly with colonoscopy if results are positive. A stool DNA test can be done every 3 years with colonoscopy if results are positive. For individuals with a first-degree relative with CRC, the ACS recommends beginning screening colonoscopy at age 40 or 10 years before the youngest case in the immediate family member and repeating the colonoscopy every 5 years. For individuals at very high risk, colonoscopy should begin at an earlier age and should be repeated every 1 to 2 years. For example, individuals with familial adenomatous polyposis should have genetic testing and colonoscopy every 1 to 2 years beginning at puberty. The American Gastroenterological Association and a consortium of other gastroenterological associations, the AAFP, and the American College of Surgeons make similar recommendations.

Fecal Occult Blood Testing

Technique

The FOBT can be performed in the examination room along with the DRE (see Chapter 4), but in-office FOBT is discouraged for screening because it is less accurate than home testing by the patient.[10] With home testing, patients are generally given three cards impregnated with guaiac and are asked to collect two specimens from three separate consecutive stool samples. The patient is given instructions to avoid eating red meat (beef, lamb, including processed meats and liver), fish, uncooked fruits, and vegetables (especially melons, radishes, turnips, and horseradish), foods or supplements containing large amounts of vitamin C, nonsteroidal anti-inflammatory agents, corticosteroids, and other medications that can cause gastritis during the week before the specimens are obtained. Evidence regarding the need for these restrictions is limited. Menstruating women and patients with active bleeding from rectal disorders (e.g., hemorrhoids) should postpone specimen collection until 3 days after the bleeding has ended. The patient should then mail or deliver the cards to the clinician's office in the provided preaddressed envelope.

When the slides are received, a drop of developer fluid is applied to the specimens, with blue discoloration representing an abnormal result. Rehydration of the dried specimens increases sensitivity at the expense of specificity, thereby increasing the likelihood of false-positive results. See page 114 regarding newer stool testing technologies.

Potential Adverse Effects

The FOBT can be distasteful and embarrassing. Some patients report that they find the FOBT unpleasant or difficult to perform. Potential harms arise when false-positive screens lead to unnecessary invasive testing or false negatives lead to false reassurance. Colonoscopy examinations precipitated by FOBT screening incur risks such as bleeding or bowel perforations. Those risks increase with therapeutic procedures, such as a polypectomy or biopsy.

Accuracy and Reliability as Screening Test

The sensitivity of FOBT varies with the frequency of testing and the method. Sensitivity and specificity for unhydrated specimens have been estimated at 40% and 96% to 98%, respectively. Hydration of the specimen increases sensitivity (60%) but reduces specificity (90%), resulting in more false-positive results. In the key studies evaluating FOBT, the PPV for detecting cancer and large polyps was 2% to 18% and 8% to 40%, respectively.

Sigmoidoscopy and Colonoscopy

Introduction

Endoscopy (sigmoidoscopy or colonoscopy) is a principal screening test for detecting adenomatous polyps and CRC. Both sigmoidoscopy and colonoscopy have the potential to be diagnostic and, by removing precancerous polyps, therapeutic. Flexible sigmoidoscopes measuring 60 to 65 cm in length can inspect the distal third of the colon, the region in which colorectal malignancies are most likely to occur. Nonetheless, more proximal lesions (which have been diagnosed more frequently in recent years) are not detectable by sigmoidoscopy, and flat malignancies within reach of the sigmoidoscope may not be visualized. Case-control studies have suggested, however, that regular sigmoidoscopy screening reduces the risk of CRC mortality within reach of the scope by 60%. Colonoscopy has the potential to inspect the entire colon—to the cecum. Although there is no direct evidence that screening colonoscopy is effective in reducing CRC mortality, the efficacy of colonoscopy is supported by its integral role in trials of FOBT as well as extrapolation of evidence from sigmoidoscopy studies. It has been hypothesized that colonoscopy screening reduces CRC mortality by 60%.

Patient Preparation

Commonly, the role of the primary care clinician is in facilitating, rather than performing, endoscopy. Endoscopy is usually performed by gastroenterologists or general surgeons, whereas the role of the primary care clinician is to identify patients who are due for screening, help patients decide whether they prefer endoscopy over FOBT, refer patients to accredited endoscopy facilities, verify that the patient obtains the study, and ensure proper interpretation and follow-up of results. The patient should provide informed consent to the procedure after being advised of the potential benefits and risks. Preparation begins on the evening before the procedure, in which the bowel is evacuated. A variety of regimens are used, typically involving some combination of magnesium citrate, polyethylene glycol, enemas, and fasting. For sigmoidoscopy, anxiolytics or sedatives may be prescribed on the day of the procedure to reduce anxiety. Colonoscopy is typically performed under conscious sedation. Endocarditis prophylaxis with antibiotics may be prescribed for those with high-risk cardiac lesions (e.g., prosthetic heart valves, congenital cardiac malformations) but is unnecessary for patients with moderate-risk lesions, such as mitral valve prolapse with regurgitation.

Technique

The techniques for performing flexible fiberoptic sigmoidoscopy and colonoscopy and for obtaining biopsies, which are learned through supervised training and practical experience, are beyond the scope of this chapter.

Definition of Abnormal Results

Large or adenomatous polyps, masses, diverticula, and areas of inflammation or bleeding are considered abnormal.

Potential Adverse Effects

A serious complication of endoscopy is bowel perforation, which occurs in approximately 0.01% of sigmoidoscopies and in up to 0.1% to 0.2% of colonoscopies. Bleeding from biopsy sites or mucosal injuries, moderate pain, and flatus are common. Transmission of infectious diseases is also possible but uncommon. Endoscopy may be inappropriate or may need reconsideration in patients with severe anal strictures or fissures, inadequate bowel preparation, recent pelvic or bowel surgery, active inflammatory bowel disease, toxic megacolon, acute diverticulitis, or immune deficiency, but many of these conditions are unlikely in asymptomatic patients undergoing screening. False-positive results are uncommon with endoscopy, but detected polyps, even if adenomatous, may not be destined to progress to cancer. Patients can incur costs, inconvenience, discomfort, and complications from the removal of these growths and for subsequent surveillance. False-negative results can occur if polyps or cancers are obscured from view or are located beyond the reach of the scope.

Accuracy and Reliability as Screening Test

Sigmoidoscopy visualizes only the lower half of the colon but has been estimated to identify 50% to 92% of all patients with significant findings in the colon and rectum, depending on whether sigmoidoscopy alone or sigmoidoscopy combined with annual FOBT is compared with colonoscopy. This is because abnormal findings ("sentinel lesions") on sigmoidoscopy or abnormal FOBTs trigger examination of the entire colon with colonoscopy. Sensitivity and detection rates vary depending on the depth of insertion. The 60 and 65 cm flexible sigmoidoscopes can reach the splenic flexure in 80% of examinations and can thereby detect 40% to 65% of CRCs. The specificity of endoscopic screening approaches 100% for detection of significant polyps and cancers.

Medical Record Documentation

The date and results of the endoscopic examination should be placed in the medical record, preferably on a health maintenance flow sheet. The appearance and location of polyps, diverticula, areas of inflammation, or other abnormalities should be carefully described. If equipment is available, a videotape recording or photograph of abnormal findings should be included. The medical record should also indicate the type and length of the endoscope, the type and adequacy of the bowel preparation and medications, depth of insertion, difficulties in advancement or visualization, reason for stopping, and discomfort or complications experienced by the patient. The record should specify whether biopsies were obtained, the specific pathology results, and the plans for follow-up and repeat testing.

Additional Colorectal Cancer Screening Methods

Stool DNA and immunochemical testing and "virtual" colonoscopy (computed tomography) are newer technologies for screening that may be more acceptable to patients. The FIT uses antibodies to detect blood in the stool. The FIT-DNA test (stool DNA test) detects altered DNA in the stool and also looks for blood in the stool. These stool tests do not require dietary restrictions, and virtual colonoscopy is noninvasive. However, there is currently limited information on accuracy, effectiveness in reducing CRC mortality, and harms of these services when performed in the general population.

Standard Counseling

Clinicians should educate patients about the options for CRC screening and their associated risks and benefits to help patients choose which test they prefer. Patients undergoing endoscopy should be advised of potential symptoms that may be experienced following the procedure (e.g., flatus, cramps). Following FOBT, endoscopy, or other forms of CRC screening, the patient should be reminded to return for repeat screening at the recommended interval, to undergo colonoscopy if their home FOBT is positive, and to contact the clinician if changes in bowel habits, stool color, or rectal bleeding occur. Patients can also be advised that reducing dietary fat and/or increasing dietary fiber intake may reduce the risk of developing CRC.

Mammography

Introduction

Breast cancer is the second leading cause of cancer deaths in women in the United States, claiming 41,211 lives in 2014. Major risk factors include age, early age of menarche, previous breast biopsies showing atypical hyperplasia, late age at first pregnancy or no pregnancy, and family history of breast cancer in first-degree relatives (mother, sister, and daughter).[11] Mammography efficacy trials have reported reductions in mortality although estimates are not statistically significant at all ages.[12]

Screening Guidelines **All women aged 50 to 74 years and older should be offered biennial mammography. Clinicians should discuss the risks and benefits of mammography screening for women between 40 and 50 years of age. The exact age to stop mammography screening is uncertain, but screening offers limited value in those patients with an average life expectancy of less than 10 years. Clinicians should screen patients to identify if they may be at increased risk for potentially harmful mutations in breast cancer susceptibility and refer them for genetic counseling if they report a family history that would put them at risk for the BRCA**

mutation (e.g., Ashkenazi Jewish women with one first-degree relative or two second-degree relatives with breast or ovarian cancer; non-Ashkenazi Jewish women with two first-degree relatives with breast cancer, one of whom received the diagnosis at 50 years or younger; a combination of three or more first- or second-degree relatives with breast cancer regardless of age at diagnosis; a combination of both breast and ovarian cancer among first- and second-degree relatives; a first-degree relative with bilateral breast cancer; a combination of two or more first-or second-degree relatives with ovarian cancer regardless of age at diagnosis; a first- or second-degree relative with both breast and ovarian cancer at any age; and a history of breast cancer in a male relative).

Official Guidelines The USPSTF recommends biennial screening mammography for women aged 50 to 74 years. The decision to start screening mammography in women before age 50 years should be an individual one. Women who place a higher value on the potential benefit than the potential harms may choose to begin biennial screening between the ages of 40 and 49 years. Beginning mammography screening at a younger age and screening more frequently may increase the risk for overdiagnosis and subsequent overtreatment. Women with a parent, sibling, or child with breast cancer are at higher risk for breast cancer and thus may benefit more than average-risk women from beginning screening in their 40s. For women 75 years and older, current evidence is insufficient to assess the balance of benefits and harms of screening mammography. For all women, current evidence is insufficient to assess the benefits and harms of digital breast tomosynthesis as a primary screening method for breast cancer. For women with dense breasts on a negative screening mammogram, the USPSTF does not recommend for or against the use of ultrasonography, magnetic resonance imaging (MRI), digital breast tomosynthesis, or other methods for adjunctive screening. The USPSTF recommends clinician screening of patients who have family members with a history of breast, ovarian, tubal, or peritoneal cancer to identify if they may be at increased risk for potentially harmful mutations in breast cancer susceptibility with referral for genetic counseling for women whose family history suggests an increased risk of *BRCA1* or *BRCA2* mutations. Multiple screening tools are available by the USPSTF (see Suggested Readings) The Task Force recommends against routine genetic counseling whose family history is not associated with an increased risk for potentially harmful mutations in *BRCA1* or *BRCA2* mutations. The AAFP agrees with the Task Force recommendations. The ACOG recommends annual screening mammography for women at average risk of breast cancer beginning at age 40 years and continuing through age 75 years. For those 75 years or older, screening mammography should be part of a shared decision-making process with their clinician. For women at average risk of breast cancer, the ACS recommends that women have the option to begin annual screening mammograms between 40 and 44 years of age. Women aged 45 to 54 years should get mammograms yearly. Women 55 years and older should continue yearly mammograms as long as they are in good health and have a life expectancy of 10 years or more. The ACS recommends yearly MRI in addition to mammography screening for women beginning at age 30 years who are determined to be at high risk for developing breast cancer.

Technique

Radiographic methods for performing mammography are the domain of the radiologist and are not discussed here. As with endoscopy screening, the role of the primary care clinician in providing mammographic screening is to identify women who are due for screening, refer patients to accredited mammographic facilities, verify that the patient obtains the study, and ensure proper interpretation and follow-up of results. In placing the requisition, the referring clinician should remember that a screening mammogram typically includes only oblique and craniocaudal views. Magnification views, spot compression films, and other special imaging techniques may be needed to evaluate abnormal screening studies and for women with palpable masses, a previous history of breast cancer, or breast augmentation. Digital mammography techniques (filmless mammography), which provide computerized acquisition and storage of mammographic images, are available at some mammography centers. Although this technology is more expensive, it allows for easier storage, transferability, and comparison of films over time. Ultrasonography and MRI of the breasts are indicated in certain circumstances; for example, MRI of the breasts has been recommended for women at very high risk of breast cancer.

Standard Counseling

Patients should be reminded to wear two-piece clothing and to not apply topical agents (e.g., deodorants) to the breasts on the day of the study. See Chapters 4 and 15 regarding CBE and breast self-examination, respectively. The patient should be advised to contact the clinician if she detects a breast lump, tenderness, or another abnormality, even if her mammogram is normal. The importance of regular breast cancer screening should be emphasized, and the patient should receive specific instructions about when to return for the next mammogram.

Definition of Abnormal Results

Radiographic features associated with malignancy include irregular margins, spiculations, and clustered microcalcifications. Indirect radiographic signs can include localized distortion of breast architecture, developing neodensities, asymmetric breast tissue, and single dilated ducts.

Potential Adverse Effects

Patients can experience discomfort from breast compression during imaging, and it is therefore preferable that they not obtain the study during menstruation. Risks from radiation exposure are minimal, totaling only a fraction of the radiation exposure used in other x-ray procedures such as lumbar spine radiography. As discussed further in Chapter 20, the potential harms of breast cancer screening include the generation of false-positive results and the overdiagnosis and overtreatment of lesions of uncertain clinical significance (e.g., ductal carcinoma in situ). Screening may also precipitate further diagnostic testing (mammography with spot views, ultrasound, invasive biopsies with either needle or open surgical procedures), anxiety, and additional medical expense. False-negative results may allow women with breast cancer to escape detection.

Accuracy and Reliability as Screening Test

The sensitivity of mammography ranges from 77% to 95% for cancers diagnosed over the following year, and specificity ranges from 94% to 97%. Recent studies report false-positive rates of 3% to 6%. Owing to increased breast tissue density, sensitivity is lower in women younger than 50 years and in women who are taking hormone replacement. Specificity increases with shorter screening intervals and access to prior mammograms for purposes of comparison.

Tuberculin Skin Testing

Introduction

An estimated 9.6 to 14.9 million persons residing in the United States have latent tuberculosis (TB) infection. Those individuals at high risk for TB include persons infected with HIV, close contacts of persons known or suspected of having TB, persons with medical conditions that increase the risk of infection (e.g., immunosuppressed patients, those with leukemia, lymphoma, diabetes, chronic renal failure), immigrants from countries with a high prevalence of TB, medically underserved low-income populations (including high-risk racial or ethnic groups), patients suffering from alcohol abuse, injection drug users, residents of long-term institutions (e.g., nursing homes, prisons), and persons who work in health care facilities. Tuberculin skin testing is most commonly performed using the Mantoux test, in which a known quantity of purified protein derivative (PPD) is injected intradermally.

Screening Guidelines **Adolescents and adults at high risk for TB.**

Official Guidelines The USPSTF, AAFP, AAP, and CDC recommend tuberculin skin testing of persons with risk factors for acquiring TB. The CDC recommends that either the TST or the IGRAs may be used for screening. The IGRAs are preferred in the evaluation of patients who have received the TB vaccine Bacille Calmette-Guérin (BCG) or for those who may not be able to return for the 48 to 72 hour follow-up of the TST. For children under the age of 5 years, the TST is preferred over IGRAs.

Technique

In the Mantoux test, a tuberculin syringe is used to inject 0.1 mL of five tuberculin units of PPD intradermally on the volar surface of the forearm. The injection should produce a skin weal measuring 6 to 10 mm. If the patient is anergic, control sites of mumps, *Candida,* or tetanus should be placed on the opposite arm. A circle should be placed around the injection site(s). The patient should return to the office or clinic in 48 to 72 hours, at which time the site is inspected for induration. (Erythema alone is an insignificant finding.) If induration is palpated, pen marks placed at the margins of induration can be helpful in measuring the diameter.

Infected persons can have false-negative TSTs because of anergy, but anergy is disproved if the control sites are indurated. Infected persons may also have negative TSTs if immunity has waned over time. In what is known as the *booster effect,* such persons may subsequently have a positive skin test if a PPD is placed a second time. In health care and other institutional settings (e.g., nursing homes), "two-step testing," in which persons with negative TSTs are retested in 1 to 2 weeks, is commonly advised to distinguish persons with booster reactions related to old infections from persons who are new converters.

The QuantiFERON-TB Gold Test, which requires a serum blood sample, is an enzyme-linked immunosorbent assay test that detects the release of interferon-γ in fresh heparinized whole blood from sensitized persons. The T-SPOT.TB test also requires a serum blood sample, which detects and enumerates effector T cells that have been specifically activated by *Mycobacterium tuberculosis* antigens.

Definition of Abnormal Results

According to the CDC and the Prevention Advisory Committee for Elimination of Tuberculosis, an induration greater than 5, 10, or 15 mm is abnormal, depending on the risk category of the patient. Induration should not be attributed to prior BCG vaccination. The QuantiFERON-TB results are reported as positive, negative, or indeterminate. The T-SPOT.TB test results are reported as positive, negative, indeterminate, or borderline.

Potential Adverse Effects

There is a small amount of discomfort and local erythema associated with PPD injection. Rarely, patients experience hypersensitivity reactions, ulcerated or vesicular eruptions, lymphadenopathy, or fever. Patients with false-positive results may receive unnecessary antibiotic therapy, with potentially serious adverse effects (e.g., hepatotoxicity), and restrictions on job and insurance eligibility. They may also undergo unnecessary diagnostic procedures (e.g., chest radiography). False-negative results may cause patients with TB to escape detection.

Accuracy and Reliability as Screening Test

For persons who have not contacted an active case, the reported probability of infection is approximately 5% for 5 to 9-mm induration, 25% for 10 to 13-mm induration, 50% to 80% for 14 to 21-mm induration, and 100% for more than 21-mm induration. The validity of these estimates depends heavily on the geographic area, the local prevalence of atypical mycobacteria, and the type of population being tested. False-positive results can be caused by improper measurement of induration (e.g., measuring erythema), cross-reactivity with atypical mycobacteria, hypersensitivity to PPD constituents, and Arthus reactions. False-negative results occur in 5% to 10% of patients owing to testing in the early stages of infection, anergy, or improper technique. The QuantiFeron test has a sensitivity of 80% and specificity of 97%. The T-Spot.TB test has a sensitivity of 90% and specificity of 97%. Compared with the tuberculin skin testing, IGRAs are unaffected by prior BCG vaccination and are less likely than the TST to be influenced by previous infection with most nontuberculous mycobacteria.

Medical Record Documentation

The patient's risk factors for TB should be described. The date, type of tuberculin test (Mantoux, QuantiFeron, T-Spot.TB), location of testing, and, if positive, the diameter of induration should be noted in the medical record. It is often helpful to use a diagram to mark the location of the tuberculin and control injections. Plans for follow-up treatment of new converters should be described.

Abdominal Ultrasonography for Abdominal Aortic Aneurysm

Introduction

Approximately 9000 people die each year from large abdominal aortic aneurysms (AAAs). Most victims are older than 65 years. Major risk factors include age greater than or equal to 65 years, smoking history, and male sex. Family history also increases the risk but to a lesser extent. The diameter of the AAA is the main risk factor for rupture. Abdominal ultrasonography offers a noninvasive and accurate means to identify AAAs. Population-based studies have shown that screening programs reduce mortality from AAAs in older men; whether screening affects all-cause mortality is uncertain. Screening studies have not shown a benefit for women.

Screening Guidelines **Males between ages 65 and 75 years with a current or past history of smoking should be offered one-time abdominal ultrasonography to screen for AAA.**

Official Guidelines The USPSTF recommends screening for AAA in men aged 65 to 75 years who have ever smoked; selective screening for AAA in men aged 65 to 75 years who have never smoked rather than routinely screening all men in this group; makes no recommendation for screening women aged 65 to 75 years who have ever smoked; and recommends against routine screening in women who never smoked. The Society for Vascular Surgery recommends one-time ultrasonography screening for AAA in men 55 years or older with a family history of AAA, all men 65 years or older, and women 65 years or older who have smoked or have a family history of AAA.

Technique

Imaging techniques for abdominal ultrasonography are the domain of the radiologist and are not discussed here. Adequate quality assurance and certification are important to ensure test accuracy. The role of the primary care clinician in providing AAA screening is to identify patients who are due for screening, refer patients to accredited ultrasonography facilities, verify that the patient obtains the study, and ensure proper interpretation and follow-up of results.

Definition of Abnormal Results

By definition, an AAA is present when the infrarenal aortic diameter exceeds 3 cm. An AAA larger than 5 cm is considered at increased risk for rupture.

Accuracy of Screening Tests

Abdominal ultrasonography is 95% sensitive and 100% specific for AAA when appropriately performed.

Adverse Effects

Screening itself can cause short-term anxiety. Those patients found to have an intermediate-sized AAA and who undergo longitudinal surveillance may experience more prolonged stress. Surgical AAA repair carries an average mortality risk of up to 5%. Furthermore, perioperative and postoperative cardiac and pulmonary complications are common in association with AAA repair.

Office and Clinic Organization for Routine Screening

Practices participating in routine screening should be properly stocked with appropriate collection instruments, culture and transport media, and storage facilities. Clinicians and staff involved with the collection, plating, and handling of specimens should be trained in proper technique, and offices that send specimens to outside laboratories should maintain transport conditions that protect the quality of the specimen.

Cervical cancer screening requires specula of varying sizes and shapes (including both Graves and Pedersen specula), specimen collection equipment (e.g., spatulas, cytobrushes, and cotton swabs); slides, fixatives, or liquid-based cytology collection vials; gloves, lubricant, and gowns or other coverings. Home FOBT screening requires a supply of preaddressed stool card packets that can be given to patients. In addition to three stool cards and a collection instrument (e.g., wooden spatula), the packet should include clearly written instructions on dietary restrictions and on how to collect the specimens. The envelopes used to mail the specimens must be approved by the U.S. Postal Service. Practices that perform or refer patients for endoscopy screening require bowel preparation kits (or standard prescriptions for the regimen). Offices and clinics that perform tuberculin testing should maintain a fresh supply of PPD and at least two controls (e.g., mumps, *Candida*, tetanus), tuberculin syringes, and a ruler that measures millimeters. A body diagram that can be inserted in the medical record may be helpful in marking the location of the injections.

Examination rooms should be outfitted with comfortable examination tables and good lighting. The practice should also provide a quiet discussion area where clinicians and patients can review the benefits and risks of tests before screening is conducted.

Reminder and referral systems should be in place to identify patients overdue for screening and to ensure that the clinician receives test results, that patients return for repeat screening at recommended intervals, and that patients with positive results receive appropriate follow-up and treatment. For practices that offer home FOBT screening, reminder systems should ensure that FOBT packets are mailed and returned to the office. For patients screened for infectious diseases, reminder systems should also ensure that infected patients receive appropriate antibiotic therapy; that potential contacts of infected patients are notified, tested, and treated according to guidelines; and that the public health department is notified of reportable cases. For patients screened for TB, reminder systems should ensure that patients return in 48 to 72 hours to have the site(s) read.

Ideally, a list of recommended preventive services should be programmed into electronic medical record systems. Appropriate data fields should automatically be populated with the dates and results of previous screening tests. Reminder letters or e-mail notices can alert patients when the next preventive service is due. Electronic medical records can automate such correspondence and can also facilitate tracking of test orders, results, and follow-up testing. Likewise, the electronic medical record can also facilitate public health department notification of reportable diseases.

The office or clinic should maintain a complete list of accredited screening facilities in the community (e.g., mammography centers), including high-quality facilities that will accept low-income or uninsured patients or that provide low-cost screening. The office should have access to the performance record and certification status of the laboratories to which specimens are sent.

CONCLUSIONS

In the face of competing demands and limited time, clinicians should focus on screening tests for which net benefit has been demonstrated in the scientific literature. As noted at the outset of this chapter, screening tests are not always beneficial. A "simple blood test" can incur harms by setting off a cascade of events. Shared decision making before ordering these tests helps to engage patients in their own care, clarify realistic expectations about the harms and benefits of completing and deferring tests, and facilitate adherence with testing and follow-up. Once the clinician is convinced that the patient is fully informed about these services, should the patient refuse the screening offered, the patient's choice to forego should be respected. At future visits, the decision to undergo screening can be revisited.

The latter point emphasizes the importance of continuity in the provision of quality preventive care. Primary care clinicians who maintain a long-term relationship with patients can provide longitudinal monitoring of the performance of screening and the follow-up of results. The broad scope of testing outlined in this chapter is too extensive to compress into a single office visit. Unlike clinicians who see patients for single consultations or time-limited relationships, or who specialize in specific disorders, primary care clinicians can organize and monitor the delivery of a range of services over time to ensure a comprehensive approach to health maintenance.

SUGGESTED RESOURCES AND MATERIALS

Decision Aids Clearinghouse

University of Ottawa
Cochrane Inventory of Patient Decision Aids
https://decisionaid.ohri.ca/AZinvent.php.

Diabetes

National Institutes of Health/National Diabetes Education Program
Learn About Diabetes
https://www.niddk.nih.gov/health-information/communication-programs/ndep/partner-community-organization-information/diabetes-alert-day.

Cholesterol and Cardiovascular Health

American Heart Association
Patient Information by Condition
http://www.heart.org/HEARTORG/Conditions/Patient-Education-Resources-for-Healthcare-Professionals_UCM_441960_SubHomePage.jsp.

HIV

Centers for Disease Control and Prevention
HIV and AIDS
http://www.cdc.gov/hiv/pubs/brochure.htm.

Syphilis

Centers for Disease Control and Prevention
Syphilis—CDC Fact Sheet
http://www.cdc.gov/std/syphilis/STDFact-Syphilis.htm.

Prostate Cancer Screening

American Cancer Society
Prostate Cancer Prevention and Early Detection
https://www.cancer.org/cancer/prostate-cancer/early-detection.html.

Centers for Disease Control and Prevention
Should I Get Screened for Prostate Cancer? http://www.cdc.gov/cancer/prostate/decisionguide/index.htm.

American Academy of Family Physicians
Prostate Cancer
https://familydoctor.org/condition/prostate-cancer/.

Cervical Cancer

American Cancer Society
Cervical Cancer
https://www.cancer.org/cancer/cervical-cancer.html.

National Institutes of Health/National Cancer Institute
Pap and HPV Testing
http://www.cancer.gov/cancertopics/pap-tests-cervical-health.

Gonorrhea

Centers for Disease Control and Prevention
Gonorrhea—CDC Fact Sheet in English and Spanish
http://www.cdc.gov/std/Gonorrhea/STDFact-gonorrhea.htm.

Chlamydia

Centers for Disease Control and Prevention
Chlamydia—CDC Fact Sheet in English and Spanish
http://www.cdc.gov/std/chlamydia/STDFact-Chlamydia.htm.

Colorectal Cancer

American Cancer Society
Colorectal Cancer
https://www.cancer.org/cancer/colon-rectal-cancer.html.

Centers for Disease Control and Prevention
Colorectal (Colon) Cancer: What Should I Know About Screening?
https://www.cdc.gov/cancer/colorectal/basic_info/screening/index.htm.

Mammography

American Academy of Family Physicians
Breast Cancer
https://familydoctor.org/condition/breast-cancer/.

American Cancer Society
Breast Cancer
https://www.cancer.org/cancer/breast-cancer.html.

National Institutes of Health/Naional Cancer Institute
What You Need to Know About Breast Cancer
https://www.cancer.gov/publications/patient-education/wyntk-breast-cancer.

Tuberculosis Screening

Centers for Disease Control and Prevention
Questions and Answers About TB; 2014
https://www.cdc.gov/tb/publications/faqs/pdfs/qa.pdf.

American Academy of Family Physicians
Tuberculosis
https://familydoctor.org/condition/tuberculosis/.

SUGGESTED READINGS

American Academy of Family Physicians. *Summary of Policy Recommendations for Clinical Preventive Services.* Available at https://www.aafp.org/dam/AAFP/documents/patient_care/clinical_recommendations/cps-recommendations.pdf. Accessed 22 February 2018.

American Cancer Society. *Guidelines for the Early Detection of Cancer.* Available at https://www.cancer.org/healthy/find-cancer-early/cancer-screening-guidelines/american-cancer-society-guidelines-for-the-early-detection-of-cancer.html. Accessed 25 February 2018.

American College of Obstetricians and Gynecologists. Primary and preventive care: periodic assessments. ACOG Committee Opinion No. 483. *Obstet Gynecol.* 2011;117(4):1008-1015.

American College of Physicians. *Clinical Guidelines and Recommendations.* Available at http://www.acponline.org/sci-policy/guidelines/recent.htm. Accessed February 2018.

Centers for Disease Control and Prevention. Sexually transmitted diseases treatment guidelines-2015. *MMWR.* 2015;64(3):1-137.

Expert Panel on Detection, Evaluation, and treatment of high blood cholesterol in adults. Executive summary of the third report of the national cholesterol education program expert panel on detection, evaluation, and treatment of high blood cholesterol in adults (ATP III). *JAMA.* 2001;285:2486-2497.

Gordis L. *Epidemiology.* 5th ed. Philadelphia, PA: Elsevier Saunders; 2014.

Lewinsohn DM, Leonard MK, LoBue PA, et al. Official American thoracic society/infectious diseases society of America/centers for disease control and prevention clinical practice guidelines: diagnosis of tuberculosis in adults and children. *Clin Infect Dis.* 2017;64(2):111-115.

Nelson HD, Fu R, Cantor A, Pappas M, Daeges M, Humphrey L. Effectiveness of breast cancer screening: systematic review and meta-analysis to update the 2009 U.S. preventive services task force recommendation. *Ann Intern Med.* 2016;164:244-255.

Nelson HD, Huffman LH, Fu R, et al. Genetic risk assessment and BRCA mutation testing for breast and ovarian cancer susceptibility. *Ann Intern Med.* 2005;143:362-379.

Taylor Z, Nolan CM, Blumberg HM, American Thoracic Society, Centers for Disease Control and Prevention, Infectious Diseases Society of America. Controlling tuberculosis in the United States: recommendations from the American thoracic society, CDC, and the infectious diseases society of America. *MMWR.* 2005;54(RR12):1-81.

U.S. Preventive Services Task Force. *The Guide to Clinical Preventive Services 2014: Recommendations of the U.S. Preventive Services Task Force. Agency for Healthcare Research and Quality.* AHRQ Pub No. 14-05158. Also Available at https://www. ahrq.gov/professionals/clinicians-providers/guidelines-recommendations/ guide/index.html. Accessed February 2018.

U.S. Preventive Services Task Force. *Genetic Testing Referral Screening Tools.* Available at https://www.uspreventiveservicestaskforce.org/Page/Document/ RecommendationStatementFinal/brca-related-cancer-risk-assessment-genetic-counseling-and-genetic-testing#table-3-referral-screening-tool. Accessed February 2018.

U.S. Preventive Services Task Force Procedure Manual. *Agency for Healthcare Research and Quality.* Rockville, Maryland; December 2016. http://www.uspreventiveser-vicestaskforce.org/Home/GetFileByID/2711. Accessed 30 June 2016.

Woolf SH, Chan EC, Harris R, et al. Promoting informed choice: transforming health care to dispense knowledge for decision making. *Ann Intern Med.* 2005;143(4):293-300.

REFERENCES

1. Schwartz LM, Woloshin S, Fowler FJ, et al. Enthusiasm for cancer screening in the United States. *JAMA.* 2004;291:71-78.

2. Sheridan SL, Harris RP, Woolf SH; and Shared Decision-Making Workgroup of the U.S. Preventive Services Task Force. Shared decision making about screening and chemoprevention: a suggested approach from the U.S. Preventive services Task Force. *Am J Prev Med.* 2004;26(1):56-66.

3. Shay LA, Lafata JE. Where is the evidence? A systematic review of shared deci-sion making and patient outcomes. *Med Decis Making.* 2015;35(1):114-131. doi:10.1177/0272989X14551638.

4. Woolf SH, Krist A. The liability of giving patients a choice: shared decision making and prostate cancer. *Am Fam Physician.* 2005;71:1871-1872.

5. *Methods and Processes.* U.S. Preventive Services Task Force. June 2018. https:// www.uspreventiveservicestaskforce.org/Page/Name/methods-and-processes. Accessed November 2018.

6. American Diabetes Association. Classification and diagnosis of diabetes. *Diabetes Care.* 2015;38(suppl 1):S8-S16.

7. Expert Panel on Detection, Evaluation, and treatment of high blood cholesterol in adults. Executive summary of the third report of the national cholesterol educa-tion program expert panel on detection, evaluation, and treatment of high blood cholesterol in adults (ATP III). *JAMA.* 2001;285:2486-2497.

8. Mulhelm E, Fullbright N, Duncan N. Prostate cancer screening. *Am Fam Physician.* 2015;92(8):683-688.

9. Centers for Disease Control and Prevention. Sexually transmitted diseases treat-ment guidelines 2002. *MMWR.* 2002;51(RR06):1-80.

10. Collins JF, Lieberman DA, Durbin TE, et al. Accuracy of screening for fecal occult blood on a single stool sample obtained by digital rectal examination: a compari-son with recommended sampling practice. *Ann Intern Med.* 2005;142:81-85.

11. Humphrey LL, Helfand M, Chan BKS, et al. Breast cancer screening: summary of the evidence. *Ann Intern Med.* 2002;137:344-346.

12. Nelson HD, Fu R, Cantor A, Pappas M, Daeges M, Humphrey L. Effectiveness of breast cancer screening: systematic review and meta-analysis to update the 2009 U.S. preventive services task force recommendation. *Ann Intern Med.* 2016;164:244-255.

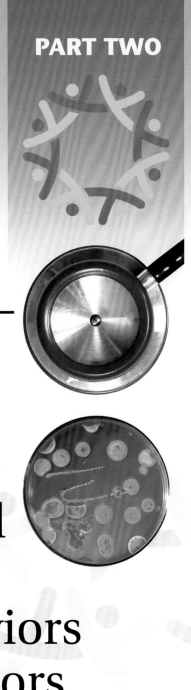

PART TWO

What to Do with the Information— Designing a Health Maintenance Plan Targeted to Personal Health Behaviors and Risk Factors

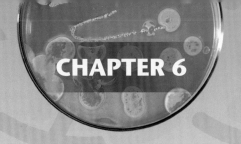

CHAPTER 6

Introduction to the Principles of Health Behavior Change

CAROLYNN SPERA BRUNO | BABETTE BIESECKER

BACKGROUND

Identifying factors associated with health and biopsychosocial processes and behavior in the United States is attributed to the Institute of Medicine (IOM) Report on Health and Behavior.[1] With increasing pressure for clinicians to conduct visits to improve health status in a short, yet efficient manner, the ability to build a trusting clinician-patient relationship, communicate patterns of caring and concern, and identify areas for health behavior change are challenging. Strategies to improve clinician-patient communication patterns from a foundationally evidence based and relevant theoretical framework will assist clinicians in collaborative goal settings of health behavior change across culturally diverse populations.

Health behavior change central to health maintenance and promotion is rooted in sociological theory, which can target effective coping mechanisms and ameliorate consequences related to existing comorbidities or promote general well-being. The health belief model, originating in social learning theory, asserts that health belief variables of perceived susceptibility and severity along with perceived benefits and barriers can regulate health behaviors.[2]

Social cognitive learning theory introduced by Bandura[3–5] and later refined proposes that psychological processes alter personal self-efficacy derived from cognitive regulation; thereby, reinterpreting these predictive cues or antecedent determinants shifts the focus of control and self-regulation to the individual. The individual must value the perceived outcome of health behavior change and cognitively endorse his or her ability to enact that behavioral change. Therefore, shifting the recognition of contextual cues to the patient and assessing his/her readiness is focal among health behavior change strategies. As such, discussion in this chapter will introduce the framework of motivational interviewing, including the "5 A's," which can assist in centering the focus of assessment and management in the visit toward setting collaborative goals that emphasize the patient's strengths and accountability in executing health change behaviors.

THEORETICAL MODELS THAT PROMOTE HEALTH BEHAVIOR CHANGE AND HEALTH BEHAVIORAL COUNSELING AND APPLICATION TO CLINICAL PRACTICE

Social Cognitive Learning Theory

There is an abundance of public health concern that addresses health risk behaviors, which prove socially persistent and seek to impair health promotion particularly among our nation's youth. The Centers for Disease Control and Prevention's Youth Risk Behavior Surveillance highlights deleterious behaviors, including unintentional injuries and violence; the use of alcohol and other substances, such as opioids and heroine; tobacco use; unhealthy dietary behaviors, obesity, and sedentary lifestyles; and high-risk sexual practices.[6,7] Other high-risk behaviors are notable, including texting while driving; persistently listening to loud noises; overexposure associated with sun tanning practices; and poor moderation of stress and anxiety. Refraining from damaging behaviors despite national campaigns to raise awareness and promote safe and health practices is challenging.

The adoption of an individual's positive health behavior change is predicated on the fluency and knowledge of inherent theoretical frameworks, and familiarity is critical for clinicians and counselors when promoting these health behaviors. Models of health behavior that are rooted in *social cognitive learning theory* or *social learning theory* assert that human motivation and behavioral action are produced by an individual's social-cognitive features. Three key expectations include (1) situation-outcome, such as those environmental influences that occur independent of the individual's own action; (2) action-outcome, beliefs linked to personal action and consequences; and (3) self-efficacy, an individual's perception that an action has the potential to generate a favorable outcome.[5,8] Bandura's social cognitive learning theory provides a view of human behavior in which the belief that individuals posit about themselves is critical to controlling their personal agency. Individuals are viewed as products of their environment, as well as construct their environment and larger social system. Working together toward collaborative goals of health, the clinician affirms an individual's self-efficacy by highlighting previous behavioral actions associated with successful change.

Bandura's *reciprocal determinism model* comprises triadic, causal factors that influence an individual's behavior, including personal, behavioral, and environmental.[5] Each of these factors operate in a bidirectional manner to influence behavior, and each may exert more independent force than the other two factors. Determinism means that each action, behavior, or decision is a consequence of past events. Therefore, people can construct their own reality and proactively moderate their environment by adjusting personal factors (thoughts, beliefs, emotions) and behavior. Personal factors involve biological and emotional components and cognitive and sensorineural processing. Anxiety arousal challenges biological protective functions as it assaults the immune system and activates autonomic reactions, whereas cognitive processes involve the construction of goals and rehearsal of anticipatory action to achieve mastery. Reflective thought evaluating one's internal environment and learning vicariously through the experiences of others assist in adopting alternative strategies that can promote health. An example of the reciprocal determinism, a principle of *social cognitive learning* model, can be seen in this smoking cessation clinical case scenario.

This 45-year-old Hispanic male, AE, comes to the clinic for an annual wellness visit. He describes a 2-ppd cigarette smoking history for 15 years. In addition, he recounts a 10-year history of using chewing tobacco daily and quit 5 years ago owing to complaints of malodorous breath by his wife. Although he continues to smoke daily outside the home, he reveals that he is embarrassed about the habit, including staining of his teeth and finger, and his two school-aged children have repeatedly asked him to stop smoking. He recounts that he has reduced his smoking by a few cigarettes per day for the last 2 weeks. During the examination, the clinician discusses the benefits and risks of cigarette smoking with AE. AE reveals that his brother-in-law quit smoking 2 years ago, and he often daydreams about quitting.

Behavioral change, grounded in the *social cognitive theory*, considers self-efficacy. This theory posits an individual's self-efficacy, the perception that an outcome can arise based on self-regulation of behavior, can exert a favorable influence.[8,9] Perceived self-efficacy influences coping abilities as a response or barrier to stress, anxiety, and depression. Active engagement and shared beliefs serve to improve capabilities and consequent behaviors. Therefore, it is advantageous for the clinician to reaffirm the recent health-promoting behavior of chewing tobacco cessation, which will enhance the patient's awareness of his self-efficacy. Personal factors (i.e., cognitive features, desire, daydreaming about smoking cessation) moderated by self-regulatory behaviors (reducing the quantity of cigarettes), and environmental factors (i.e., positive role models for smoking cessation; family requesting that the patient stop) will favor smoking cessation. Based on the scientific evidence, it is widely accepted that concurrent modalities (smoking cessation aids and behavioral therapy) will support self-regulatory efforts to optimize cessation.

Health Belief Model

The Health Belief Model (HBM) was initially conceptualized in the 1950s by social psychologists Hochbaum, Rosenstock, and Kegels as a method to explain health motivation and the prediction of health behaviors.[10] Origins of the model were based on Lewin's field theory, which explicated the concept of barriers to and facilitators of behavioral change. Becker offered further modification to *the HBM*.[11]

Two major influences from the learning theory was the stimulus response theory and cognitive theory. *The HBM* is a value-expectancy theory that examines intrapersonal psychological antecedents and motivators. Underlying assumptions to the theory posit that individuals desire to avoid illness and seek to adopt a specific health action to support their health. In so doing, readiness to change lifestyle and modifiable risk factors is enhanced. The model proposes that the individual is likely to alter behavior that is inconsistent with health and well-being when he or she perceives that the potential for illness or disease poses a viable threat to health. We can consider the constructs of the HBM using a clinical case scenario.

Mary is a 52-year-old postmenopausal Caucasian female with a past medical history of deep vein thrombosis 2 years ago for which she was given anticoagulant warfarin for 3 months with resolution; no past surgical history; and family history of coronary artery disease and dyslipidemia. NKDA, NKEA, NKFA; medications: ibuprofen (Motrin) 400 mg po every 6 to 8 hours prn for occasional headaches. Mary's mother, Susan, is 74 years old, alive and well with history of diabetes mellitus (DM) type 2. Mary's father, John, died at the age of 47 years from an acute myocardial infarction. Mary presents to the primary care provider today with reports of feeling "twinges" in the center of her chest after walking the dog one city block and when climbing up one flight of stairs to return to her apartment. The chest sensations are intermittent, occur with exercise, and last for several minutes. She has experienced these three or four times this past month. She slows down her pace or alternatively sits down when these symptoms occur, and the symptoms resolve within 2 to 3 minutes. There are no associated symptoms, no lightheadedness, syncope, palpitations, or radiation of the pain to the arm or neck. During the visit, Mary expresses concern that she may be having "heart attack symptoms" like her father experienced the year before his death.

One construct in *the HBM* is **perceived susceptibility**, the belief that the person is susceptible to the condition of risk, such as a myocardial infarction evidenced in the clinical case scenario. Personal vulnerability is inherent to the construct and a prime motivator in seeking medical treatment, deterring symptom presentation, and reducing the risk of future cardiovascular events. **Perceived severity**, a second construct in *the HBM*, relates to cognition and emotion based on the likelihood of developing illness or disease if the condition is left untreated.[9,10,12] Consequent to behavioral action, repercussions may include medical, emotional, or social effects. In the clinical case, Mary cognitively associates the potential severity of her "twinges" to her father's cardiovascular disease and premature death from a myocardial infarction. The combination of her perceived susceptibility to and perceived severity of disease is known as perceived threat.[9,10,12] The third construct, ***perceived benefits***, is based on the person's belief that personal susceptibility to a health threat and subsequent behavioral change will provide a reward, such as reducing the nature of the threat. Mary's health-seeking behavior with the primary care clinician can ameliorate the presence of related symptoms. Given Mary's symptoms, diagnostic testing will be ordered and a management plan constructed to promote her health and reduce her risk of cardiovascular sequelae. Her perceived benefit of improved cardiovascular health is likely to enhance compliance with diet, exercise, and future medication or holistic regimes. ***Perceived barriers***, a fourth construct, represents the individual's own appraisal of factors that prohibit her from constructive change or adopting a positive behavior. Perceived barriers are moderated by the individual's subconscious evaluation of expected benefits versus self-apparent barriers. Janz and Becker consider this construct to be the most influential in determining whether behavior will change in a favorable manner.[11] Modifying variables present in the model influence the major constructs, including educational level, experiences, skill, personality, and demographic variables, such as age, gender, and ethnicity. Demographic, psychological, genetic, and structural features of an individual introduce variability in the model's outcome because individual beliefs and motivation to act are distinct.

The HBM proposes an additional construct, ***cues to action***, which influences behavior by initiating action.[9,10,12] Cues represent triggers that heighten the pace of the person to take action related to his or her perceived susceptibility and benefits.[9,10,12] Examples of cues to action are bodily symptoms, such as, in this case, chest pain, or dyspnea in older individuals, that mitigate their ability to perform instrumental activities of daily living. Other examples include news reports on cardiovascular disease, current trends, or a cardiovascular-related event of a family member or friend. In their study, Katz et al. found cues to action were critical antecedents in renovating attitudinal change.[13]

Self-efficacy was not originally embedded in *the HBM*, rather it was added by Rosenstock, Strecher, and Becker in 1998.[9,10] Bandura regards self-efficacy as an individual's own belief regarding his or her ability to perform the above-mentioned influences that would otherwise affect his or her behavior.[9] These self-perceptions about behavior help to regulate decision making and consequently determine action. In the clinical scenario, Mary exerted health-seeking behaviors to moderate cognitive concerns about her recent chest-related symptoms. She expresses the association between her chest-related symptoms and her father's fatal myocardial infarction in middle adulthood, which is 5 years younger than Mary's present age.

The Transtheoretical Model

The transtheoretical model (TTM)[14] is an integrative model of change that conceptualizes a series of progressive stages inherent to intentional change behavior. The model, developed by Prochaska and Diclemente, proposes core constructs including **stages of change** representing a temporal dimension of decision making (weighting the pros and cons), **self-efficacy**, and **temptations** (intensity of urges).[15] Stages of change are a series of five successive steps of readiness to change behavior, including precontemplation, contemplation, preparation, action, and maintenance. In the precontemplation phase, individuals are not yet ready to change in the near future. Precontemplation occurs either when individuals are uninformed about the need to change their health behavior or when change attempts have not met with prior success, which can lead to a negative self-concept about the ability to change. Contemplation may represent some ambivalence or reevaluation related to the actual change behavior, so thought about change is apparent at this juncture. Once the individual commits to a perceived change of behavior, he or she begins preparations within 4 weeks of time and action will ensue[15] Action occurs once the individual not only commits to the change but also takes an active role in ensuring this course of behavior. The last stage of change is maintenance, whereby the individual has already made the change behavior and needs to be diligent to maintain the goal. Maintenance is the key to guard against relapse of negative behaviors that undermine health. Regression to a previous stage can occur along the continuum and represents a return from action or maintenance.[15] Let us consider a clinical case scenario that explicates the concepts.

Kivon is a nonsmoking 38-year-old African American man who comes to the primary care provider for a 1-month follow-up of his recently diagnosed hypertension and DM type 2. He works as an accountant and is recently separated from his wife with whom he shares a 6-year-old son with autism. Kivon shares coparenting responsibilities with his wife, and they live in nearby residences. They have an amicable relationship since their marital separation and enjoy many social supports including family and friends. Kivon's past medical history includes obesity, hypertension, dyslipidemia, and DM type 2. Past surgical history is a right knee meniscus repair 2 years ago. He has NKDA and NKFA. Medications include metformin, angiotensin-converting enzyme inhibitor (ACE1), and a statin. Since his visit 1 month ago, the primary care clinician discussed with Kivon the need for weight control, exercise, and stress management. At that visit, Kivon said he was thinking about "eating healthier" to care for his son over the long term but realizes this will be a challenge because he does not cook. He states he feels less stressed recently.

According to *the TTM*, Kivon's nutritional goals during the primary care visit last month were in the precontemplation phase. The primary care clinician in this visit readdresses the health behavioral goals, including weight loss, exercise, and proper nutrition, using the dietary approach to stop hypertension (DASH) eating plan.[16] Consciousness raising, an element of the change process, increases awareness about the trajectory of health decisions providing information about consequences to certain behaviors.[15] The key to the clinician-patient communication is first recognizing the phase of readiness to change the behavior of "eating healthier" as prioritized by the patient. There is clear evidence of temporal decision making. In fact, you can hear the patient evaluating the pros and cons of this behavioral change—he wants to care for his son long term, but he does not cook. The patient is moving to the contemplation phase considering his current health status and short-term goal of weight loss. How can the clinician move the communication forward to facilitate the change behavior?

> Clinician: "I hear that you are considering adopting a healthy diet, such as the DASH eating plan, in order to eat and be healthier for your son's continued care. Am I understanding that correctly?"
>
> Patient: "Yes, I've been thinking that this extra weight is not good for my diabetes and heart, and I need to be around to see my son grow."
>
> Clinician: "I agree that healthy eating will help to meet those goals-helping with your diabetes and your hypertension. Is there anything preventing you from starting the DASH eating plan?"
>
> Patient: "Well, no. I don't cook though."
>
> Clinician: "There are many healthy foods that you can consume on the plan, so cooking isn't required. I have a handout of the DASH eating plan. Let's review it together."
>
> Patient: "Okay. I have to read it and then see if I can buy these foods at the local market."

A revision of the management plan may be necessary if the patient is not yet ready to consider the change behavior. However, in this clinical scenario there is contemplation moving toward preparation as the advantages and disadvantages of adopting the healthy eating plan are considered. The next follow-up appointment will be scheduled in 1 month and additional counseling and self-management support provided. At that time, the clinician will review blood pressure and weight loss goals, specifically the adoption of the DASH eating plan to evaluate and increase self-control. Depending on the level of commitment, the clinician may address healthy exercise behaviors next.

Central to *the TTM* is the construct of self-efficacy. *Self-efficacy*, the ability of an individual to have confidence in his or her ability to self-regulate with a situation-specific high-stake health behavior believing that he or she can overcome the behavior.[9,10,15] Although there is no specific evidence of self-efficacy in the clinical case scenario, further patient-clinician discussion is likely to reveal the thought process and confidence to surmount dietary habits incongruent with cardiovascular health.

Underlying assumptions in *the TTM* concedes that behavior change develops sequentially in stages and is a process occurring over time. No single theory accounts for the comprehensiveness of behavior change. Planned interventions are necessary to facilitate change behavior as most at-risk individuals are unprepared to take action or chronic behavior patterns embedded in biopsychosocial processes combined with self-control mechanisms represent barriers to change.[15]

PRINCIPLES OF EFFECTIVE CLINICIAN-PATIENT COMMUNICATION

Effective clinician-patient communication in primary care is critical to unmasking underlying health concerns and comorbidities, as well as developing collaborative action plans sentinel to health promotion and disease prevention. The IOM's Roundtable on Value and Science-Driven Health Care prioritizes that by 2020, evidence-based clinical decisions will support accurate, safe, efficient, and up-to-date clinical evidence that is transparent to its stakeholders.[17] In an effort to support that goal, the IOM convened the Evidence Communication Innovation Collaborative to explore collaborative communication between clinicians and their patients, which promotes shared decision making. Guiding principles are founded upon basic expectations that are essential to promote engagement of patients in their health decisions. These principles include developing communication strategies that guide best evidence and can afford improved health, greater satisfaction, and reduced financial burden.[18] Best medical evidence, such as screening guidelines, clinician expertise, and patients' preferences (i.e., goals or concerns) account for essential elements in this model[18] (see Chapter 22).

Evidence-based guidelines for clinical preventive and health promotion strategies, such as those published by the U.S. Preventive Services Task Force require dissemination. Many of these recommendations not only address primary and secondary prevention but also serve to guide public policy, managed care, quality improvement strategies, and medical research.[19] Communication of these recommendations occurs via social health campaigns in the public sector, as well as between clinicians and patients in clinical practice settings. It is incumbent upon the primary health clinicians to discuss recommendations with their patients in an open and nonbiased manner, advising benefits and risks of adopting certain health promotion and disease prevention strategies. In the light of patients' health status, clinicians present these health promotion options in a professional manner, which respectfully communicates and affirms that the patients' sociocultural beliefs are central to shared decision making. Clinician-patient communication that prioritizes individuals' health behavior, offers counseling, and promotes self-management are paramount. The utilization of strategies that promote adoption of these health behaviors will be further discussed in the context of motivational interviewing and the 5 A's framework.

MOTIVATIONAL INTERVIEWING

A very effective way to foster patients' healthy behavior changes is motivational interviewing, a guiding, person-centered, and relationship-centered style of communication developed by William R. Miller, PhD, and Stephen Rollnick, PhD.

> Motivational interviewing is a collaborative, goal-oriented style of communication with particular attention to the language of change. It is designed to strengthen personal motivation for and commitment to a specific goal by eliciting and exploring the person's own reasons for change within an atmosphere of acceptance and compassion.[20,p. 29]

The spirit of motivational interviewing is founded on core aspects of collaboration, acceptance, compassion, and evocation.[20] Each of these core aspects will be explicated further in the following paragraphs.

Collaboration entails an active partnership between the patient and clinician who work together as two experts to achieve change.[20,21] Motivational interviewing is conducted *with* the patient not done *to* the patient.[20,22] The patient is recognized as the expert on self. The clinician's role is to explore in an interested, respectful, and supportive way the patient's own motivations and resources for change.[20,21] Through collaboration, there is activation and mobilization of the patient's inner resources for change. The clinician is an empathetic facilitator who does not try to manipulate or trick the patient into behavior change.[23]

Acceptance, in the spirit of motivational interviewing, entails four aspects: absolute worth, accurate empathy, autonomy, and affirmation.[20] Absolute worth is unconditional positive regard for the patient, belief in the patient's inherent worth, and respect for the patient as a unique person, as described by Carl Rogers.[24] Accurate empathy is depicted by the clinician's active attention and endeavors to understand the patient's inner perspective and to see life through the patient's eyes.[25] Respecting and honoring patient autonomy is an essential part of acceptance in motivational interviewing. The clinician recognizes and supports the patient's complete freedom and capacity to choose, which in turn decreases the patient's defensiveness and resistance to change.[25] Affirmation, the fourth essential aspect of acceptance, entails exploring, recognizing, and highlighting the patient's strengths and endeavors.[20] It is an intentional lens through which the clinician views what is right rather than what is wrong and needs to be fixed in the patient.[24] Acceptance in motivational interviewing, as described by these four facets, creates a therapeutic milieu for growth and positive behavior changes to transpire.[24]

Compassion, in the spirit of motivational interviewing, is the clinician's "deliberate commitment to pursue the welfare and best interests of the other."[20,p. 20] Compassion is not sympathy or the experience of suffering with another. Compassion underlies the inspirations for clinicians to become health professionals initially and to continue to benevolently and actively promote the well-being and health of others throughout their careers.[20]

Evocation, in the spirit of motivational interviewing, is the intentional act of eliciting, recognizing, and reinforcing the patient's own motivations for healthy behavior change, which are expressed as change talk.[20,21] The clinician recognizes that a patient's ambivalence about changing behavior is a normal part of the process; one part of the patient wants to change, whereas the other part wants to sustain the status quo.[20,21] Often this ambivalence is stated by the patient as a "but," with change talk on one side and sustain talk on the other side of the "but." "I want to eat healthy *(change talk)* but fruits and vegetables cost too much *(sustain talk).*" By skillfully using language that evokes the patient's values, develops discrepancy between those values and the status quo behavior, and elicits and strengthens the patient's own motivations for change, the decisional balance tips in the direction of change. This can be heard during the interview as increasing expression of change talk on the patient's part. In motivational interviewing, clinicians avoid trying to "fix" the problem by advising or telling the patient what to do, because, although well intentioned, this so-called righting reflex often triggers the opposite effect, with the patient defending the behavior and expressing sustain talk.[20,21,26]

> Clinician: "You must quit smoking." *(righting reflex)*
> Patient: "Smoking is the only thing that makes me happy." *(sustain talk)*

Rather, in motivational interviewing, the patient's autonomy is honored, which communicates respect and increases the patient's self-efficacy and confidence in making change.

> Patient: "I know you're going to tell me to quit smoking."
> Clinician: "Only you can decide whether quitting smoking is right for you or not." *(reflection that affirms autonomy)* "What are your thoughts about smoking?" *(open question to evoke patient's own motivations for change)*

The following is another example of a reflection that honors patient autonomy is:

> Clinician: "It's your choice if you change your way of eating now or not."

Key Skills: OARS

As previewed in the previous section, there are several key skills in motivational interviewing that are utilized within the spirit of motivational interviewing to facilitate positive behavior change. **OARS** is a useful acronym for remembering the key skills of motivational interviewing. **OARS** represents asking **O**pen questions, **A**ffirming, **R**eflective listening, and **S**ummarizing.

Open Questions

Open questions are utilized to evoke and elicit the patient's own motivations for change.[20,21] In motivational interviewing, the patient is the expert on his or her behavior and motivations for change. Some examples of open questions include "What are some of the good things about exercising for you?" "Where do you see yourself in 10 years if you don't stop drinking?" "How did you quit smoking in the past?" "What concerns you most about taking medications?"

Affirming

Affirming is a powerful skill in motivational interviewing that reflects recognition on the clinician's part of the inherent positive qualities, goodness, and potential for growth in each person. The clinician notices and then actively affirms each patient's strengths and values. The clinician's positive regard communicates respect, enhances self-efficacy, and broadens the patient's awareness of possibilities and personal merits that may have been previously overlooked.[20] Affirming reflections may be used to positively reframe the patient's behavior, past actions, or current state of affairs. This is particularly helpful if the patient is self-blaming, discouraged, or holds a negative self-image.[20]

> Patient: "I can't believe I started smoking again when my mother got sick. It was the only thing that helped with the stress."
> Clinician: "When caring for your dying mother, smoking helped you through a very painful time. Now, you are focusing on your health and in a better place to quit."

Some other examples of affirming reflections include "You have really been working hard at losing weight." "Spending time with your family is very important to you." "You don't give up, even when the going gets tough." "You want to eat healthy so your children follow your good habits." "You were really there for your brother when he needed you."

Reflective Listening

Reflective listening is an essential skill in motivational interviewing.[20] Reflecting back the patient's evoked change talk through statements that communicate active listening, compassion, nonjudgmental acceptance, and genuine caring is powerfully motivating.[27] Change talk is expressed by patients in different forms. The acronym **DARN CAT** includes change talk expressed as the patient's **D**esire, **A**bility, **R**easons, **N**eed, **C**ommitment, **A**ctivation, and/or **T**aking Steps.[20,21] Examples of **D**esire change talk are "I wish I could stop smoking" and "I want to lose weight." **A**bility change talk examples are "I could go to the gym before work every day" and "I can cut back on how much marijuana I smoke." **R**easons change talk examples are "If I don't stop drinking and driving, I might lose my license or get in an accident" and "I might have a stroke if I don't take my medications every day." Need change talk examples are "I've got to get my diabetes under better control" and "I have to get my kids back." Examples of **C**ommitment change talk are "I will go to a 12-step meeting this weekend" and "I will buy exercise shoes on the way home today." Examples of **A**ctivation change talk are "I am prepared to quit smoking in two weeks" And "I am ready to start a diet." Examples of **T**aking Steps change talk are "I bought a scale to measure my food" and "I got a sponsor from AA."

Reflections can be expressed by the clinician in many ways. Simple reflections paraphrase the person's statements without changing the meaning and can be effective at communicating active listening without judgment when the person is angry or resistant.[20,21]

> Patient: "I wouldn't be here if the court hadn't ordered it." *(sustain talk)*
> Clinician: "Getting treatment isn't your idea." *(simple reflection)*
> Patient: "I wish I could quit drinking *(desire change talk)* but being a stay-at-home mother is really stressful and having a few glasses at night is the only thing that relaxes me." *(sustain talk)*
> Clinician: "Drinking is relaxing." *(simple reflection)*

However, repeated use of simple reflections throughout the interview can be tiresome for the patient and provider alike. Complex reflections go further, hypothesizing or guessing about the meaning of the patient's statements. It does not matter if the clinician's hypothesis is correct or not, as through the process of responding to and clarifying the clinician's guess, the patient's motivations and understanding of his or her behavior are further evoked.[20,21]

> Clinician: "What are some of the not so good things about drinking?" *(open question)*
> Patient: "If I don't quit drinking, I might die young, like my father." *(change talk)*
> Clinician: "You want to live a long and healthy life and be present for your children." *(complex reflection)*
> Patient: "I've smoked for fifty years." *(sustain talk)*
> Clinician: "It's hard for you to imagine what life would be like if you didn't smoke." *(complex reflection)*

Agreeing with a twist is a complex reflection of the patients meaning with additional content added to reframe the patient's assessment of his or her situation and abilities.[20,21,23]

> Patient: "I tried to quit before and always end up drinking again." *(sustain talk)*
> Clinician: "You haven't found the best way to stay sober yet." *(complex reflection that reframes)*

Double-sided reflections include both sides of the patient's ambivalence about changing behavior.

Clinician: "You would like to work out at the gym to lose weight and improve your blood pressure but you can't see how exercise could fit into your busy schedule."

Clinician: "On one hand you know that quitting smoking would improve your breathing and save money but on the other hand, you don't want to gain weight and to be the only one who doesn't smoke at work."

Amplified reflections accurately depict but overstate the person's meaning in an effort to elicit more change talk. The tone of the practitioner using amplified reflection communicates nonjudgmental acceptance and compassion rather than sarcasm.

Patient: "I don't know why my wife is always nagging at me about drinking too much." *(sustain talk)*

Clinician: "Your drinking hasn't caused any problems." *(amplified reflection)*

Patient: "Well, I wouldn't say that. We do fight more when I drink." *(change talk)*

Framing reflections as similes or metaphors is another way to express understanding and empathy.

Patient: "Everyone is on my back about my DUI; my husband, my boss, my kids. I wish they would just leave me alone."

Clinician: "It feels like everyone is ganging up on you." *(complex reflection as a simile)*

Patient: "I try to lose weight and honestly don't eat much at all. My sisters eat so much more than me and they are all skinny."

Clinician: "It's a real puzzle to you." *(complex reflection as a metaphor)*

Summarizing is an important skill in motivational interviewing that communicates active listening and underscores the patients' verbalizations toward behavior change.[20,27,28] Summarizing reflections are given by the clinician intermittently throughout the motivational interview and always at the end of the interview. In summarizing reflections, the patient's change talk, and plan, if already discussed, are gathered and reflected back to the patient by the clinician in the form of a longer statement. Hearing his or her change talk and plan reflected back again is powerfully motivating for the patient, who then has the opportunity to respond to and perhaps clarify or augment what has been summarized. Some examples of summarizing reflections follow.

Clinician: "What you've said so far is that you've been concerned about your drinking for a few months now. You don't like that you've gained weight. You recently let some work assignments slip, which isn't like you. You're fighting with your fiancé when you drink, which makes you feel guilty. And the next day, you wake up with a bad headache, fuzzy thinking, and feel really miserable for a few hours. You're also concerned that the alcohol may be damaging your liver and brain. While you would like to cut back, you aren't sure if you can." (summarizing reflection)

Clinician: "You've been thinking about quitting smoking for some time. Lately it's really on your mind because you noticed that you're more short of breath when you climb the stairs to your apartment which worries you because of your father's history of COPD and continuous need for oxygen. You are also concerned about the cost of cigarettes. Most of all you want to set a good example for your children." (summarizing reflection)

Putting Motivational Interviewing Into Practice

Although motivational interviewing may appear deceptively simple when done by an expert practitioner, learning motivational interviewing is a process that requires not only knowledge but guided practice.[20] The amount of guided practice necessary to learn the integrated set of core motivational interviewing skills and to embody the spirit of motivational interviewing varies. Guided practice includes feedback from an expert coach or trainer based on the direct observation of the learner's motivational interviewing sessions. Direct observation can occur in person, through audio recordings, or through video recordings. Miller and Rollnick[20] recommend that training in motivational interviewing includes initial training through self-study or a workshop, follow-up training with continued guided practice and feedback based on direct observation, and maintenance of skills via further direct observation and guided practice.

FIVE MAJOR STEPS TO INTERVENTION IN TOBACCO USERS—THE 5 A'S FRAMEWORK

Tobacco continues to be the major cause of preventable death in the United States.[29,30] Smokers die an estimated 10 years earlier than nonsmokers.[29] An estimated 70% of smokers want to quit smoking.[29,31] More than 55% of adult smokers tried to quit in the past year.[29,32]

It is therefore vitally important for clinicians to effectively address the behavior change of smoking cessation to prevent illness, disease, disability, and unnecessary death. The U. S. Department of Health and Human Services and the Agency for Healthcare Research and Quality recommend smoking cessation interventions by clinicians based on the 5 A's framework. Similar to motivational interviewing, the 5 A's utilize integrated communication strategies to evoke the patient's own internal motivation for behavior change (smoking cessation), However, the 5 A's contrast from motivational interviewing in that clinicians always advise patients to quit smoking. In motivational interviewing, clinicians offer advice discriminately and only after permission for advice has been granted by the patient, as telling the patient what to do is a potential roadblock for behavior change.[20,21,23,26] However, the tone for advising smoking cessation in the 5 A's framework is still one of empathetic, non-judgmental caring and couched in a collaborative, respectful, relationship-centered approach.

The five A's in this framework represent **A**sk, **A**dvise, **A**ssess, **A**ssist, and **A**rrange. It is very important that clinicians systematically identify all users of tobacco to intervene and treat. In an empathetic, nonjudgmental manner, clinicians *ask every* patient at *every* visit about tobacco use and document the patient's tobacco use status in the electronic health record. For those patients who do smoke, clinicians *advise* them to quit using clear-cut, compelling, and individualized messaging. Clinicians *assess* and document the patient's willingness to quit at every visit.

For patients who are precontemplative to the behavior change of smoking cessation, clinicians utilize motivational statements that roll with his or her resistance. The **5 R's** is an effective framework to motivate patients who are presently unwilling to quit. In this framework, the **five R's** represent **R**elevance, **R**isks, **R**ewards, **R**oadblocks, and **R**epetition.

Clinicians evoke motivation by assessing the *relevance* of smoking cessation for the patient. What does the patient see as effects of smoking relative to his or her health status, disease risks, and current illnesses or diseases? What are the patient's family and social circumstances? Examples may include being smoking parents of children or living, working, or socializing with nonsmoking adults. What is the status of smoking within his or her sociocultural group? What relevance does the patient's age, gender, and other pertinent individualities bear on the importance of smoking cessation for him or her at this time?

Clinicians next ascertain what the patient perceives as his or her *risks* related to smoking to further evoke individualized motivations for change. Where does the patient see himself or herself in 5, 10, and 20 years if he or she continues smoking? What most concerns the patient about his or her smoking? Answers may include acute health risks such as exacerbation of asthma, respiratory illnesses, or infertility or long-term health risks such as cancer, cardiovascular disease, and pulmonary diseases, and environmental risks for those people exposed to the patient's smoke, such as fetuses, infants, children, and spouses.

The clinician should also ascertain what the possible *rewards* of smoking cessation would be for the patient. Asking the patient to voice personal benefits of being tobacco free is a way to evoke more change talk. Economic savings, better taste and smell, improved health, enhanced physical appearance, increased physical activity endurance, greater self-esteem, and being a positive role model for children are all possible rewards the patient may express.

Exploring what the patient perceives as ***roadblocks*** to smoking cessation is another important strategy for success. What does the patient see as impediments to quitting? Roadblocks could include concern about nicotine withdrawal, weight gain, depression, fear of failure, close contact with other smokers, insufficient support for smoking cessation efforts, and lack of other ways to relax or enjoy oneself. Discussing perceived roadblocks and how the patient could best overcome optimizes success.

Repetition of smoking cessation counseling using the 5 R's *every* time a patient is seen increases the likelihood of successful quitting. Repeatedly using motivational strategies when communicating collaboratively at each visit meets patients where they are in terms of stages of change while best optimizing movement forward. Smoking cessation counseling efforts are like seeds planted by the clinician during brief interventions that may germinate when the patient experiences a novel relevant motivation such as a new diagnosis, harmful consequence, or other compelling incentive for change.

Clinicians ***assist*** patients interested in quitting by collaboratively developing a smoking cessation plan. Counseling that includes both behavioral strategies for success and pharmacotherapeutic options, if applicable, are conducted. Encouraging patients to select a quit date, to prepare successfully for that date, to think through and address any barriers that may emerge, and to utilize resources such as the 1-800-quit-now are important assist efforts.

Finally, clinicians ***arrange*** follow-up for patients who have developed a plan for cessation. Optimal follow-up is contacting the patient via a phone call or office visit within one week of the quit date. Topics at follow-up include success so far, discussion of challenges that have occurred since the quit date, reframing of relapses as part of the quitting process, response and side effects to medications, weight gain, depression, and other issues that may have emerged. Ongoing support and interventions, if needed, from the clinician during this pivotal time are instrumental in optimizing smoking cessation success.

For additional information on tobacco use, substance abuse, and weight management see Chapters 9–11.

CONCLUSIONS AND FUTURE DIRECTIONS

The need for clinicians who provide patient-centered and relationship-centered care that effectively addresses patients' health risk behaviors and facilitates positive behavior change has never been more pressing.[33] Chronic diseases account for an estimated 86% of health care expenditures in the United States and are largely preventable.[34] Health risk behaviors, including smoking, excess alcohol use, poor nutrition, and physical inactivity, are major drivers of chronic disease.[34]

Traditionally, payment structures for clinician services incentivized treatment rather than prevention of disease.[35] However, the Centers for Medicare and Medicaid Services[35] is progressively linking health care payments to quality and alternative payment models with an increased focus on population health management.[35] Value-based payment structures, such as fee for performance, support preventive, relationship-centered, patient-centered care, incentivizing clinicians to meet benchmarks for important drivers of chronic disease, such as smoking cessation.

Moving forward, further measurement of the impact that clinicians' relationship-centered, patient-centered communication has on improving health behaviors and health outcomes is needed. Research with diverse and vulnerable populations is a vital priority. Studying the effectiveness of applications of motivational interviewing, which have mushroomed beyond the initial alcohol and substance use foci to all arenas of primary care where healthy patient behaviors lead to better long-term outcomes, is necessary.[20] Because the benefits of health behavior changes are not always evident in the short-term, but rather over the course of patients' lifetimes, long-term, longitudinal research is also called for. In conclusion, although challenging, this is a very promising time for clinicians and researchers alike to effectively endorse styles of communication that promote health and wellness and prevent disease.

REFERENCES

1. Institute of Medicine. *Health and Behavior: The Interplay of Biological, Behavioral, and Societal Influences.* Washington, DC: National Academies Press; 2001.
2. Rosenstock I, Stretcher V, Becker M. Social learning theory and the health belief model. *Health Educ Behav.* 1988;15(2):175-183.
3. Bandura A. Self-efficacy: toward a unifying theory of behavior change. *Psychol Rev.* 1977;84:191-215.
4. Bandura A. *Social Learning Theory.* Englewood Cliffs, NJ: Prentice-Hall; 1977.
5. Bandura A. *Social Foundations of Thought and Action: A Social-cognitive Theory.* Englewood Cliffs, NJ: Prentice Hall; 1986.
6. Center for Disease Control and Prevention, Summary of Youth Surveillance Activities. Division of Adolescent and School Health (DASH). https://www.cdc.gov/healthyyouth/data/pdf/2017surveillance_summary.pdf.
7. Centers for Disease Control and Prevention. Youth Risk Behavior Surveillance-United States 2017. *MMWR.* 2017;67(8):1-114.
8. Bandura A. *Self-Efficacy in Changing Societies.* Cambridge, UK: Cambridge University Press; 1995.
9. Bandura A. Self-efficacy. In: Ramachandran VS, ed. *Encyclopedia of Human Behavior.* New York: Academic Press; 1994. Reprinted in Friedman H, ed. *Encyclopedia of Mental Health.* San Diego: Academic Press; 1998.
10. Hochbaum G, Rosenstock I, Kegels S. *Health Belief Model.* United States Public Health Service; 1952.
11. Janz N, Becker M. The health belief model: a decade later. *Health Educ Q.* 1984;11(1):1-47.

12. Champion V, Skinner C. The health belief model. In: Glanz K, Rimer B, Viswanath K, eds. *Health Behavior and Health Education: Theory, Research, and Practice*. 4th ed. San Francisco, CA: Jossey-Bass; 2008.

13. Katz D, Graber M, Birrer W, et al. Health beliefs toward cardiovascular risk reduction in patients admitted to chest pain observation units. *Acad Emerg Med.* 2009;16(5):379-387.

14. Prochaska JO, DiClemente CC. Toward a comprehensive model of change. In: Miller W, Heather N, eds. *Treating Addictive Behavior*. New York: Plenum Publishing; 1986.

15. Prochaska JO, Velicer W. The transtheoretical model of behavior change. *Am J Health Promot.* 1997;12(1):38-48.

16. National Heart, Lung, and Blood Institute (NIH). *DASH Eating Plan*; 2018. https://www.nhlbi.nih.gov/health-topics/dash-eating-plan.

17. Institute of Medicine. *Value in Health Care: Accounting for Cost, Quality, Safety, Outcomes, and Innovation: Workshop Summary*. Washington, DC: The National Academies Press. doi:10.17226/12566.

18. Alston CL, Paget GC, Halvorson B, et al. *Communicating With Patients on Health Care Evidence. Discussion Paper*. Washington, DC: Institute of Medicine; 2012. http://nam.edu/wp-content/uploads/2015/06/evidence.

19. U.S. Preventive Services Task Force. *Current Processes: Refining Evidence-based Recommendation Development*. U.S. Preventive Services Task Force; January 2014. https://www.uspreventiveservicestaskforce.org/Page/Name/current-processes-refining-evidence-based-recommendation-development.

20. Miller WR, Rollnick S. *Motivational Interviewing: Helping People Change*. 3rd ed. New York: Guilford Press; 2013.

21. Rollnick S, Miller WR, Butler CC. *Motivational Interviewing in Health Care: Helping Patients Change Behavior*. New York: Guilford Press; 2008.

22. Levounis P, Aranout B. *Handbook of Motivation and Change: A Practical Guide for Clinicians*. Washington, DC: American Psychiatric Publishing; 2010.

23. Nair-King S, Suarez M. *Motivational Interviewing With Adolescents and Young Adults*. New York: Guilford Press; 2011.

24. Rogers CR. *A Way of Being*. Boston: Houghton Mifflin; 1980.

25. Rogers CR. *Client-Centered Therapy*. London: Constable; 1951.

26. Rosengren DB. *Building Motivational Interviewing Skills: A Practitioner Workbook*. New York: Guilford Press; 2009.

27. Miller WR, Rollnick S. *Motivational Interviewing: Professional Training Videotape Series*. Directed by Theresa B Moyers; 1998.

28. Hettama J. *Motivational Interviewing Training Video: A Tool for Learners*. Directed by Lawrence L Langdon; 2009.

29. Centers for Disease Control and Prevention (CDC). *Smoking and Tobacco Use: Fast Facts and Fact Sheets*; 2017. https://www.cdc.gov/tobacco/data_statistics/fact_sheets/cessation/quitting/index.htm.

30. U.S. Department of Health and Human Services. *The Health Consequences of Smoking – 50 Years of Progress: A Report of the Surgeon General*. Atlanta: U.S. Department of Health and Human Services, Centers for Disease Control and Prevention, National Center for Chronic Disease Prevention and Health Promotion, Office on Smoking and Health; 2014.

31. Fiore MC, Jaén CR, Baker TB, et al. *Treating Tobacco Use and Dependence, 2008 Update: Clinical Practice Guideline*. Rockville: U.S. Department of Health and Human Services, Public Health Service, Agency for Healthcare Research and Quality; 2008.

32. Jamal A, Phillips E, Gentzke AS, et al. Current cigarette smoking among adults – United States. *MMWR.* 2018;67:53-59.

33. Institute of Medicine. *Crossing the Quality Chasm: A New Health System for the 21st century.* Washington, DC: National Academy Press; 2001.
34. Centers for Disease Control and Prevention, *National Center for Chronic Disease Prevention and Health Promotion.* Chronic Disease Overview; 2017.
35. Center for Medicare & Medicaid Services. *Better Care, Smarter Spending, Healthier People. Paying Providers for Value, Not Volume Fact Sheet;* 2015.

Please see Online Appendix: Apps and Digital Resources for additional information.

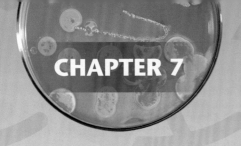

CHAPTER 7

Regular Exercise

LINDA T. GOTTLIEB

INTRODUCTION

The goal of this chapter is to provide current insight into the topic of regular exercise. Its purpose is to update and guide clinicians on how to provide exercise counseling to their otherwise healthy patients; the sedentary person who wants to exercise; the sedentary person who needs to exercise for risk factor modification; and the exerciser who is looking for advice because of injury, burnout, or a need for consultation and reinforcement. This chapter presents a practical guide. It is a compilation based on decades of experience in the field and review of an extensive lay literature on how to effectively offer physical activity counseling. The approach presented in the subsequent text reflects an experience-based consensus on fostering leisure-time, health-promoting, regular exercise, for its own sake.

First Thoughts

Regular exercise provides many health benefits to those who engage in the activity.[1-3] In addition to its direct benefits of muscular strength, flexibility, and cardiovascular health, regular exercise is an essential part of healthy weight management and any effective program to lose weight. The broad public health implications of exercise therefore include its pivotal importance in dealing with the obesity epidemic (see Chapter 9 for more details).

The following definitions apply to the commonly used term *exercise*.

Physical activity is any body movement produced by skeletal muscles that results in a substantive increase over the resting energy expenditure.[1] Activities of daily living fall into this category.

Leisure-time physical activity, another component of physical activity, is an activity undertaken in the individual's discretionary time that leads to any substantial increase in the total daily energy expenditure.[1]

Exercise, another subcategory of physical activity, is a form of leisure-time physical activity that is usually performed on a repeated
basis over an extended period of time (exercise training) with a specific external objective such as the improvement of fitness, physical
performance, or health.[1]

It is important to note that "regularity," exercising on a repeated basis
over an extended period of time, is included in the standard definition for
exercise. *Sessions, workouts,* and *going to the gym* are terms that are used
interchangeably with regular exercise throughout this chapter.

Counseling and Vital Signs

The most recent U.S. Preventive Services Task Force (USPSTF) recommendation on counseling for regular exercise, issued in 2012,[4] states that based
on the current evidence, providing patients (without prevalent chronic
disease) with behavioral counseling pertaining to increased physical activity in primary care will only result in a small net benefit, whereas there
is a higher level of evidence regarding the benefits of this counseling to
patients with cardiovascular disease risk factors, obesity, and abnormal
glucose levels. Therefore, clinicians may choose to selectively counsel
patients rather than incorporate counseling into the care of all adults in
the general population. Other controlled studies suggest that counseling
for regular exercise in clinical practice may be effective in helping patients
to become regular exercisers.[5-7] Whether there exists high-quality evidence
to support exercise counseling in the primary care setting or not, patients
may request advice on how to become more physically active.

It is important to note that there has recently been a strong call for
a physical activity vital sign (PAVS) to be utilized in clinical practice and
added to the patient's health care record. Because physical activity has
been established as having wide-ranging health benefits, and elevated
risk factors for several diseases result from a sedentary lifestyle, it is essential that the clinician assess and stay abreast of the patient's exercise and
physical activity history. Current measures of weight and blood pressure
as well as calculation of body mass index are customary at a patient visit;
adding a question or two about a patient's regular physical activity (added
to their health record) will provide history and may also put the importance of physical activity on the patient's agenda. It is recommended that
in the future, health care providers may review the PAVS and offer one
or two recommendations to patients to help them meet physical activity
guidelines.[8-10]

This chapter does not specifically address the role of regular exercise
in either the treatment or management of diseases or pathologic conditions (such as hypertension), or rehabilitation, although many of the basic
principles for helping any patient to become a regular exerciser would
hold true.

BASIC CONCEPTS IN EXERCISE

Epidemiology of Exercise

Epidemiologic data show that regular exercise promotes general health, whereas its lack, known variously as *physical inactivity* or *sedentary lifestyle*, increases the risk of a variety of diseases and negative health conditions. Building on three generations of foundational work, the fourth generation, *Healthy People 2020*,[3] reinforces its message:

> Research has demonstrated that virtually all individuals will benefit from regular physical activity ... Moderate physical activity can reduce substantially the risk of developing or dying from heart disease, diabetes, colon cancer, and high blood pressure. Physical activity may also protect against lower back pain and some [other] forms of cancer (for example, breast cancer). On average, physically active people outlive those who are inactive. Regular physical activity also helps to maintain the functional independence of older adults and enhances the quality of life for people of all ages.

The 2004 "Best Practices" of the American College of Sports Medicine (ACSM)[11] states:

> Physical activity offers one of the greatest opportunities for people to extend years of active independent life and reduce functional limitations ... A substantial body of scientific evidence indicates that regular physical activity can bring dramatic health benefits to people of all ages and abilities, with these benefits extending over the life span ... and improve the quality of life ...

The position taken in these and many other reports, since exercise science research returned to the medical arena in the 1960s, emphasizes the confirmation that regular exercise leads to prevention and improvement of several chronic diseases. The major challenge remains in how to use our knowledge and understanding to actually help patients become regular exercisers at a level that is both comfortable and useful to them. Because 80% of Americans cite their clinician as their primary source of information about health,[12] sound clinical advice, provided in an appropriate way by clinicians, may help patients unleash their own motivational process to become regular exercisers.

Over the last decade, clinical trials have begun to study the effectiveness of specific leisure-time exercise; however, they prove to be difficult to design and expensive to conduct. On the other hand, there is considerable and growing research on various exercise programs used as therapeutic interventions for the treatment of specific diseases and disorders. Therapeutic exercise regimens (and there are many very useful ones) are beyond the scope of this chapter.

Exercise: Aerobic and Nonaerobic

There are two types of regular exercise based on the level of intensity: "aerobic" and "nonaerobic." Exercise is considered aerobic when it is intense enough to lead to a significant increase in muscle oxygen uptake. Nonaerobic exercise is any physical activity above the normal resting state involving one or more major muscle groups that is sustained but not so intense as to cause a significant increase in muscle oxygen uptake.

(Anaerobic exercise is intense physical activity, necessarily of very short duration [usually measured in seconds], fueled by energy sources within the contracting muscles, without the use of inhaled oxygen, most often incurred in competitive sports. It is not a factor in regular exercise.)

The heart rate is a simple measure to distinguish aerobic exercise from nonaerobic exercise. The exercise is considered to be aerobic when the pulse reaches or exceeds a level of 60% of the theoretical maximum normal, age-adjusted heart rate (220 − the person's age); 0.6 (220 − age). This commonly used formula roughly approximates the true degree of increased oxygen uptake by the muscles[10] and is more accurate for measuring the intensity of exercise in beginners than in conditioned athletes. Most regular exercisers do not routinely measure their heart rate during their workouts, relying instead on subjective measures, such as deep breathing and sweating, to know when they are *in the zone*. Patients who are subject to extreme tachycardia should take their pulse while exercising. To assure that exercise intensity remains at a safe level, the pulse rate should remain below 85% of the person's theoretical maximum age-adjusted heart rate (220 − age).

Although evidence to date shows that exercise must be aerobic or at high levels of physical activity to be most beneficial in reducing long-term risk for coronary artery disease, recent studies demonstrate that exercise at *any* level, even modest changes in physical activity above the sedentary state is associated with reducing all-cause mortality.[13,14] Substantial evidence demonstrates that high levels of physical activity, exercise training, and overall fitness helps with prevention of cardiovascular disease.

Objectives for Regular Exercise

Given the known benefits of regular exercise and the harmful consequences of a sedentary lifestyle, the objectives for the activity can be set out in a straightforward manner. Regardless of volumes of accumulated data about the long-term health benefits of regular exercise, most regular exercisers engage in the activity because of the immediate benefits of feeling good and feeling better about themselves. When counseling patients about regular exercise, it is very important to bear this in mind. Most regular exercisers do not engage in the activity to reduce their risk for future disease. Risk reduction does not motivate most nonexercisers to start exercising either, unless a negative health event such as a heart attack shocks them into appropriate action or they are exercising to promote weight loss. When patients ask about the benefits of regular exercise, the clinician should stress the short-term gains: feeling good, improved personal appearance, and increased self-esteem. The clinician should point out, however, that most but not all sedentary people who become regular exercisers experience these gains. Long-term benefits will also motivate some patients and should be noted.

Risks of Regular Exercise in the Otherwise Healthy Patient

Regular exercise has its risks as well as its benefits. Virtually all of the risks are preventable or modifiable. The most common risk of exercise is injury. There are three types of injuries: intrinsic, extrinsic, and overuse. Intrinsic injury is that caused by the nature of the activity or sport, for example, shin splints in running. Extrinsic injury is that caused by an external factor, for example, a cyclist hit by an automobile. Overuse injury results from exercising too far, too fast, too frequently. The latter is the most common cause of injury in most of the activities and sports used for regular exercise, such as running, fast walking, cycling, and swimming.

Intrinsic injury can be prevented by the use of proper equipment and correct technique. The risk of extrinsic injury can be significantly diminished by taking certain, mainly common sense, safety precautions, such as always wearing a helmet and never wearing headphones while riding a bicycle on the street. Overuse injury can be prevented by choosing a sport along with a workout schedule, including appropriate stretching, suitable to the exerciser, and by maintaining moderation in distance, intensity, and speed. The risk of a variety of pathologic problems is increased when a previously sedentary person engages suddenly in intense exercise or when a regular exerciser suddenly increases exercise intensity. Therefore, moderation and gradual change, if changes are to be made, are as always, good counsel.

EXERCISE AS MEDICINE

"Recommendation" Versus "Prescription"

The term "exercise prescription" has gained greater acceptance since the launch of the Exercise is Medicine (EIM) health initiative coinitiated by the ACSM and American Medical Association in 2007.[15]

The term, when used in the Exercise is Medicine approach, commonly refers to a specific plan of physical activity–related activities that are designed for a patient to meet a specific goal. An exercise prescription is created to address the unique needs and interests of the patient, with goals established to assist in achievement and maintaining momentum.

Some practitioners may not feel the term "prescription" as appropriate because it hails from the disease and medical models and usually means telling a patient to do something for a limited period of time. Regular exercise is by its very nature voluntary. No one can be forced to do it.

Regular exercise requires more than just the temporary extra expenditure of time required to establish most other positive lifestyle changes such as engaging in healthy eating, achieving weight loss, and stopping cigarette smoking. For example, all people spend time food shopping, cooking, and eating. After learning about what changes to make, healthy eating requires only that the time be spent differently. After undergoing smoking cessation counseling and quitting tobacco use, no extra time need be spent again, unless relapse occurs. In contrast, regular exercise requires a permanent commitment of time that would be otherwise spent doing something else. Of course, the maintenance of any successful behavior change requires constant attention for the rest of one's life, to a greater or lesser extent. However, to be most effective in counseling their patients to become regular exercisers, clinicians need to recognize the ongoing time commitment that regular exercise requires.

Because of its special nature, exercise cannot be prescribed exactly like a drug. Rather, the clinician *recommends* the effort to become a regular exerciser. The clinician's goal should be to develop a respectful and supportive partnership with the patients, using advice and counseling to assist them in the decision-making process. The primary need is for the clinician to spend time with patients communicating about regular exercise, recognizing obstacles to success, and equipping patients with the tools to overcome them.

WEARABLE DEVICES AND SMART PHONE TECHNOLOGY

In the past 10 years, a significant trend in consumer wearable devices has emerged, feeding the popular and growing market for self-monitoring of physical activity (mostly steps), sleep, and other behaviors. These tools may offer a powerful opportunity to engage those who wish to track their personal data to optimize health behaviors.[16] It has been established that 7 in 10 U.S. adults track a health indicator. About 60% of those track weight, diet, or exercise routines. When it comes to health apps utilizing smart phone technology, 38% of health app users track exercise, fitness, pedometer, or heart rate monitoring.[17] Clinicians may wish to inquire about these tools with their patients and have discussions around regular exercise statistics acquired by these devices.

GETTING UNDERWAY

Risk Assessment

The clinician should assess every patient before recommending a regular exercise program. There is no single widely accepted or implemented instrument for measuring physical activity in the clinical setting; however, several studies have been initiated to establish PAVS assessments to be used at every patient appointment.[18] Some patients will need a full medical examination (see subsequent text). Many otherwise healthy patients will not. According to the USPSTF, neither a resting electrocardiogram nor an exercise stress test provides information helpful in reducing the risk of an adverse outcome from regular exercise among asymptomatic persons. Although the USPSTF does not endorse them, these tests may be clinically indicated for men older than 40 years with two or more risk factors for coronary artery disease other than sedentary lifestyle. Coronary artery disease risk factors include elevated serum cholesterol, history of cigarette smoking, hypertension, diabetes, or a family history of early-onset coronary artery disease.

Furthermore, the clinician should conduct a thorough clinical evaluation of patients for whom regular exercise presents a *definite* risk, before advising these patients to start exercising. These high-risk patients may have a history of one or more of the following diseases or conditions:

- Previous myocardial infarction
- Exertional chest pain or pressure, or severe shortness of breath
- Pulmonary disease, especially chronic obstructive pulmonary disease
- Bone, joint, or other musculoskeletal diseases or other limitations

These conditions are not necessarily contraindications to regular exercise, but each patient's risk must be assessed on an individual basis.

Patients for whom regular exercise presents *a possible* risk may have a history of one or more of the following diseases or conditions:

- Hypertension
- Cigarette smoking
- Elevated serum cholesterol
- Prescription medication used on a regular basis
- Abuse of drugs or alcohol
- Any other chronic illness, such as diabetes
- Family history of heart disease
- Overweight in excess of 20 lb
- Current sedentary lifestyle

Regular exercise is very useful in the management of a number of these diseases and conditions.[3] For example, regular physical activity has been shown to reduce the rate of progression of diabetes by more than 50%.[19] In fact, regular exercise may be a pivotal force in changing the natural history of a number of disease processes and possibly even obviate the need for therapeutic interventions. As mentioned earlier, the presence of these diseases may well become a motivational factor in convincing a nonexerciser to get started. Regular exercise in high-risk patients is beyond the scope of this chapter. However, it is important to stress that, in initiating exercise, such patients must follow a slow, gradual, and careful regimen with close medical supervision. Referral to qualified health and fitness professionals can offer the patient both supervision and motivation as well as recommendations for appropriate exercise.

COUNSELING

Getting Started

Goal Setting

In most cases, the first subject to discuss with patients is goal setting: why is the patient thinking about regular exercise? It may be because the clinician suggested it, but virtually no one becomes and remains a regular exerciser simply because they are told to do so. To succeed, the patient must mobilize internal motivation. What goals does the patient want to achieve, and why? Specifically, does the patient want to become fit, lose weight, look better and feel better, reduce future risk of various diseases and conditions, or join a friend or family member in a race? In both starting and staying with a regular exercise program, it is very helpful if patients have a good grasp of just why they are doing it in the first place. The same list can be used in the process of motivational interviewing with patients who are not yet prepared to make health-promoting lifestyle changes. Chapter 6 provides additional information about motivational interviewing and also discusses the "stages of change" delineated in Prochaska's transtheoretical model: *precontemplation, contemplation, preparation, action*, and *maintenance* (see page 164). For patients currently in the precontemplation or contemplation stages of change, addressing the questions mentioned earlier may be helpful to patients in advancing to the next stage.

Realism

The clinician should counsel patients to set realistic goals and define success for themselves. A good formulation of this concept is to "explore your limits and recognize your limitations." Consider the example of endurance versus speed. After some reasonable period of training, say 3 to 4 months, most people can improve endurance, but they may not be able to improve their speed. Speed is the product of speed-specific training plus natural ability. Many people will be able to train fairly easily for endurance, because for most people endurance is not simply the product of natural ability. On the other hand, because natural ability is such an important element in speed, many exercisers will not be able to improve their speed no matter how hard they try. Clinicians should stress this point to their patients to avoid frustration, injury, and quitting. On the other hand, if patients are encouraged to explore their limits gradually and carefully, they may discover abilities they never knew they had.

Inner Motivation

As noted in Chapter 6, the literature regarding positive lifestyle and behavior change clearly shows that the only kind of motivation that works in the long run comes from within. The patient says, "*I want to do this for me, because I want to look better, feel better, and feel better about myself, not for anyone else.*" In contrast, a patient who is externally motivated says, "*I'm doing this to make my [spouse, boy/girlfriend, children/parents, employer/coworkers] feel better, but I don't anticipate getting much out of it for me.*" External motivation almost invariably leads to guilt, anxiety, anger, frustration, and quitting and possibly even injury.

Taking Control

"Taking control" is an important concept to stress with patients. In this formulation, patients decide to engage in physical activity on a regular basis, perhaps in a physical activity that they have never done before or even contemplated doing. Many people find that "taking control" of the process for themselves, thinking "yes I can, because yes, *I* can do this" is an important motivator, both in starting a regular exercise program and sticking with it.

Gradual Change

"Gradual change leads to permanent changes" is another basic element leading to success in becoming a regular exerciser, losing weight (see Chapter 9), and making other lifestyle changes. It is recommended that the previously sedentary person should start with ordinary walking, at a normal pace, for 10 minutes or so, three times a week (see Table 7.1). After a couple of weeks, the patient can increase the length of each session. After several more weeks, the patient can increase the frequency of sessions and the speed with which the exercise is performed. The hardier soul may move through this program more quickly, but all should be counseled against going out for an hour, at full tilt at the beginning. "Too much, too soon" may lead to muscle pain, injury, and an increased likelihood of quitting. Once again, a *gradual* increase in time spent, distance covered, and speed are the proven formula for adherence.

Getting Started: "It Is the Regular, Not the Exercise"

Furthermore, the clinician should recognize that, for most people, the first challenge of becoming a regular exerciser is the "regular" and not the "exercise." Indeed, for most people who are regular exercisers, the hard part remains the regular, not the exercise. Most people are aware that exercise is *good for them* and that they will feel better and increase their self-esteem if they begin exercising. Despite these positive reinforcements, most people have busy schedules and other demands that make it difficult for them to make room in their lives for exercise on a regular basis.

			Day					
Week	M	T	W	Th	F	S	S	Total	Comments
1	Off	10	Off	10	Off	Off	10	30	Ordinary walking
2	Off	10	Off	10	Off	Off	10	30	Ordinary walking
3	Off	20	Off	20	Off	Off	20	60	Ordinary walking
4	Off	20	Off	20	Off	Off	20	60	Ordinary walking
5	Off	20	Off	20	Off	Off	20	60	Fast walking
6	Off	20	Off	20	Off	Off	20	60	Fast walking
7	Off	20	Off	20	Off	Off	30	70	Fast walking
8	Off	20	Off	20	Off	Off	30	70	Fast walking
9	Off	20	Off	20	Off	Off	20	60	Pace walking
10	Off	20	Off	20	Off	Off	30	70	Pace walking
11	Off	20	Off	30	Off	Off	30	80	Pace walking
12	Off	20	Off	30	Off	Off	30	80	Pace walking
13	Off	30	Off	30	Off	Off	30	90	Pace walking

TABLE 7.1 The Pace Walking Plan (Phase I: Introductory Program)

Times in minutes.

The correct first step for many patients who are motivated to start exercising is to discover that they can indeed find and make the time in their lives for exercise on a regular basis. They should define success for themselves by setting reasonable goals, recognizing that change will not occur overnight, and placing themselves in control of the process. For most people, the focus of the first 2 to 4 weeks of an exercise program (Table 7.1) should include making the time to exercise and walking instead of learning a new sport or athletic activity.

Patients who live in poor neighborhoods or who have limited resources face special challenges in becoming physically active. They often lack a conducive and convenient place in their built environment or safe surroundings to engage in regular exercise of the type discussed here. Researchers and urban planners are beginning to deal with this important issue.

Duration and Frequency

The original regular exercise recommendation of the ACSM dates back to the early 1980s and stated that for exercise to have a health benefit, it should be performed continuously for a minimum of 20 to 60 minutes at least three times per week. As of 2011, the ACSM recommendation was for

30 to 60 minutes of moderate intensity exercise five times per week or 20 to 60 minutes of vigorous intensity exercise three days per week.[20] They further stated that one's daily exercise can be effectively accumulated in 10 minutes or longer or shorter accumulating bouts. These new guidelines acknowledge the health benefits of shorter bouts of exercise. Some guidelines encourage even greater duration for daily exercise (e.g., 60 or more minutes). However, they are problematic in terms of patient adherence and the heightened risk of overuse injuries. In the tables for regular exercise schedules presented in this chapter (Tables 7.1–7.4), the recommended duration and periodicity are also based on the assumption that the exercise will be done at the aerobic level of intensity.

As previously noted, since the early 1990s it has been recognized that physical activity, even at a moderate level of intensity, can also be beneficial to health. The Centers for Disease Control and Prevention and the ACSM[21] recommended that, for persons not engaging in regular aerobic exercise at the ACSM standard, an accumulated 30 minutes daily of moderate-intensity physical activity (below the aerobic level) should be performed on as many days of the week as possible. The so-called lifestyle approach to exercising regularly includes activities such as ordinary walking, gardening, and

TABLE 7.2   The Pace Walking Plan (Phase II: Developmental Program)

Week	M	T	W	Th	F	S	S	Total
				Day				
1	Off	Off	Off	Off	Off	Off	Off	Off
2	Off	20	Off	20	Off	Off	20	60
3	Off	20	Off	20	Off	20	20	80
4	Off	20	Off	20	Off	20	30	90
5	Off	20	Off	30	Off	20	30	100
6	Off	20	Off	30	Off	20	40	110
7	Off	30	Off	30	Off	30	30	120
8	Off	30	Off	30	Off	30	40	130
9	Off	30	Off	40	Off	30	40	140
10	Off	30	Off	40	Off	30	50	150
11	Off	40	Off	30	Off	30	60	160
12	Off	40	Off	30	Off	40	60	170
13	Off	30	Off	40	Off	50	60	180

Times in minutes.

TABLE 7.3 The Pace Walking Plan (Phase III A: Maintenance— 2 hr/wk)

Week	M	T	W	Th	F	S	S	Total
				Day				
1	Off	Off	Off	Off	Off	Off	Off	Off
2	Off	30	Off	30	Off	40	Off	100
3	30	Off	40	Off	20	Off	40	130
4	Off	40	Off	30	Off	40	Off	110
5	30	Off	40	Off	20	Off	40	130
6	Off	40	Off	30	Off	60	Off	130
7	20	Off	30	Off	30	Off	40	120
8	Off	40	Off	30	Off	50	Off	120
9	20	Off	40	Off	20	Off	60	140
10	Off	30	Off	30	Off	40	Off	100
11	20	Off	30	Off	20	Off	40	110
12	Off	40	Off	30	Off	60	Off	130
13	20	Off	30	Off	30	Off	40	120

Times in minutes.

housecleaning for a minimum of 10 minutes per session.[22] The "lifestyle" approach can help some people get started exercising regularly. Counting and recording short sessions and trying to figure what does and does not "count" as exercise can become confusing and time consuming. Therefore, it is likely that most people who commit to exercising regularly will prefer the leisure-time, scheduled approach. Nevertheless, for some, the lifestyle approach can be a very good way to get started.

Current research continues to emphasize that any amount of regular exercise at any level of intensity is better than no exercise at all. Whatever the recommendations suggest, the amount of time that an individual devotes to regular exercise must fit comfortably into that individual's overall lifestyle, whether it is 2 hours a week or 12. Otherwise, success is doubtful.

Choosing the Activity or Sport

Once the patient deals successfully with the problem of making exercise a *regular activity*, the patient will need to focus on choosing a specific sport or activity. Please see the list of suggested readings at the end of this chapter for details on a variety of sports options. The first point the clinician

TABLE 7.4   The Pace Walking Plan (Phase III B: Maintenance Plus—3 hr/wk)

Week				Day				
	M	T	W	Th	F	S	S	Total
1	Off	Off	Off	Off	Off	Off	Off	Off
2	Off	30	Off	40	Off	30	50	150
3	Off	30	Off	50	Off	40	60	180
4	Off	40	Off	40	Off	50	80	210
5	Off	30	Off	50	Off	40	60	180
6	Off	50	Off	30	Off	50	70	200
7	Off	40	Off	30	Off	30	60	160
8	Off	30	Off	50	Off	40	60	180
9	Off	30	Off	40	Off	30	50	150
10	Off	30	Off	50	Off	40	50	170
11	Off	40	Off	30	Off	50	70	190
12	Off	40	Off	40	Off	50	80	210
13	Off	30	Off	50	Off	40	60	180

Times in minutes.

should stress is that regular aerobic exercise is not limited to running and aerobic dance. There is a wide range of activities or sports that can be used for regular exercise, whether aerobic or nonaerobic.

There are the "tried and true" sports, such as running, fast walking, bicycling, and aerobic dance. These are sports to which most people have ready access at home, where they may even exercise to the accompaniment of a video, internet streaming workouts, or television. Less widely available are activities that often require an athletic facility, such as running and walking on a treadmill or indoor track, swimming, and group exercise classes. Exercise machines, such as treadmills, stair climbers, ellipticals, and stationary bicycles, can be purchased for home use. For cycling, there are compact spin bikes and "indoor trainer" devices on which road bicycles can be mounted for riding in place. Certain individual and team skill sports are often played at aerobic intensity and are useful for regular exercise. These sports include singles tennis, squash, racquetball, handball, and full-court basketball. They require an athletic facility with courts and at least one partner. Weight training, with body weight, free weights, or a machine, can be done at home or in the gym and can also be performed aerobically. As contrasted with weight training for strength and bulk, aerobic routines stress lighter resistance, more repetitions and sets (groups of repetitions) of each program component, and less time between sets to keep the heart rate in the training range. Some health clubs feature "circuit training," utilizing a set of machines and stations offering different muscle resistance levels. Aerobic exercises are performed by participants in a series, following a timed schedule established by a prerecorded set of instructions broadcast in the circuit training room over the sound system, or via virtual screen units.

The choice of sports and activities for regular exercise is therefore very broad. No one sport is "better" than any other sport for regular exercise. The "best" sport or other physical activity is the one that gets the exerciser into a long-term regular schedule while hopefully achieving some level of enjoyment. The heart and muscles do not "know" what sport the exerciser is performing. If the activity increases heart rate and muscle oxygen uptake to a given level, the benefit will be the same, regardless of the sport. For example, pace walking—fast walking with a strong arm swing (see Fig. 7.1)—is equivalent to running if each is done to the same level of aerobic intensity. Pace walking with a strong arm swing at a rate of 11 to 12 minutes per mile is usually as demanding on the cardiovascular system as running 8 to 9 minutes per mile.

After learning the "regular" part by engaging in ordinary walking, it is then time for the patient to choose a sport or other physical activity that he or she will enjoy. In fact, the likelihood of remaining a regular exerciser will be increased if the patient chooses two different sports or activities (e.g., going to the health club once or twice a week for low-impact aerobic dance and pace walking once or twice a week). Once the exerciser is in a routine, the activities can be varied over the course of the year to further decrease the chance of boredom.

Making Exercise "Fun"

When contemplating regular exercise, many patients will say, "*Well, I know I should exercise, but I know it just isn't going to be fun.*" In fact, some people find to their surprise that exercise is enjoyable, in and of itself. For those exercisers whose enjoyment from exercise lie in between, there are some techniques for making exercise more fun. Over the long run, the following techniques may also help all exercisers maintain the fun level:

- Let it be fun: positive anticipation is very important.
- Set appropriate goals, and avoid doing too much, too soon, as discussed previously.
- For the distance sports, train by minutes, not miles (see later in this chapter).
- Recognize that, in those distance sports in which concentration on technique is not required, exercise time is uniquely private and great for thinking. (For safety considerations, road bicycling should not be viewed this way.)

- Listen to music, a book, or podcast through headphones. (Appropriate safety measures must be taken, however. Outdoor use of in-the-ear headphones can block out the sounds of traffic, animals, and other individuals approaching. Rather, sponge phones mounted on the temple in front of the auditory canal should be used. Outdoor cyclists should never use headsets.)
- Set non–exercise-related goals such as getting an errand or two completed in the course of a workout.
- Periodically, reward oneself with a new piece of clothing or a movie night out.
- Enjoy the rhythm, being outdoors, and the seasonal variation that is part of many of the sports done for aerobic exercise.
- Many regular exercisers find that a very useful way to stay on a program and enjoy it is to engage occasionally in racing, not for speed but for participation and feelings of personal achievement in terms of distance covered or time spent. Participating in a fund-raising run or walk for charity can combine personal accomplishment with a way to contribute to the community.
- Be sure to take a week or two off when needed, at least one to two times per year.

Generic Training Program

Tables 7.1–7.4 present a generic training program from the beginning phase through regular maintenance, at all levels up to the training level required for racing on a regular basis. This Physician-based Counseling for Exercise (PACE) program was provided in less than 5 minutes by 70% of clinicians, and most patients reported following the recommendations.[23] Note that the workouts are measured in minutes instead of miles. Time rather than distance is a better way to define the workout because, in the end, what counts is the duration and not the speed: the mental and physical stressor of speed is not a factor for distance sports.

Psychologically, it is much easier to pace walk regularly for 40 minutes at a stretch than it is to cover three or four measured miles. If the person is feeling good and the weather is nice, he or she will go faster and cover more ground. A bit of stiffness on a given day will lead to a slower workout and therefore less distance covered. The benefit of focusing on time is that the workouts can be used for any sport or activity the patient decides to undertake. The minutes formula allows the person to easily mix and match sports or activities in a single program. The periodicity and duration of the sessions comprising the program recommended in these tables are based on the assumption that the person will be engaging in a *regular exercise* program, at a level of intensity eventually reaching the aerobic range. The objective is to help patients become regular exercisers at a comfort level that works for them.

The Introductory Program (Table 7.1) starts with ordinary walking and concludes with pace walking (see page 193 for a brief description of the technique). This program leads up to engaging in 1.5 hours of exercise per week. The Developmental Program (Table 7.2) provides for up to 3 hours of exercise per week. There are two Maintenance Programs: the program in Table 7.3 provides an average of 2 hours per week over a 13-week period, whereas that in Table 7.4 provides an average of 3 hours per week. The latter is the equivalent of 15 to 20 miles of running per week, which is all that is required to gain the maximum health benefits from regular exercise. Musculoskeletal fitness increases with exercise intensity, time, and distance, up to approximately 75 miles of running per week.

As noted, the current (2011) ACSM recommendation encourages working out 5 days per week. The total weekly allotted time for each pace walking program in the tables is distributed over 3 to 4 days per week. Obviously, the suggested times can be redistributed over 4 to 5 days per week, with shorter sessions for each workout. Some stretching after a brief warm-up is recommended. There are books devoted entirely to stretching (see "Resources" at the end of this chapter). Some sport-specific books also contain a section on stretching. Note that, once a 4-day-per-week level is reached, in either phase II or phase III B, more than half of the total workout time is scheduled for the weekends, making the program more convenient for most people. Phase III A is an every-other-day program, requiring an average of only 2 hours per week. These programs provide the framework in which virtually any motivated patient can become a regular exerciser—slowly, gradually, and without the need to make an overwhelming time commitment.

Technique

The clinician need not be a technical expert in the sports or activities suitable for regular exercise. There are many good books written for the layman on the subject (see "Resources" for some examples). If exercise counseling becomes a regular part of the practice, the clinician may benefit from periodic visits to local bookshops and/or the popular Web-based booksellers for an update on available books.

The technique for pace walking (Fig. 7.1), the recommended starting sport, is very simple. The following are sample instructions for the patient.

How to Pace Walk: Walk fast with a purposeful stride of medium length. With each step, land on your heel, then roll forward along the outside (lateral aspect) of your foot, and push off with your toes. Try to keep your feet pointed straight ahead, walking along an imaginary white line. This will help your balance and rhythm and will allow you to increase your speed. Your back should be comfortably straight, but not rigidly so. Your shoulders should be dropped and relaxed, your head up. Swing your arms forward and back, strongly, with your elbows comfortably bent. (The elbow bend prevents the accumulation of fluid in the hands, which will happen if you swing your arms strongly while keeping them straight.) At the end of the back swing, you should feel a tug in your shoulder. On the fore swing, your hand should come up no further

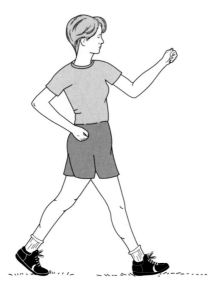

Figure 7.1   Correct pace walking gait and arm swing.

than mid-chest level. To stay in balance and maintain a smooth forward motion from the hips down, concentrate on the back swing, not the fore swing.

For most people, it is the strong arm swing that makes pace walking aerobic. If a person has been completely sedentary for some time, just walking quickly without the strong arm swing will most likely raise the heart rate into the aerobic range. When the exerciser has been working out more regularly, however, walking fast alone will not be sufficient to raise the heart rate into the aerobic range. That is why if walking is to be used as the aerobic exercise on an ongoing basis (and many regular exercisers do so use it), a second major muscle group must be brought into play (i.e., swinging the arms strongly as in pace walking).

Equipment

As with technique, details on equipment can be found in various sport-specific books. Common to most regular exercise sports or activities is the need for properly fitting shoes to achieve success and avoid injury. Proper fit means that the shoe should conform to the shape of the exerciser's foot by touching the foot in as many places as possible, except over the toes. The shoe should be flexible under the ball of the foot, and it should have a firm vertical "heel counter" at the back end of the shoe to keep the heel down in the shoe. The design should be suited to the sport for which it will be used, that is, shoes for pace walking or running should facilitate forward motion, shoes for tennis or aerobic dance should facilitate lateral motion. Referral to a sports medicine orthopedist or podiatrist may be necessary for orthotics or special shoes in patients with a lower-extremity disorder or a known foot deformity such as hallux valgus. In general, a person should be advised to buy equipment in a "pro shop" rather than in a department store. A pro shop is a store other than a sports "superstore" that is dedicated to sports equipment. In general, the more sport specific the focus of the store, the more likely the buyer will come away with suitable equipment. In a pro shop, the buyer is more likely to find salespeople who are knowledgeable about the sport for which they are selling equipment and more likely to actually engage in the sport themselves. Although "good buys" and high-quality equipment can be found at sports "superstores," the quality of the advice received can be highly variable, if available at all. The cost of equipment for the regular exerciser can range from nothing (the person decides to pace walk or jog, and their wardrobe already includes an adequate pair of shoes and the necessary clothing) to hundreds or even several thousand dollars for a health club membership, high-performance athletic shoes, or a top-of-the-line road or racing bicycle. The best recommendation for beginners is to spend as little as possible, except on buying a good pair of shoes if they lack a pair, until they are convinced they are going to stay with the sport.

OFFICE AND CLINIC ORGANIZATION

These principles must be reduced to a counseling package that can be used successfully in clinical practice. First, of course, clinicians must decide whether exercise counseling is important for some or all of their patients. To do that, the clinician should follow the same goal-setting process that the potential exerciser undertakes as his or her first step. It will also be necessary for the clinician to answer the following questions:

- Is exercise promotion important in my practice? Why? For which patients?
- What are the goals, for the patients, the practice, and the clinician?
- Who should do the counseling: medical professionals, staff members, or a referred professional?
- How is exercise counseling going to be paid for?
- Is counseling groups of patients (group visits) a strategy worth trying?
- If so, when will they be offered and under what fee arrangements?
- How should the practice use community resources (e.g., classes offered by health systems and community centers, health clubs, sports clubs, gyms, pools, tracks, bicycle routes, walking or running trails, courts, and pro shops), if at all?
- Are there other resources, such as the Internet or telephone coaching services, which can be used in concert with the clinician?
- Is role modeling important?

- How should I learn the specifics of regular exercise counseling and incorporate them into my own knowledge base and skills?
- How much time am I willing to invest in developing an exercise promotion component in my practice?

It should be noted that asking and answering these questions for oneself, with certain variations to be sure, applies to the consideration of adding any health behavior counseling program/protocol to one's practice. In particular, the list applies to weight management efforts for which a regular exercise component should surely be included. In many practices, group programs for promoting both regular exercise and healthy weight management will be at least in part integrated. Practices face opportunity costs in setting up a group class for every behavior, and therefore some parsimony is required. Although a practice would likely run separate group classes for smoking cessation or healthy sexual practices, an integrated program for exercise and weight management might come naturally because regular exercise is so central to effective weight management and because so many persons who first seek help with regular exercise are trying to lose weight. Indeed, it would make sense for a practice to have an integrated approach to the triad of exercise, diet, and weight management, at least for "beginners." More advanced classes that focus on exercise might be considered for patients going on to higher levels of regular exercise for its own sake and perhaps competitive sports (e.g., racing).

Furthermore, if it is decided to incorporate exercise promotion into one's routine clinical practice, it is worth spending time to learn about and evaluate the various community resources for promoting both regular exercise and weight management. This will save time and provides substantive assistance to patients. The clinician can consider setting up a formal referral relationship with respected community facilities and establishing convenient in-office systems (e.g., fax referral forms, automated referrals using an electronic health record) to facilitate the process. By whatever method exercise counseling is accomplished, the clinician should make it a regular part of the practice and be sure to document the exercise counseling in the patient's medical record. Finally, although not essential, clinicians who regularly exercise themselves can set examples for patients. Such clinicians can draw on their own experiences to counsel patients on the benefits and the drawbacks of being a regular exerciser.

SUGGESTED RESOURCES AND MATERIALS

Organizations

American Academy of Family Physicians
http://www.aafp.org/

EXERCISE – HOW TO GET STARTED

American College of Sports Medicine
http://www.acsm.org/

REDUCE SEDENTARY BEHAVIORS – SIT LESS AND MOVE MORE

http://www.acsm.org/docs/default-source/brochures/reducing-sedentary-behaviors-sit-less-and-move-more.pdf?sfvrsn=4

American Diabetes Association
http://www.diabetes.org/

STARTER WALKING PLAN

http://main.diabetes.org/dorg/PDFs/walking-plan.pdf

American Heart Association
http://www.americanheart.org

GETTING STARTED – TIPS FOR LONG-TERM EXERCISE SUCCESS

http://www.heart.org/HEARTORG/HealthyLiving/PhysicalActivity/GettingActive/Getting-Started--Tips-for-Long-term-Exercise-Success_UCM_307979_Article.jsp#.WmpWra6nGM8

Centers for Disease Control and Prevention
http://www.cdc.gov/

PHYSICAL ACTIVITY BASICS

https://www.cdc.gov/physicalactivity/basics/adding-pa/

National Institute on Aging
http://www.nia.nih.gov/

GO FOR LIFE

https://go4life.nia.nih.gov/

Books

GENERAL

Jonas, S. *Regular Exercise: A Handbook for Clinical Practice.* New York City: Springer-Verlag New York; 1996.

Jonas, S, Phillips, EM. *ACSM's Exercise is Medicine. A Clinician's Guide to Exercise Prescription.* Philadelphia: Lippincott, Williams and Wilkins; 2009.

Thompson, W, Jonas, S, Bernadot, D. *American College of Sports Medicine. ACSM Fitness Book.* Champaign: Human Kinetics Publishers; 2003.

WALKING

Ikonian, T. *Fitness Walking.* 2nd ed.Champaign: Human Kinetics Publishers; 2005.

Jonas, S. *Pace Walking.* New York City: Crown; 1988.

RUNNING

Bingham, J. *No need for speed. A Beginner's Guide to the joy of Running.* Pennsylvania: Rodale Books; 2002.

Brown, RL, Henderson, JK. *Fitness Running.* 2nd ed.Champaign: Human Kinetics Publishers; 2003.

Burfoot, A. *Runner's World Complete Book of Running: Everything You Need to Run for Weight Loss, Fitness, and Competition;* 2009.

Fixx, J. *The Complete Book of Running.* New York: Random House; 1977.

Sheehan, G. *Running and Being: The Total Experience, 2nd Wind II.* New Jersey: Simon and Schuster; 1998. (This is a reissue of this classic work).

BICYCLING

Barry, DD, Barry, M, Sovndal, S. *Fitness Cycling.* Champaign: Human Kinetics Publishers; 2006.

HEART RATE MONITORING

Edwards S. *Heart Rate Monitor Guidebook.* Sacramento: Heart Zones Publishing; 2005.

SWIMMING AND WATER WORKOUTS

Brems M. *The Fit Swimmer.* Chicago: Contemporary Books; 1984.

Katz J. *Swimming for Total Fitness, Updated.* New York: Broadway Books; 2002.

STRETCHING

Walker B. *Ultimate Guide to Stretching and Flexibility (Handbook).* 3rd ed.New York: The Stretching Institute; 2013.

TRIATHLONING

Jonas S. *Triathloning for Ordinary Mortals, and Doing the Duathlon Too, 20th Anniv.* 2nd ed. New York: W.W. Norton; 2006.

WEIGHT TRAINING

Baechle TR, Earle, RW. *Fitness Weight Training.* Champaign: Human Kinetics Publishers; 2005.

SUGGESTED READINGS

American College of Sports Medicine. New Recommendations on quantity and quality of exercise. http://www.acsm.org/about-acsm/media-room/news-releases/2011/08/01/acsm-issues-new-recommendations-on-quantity-and-quality-of-exercise.

Blair SN, Kohl HW, Paffenbarger RS, et al. Physical fitness and all-cause mortality. *JAMA.* 1989;262:2395-2401.

Harris SS, Caspersen CJ, De Friese GH, et al. Physical activity counseling for healthy adults. *JAMA.* 1989;261:3590-3598.

Jonas S, Phillips EM. *ACSM's Exercise Is Medicine™: A Clinicians Guide to Exercise Prescription.* Philadelphia PA: Lippincott, Williams & Wilkins; 2009.

Paffenbarger RS, Hyde RT, Wing AL, et al. The association of changes in physical-activity level and other lifestyle characteristics with mortality among men. *N Engl J Med.* 1993;328:538-545.

Pate RR, Pratt M, Blair SN, et al. Physical activity and public health: a recommendation from the centers for disease control and prevention and the American college of sports medicine. *J Am Med Assoc.* 1995;273:402-407.

Rahl RL. *Physical Activity and Health Guidelines.* Champaign: Human Kinetics Publishers; 2010.

Sandvik L, Erikssen J, Thaulow E, et al. Physical fitness as a predictor of mortality among healthy, middle-aged Norwegian men. *N Engl J Med.* 1993;328:533-537.

U.S. Department of Health and Human Services, Public Health Service. *Healthy People 2020.* Washington, DC: U.S. Department of Health and Human Services, Office of Disease Prevention and Health Promotion. ODPHP Publication No. B0132; November 2010. www.healthypeople.gov.

REFERENCES

1. Caspersen CJ, Powell KE, Christenson GM. Physical activity, exercise and physical fitness: definitions and distinctions for health-related research. *Public Health Rep.* 1985;100(2):126-131.

2. Blair SN, LaMonte MJ. How much and what type of physical activity is enough? *Arch Intern Med.* 2005;165:2324-2325.

3. U.S. Department of Health and Human Services. *Healthy People 2020.* Washington, DC: U.S. Department of Health and Human Services, Office of Disease Prevention and Health Promotion. ODPHP Publication No. B0132; November 2010. www.healthypeople.gov.

4. Patnode CD, Evans CV, Senger CA, et al. *Behavior Counseling to Promote a Healthful Diet and Physical Activity for Cardiovascular Disease Prevention in Adults without Known Cardiovascular Disease Risk Factors: Updated Systematic Review for the U.S. Preventive Services Task Force.* Evidence Synthesis No. 152. AHRQ Publication No.15-05222-EF-1. Rockville, MD: Agency for Healthcare Research and Quality; 2017.

5. Petrella RJ, Koval JJ, Cunningham DA, et al. Can primary care doctors prescribe exercise to improve fitness? *Am J Prev Med.* 2003;24(45):316-322.

6. Elley CR, Kerse N, Arroll B, et al. Effectiveness of counseling in patients on physical activity in general practice: cluster randomized controlled trial. *Br Med J.* 2003;326:793-799.

7. Pinto BM, Goldstein MG, Ashba J, et al. Randomized controlled trial of physical activity counseling for older primary care patients. *Am J Prev Med.* 2005;29(4):247-255.

8. Sallis R Franklin B, Joy L, et al. Strategies for promoting physical activity in clinical practice. *Prog Cardiovas Dis.* 2015;57(4):375-386.

9. Whitehead JR, Franklin BA, Sallis RE, et al. The call for a physical activity vital sign in clinical practice. *Am J Med.* 2016;129(9):903.

10. Blair SN. Physical Activity: the biggest health problem of the 21st century. *Br J Sports Med.* 2009:43:1-2.

11. Wojtek CZ, Buchner, DM, Cress, ME, et al. Best practices for physical activity programs and behavior counseling in older adult populations. *J Aging Phys Act.* 2005;13(1):61.

12. Stafford RS, Alehegan, T, Ma, J, et al. Diet and physical activity counseling during ambulatory care visits in the United States. *Prev Med.* 2004;39(4):815.

13. Paffenbarger RS, Hyde, RT, Wing, AL, et al. The association of changes in physical-activity level and other lifestyle characteristics with mortality among men. *N Eng J Med.* 1993;328:538-545.

14. Gregg EW, Cauley, JA, Stone, K, et al; and Study of Osteoporotic Fractures Research Group. Relationship of changes in physical activity and mortality among older women. *JAMA.* 2003;289:2379-2386.

15. Berryman JW. Exercise is medicine: a historical perspective. *Curr Sports Med Rep.* 2010;9(4).

16. Evenson KR, Coto MM, Furberg RD. Systematic review of the validity and reliability of consumer-wearable activity trackers. *Int J Behav Nutr Phys Act.* 2015; 12:159.

17. Fox S, Duggan T. *Tracking for Health.* Pew Research Center. Pew Internet & American Life Project; 2013. http://www.pewinternet.org/2013/01/28/tracking-for-health/.

18. Greenwood JLJ, Joy EA, Stanford, JB. The physical activity vital sign: a primary care tool to guide counseling for obesity. *J Phys Act Health.* 2010;7:571-576.

19. Diabetes Prevention Program Research Group. Reduction in the incidence of type 2 diabetes with lifestyle intervention or metformin. *N Engl J Med.* 2002;346: 393-403.

20. Garber CE, Blissmer B, Deschenes MR, et al. Position stand: quantity and quality of exercise for developing and maintaining cardiorespiratory, musculoskeletal, and neuromotor fitness in apparently healthy adults: guidance for prescribing exercise. *Med Sci Sports Exerc.* 2011;43(7) 1334-1359.

21. Pate RR, Pratt M, Blair SN, et al. Physical activity and public health: a recommendation from the centers for disease control and prevention and the American college of sports medicine. *J Am Med Assoc.* 1995;273:402-407.

22. Fogelholm M, Suni, J, Rinne, M, et al. Physical activity pie: a graphical representation integrating recommendations for fitness and health. *J Phys Act Health.* 2005;2(4):391-396.

23. Long BJ, Calfas KJ, Wooten W, et al. A multisite field test of the acceptability of physical activity counseling in primary care: project PACE. *Am J Prev Med.* 1996;12(2):73-81.

⊕ Please see Online Appendix: Apps and Digital Resources for additional information.

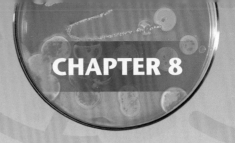

CHAPTER 8

Nutrition

LISA KIMMEL

BACKGROUND

The goal of this chapter is to provide evidence-based information to help clinicians counsel patients regarding the latest nutritional approaches to disease prevention and health promotion. It also attempts to clarify the strong relationships between nutrition and the prevention of chronic disease and the important influence of nutrient deficiencies and excesses.

For a large majority of the population, the food choices made daily, over time, will either benefit or impair health. Food choices and habits are very complex and personal issues that reflect preferences developed through association with family and friends, as well as habits developed through one's culture, traditions, ethnicity, religion, and social interactions. Food is used for celebrations of all aspects of life and therefore can serve as "comfort foods," especially at emotionally stressful times. In the current rushed environment, the availability, convenience, and economy of food often sway personal choices. Individuals select foods for a variety of reasons, but the diet ingested over time can make important contributions to health.

Nutrient effects are a common thread that run through many of the chronic diseases that affect populations. Consuming a diet high in refined carbohydrates and fat, along with a low-fiber intake, high caloric density, low nutrient density, and inadequate physical activity, are common risk factors for cardiovascular disease, diabetes, obesity, and hypertension among other diseases and negative health conditions. As discussed in Chapter 9, the prevalence of overweight and obesity is increasing in the United States, which in turn increases the risk of many chronic diseases (e.g., hypertension, diabetes, and some forms of cancer) and of premature death. See Chapter 9 for further details on the assessment and treatment of overweight and obesity.

According to the Academy of Nutrition and Dietetics Position Statement on the role of nutrition in health promotion and chronic disease prevention[1]:

> …primary prevention is the most effective and affordable method to prevent chronic disease and that dietary intervention positively impacts health outcomes across the life span.

This chapter focuses on the components of a healthy diet throughout the lifecycle. It includes a practical discussion of the influence of macronutrients, vitamins, and minerals upon health, with special emphasis on nutrition's effect on lipoproteins, blood pressure, and diabetes. Chapter 6 discusses the important role of physical activity, which must generally be combined with the nutrition interventions discussed here to promote well-being and weight maintenance.

NUTRITION SCREENING AND ASSESSMENT

Nutrition Screening

Nutrition screening is the process of differentiating those at high risk for nutrition problems who would benefit from a comprehensive nutrition assessment and intervention by qualified health care professional, such as a registered dietitian (RD). Screening can be conducted in any practice setting as appropriate with tools that are easy to use, valid, and reliable for the patient population or setting.[2]

Nutrition Screening of Older Adults

Although routinely conducted in an inpatient setting, a comprehensive nutrition-focused physical examination and the use of nutrition screening tools, particularly for seniors, can be utilized in an outpatient setting to identify individuals who are at nutritional risk and need further intervention. The Nutrition Screening Initiative, a project of the American Academy of Family Physicians, Academy of Nutrition and Dietetics, and the National Council on Aging, is targeted for identifying elderly individuals who are at nutritional risk. The "Determine Your Nutrition Health" checklist uses the mnemonic D-E-T-E-R-M-I-N-E, which includes a list of warning signs for malnutrition that should be addressed (see Tables 8.1 and 8.2).

Subjective Global Assessment

The Subjective Global Assessment of Nutritional Status (see Table 8.3) does not employ objective biochemical and anthropometric measurements. It is a screening tool that requires clinical judgment to interpret information collected by interviews and observations. The instrument correlates well with other more objective measures and is cost-effective.[3]

Nutrition Assessment

Nutrition assessment involves a comprehensive, detailed assessment (anthropometric, biochemical, clinical, and dietary) and physical

TABLE 8.1   Checklist to Help Older Adults Assess Their Nutritional Health

The warning signs of Poor Nutritional health are often overlooked

	Yes
I have an illness or condition that made me change the kind and/or amount of food I eat	2
I eat fewer than two meals per day	3
I eat few fruits or vegetables, or milk products	2
I have three or more drinks of beer, liquor, or wine almost every day	2
I have tooth or mouth problems that make it hard for me to eat	2
I do not always have enough money to buy the food I need	4
I eat alone most of the time	1
I take three or more different prescribed or over-the-counter drugs a day	1
Without wanting to, I have lost or gained 10 lb in the last 6 mo	2
I am not physically able to shop, cook, and/or feed myself	2
	Total

Total your nutritional score. If it is:

0–2	**Good!** Recheck your nutritional score in 6 mo
3–5	**You are at moderate nutritional risk.** See what can be done to improve your eating habits and lifestyle. Your area's office on aging, senior nutrition program, senior citizens center, or health department can help. Recheck your nutritional score in 3 mo
6 or more	**You are at high nutritional risk.** Bring this checklist the next time you see your doctor, dietician, or other qualified health or social service professional. Talk with them about any problems you may have. Ask for help to improve your nutritional health

Remember that warning signs suggest risk but do not represent diagnosis of any condition.

The "Determine Your Nutritional Health" checklist was developed by the Nutrition Screening Initiative, a project of the American Academy of Family Physicians, the American Dietetic Association, and the National Council on the Aging, Inc. Firstpublished: June 1998. Revised: April 2005.

examination to diagnose patients with malnutrition; however, it is too time consuming to complete this process during a clinician visit. Using one of the aforementioned screening tools is a feasible alternative to identify at-risk patients. Patients identified as being at risk for malnutrition by nutrition screening can then undergo a comprehensive nutrition assessment by an RD to confirm the diagnosis. Many RDs are also trained to conduct nutrition-focused physical examinations, assessing for muscle or subcutaneous fat loss,

TABLE 8.2   D-E-T-E-R-M-I-N-E Checklist to Help Older Adults Identify Symptoms of Nutritional Problems

The nutrition checklist is based on the warning signs described below. Use the word D-E-T-E-R-M-I-N-E to remind you of the warning signs

☐ *Disease* Any disease, illness, or chronic condition that causes you to change the way you eat, or makes it hard for you to eat, puts your nutritional health at risk. Four of five adults have chronic diseases that are affected by diet. Confusion or memory loss that keeps getting worse is estimated to affect one of five or more of older adults. This can make it hard to remember what, when, or if you have eaten. Feeling sad or depressed, which happens to about one in eight older adults, can cause big changes in appetite, digestion, energy level, weight and well-being

☐ *Eating poorly* Eating too little and eating too much both lead to poor health. Eating the same foods day after day or not eating fruit, vegetables, and milk products daily will also cause poor nutritional health. One in five adults skip meals daily. Only 13% of adults eat the minimum amount of fruit and vegetables needed. One in four older adults drink too much alcohol. Many health problems become worse if you drink more than one or two alcoholic beverages per day

☐ *Tooth loss/mouth pain* A healthy mouth, teeth, and gums are needed to eat. Missing, loose, or rotten teeth or dentures that do not fit well or cause mouth sores make it hard to eat

☐ *Economic hardship* As many as 40% of older Americans have incomes of less than $6,000 per year. Having less—or choosing to spend less—than $25–$30 per week for food makes it very hard to get the foods you need to stay healthy

☐ *Reduced social contact* One-third of all older people live alone. Being with people daily has a positive effect on morale, well-being, and eating

☐ *Multiple medicines* Many older Americans must take medicines for health problems. Almost half of older Americans take multiple medicines daily. Growing old may change the way we respond to drugs. The more medicines you take, the greater the chance of side effects, such as increased or decreased appetite, change in taste, constipation, weakness, drowsiness, diarrhea, nausea, and others. Vitamins or minerals, when taken in large doses, act like drugs and can cause harm. Alert your doctor to everything you take

☐ *Involuntary weight loss/gain* Losing or gaining a lot of weight when you are not trying to do so is an important warning sign that must not be ignored. Being overweight or underweight also increases your chance of poor health

☐ *Needs assistance in self-care* Although most older people are able to eat, one of every five has trouble walking, shopping, or buying and cooking food, especially as they get older

☐ *Elderly, age above 80 yr* Most older people lead full productive lives. But as age increases, the risk of frailty and health problems increases. Checking your nutritional health regularly makes good sense

Adapted from materials developed by the Nutrition Screening Initiative. Washington, DC; 2007.

TABLE 8.3 Subjective Global Assessment Summary

History

1. Weight change

   Overall loss in past 6 mo: amount = _____ kg _____%

   Change in past 2 wk: _____ increase

   _____ no change

   _____ decrease

2. Dietary intake change (relative to normal)

   _____ no change

   _____ change

   Duration: _____ wk

   Type: _____ suboptimal solid diet

   _____ full liquid diet

   _____ hypocaloric liquids

   _____ starvation

3. Gastrointestinal symptoms (persisting for >2 wk)

   _____ none _____ nausea _____ vomiting _____ diarrhea _____ anorexia

4. Functional capacity

   _____ no dysfunction (e.g., full capacity)

   _____ dysfunction

   Duration: _____ wk

   Type: _____ working suboptimally

   _____ ambulatory

   _____ bedridden

Physical Examination

For each trait, specify a rating as follows:

0 = normal, 1+ = mild, 2+ = moderate, 3+ = severe

_____ loss of subcutaneous fat (triceps, chest)

_____ muscle wasting (quadriceps, deltoids)

_____ ankle edema

_____ sacral edema

_____ ascites

(Continued)

TABLE 8.3   Subjective Global Assessment Summary   (Continued)
Subjective Global Assessment Rating (select one)
_____ A = well nourished
_____ B = moderately (or suspected of being) malnourished
_____ C = severely malnourished

From Detsky AS, McLaughlin JR, Baker JP, et al. What is subjective global assessment? *J Parent Ent Nutr.* 1987;11(1):8.

localized or generalized fluid accumulation, or decrease in functional status. Chapter 3 discusses screening and exploratory questions that clinicians can use in the periodic health examination to quickly assess a patient's dietary habits. A nutrition history should include the following:

- Sample 24-hour food recall
- Food preferences, intolerances, allergies, altered taste perceptions, and so on
- Changes in weight and muscle mass
- Symptoms and alterations in the ability to consume an adequate intake (e.g., anorexia, early satiety, diarrhea)
- Intake of nutritional products, vitamin, mineral and herbal supplements, and alternative agents

Anthropometric Assessments

See Chapter 4 regarding the measurement of height and weight to calculate the body mass index (BMI). Waist circumference is also recommended to assess abdominal obesity in overweight and obese adults.[4] A waist circumference of ≥40 in (102 cm) for men and ≥35 in (88 cm) for women is considered elevated and indicative of increased cardiometabolic risk. A waist circumference measurement is unnecessary in patients with BMI >35 kg/m², as almost all individuals in this BMI range also have an abnormal waist circumference and are already at a high risk from their adiposity.

THE IMPORTANCE OF NUTRITION COUNSELING

A clinician's advice on nutrition is of great importance in helping patients to modify dietary practices. This section provides guidance, but the science of healthy living needs to be made practical and sustainable for patients. The U.S. Preventive Services Task Force recommends *"that primary care professionals individualize the decision to offer or refer adults without obesity who do not have hypertension, dyslipidemia, abnormal blood glucose levels, or diabetes to behavioral counseling to promote a healthful diet and physical activity. Existing evidence indicates a positive but small benefit of behavioral counseling for the prevention of CVD in the population. Persons who are interested and ready to make behavioral changes may be more likely to benefit from behavioral counseling."*[5]

Adopting a healthy diet can be simple but is not always easy. There is no one educational technique that works best for all patients. Choosing the best strategy requires an understanding of the patient's current knowledge and practices, learning needs, literacy, motivation, interest in meal planning, and readiness to change. Using motivational interviewing and asking questions such as, "How ready do you feel to change your eating patterns and/or lifestyle behaviors?" allows for an interactive discussion and enhances self-efficacy and personal control for behavior change.

Patients can easily become discouraged when they attempt to change too many eating habits at once. Clinicians can advocate small steps, such as adding one fruit or vegetable to a meal or replacing sugar-sweetened beverages with water, and remind them that healthy living is not defined by perfection. Success is not dependent on a single meal or day but the accumulation of small changes that become habits over time. Table 8.4 includes actionable behavioral steps for a healthy diet.

TABLE 8.4 Behavioral Strategies for a Healthy Diet
Food Preparation
Preplan meals Learn to cook Include high-volume, low-calorie foods at each meal Show when you are not hungry and have a list
Mealtime
Preload your stomach with calorie-free liquids, such as water, and drink throughout your meal Fill half your plate with vegetables and fruit and split the other half between a lean protein and whole grain Use smaller plates, bowls, glasses, and serving utensils Keep serving dishes off of the table Put your utensils down while you're chewing Leave a little food on your plate
Snacking
Build balanced snacks with lean protein, whole grains, and heart healthy fats Preplan snacks into your eating plan Keep tempting foods out of the house, out of reach, or store in opaque containers Ask family and friends for support and not offer you extra food
Emotional and Stress Eating
Practice mindful eating, breath, meditate HALT: Ask yourself if you are Hungry, Angry, Lonely, or Tired. If you note that you are not hungry, pay attention to what you really need Be kind to yourself If you eat for emotional or stress reasons, do not beat yourself up. Learn from it and make a plan to change the behavior next time

Dietary Reference Intake and Dietary Guidelines for Americans

The Institute of Medicine (IOM) and Health Canada developed the Dietary Reference Intakes (DRIs), which are a set of nutrient reference values related to both adequate and upper levels of intakes. Since July 1, 2015, the National Academies of Sciences, Engineering, and Medicine have continued the consensus studies and convening activities previously carried out by the IOM. The DRIs are based on scientific relationships between nutrient intake, chronic disease, and health status. They provide the scientific basis for the development of food guidelines in the United States and Canada.[6]

Every 5 years, the U.S. Departments of Health and Human Services (HHS) and Agriculture (USDA) publish a joint report containing nutritional and dietary information and guidelines for the general public. The 2015–2020 Dietary Guidelines for Americans provide evidence-based nutritional guidance for ages 2 years and older with the goals of inspiring individuals to seek more information about healthy eating, communicating scientifically accurate but understandable information, and guiding federal policy and programs.[7] The eighth edition's five overarching guidelines acknowledge that a healthy eating pattern exists within an adaptable framework where food can be enjoyed and fit within one's budget. It is not a rigid prescription, rather a personalized approach that embodies personal, cultural, and traditional preferences. Clinicians can access the 2015–2020 Toolkit, which compiles the latest evidence-based nutrition and physical activity recommendations. https://health.gov/dietaryguidelines/2015/resources.asp.

The Guidelines:

Follow a healthy eating pattern across the life span.

All foods and beverage choices matter. Choose a healthy eating pattern at an appropriate calorie level to help achieve and maintain a healthy body weight, support nutrient adequacy, and reduce the risk of chronic disease.

Focus on variety, nutrient density, and amount.

To meet nutrient needs within calorie limits, choose a variety of nutrient-dense foods across and within all food groups in recommended amounts.

Limit calories from added sugars and saturated fats and reduce sodium intake.

Consume an eating pattern low in added sugars, saturated fats, and sodium. Cut back on foods and beverages higher in these components to amounts that fit within healthy eating patterns.

Shift to healthier food and beverage choices.

Choose nutrient-dense foods and beverages across and within all food groups in place of less healthy choices. Consider cultural and personal preferences to make these shifts easier to accomplish and maintain.

Support healthy eating patterns for all.

Everyone has a role in helping to create and support healthy eating patterns in multiple settings nationwide, from home to schools to work to communities.

Taken from the Office of Disease Prevention and Health Promotion. The full document is available at https://health.gov/dietaryguidelines/2015/guidelines/.

Key Recommendations

Key recommendations provide practical guidance on how individuals can implement the five guidelines. Understanding the following key terms is essential to operationalizing the principles and recommendations.

Eating pattern: *"The combination of foods and beverages that constitute an individual's complete dietary intake over life. May describe a customary way of eating or a combination of foods recommended for consumption."*

Nutrient dense: *"A characteristic of foods and beverages that provide vitamins, minerals and other substances that contribute to adequate nutrient intakes or may have positive health effects, with little or no solid fats and added sugars, refined starches and sodium."*

Variety: *"A diverse assortment of foods and beverages across and within all food groups and subgroups selected to fulfill the recommended amounts without exceeding the limits for calories and other dietary components."*

Acknowledging that foods and nutrients are consumed in combination and not in isolation, key recommendation for healthy eating patterns should be applied in their entirety.

A key theme in the guidelines is the consumption of a healthy eating pattern that accounts for all foods and beverages within an appropriate calorie level. This can be accomplished by including the following:

- A variety of vegetables, including dark green, red, and orange, starchy (sweet potatoes), and other
- Fruits, especially whole
- Grain, with at least half being whole
- Fat-free and low-fat dairy, including milk, yogurt, cheese, and/or fortified soy beverages
- A variety of lean protein foods, including seafood, lean meats and poultry, legumes (beans and peas), nuts, seeds, and soy products
- Unsaturated fats

Healthy eating patterns limit saturated and trans fats, added sugar, and sodium:

- Consume less than 10% of calories per day from added sugar.
- Consume less than 10% of calories per day from added saturated fats.

- Consume less than 2300 mg of sodium per day.
- If alcohol is consumed, it should be done so in moderation—up to one drink a day for women and up to two drinks a day for men, both of legal drinking age.

Tools such as Choose My Plate (https://www.choosemyplate.gov/) are available for translating these recommendations into practical meals for patients of all ages. Printable materials are also available on a variety of topics including eating on a budget, dining out, and meal planning (https://www.choosemyplate.gov/printable-materials) (Fig. 8.1). Figure 8.2 is an example of daily serving recommendations for a 2000-calorie diet.

General Healthful Diet

Building off of the Dietary Guidelines and DRIs, a general healthful diet can be individualized to meet the needs of patients with a variety of diseases or conditions, such as diabetes, cardiovascular disease, and obesity. It can also be used as part of an eating pattern intended for chronic disease prevention.

Caloric Balance

The maintenance of caloric balance over time is critical for maintaining a healthy weight. Excess caloric intake leading to overweight and obesity is the single most important dietary factor associated with poor health outcomes, including premature mortality and an increased incidence of chronic conditions such as cardiovascular disease, diabetes, and hypertension and cancer. Overconsumption continues to be a public health challenge. Balancing caloric intake requires awareness of calories consumed and expended during physical activity. Adhering to a nutrient-dense diet pattern that leads to healthy weight maintenance is critical for meeting food-based dietary recommendations. Calculations for daily caloric intake are based on age, sex, weight, and activity level. The My Plate Checklist Calculator is a useful tool for assessing caloric needs and daily recommended servings from each food group. https://www.choosemyplate.gov/MyPlate-Daily-Checklist-input.

Macronutrients

Macronutrients, carbohydrates, protein, and fat are the compounds that provide the majority of energy in the diet. General guidelines for incorporating each macronutrient into the diet are summarized in the following discussion.

Carbohydrates. Carbohydrates should provide 45% to 65% of total daily calories and should emphasize complex carbohydrates that include dietary fiber. Carbohydrates come from a variety of food sources. The quantity, type, and combination with other macronutrients have differential effects on postprandial glucose levels (i.e., whole grain versus refined grain). Starch and sugar contribute the major types of carbohydrates. Grains and

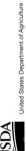

United States Department of Agriculture

MyPlate Plan

Find your Healthy Eating Style

Everything you eat and drink matters. Find your healthy eating style that reflects your preferences, culture, traditions, and budget—and maintain it for a lifetime! The right mix can help you be healthier now and into the future. The key is choosing a variety of foods and beverages from each food group—*and making sure that each choice is limited in saturated fat, sodium, and added sugars.* Start with small changes—"MyWins"—to make healthier choices you can enjoy.

Food Group Amounts for 2,000 Calories a Day

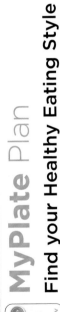
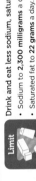

Fruits	Vegetables	Grains	Protein	Dairy
2 cups	**2 1/2 cups**	**6 ounces**	**5 1/2 ounces**	**3 cups**
Focus on whole fruits	Vary your veggies	Make half your grains whole grains	Vary your protein routine	Move to low-fat or fat-free milk or yogurt
Focus on whole fruits that are fresh, frozen, canned, or dried.	Choose a variety of colorful fresh, frozen, and canned vegetables—make sure to include dark green, red, and orange choices.	Find whole-grain foods by reading the Nutrition Facts label and ingredients list.	Mix up your protein foods to include seafood, beans and peas, unsalted nuts and seeds, soy products, eggs, and lean meats and poultry.	Choose fat-free milk, yogurt, and soy beverages (soy milk) to cut back on your saturated fat.

Limit Drink and eat less sodium, saturated fat, and added sugars. Limit:

- Sodium to **2,300 milligrams** a day.
- Saturated fat to **22 grams** a day.
- Added sugars to **50 grams** a day.

Be active your way: Children 6 to 17 years old should move **60 minutes** every day. Adults should be physically active at least **2 1/2 hours** per week.

Figure 8.1 Myplate plan: find your healthy eating style. Taken from the Office of Disease Prevention and Health Promotion (ODPHP). Available at https://choosemyplate-prod.azureedge.net/sites/default/files/myplate/checklists/MyPlatePlan_2000cals_Age14plus.pdf.

MyPlate Plan

Write down the foods you ate today and track your daily MyPlate, MyWins!

Food group targets for a 2,000 calorie* pattern are:	Write your food choices for each food group	Did you reach your target?
Fruits **2 cups** 1 cup of fruits counts as • 1 cup raw or cooked fruit; or • 1/2 cup dried fruit; or • 1 cup 100% fruit juice.		Y N
Vegetables **2 1/2 cups** 1 cup vegetables counts as • 1 cup raw or cooked vegetables; or • 2 cups leafy salad greens; or • 1 cup 100% vegetable juice.		Y N
Grains **6 ounce equivalents** 1 ounce of grains counts as • 1 slice bread; or • 1 ounce ready-to-eat cereal; or • 1/2 cup cooked rice, pasta, or cereal.		Y N
Protein **5 1/2 ounce equivalents** 1 ounce of protein counts as • 1 ounce lean meat, poultry, or seafood; or • 1 egg; or • 1 Tbsp peanut butter; or • 1/4 cup cooked beans or peas; or • 1/2 ounce nuts or seeds.		Y N
Dairy **3 cups** 1 cup of dairy counts as • 1 cup milk; or • 1 cup yogurt; or • 1 cup fortified soy beverage; or • 1 1/2 ounces natural cheese or 2 ounces processed cheese.		Y N

Limit:
• Sodium to **2,300 milligrams** a day.
• Saturated fat to **22 grams** a day.
• Added sugars to **50 grams** a day.

Y N

Be active your way:
Adults:
• Be physically active at least 2 1/2 hours per week.

Children 6 to 17 years old:
• Move at least **60 minutes** every day.

Y N

MyWins   Track your MyPlate, MyWins

_____

_____

* This 2,000 calorie pattern is only an estimate of your needs. Monitor your body weight and adjust your calories if needed.

Center for Nutrition Policy and Promotion
January 2016
USDA is an equal opportunity provider and employer.

Figure 8.2A   Myplate plan. Taken from the Office of Disease Prevention and Health Promotion (ODPHP). Available at https://choosemyplate-prod.azureedge.net/sites/default/files/myplate/checklists/MyPlatePlan_2000cals_Age14plus.pdf.

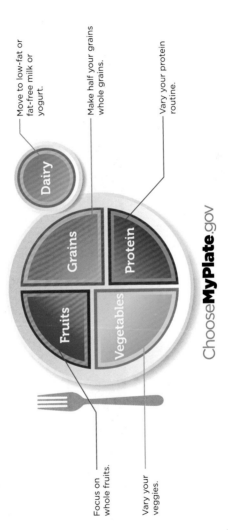

MyPlate, MyWins: Make it yours

Find your healthy eating style. Everything you eat and drink over time matters and can help you be healthier now and in the future.

Move to low-fat or fat-free milk or yogurt.

Make half your grains whole grains.

Vary your protein routine.

Focus on whole fruits.

Vary your veggies.

Choose**MyPlate**.gov

Limit the extras.
Drink and eat beverages and food with less sodium, saturated fat, and added sugars.

Create 'MyWins' that fit your healthy eating style.
Start with small changes that you can enjoy, like having an extra piece of fruit today.

United States Department of Agriculture

Figure 8.2B MyPlate, MyWins. Taken from the Office of Disease Prevention and Health Promotion (ODPHP). Available at https://choosemyplate-prod.azureedge.net/sites/default/files/printablematerials/mini_poster.pdf.

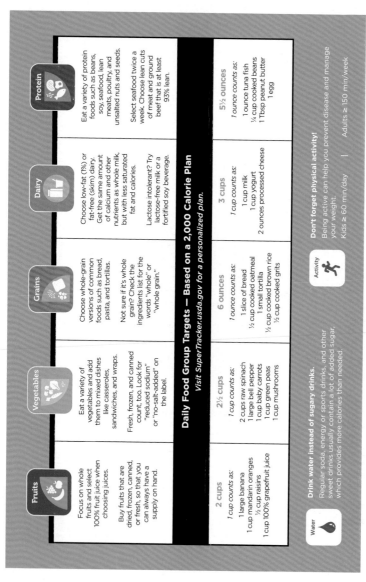

Figure 8.2C Daily food group targets. Taken from the Office of Disease Prevention and Health Promotion (ODPHP). Available at https://choosemyplate-prod.azureedge.net/sites/default/files/printablematerials/mini_poster.pdf.

some vegetables (corn, peas, potatoes) are sources of starch. Natural sugars are found in fruits and juice. Added sugars are found in concentrated sweets, such as sugar-sweetened beverages, candy, fruit drinks, and many desserts, and should comprise no more than 10% of total calories consumed. Healthful diets emphasize whole grains, fruits, and vegetables. The intake of refined carbohydrates and sugars should be limited not only for their limited nutritional value but also to help reduce the risk of caries.

Fiber. The recommended amount of dietary fiber is 14 g per 1000 cal (Table 8.5). That translates into 25 to 36 g/d for moderately active adults. Fiber includes two main types: soluble and insoluble. *Insoluble fiber*, an important aid in normal bowel function, is provided in high concentrations in whole wheat breads and cereals, wheat bran, rye, rice, barley, cabbage, beets, carrots, brussels sprouts, turnips, cauliflower, and apple skins. Sources of *soluble fiber* include oat bran, oatmeal, beans, peas, rice bran, barley, citrus fruits, apple pulp, psyllium, carrots, strawberries, peaches with skin, and apples with skin. Most fiber-rich foods contain a mixture of both soluble and insoluble fibers.

Fiber, especially insoluble fiber, helps promote bowel regularity. Individuals should start slowly and gradually increasing their fiber intake over time, while also making sure to increase their intake of fluids. Patients

TABLE 8.5 Recommended Fiber Intake (g/d)

Children		
1–3 yr	Boys and girls	19
4–8 yr	Boys and girls	25
9–13 yr	Boys	31
	Girls	26
14–18 yr	Boys	38
	Girls	26
Adults		
19–50 yr	Men	38
	Women	25
>50 yr	Men	30
	Women	21

Institute of Medicine: Dietary Reference Intakes for Energy, Carbohydrate, Fiber, Fat, Fatty Acids, Cholesterol, Protein, and Amino Acids. Washington, DC: National Academy of Sciences; 2002.

should be encouraged to replace refined grains (white rice, white bread) with whole grains. Foods high in fiber tend to be lower in total calories, saturated fat, and cholesterol. Fiber may also help to curb appetite and can be an important adjunct to weight management plans.

Protein. Protein should make up 10% to 35% of total caloric intake. Dietary guidelines recommend a variety of protein-rich foods, including fish, lean meats, poultry, eggs, beans, soy products, seeds, and nuts. Protein needs may be higher for more active individuals.

Fats. Total fat intake should make up 20% to 35% of total calories, with less than 10% of calories coming from saturated fats. The American Heart Association (AHA) recommends reducing saturated fat intake to less than 7% of total calories and <6% for patients with cardiovascular risk.[8] Dietary fats are found in both plant and animal foods. In addition to providing calories, they assist with the absorption of fat-soluble vitamins, including A, D, E, and K. All dietary fats consist of different proportions of polyunsaturated, monounsaturated, and saturated fatty acids. Trans fats are primarily found in stick margarines and partially hydrogenated vegetable fats and in many processed and fast foods. Trans fatty acids contribute to heart disease, and consumption should be minimal, whereas omega-3 fatty acids have a protective effect. Oils contain a high percentage of polyunsaturated and monounsaturated fats. The type of fat, its primary food sources, and impact on cholesterol and heart disease are outlined in Table 8.6.

Triglycerides. Factors that increase triglyceride levels include excess body weight and reduced physical activity; increased intake of sugar and refined carbohydrates, particularly in the setting of insulin resistance and glucose intolerance; and increased alcohol intake. High levels of triglycerides are often associated with low levels of high-density lipoprotein cholesterol, obesity, diabetes, and high blood pressure (see Table 8.7).

Alcoholic Beverages

For those who choose to drink alcoholic beverages, the U.S. Dietary Guidelines recommend doing so sensibly and in moderation, defined as the consumption of up to one drink per day for women and up to two drinks per day for men. These calories should be accounted for within the limits of the individual's healthy eating pattern and consumed only by those of legal drinking age. The Guidelines do not recommend that those who do not drink begin drinking for any reason. A standard drink is considered to be 12 oz of beer, 1.5 oz of distilled spirit, or 5 oz of wine. Alcohol should not be consumed by some individuals, including pregnant women, and should be avoided by individuals engaging in activities that require attention, skill, or coordination.

TABLE 8.6	Types of Fat and Primary Effect on Blood Lipids	
Type of Fat	**Food Sources**	**Effects on Lipids**
Trans	Stick and full fat margarines Processed sweets, packaged foods made with hydrogenated oils, deep-fried foods	Increases LDL-C Lowers HDL-C
Saturated	Animal proteins, whole fat dairy foods, fatty/marbled beef and pork, poultry with skin, tropical oils (coconut, palm)	Increases total cholesterol
Monounsaturated	Vegetable oils (canola, olive), also found is some meats and dairy products	Lowers LDL-C and triglycerides Maintains HDL-C
Polyunsaturated/ omega-6	Safflower, sunflower, and corn oils	Lowers LDL-D, HDL-C, and triglycerides
Polyunsaturated/ omega-3	Canola, soybean, flaxseed, and walnut oils, wheat germ	Lowers LDL-C and triglycerides Maintains HDL-C

Adapted by author from materials developed by Up To Date. Available at https://www.uptodate. com/contents/image?imageKey=PC%2F75539&topicKey=PC%2F5364&rank=1~150&source=- see_link&search=healthy%20diet. Accessed December 2017.
HDL-C, high-density lipoprotein cholesterol; LDL-C, low-density lipoprotein cholesterol.

TABLE 8.7	Lifestyle Methods to Lower Triglyceride Levels

- Lose weight if you are overweight. Even a small loss of 5%–10% can be helpful
- If you are at a healthy weight, stay there
- Limit foods high in sugar and refined carbohydrates that have little fiber, such as white bread, crackers, white rice, pasta, noodles, and some cereals
- Eat more vegetables, whole fruits, and fiber-rich whole grains
- Exercise regularly
- Limit or avoid alcohol
- Choose healthy fats, especially omega-3 fatty acids, which are found in fish and seafood
- Limit saturated fats found in animal foods and tropical oils such as coconut and palm kernel
- Avoid trans fats found in foods made with hydrogenated oils, such as stick margarine, packaged foods, and fried foods
- Limit the cholesterol you eat
- Choose lean meats, fish, and vegetable protein foods, such as beans, lentils, nut, seeds, and soy
- Choose foods low in salt and avoid processed foods

Adapted from Academy of Nutrition and Dietetics Nutrition Therapy for High Triglyceride Levels.

Additional Heart-Healthy Dietary Practices

Aligned with the Dietary Guidelines, the AHA and American College of Cardiology evidence-based diet and lifestyle recommendations support their 2020 Strategic Impact Goals for cardiovascular health promotion and disease reduction.[9] These recommendations offer practical tools and approaches to assist clinicians in helping their patients adapt these guidelines into their dietary patterns. The committee concluded that a dietary pattern that emphasizes vegetables, fruits, and whole grains; includes low-fat dairy products, poultry, fish, legumes, nontropical oils, and nuts; and limits sweets, sugar-sweetened beverages, red meat, and processed foods is advantageous for adults who need to lower their low-density lipoprotein cholesterol and blood pressure. In addition to meeting appropriate caloric requirements, this dietary pattern should also account for cultural food preferences and incorporate other medical nutrition therapy needs, such as type 2 diabetes. Extensive evidence supports that these goals can be accomplished by following the Dietary Approaches to Stop Hypertension (DASH) diet, the USDA Dietary Guidelines, a traditional Mediterranean style diet, or the AHA dietary pattern. These patterns share many commonalities and can be adapted to a patient's cultural food preferences and tastes.

Dietary Approaches to Stop Hypertension Diet

The DASH diet emphasizes 4 to 5 servings of fruits, 4 to 5 servings of vegetables, and 2 to 3 servings of low-fat dairy products; includes whole grains, poultry, fish, and nuts; and is limited in saturated fats, red meat, sweets, and sugar-sweetened beverages (Table 8.8). This pattern is effective in lowering blood pressure, particularly among blacks and individuals with hypertension.[10] When coupled with sodium reduction up to 1500 mg of sodium per day, the greatest blood pressure reductions were seen. The DASH diet contains higher amounts of magnesium, potassium, calcium, protein, and fiber as compared with the average American diet. Owing to its relatively high content of potassium, phosphorus, and protein, the DASH diet is not recommended for those individuals with chronic kidney disease, that is, an estimated glomerular filtration rate lower than 60 mL/min/1.73 m².

The National Heart, Lung, and Blood Institute Health Information Center has developed various patient tools for following the DASH diet, including *Your Guide for Lowering Your Blood Pressure with DASH*. The guide provides examples of the DASH diet on a daily basis; information on lowering calories, finding sodium in the diet, and reducing use of sodium in food preparation and when dining; and a week's worth of DASH eating plans to help guide patients through the process (www.nhlbi.nih.gov).

The Mediterranean Diet

The Mediterranean-type diet includes an increased amount of vegetables, legumes, fruits, and cereals (mostly unrefined); a low to moderate intake of dairy products; a moderate to high intake of fish; a meal pattern

TABLE 8.8   The DASH Eating Style

Food Group	Daily Servings	1 Serving Equals
Low-fat or fat-free dairy	2–3	1 cup milk or yogurt 1½ oz cheese
Fruits	4–5	1 medium fruit ¼ cup dried fruit ½ cup frozen or canned ½ cup fruit juice
Vegetables	4–5	1 cup raw leafy ½ cup cooked or cut-up raw ½ cup vegetable juice
Grain Foods (whole grain encouraged)	6–8	1 slice bread ½ cup dry or hot cereal, cooked rice or pasta 1 oz dry cereal
Lean meat, fish poultry	6 or less	1 oz cooked meat poultry, or fish 1 egg (limit whole to no more than 4/wk)
Nuts, seeds, legumes	4–5 per wk	1/3 cup nuts 2 tbsp nut butter or seeds ½ cup cooked legumes
Fats and oil	2–3	1 tbsp soft margarine or vegetable oil 1 tbsp mayonnaise 2 tbsp salad dressing
Sweets and added sugars	5 or less per wk	1 tbsp sugar, jelly, or jam ½ cup sorbet, gelatin 1 cup lemonade

characteristically low in saturated fats and high in unsaturated fats (olive oil); relatively low meat intake; and moderate intake of ethanol, usually in the form of wine. Such dietary patterns—emphasizing plant foods and unsaturated fats—are associated with a lower risk of developing cardiovascular disease and longer life expectancy. The Mediterranean diet also utilizes foods high in omega-3 fatty acids, specifically eicosadienoic acid and docosahexaenoic acid, which confer cardioprotective effects.

VITAMINS AND MINERALS

Sodium and Potassium

Sodium intake should be limited to less than 2300 mg (approximately one teaspoon of salt) a day. This can be accomplished by choosing and preparing foods with little salt and at the same time consuming potassium-rich foods, such as fruits and vegetables. Table 8.9 lists the top 10 foods high in sodium.

TABLE 8.9   Top 10 Sources of Sodium

Breads and rolls
Pizza
Sandwiches
Cold cuts and cured meats
Soups
Burritos and tacos
Savory snacks (chips, popcorn, pretzels, snack mixes, crackers)
Chicken
Cheese
Eggs and omelets

Hoy MK, Goldman JD, Murayi T, Rhodes DG, Moshfegh AJ. *Sodium Intake of the U.S. Population: What We Eat in America, NHANES 2007–2008. Food Surveys Research Group Dietary Data Brief No. 8*; October 2011. Available at http://arsusdagov/Services/docshtm?docid=19476.

The AHA recommends limiting sodium intake to approximately 1500 mg/d for those with or without hypertension. The reduction of salt intake is most effective in lowering blood pressure in older individuals and in those with hypertension, diabetes, or chronic kidney disease. The AHA recommends eating 8 to 10 servings of fruits and vegetables daily to increase potassium intake, which effectively reduces blood pressure in both normotensive and hypertensive individuals.

Calcium and Vitamin D

The National Osteoporosis Foundation estimated in 2014 that 10.2 million Americans are affected by osteoporosis and 43.4 have low bone mass[11] (https://www.nof.org/news/54-million-americans-affected-by-osteoporosis-and-low-bone-mass/).

Risk factors that can be altered include inadequate intake of calcium, vitamin D, fruits, and vegetables; excessive protein, sodium, caffeine, and alcohol; and smoking as well as inadequate weight-bearing exercise (see Chapter 7). Weight-bearing exercises done on a regular basis, working against gravity, contribute to the development of a higher peak bone mass and may reduce the risk of falls because of increased strength in muscle, bone, and balance. The age groups with mean intakes of inadequacy in excess of 50% include boys and girls aged 9 to 13 years, girls aged 14 to 18 years, women aged 51 to 70 years, and both men and women older than 70 years. Other groups at risk for deficiency include amenorrheic women, those with cow's milk allergy or lactose intolerance, and vegetarians. Calcium needs are outlined in Table 8.10.

Rich, natural sources of calcium include milk, cheese, and yogurt, whereas broccoli, kale, and Chinese cabbage are nondairy sources. Although spinach contains calcium, it is not well absorbed. Fortified calcium products include fruit juices and drinks, some cereals, and soy products. Fortified rice and nut (such as almond and cashew) milks are options. Other sources of calcium are listed in Table 8.11.

TABLE 8.10   Calcium Recommendations

Age	Calcium (mg/d)
0–6 mo	200
7–12 mo	260
1–3 yr	700
4–8 yr	1000
9–13 yr	1300
14–18 yr	1300
19–50 yr	1000
51–70 yr	1000 (male); 1200 (female)
71 yr and over	1200
Pregnant or Lactating	
14–18 yr	1300
19–50 yr	1000

Committee to Review Dietary Reference Intakes for Vitamin D and Calcium, Food and Nutrition Board, Institute of Medicine. *Dietary Reference Intakes for Calcium and Vitamin D*. Washington, DC: National Academy Press; 2010.

Based on the MyPlate guidelines, 3 cups of foods from the dairy group are recommended a day. A cup is equal to 1 cup (8 oz) of milk, 1 cup of yogurt, 1.5 oz of natural cheese (such as Cheddar), or 2 oz of processed cheese (such as American).

Patients who do not consume sufficient calcium in foods may consider taking calcium supplements. The two main sources of supplemental calcium are carbonate and citrate. Calcium carbonate is more commonly available and inexpensive. Because it depends on stomach acid for absorption, calcium carbonate is absorbed most efficiently when taken with food, whereas calcium citrate is absorbed equally well when taken with or without food. If calcium supplementation is needed, an additional calcium supplement should be taken in addition to the low amount provided in most multivitamin and mineral supplement preparations. Absorption is maximized at 500 mg, so patients requiring 1000 mg of supplemental calcium should divide the dose into 500 mg/d at two separate times during the day. Not all calcium consumed is actually absorbed in the gut. Humans absorb about 30% of the calcium in foods, but this varies depending on the type of food consumed. Other factors also affect calcium absorption, including the following:

- Amount consumed: the efficiency of absorption decreases as calcium intake increases.

TABLE 8.11   Selected Food Sources of Calcium

Food	Milligrams per Serving	Percent DV[a]
Yogurt, plain, low fat, 8 oz	415	42
Mozzarella, part skim, 1.5 oz	333	33
Sardines, canned in oil, with bones, 3 oz	325	33
Yogurt, fruit, low fat, 8 oz	313–384	31–38
Cheddar cheese, 1.5 oz	307	31
Milk, nonfat, 8 oz**	299	30
Soymilk, calcium fortified, 8 oz	299	30
Milk, reduced fat (2% milk fat), 8 oz	293	29
Milk, buttermilk, low fat, 8 oz	284	28
Milk, whole (3.25% milk fat), 8 oz	276	28
Orange juice, calcium fortified, 6 oz	261	26
Tofu, firm, made with calcium sulfate, 1/2 cup***	253	25
Salmon, pink, canned, solids with bone, 3 oz	181	18
Cottage cheese, 1% milk fat, 1 cup	138	14
Tofu, soft, made with calcium sulfate, 1/2 cup***	138	14
Ready-to-eat cereal, calcium fortified, 1 cup	100–1,000	10–100
Frozen yogurt, vanilla, soft serve, 1/2 cup	103	10
Turnip greens, fresh, boiled, 1/2 cup	99	10
Kale, fresh, cooked, 1 cup	94	9
Ice cream, vanilla, 1/2 cup	84	8
Chinese cabbage, bok choy, raw, shredded, 1 cup	74	7
Bread, white, 1 slice	73	7
Pudding, chocolate, ready to eat, refrigerated, 4 oz	55	6
Tortilla, corn, ready-to-bake/try, one 6″ diameter	46	5
Tortilla, flour, ready-to-bake/fry, one 6″ diameter	32	3
Sour cream, reduced fat, cultured, 2 tbsp	31	3
Bread, whole wheat, 1 slice	30	3
Kale, raw, chopped, 1 cup	24	2

TABLE 8.11 Selected Food Sources of Calcium (Continued)

Food	Milligrams per Serving	Percent DV[a]
Broccoli, raw, 1/2 cup	21	2
Cheese, cream, regular, 1 tbsp	14	1

U.S. Department of Agriculture, Agricultural Research Service. *USDA National Nutrient Database for Standard Reference, Release 24.* Nutrient Data Laboratory Home Page; 2011. http://www.ars.usda.gov/ba/bhnrc/ndl.

[a]DV, daily value. DVs were developed by the U.S. Food and Drug Administration to help consumers compare the nutrient contents among products within the context of a total daily diet. The DV for calcium is 1000 mg for adults and children aged 4 years and older. Foods providing 20% of more of the DV are considered to be high sources of a nutrient, but foods providing lower percentages of the DV also contribute to a healthful diet.

**Calcium content varies slightly by fat content; the more fat, the less calcium the food contains.

***Calcium content is for tofu processed with a calcium salt. Tofu processed with other salts does not provide significant amounts of calcium.

TABLE 8.12 Vitamin D Recommendations

Life Stage	Recommended Amount (IU)
Birth to 12 mo	400
Children 1–13 yr	600
Teens 14–18 yr	600
Adults 19–70 yr	600
Adults 71 yr and older	800
Pregnant and breast-feeding women	600

- Age and life stage: net calcium absorption is as high as 60% in infants and young children, who need substantial amounts of the mineral to build bone. Absorption decreases to 15% to 20% in adulthood (although it is increased during pregnancy) and continues to decrease as people age; compared with younger adults, recommended calcium intakes are higher for females older than 50 years and for both males and females older than 70 years.
- Vitamin D intake: this nutrient, obtained from food and produced by skin when exposed to sunlight of sufficient intensity, improves calcium absorption. Average recommended daily amounts of vitamin D are listed in Table 8.12.
- Other components in food: phytic acid and oxalic acid, found naturally in some plants, bind to calcium and can inhibit its absorption. Foods with high levels of oxalic acid include spinach, collard greens, sweet potatoes, rhubarb, and beans. Among the foods high in phytic acid are fiber-containing whole-grain products and wheat bran, beans, seeds, nuts, and soy isolates.

Magnesium

More than 300 enzyme systems require magnesium to regulate diverse bio-chemical reactions in the body, including energy production, protein synthe-sis, muscle and nerve function, blood glucose control, and blood pressure regulation. Some studies suggest that magnesium consumption may improve bone density and reduce fracture rates. Magnesium is widely distributed in plant and animal foods and in beverages. Generally, magnesium is found in foods containing dietary fiber, including whole grains, legumes, nuts, and seeds. It is also found in green leafy vegetables, such as spinach. Magnesium is also added to some breakfast cereals and other fortified foods.

Iron

Iron plays an important role in hemoglobin synthesis and in supporting immune responses. Needs throughout the lifecycle are listed in Table 8.13. Inadequacies may occur in certain high-risk subgroups. Anemia, the most common hematologic disorder, is usually caused by inadequate iron intake. If patients do not consume sufficient iron from good food sources (see Table 8.14), the clinician can prescribe iron sulfate (325 mg three times daily).

For persons with poor digestive-tract iron absorption due to low gas-tric acidity, serum iron levels can drop if dietary sources are mainly "non-heme" iron (from vegetables and fruits). *Heme iron* derives from animal products (meat, fish, and poultry); its absorption does not require stomach acid and is therefore unaffected by higher gastric pH. Although heme iron is more readily absorbed, nonheme iron contributes the larger portion of available iron in the average diet.

TABLE 8.13	Iron Requirements			
Age	Males (mg/d)	Females (mg/d)	Pregnancy (mg/d)	Lactating (mg/d)
0–6 mo	0.27	0.27		
6–12 mo	11	11		
1–3 yr	7	7		
4–8 yr	10	10		
9–13 yr	8	8		
14–18 yr	11	15	27	10
19–30 yr	8	18	27	9
31–50 yr	8	18	27	9
51–70 yr	8	8		
71 yr and older	8	8		

TABLE 8.14 Food Sources of Iron		
Food	Milligrams per Serving	Percent DV[a]
Breakfast cereals, fortified with 100% of the DV for iron, one serving	18	100
Oysters, eastern, cooked with moist heat, 3 oz	8	44
White beans, canned, 1 cup	8	44
Chocolate, dark, 45%–69% cacao solids, 3 oz	7	39
Beef liver, pan fried, 3 oz	5	28
Lentils, boiled and drained, 1/2 cup	3	17
Spinach, boiled and drained, 1/2 cup	3	17
Tofu, firm, 1/2 cup	3	17
Kidney beans, canned, 1/2 cup	2	11
Sardines, Atlantic, canned in oil, drained solids with bone, 3 oz	2	11
Chickpeas, boiled and drained, 1/2 cup	2	11
Tomatoes, canned, stewed, 1/2 cup	2	11
Beef, braised bottom round, trimmed to 1/8″ fat, 3 oz	2	11
Potato, baked, flesh and skin, 1 medium potato	2	11
Cashew nuts, oil roasted, 1 oz (18 nuts)	2	11
Green peas, boiled, 1/2 cup	1	6
Chicken, roasted, meat and skin, 3 oz	1	6
Rice, white, long grain, enriched, parboiled, drained, 1/2 cup	1	6
Bread, whole wheat, 1 slice	1	6
Bread, white, 1 slice	1	6
Raisins, seedless, 1/4 cup	1	6
Spaghetti, whole wheat, cooked, 1 cup	1	6
Tuna, light, canned in water, 3 oz	1	6
Turkey, roasted, breast meat and skin, 3 oz	1	6
Nuts, pistachio, dry roasted, 1 oz (49 nuts)	1	6
Broccoli, boiled and drained, 1/2 cup	1	6
Egg, hard boiled, 1 large	1	6

(Continued)

TABLE 8.14   Food Sources of Iron   (Continued)

Food	Milligrams per Serving	Percent DV[a]
Rice, brown, long or medium grain, cooked, 1 cup	1	6
Cheese, Cheddar, 1.5 oz	0	0
Cantaloupe, diced, 1/2 cup	0	0
Mushrooms, white, sliced and stir fried, 1/2 cup	0	0
Cheese, cottage, 2% milk fat, 1/2 cup	0	0
Milk, 1 cup	0	0

From the Office of Dietary Supplements. https://ods.od.nih.gov/factsheets/Iron-Health Professional/#h3.

[a]DV, daily value. DVs were developed by the U.S. Food and Drug Administration (FDA) to help consumers compare the nutrient contents of products within the context of a total diet. The DV for iron is 18 mg for adults and children aged 4 year and older. Foods providing 20% or more of the DV are considered to be high sources of a nutrient.

Zinc

Sources of zinc are listed in Table 8.15. Zinc intake declines with age and among those who avoid meats. Some evidence suggests that zinc improves immune function and, in the elderly, reduces pressure ulcers. After 50 years of age, the recommended daily allowance for zinc is 8 mg for women and 11 mg for men, but most persons older than 70 years have inadequate intake. High-dose zinc supplementation can induce copper deficiency and suppress the immune system. Unless an individual is being monitored closely for copper status, doses of zinc supplements should be 40 to 50 mg/d.

Nutritional Supplements

A large proportion of persons in the United States use vitamins and other nutrient supplements. When patients report current medications to their clinician, they often do not mention the use of such supplements. A vitamin/mineral supplement that does not exceed 100% of the DRI for any components may be helpful if an individual is on a very-low-calorie weight loss diet; elderly and not eating as much as needed; a strict vegetarian; or does not consume milk, cheese, or yogurt. They should check for the United States Pharmacopeia Verified Mark on the product label, indicating that the product contains the advertised amount of the nutrient. Patients should also be aware that many supplements now have added herbs, enzymes, or amino acids that may interfere with medications such as anticoagulants. Patients should be reminded that supplements can be helpful to complement their diet, rather than compensate for a poorly balanced diet.

TABLE 8.15 Food Sources of Zinc

Food	Milligrams (mg) per Serving	Percent DV[a]
Oysters, cooked, breaded and fried, 3 oz	74.0	493
Beef chuck roast, braised, 3 oz	7.0	47
Crab, Alaska king, cooked, 3 oz	6.5	43
Beef patty, broiled, 3 oz	5.3	35
Breakfast cereal, fortified with 25% of the DV for zinc, 3/4 cup serving	3.8	25
Lobster, cooked, 3 oz	3.4	23
Pork chop, loin, cooked, 3 oz	2.9	19
Baked beans, canned, plain or vegetarian, 1/2 cup	2.9	19
Chicken, dark meat, cooked, 3 oz	2.4	16
Yogurt, fruit, low fat, 8 oz	1.7	11
Cashews, dry roasted, 1 oz	1.6	11
Chickpeas, cooked, 1/2 cup	1.3	9
Cheese, Swiss, 1 oz	1.2	8
Oatmeal, instant, plain, prepared with water, 1 packet	1.1	7
Milk, low fat or nonfat, 1 cup	1.0	7
Almonds, dry roasted, 1 oz	0.9	6
Kidney beans, cooked, 1/2 cup	0.9	6
Chicken breast, roasted, skin removed, 1/2 breast	0.9	6
Cheese, Cheddar or mozzarella, 1 oz	0.9	6
Peas, green, frozen, cooked, 1/2 cup	0.5	3
Flounder or sole, cooked, 3 oz	0.3	2

From the Office of Dietary Supplements. https://ods.od.nih.gov/factsheets/Zinc-HealthProfessional/.
[a]DV, daily value. DVs were developed by the U.S. Food and Drug Administration to help consumers compare the nutrient contents of products within the context of a total diet. The DV for zinc is 15 mg for adults and children aged 4 year and older. Food labels, however, are not required to list zinc content unless a food has been fortified with this nutrient. Foods providing 20% or more of the DV are considered to be high sources of a nutrient.

Overuse of multivitamin and mineral preparations is a policy concern. For example, excessive vitamin A intake can increase the risk of hip fractures, and high iron intake can aggravate hemochromatosis. Large amounts of folate can mask vitamin B_{12} deficiency. Supplementation of single nutrients can sometimes have adverse effects on the absorption and utilization of other nutrients. Treatment with beta-carotene, vitamin A, and vitamin E may increase mortality. The National Institutes of Health Office of Dietary Supplements provides information and fact sheets for consumers and health professionals.[12]

In 2007, the U.S. Food and Drug Administration established a final rule requiring "good manufacturing practices" for dietary supplements to ensure that supplements contain what is on the label and no contaminants or impurities. The rule requires manufacturers to evaluate the identity, strength, purity, and composition of the supplements.

LIFECYCLE NUTRITION

Prepregnancy and Pregnancy

Nutritional status before and during pregnancy can affect the health of the mother, the growth and development of the fetus, and the risk of birth defects and future health in the parturient. Risk factors that may be apparent before pregnancy include poor eating habits and an increased need for nutrients (a special concern with adolescent mothers) and a history of three or more pregnancies in the last 2 years (especially miscarriages) or of poor obstetrical outcomes. Overweight and obese mothers are at higher risk for gestational diabetes and its complications (e.g., macrosomia); see Chapter 9 for guidance on weight management. Nutritional issues of concern during pregnancy include poor intake of energy and important nutrients (especially magnesium, zinc, calcium, iron, vitamin A, vitamin D, iodine, and magnesium) and those on a poorly managed vegetarian diet. As noted in the preceding text, pregnant women should also avoid alcoholic beverages.

In 1990, the IOM published weight gain recommendations for pregnancy based on prepregnancy BMI[13] (see Table 8.16). Folic acid supplementation is important before and during pregnancy to reduce the risk of neural tube and other birth defects. The dose is 400 μg/d of folate from supplements or fortified food in addition to the folate provided through foods. Because many pregnancies are unplanned, it is recommended that women of reproductive age increase the folic acid content of their diet, "just in case." Pre-existing chronic diseases such as diabetes increase the risk of birth defects, especially those involving the heart and central nervous system. Vegan vegetarians will most likely need a vitamin B_{12} supplement and perhaps zinc, calcium, and vitamin D. Women with phenylketonuria must resume a low-protein amino acid modified diet during pregnancy.

Breast-feeding

Breast-feeding is strongly endorsed by the world's health and scientific community. Benefits for children include fewer infectious illnesses (e.g., diarrhea, otitis media, and respiratory tract infections), and urinary tract

TABLE 8.16 Weight Gain Recommendations for Pregnancy Based on Prepregnancy Body Mass Index

Prepregnancy Body Mass Index (kg/m²)	Recommended Total Gain (lb)	Recommended Rate of Gain during 2nd and 3rd Trimester (lb/wk)
<18.5	28–40	1.0–1.3
18.5–24.9	25–35	0.8–1.0
25.0–29.0	15–25	0.5–0.7
30 and above	11–20	0.4–0.6

Modified from Institute of Medicine (US). *Weight Gain During Pregnancy: Reexamining the Guidelines.* Washington, DC: National Academies Press; 2009. © 2009 National Academy of Sciences.

infections, necrotizing enterocolitis and lower incidence of sudden infant death syndrome, asthma, and eczema.[14] There is also evidence that breast-fed infants are at lower risk of childhood obesity, diabetes, and leukemia. The breast-feeding mother benefits from a greater feeling of bonding with the child, a reduced risk of postpartum bleeding, more rapid uterine involution, an earlier return to prepregnancy weight, and earlier resumption of the menstrual cycle with decreased menstrual blood loss and anemia.

The AAP recommends exclusive breast-feeding for about the first 6 months of life with continued breast-feeding as solid foods are introduced, with the continuation for 1 year or longer as desired between mother and infant. Gradual introduction of complementary foods rich in iron and other micronutrients at about 6 months is preferred. The AAP recommends delaying the introduction of solid food until 4 to 6 months of age until the infant shows developmental signs of readiness and avoiding any milk (including cow's milk, rice milk, soy milk, almond milk, or goat's milk) until after 12 months of age.[15] Starting within the first few days of birth, all breast-fed and partially breast-fed infants should receive a supplement of 400 IU vitamin D per day. Formula-fed infants consuming less than 1 L of formula should receive a supplement of 400 IU vitamin D per day.[16] Table 8.17 lists the WHO/UNICEF Ten Steps to Successful Breastfeeding.

Infants and Toddlers

Rapid growth and development of infants and children provide a higher turnover of nutrients and a unique set of nutrient needs for growth and development. Dietary patterns established during infancy set the stage for lifelong eating habits. Caloric needs during childhood are approximately 90 to 102 kcal/kg of body weight and 1.1 g/kg of protein.[17]

For toddlers under the age of 2 years, it is important not to restrict dietary fat and cholesterol, as they are important for brain and nerve development. After the age of 2 years, aim for 30% of total calories from fat, with

TABLE 8.17   WHO/UNICEF Ten Steps to Successful Breastfeeding
1. Have a written breast-feeding policy that is routinely communicated to all health care staff
2. Train all health care staff in skills necessary to implement this policy
3. Inform all pregnant women about the benefits and management of breast-feeding
4. Help mothers initiate breast-feeding within the first hour of birth
5. Show mothers how to breast-feed and how to maintain lactation even if they should be separated from their infants
6. Give newborns no food or drink other than breast milk unless medically indicated
7. Practice rooming-in. Allow mothers and infants to remain together 24 hr a day
8. Encourage breast-feeding on demand
9. Give no artificial nipples or pacifiers to breast-feeding infants
10. Foster the establishment of breast-feeding support groups and refer mothers to them on discharge from the hospital or clinic

less than 10% of total energy from saturated fat. A varied diet including all food groups can help meet the DRIs for vitamins and minerals and the recommended 19 g of fiber a day. If there is difficulty tolerating or accepting meats or cow's milk, there is risk of iron, zinc, or calcium deficiencies. Cooking in a cast iron skillet, grinding meats, and combining with acidic foods such as tomato sauce can increase iron absorption. As a toddler is weaned from breast-feeding or formula, usual cow's milk consumption is 24 oz/d. Calcium-fortified nondairy beverages (such as almond or soy milk) can be helpful for those who experience lactose intolerance. If fruit juice is offered, it should be limited to 4 to 6 oz/d and diluted 50% with water. All other sugar-sweetened beverages should be limited. Good oral health habits should be established early to prevent the formation of dental caries. Only water should be offered for nighttime, especially in a bottle.

Adolescence

Nutritional needs increase during this stage of significant growth and development. More autonomy in decision making around food choices and the influence of peers and the media can pose a nutritional risk. Because 90% of bone mass is accrued by age 18 years, meeting the recommended 1300 mg of calcium a day is critical. Nutritional needs remain similar for boys and girls up until puberty, when changes in body composition and menarche prompt the need for sex-specific recommendations as previously noted. Energy needs depend on the stage of maturation along with physical activity. Daily nutrient intakes can be calculated using the USDA's Interactive DRI for Healthcare Professionals.[18] Nutrients often inadequately consumed include vitamins A and E, folate, iron, zinc, magnesium, and calcium. Vegetarians should be encouraged to consume adequate sources of protein, iron, zinc, omega-3 fatty acids, vitamin D, and vitamin B_{12}. Adolescent pregnancy, substance use, and disordered eating and nutritional needs for the teen athlete are all issues to consider.

Older Adults

Although successful aging begins early in life by committing to eating well and being physically active, the goals of good nutrition in the elderly are to maintain adequate weight and appetite and to avert complications from nutrition-related disorders (e.g., osteoporosis, fractures, anemias, obesity, diabetes, heart disease, and cancers). Older individuals are the largest demographic group at disproportionate risk for nutritional deficiencies, inadequate diet, and malnutrition. Poor nutritional status may often go unrecognized until pronounced changes are evident. Unintended weight loss, in particular, may herald a terminal downward spiral if weight loss is not identified and addressed.

Nutritional deficiencies occur among older adults because of chronic medical conditions, physical health problems, altered taste, medications, poverty, food insecurity, depression, grief, and dementia. Nutrition labels that are difficult to read or interpret can contribute to inappropriate food purchases. The elderly are also susceptible to the misleading claims of advertisers, and many unnecessarily use nutritional supplements and other over-the-counter therapies, which can be costly and may lead to adverse effects.

Seniors' diets also reflect their environment and social support system: who shops and cooks, finances, the number of meals per day, and where they are eaten. Social isolation, lack of family support, loss of a significant other or caregiver, and the decreased mobility that results from physical disabilities or from social isolation can lessen the availability of foods. The elderly at high risk are most often dependent on others for care, and this dependency may result in the potential for abuse. Home visits and direct conversations with caregivers often provide a different picture of the ability to care for the patient than that reported in the office visit. Physical activity, especially resistance training, is an important objective to maintain lean body mass and muscle tone and to help constipation.

Reduction in resting metabolic rate is associated with sarcopenia and decreased exercise volume and energy intake. Assessing energy needs in this population is very challenging, as reductions may be due to the factors above but increase during times of infection and stress. A reliable means is regularly monitoring body weight while giving consideration to the input and output of fluids.[19] Because their caloric needs diminish but nutrient requirements do not, older adults are in greater need of high nutrient density in their diets. Nutrition is affected further by the complications of chronic illness. Dysphasia, slow eating, low protein intake, and anorexia (often accompanying depression) can also compromise nutrition. Of those 75 years and older, two-thirds are edentulous. The elderly often have decreased salivation and absorption accompanied with changes in taste and smell acuity.

Older patients are at high risk of adverse food-drug interactions. Seniors often take multiple medications (engaging in "polypharmacy") for multiple chronic medical conditions. Aging alters drug absorption, distribution, metabolism, and excretion. Aging affects gastric emptying and intestinal motility, lowers the ratio of lean body weight to body fat, diminishes binding of drugs by serum protein, and reduces renal and hepatic function.

Food interactions can further potentiate these drug effects. Drugs may also reduce appetite, taste, or smell. Polypharmacy, depression, and underlying medical illnesses may produce a situation very similar to "failure to thrive" in infants. When assessing nutritional status, clinicians should therefore be careful to obtain an accurate drug history. They should also ask about vitamin, mineral, and other dietary supplements, which are widely used by seniors as a form of "nutritional insurance" and perceived by them as safe. Clinicians should consider potential interactions between these supplements and prescribed medications.

Liberalization of the diet prescription can enhance the quality of life and nutritional status of older residents in long-term care. An unacceptable or unpalatable diet can lead to lessened food and fluid intake. It may not be advantageous to initiate a medically or self-imposed restrictive nutrition prescription if it may suppress appetite and cause substantial, unintentional weight loss. Foods offered to the elderly may often need enhancements to achieve proper consistency and to accommodate their taste acuity.

Clinicians should monitor older patients for both laxative and alcohol abuse and for major changes in body weight, as well as the maintenance of adequate hydration. Fluid intake is essential for good health and is an important dietary component to consider when working with this population. A minimum of 1.5 L/d or 30 mL/kg of body weight, which includes fluids from food, beverages, and water, is recommended unless medically contraindicated.

OFFICE AND CLINIC ORGANIZATION

The practice should display health literate patient education materials and/or posters that may stimulate questions about healthy diets. These materials should be readily available to reinforce discussions and provide an opportunity for the patient to learn more at a later time. The reception area and waiting rooms are an excellent place to educate patients.

Clinics that do not have the services of an RD should develop a referral system so that patients can obtain the help they need to meet the dietary goals.

SUMMARY

A healthy diet coupled with appropriate food choices is an essential component of health promotion and disease prevention. Eating well and physical activity help slow the progression of chronic disease. Substantial amounts of health care resources could be saved by expanding health promotion and disease prevention programs that target dietary changes.

SUGGESTED RESOURCES AND MATERIALS

Choose My Plate
https://www.choosemyplate.gov/

The Academy of Nutrition and Dietetics
http://www.eatright.org/

The American Heart Association
http://www.heart.org/HEARTORG/HealthyLiving/HealthyEating/Healthy-Eating_
    UCM_001188_SubHomePage.jsp

Office of Disease Prevention and Health Promotion
http://www.heart.org/HEARTORG/HealthyLiving/HealthyEating/Healthy-Eating_
    UCM_001188_SubHomePage.jsp

Tools for assessing and achieving recommended dietary patterns
https://www.choosemyplate.gov/tools-supertracker.
https://www.myfitnesspal.com/
http://www.sparkpeople.com/

Eat Right Now: an app to improve your relationship with food and strengthen your
    control over cravings
https://goeatrightnow.com/

stickK.com: create commitment contracts to set goals and achieve them
http://www.stickk.com/

REFERENCES

1. Slawson DL, Fitzgerald N, Morgan KT. Position of the academy of nutrition and dietetics: the role of nutrition in health promotion and chronic disease prevention. *J Acad Nutr Diet.* 2013;113:972-979.
2. Academy of Nutrition and Dietetics. Nutrition Terminology Reference Manual (eNCPT): Dietetics Language for Nutrition Care 2014, Nutrition Assessment Introduction, page-001. http://ncpt.webauthor.com. Accessed 14 December 2017.
3. Detsky AS, McLaughlin JR, Baker JP, et al. What is subjective global assessment of nutritional status? *JPEN J Parenter Enteral Nutr.* 1987;11:8-13.
4. National Heart, Lung and Blood Institute. *The Practical Guide Identification, Evaluation and Treatment of Overweight and Obesity in Adults.* NIH Publication Number 00-4084; 2000.
5. David G, Bibbins-Domingo K, Curry SJ, et al. Behavioral counseling to promote a healthful diet and physical activity for cardiovascular disease prevention in adults without cardiovascular risk disease, the U.S. preventive services task force recommendation statement. *JAMA.* 2017;318(2):167-174.
6. The National Academies of Sciences. Engineering, Medicine. Dietary Reference Intakes. Available at http://nationalacademies.org/HMD/Activities/Nutrition/SummaryDRIs/DRI-Tables.aspx. Accessed 18 December 2017.

7. U.S. Department of Health and Human Services and U.S. Department of Agriculture. *2015–2020 Dietary Guidelines for Americans.* 8th ed. December 2015. Available at https://health.gov/dietaryguidelines/2015/guidelines/. Accessed 18 December 2017.

8. Horn LV, Carson JS, Appel LJ, et al. Recommended dietary pattern to achieve adherence to the American heart association/American college of cardiology (AHA/ACC) guidelines a scientific statement from the American heart association. *Circulation.* 2016;134:e505-e529.

9. Jensen MD, Ryan DH, Apovian CM, et al. 2013 AHA/ACC/TOS guideline for the management of overweight and obesity in adults: a report of the American college of cardiology/American heart association task force on practice guidelines and the obesity society. *Circulation.* 2014;129(25 suppl 2):S102.

10. National Heart, Lung and Blood Institute. *Your Guide to Lowering Your Blood Pressure with DASH.* NIH Publication No. 06-5834; 2015.

11. *National Osteoporosis Foundation NOF Releases Updated Data Detailing the Prevalence of Osteoporosis and Low Bone Mass in the US.* NOF; 2014. Available at https://www.nof.org/news/54-million-americans-affected-by-osteoporosis-and-low-bone-mass/. Accessed 18 December 2017.

12. Office of Dietary Supplements. https://ods.od.nih.gov/. Accessed 18 December 2017.

13. *The American College of Obstetricians and Gynecologists Committee Opinion Weight Gain during Pregnancy;* January 2013 Number 548.

14. American Academy of pediatrics policy statement breastfeeding and the use of human milk. *Pediatrics.* 2012;129(3):e827-e841.

15. American Academy of Pediatrics. Complementary foods. In: *American Academy of Pediatrics Pediatric Nutrition Handbook.* 7th ed. Elk Grove Village, IL: American Academy of Pediatrics; 2014:123-134.

16. Misra M, Pacaud D, Petryk A, Collett-Solberg PF, Kappy M. Vitamin D deficiency in children and its management: review of current knowledge and recommendations. *Pediatrics.* 2008;122:398-417

17. Center for Nutrition Policy and Promotion. USDA Food Guidance System. Health and Nutrition Information for Preschoolers; Daily Food Plan. Available at https://www.choosemyplate.gov/health-nutrition-information-preschoolers/daily-food-plan-preschoolers.html. Accessed 18 December 2017.

18. USDA Food and Nutrition Center Interactive DRI. Available at https://www.nal.usda.gov/fnic/interactiveDRI/. Accessed 18 December 2017.

19. Harris NG. Nutrition in aging. In: Mahan LK, Escott-Stump S, eds. *Krause's Food, Nutrition and Diet Therapy.* Philadelphia, PA: WB Saunders; 2004:318-339.

Please see Online Appendix: Apps and Digital Resources for additional information.

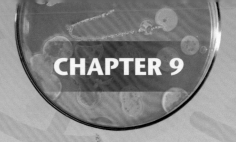

CHAPTER 9

Weight Management

MARY SAVOYE

BACKGROUND

There are now more obese U.S. adults than those classified as just over-weight.[1] In 2015–2016, almost 40% of adults and 19% of youth were consid-ered obese.[2] In adults, the rates are higher in women than in men, whereas in youth there is no difference between boys and girls; however, non-His-panic blacks and Hispanics have the highest obesity rates in both adults and children.[2]

Although obesity is associated with a host of diseases such as type 2 diabetes, hypertension, hyperlipidemia, coronary artery disease, polycys-tic ovarian syndrome, some forms of cancer, sleep apnea, and depression, it is also considered one of the most preventable morbidities and mortal-ities in the United States.[3] Paradoxically, although deemed preventable, obesity is difficult to treat and is usually chronic.[4,5]

In 2013, the American Medical Association recognized obesity as a disease, and shortly after, other professional organizations such as the American Association of Clinical Endocrinologist and the American Academy of Family Physicians followed suit.[4] Its continued growth as a risk factor puts obesity on track to replace smoking as the leading cause of death in the United States sometime in the future. More than 100,000 excess deaths are thought to occur annually because of obesity.[6]

OVERWEIGHT, OBESITY, AND HEALTH

Assessment and Definition of Overweight and Obesity

Body mass index (BMI) is the standard method used clinically to assess the degree of excess weight and is used to determine the health risk associ-ated with body weight as well. Its formula is weight in kilograms/height in square meters; however, online calculators such as http://www.hblbi.hih.gov/guidelines/obesity/BMI/bmicalc.htm and smart phone apps such as http://apps.usa.gov/bmi-app.shtml are often used for convenience.

The definitions of overweight and obesity in current use (2018) were established by the World Health Organization in 1997.[7] An adult is *overweight* if the BMI is 25 to 29.9 kg/m². *Mild or class I obesity* is defined as a BMI of 30 to 34.9 kg/m², *moderate or class II obesity* as a BMI of 35 to 39.9 kg/m², and *extreme, morbid, or class III obesity* as a BMI of >40 kg/m².[7]

BMI is the most widely accepted assessment guideline clinically for weight and health risk[8]; however, it is limited because it is an indirect measure of body fatness.[9] Research on the relationship of body composition and fat distribution suggests that visceral body fat or intra-abdominal fat percentage may be a better predictor of poor health than weight or percentage of body fat alone.[9] Methods such as computed tomography scans, magnetic resonance imaging, or dual energy X-ray absorptiometry are sophisticated techniques usually reserved for research and not practical in the clinical setting. Although bioelectrical impedance methods can be used clinically because of portability and convenience, they are less accurate for various reasons such as age, sensitivity to hydration, and degree of obesity.[10,11] Ironically, central body fat tends to overestimate fat-free mass.[11] Nonetheless, bioelectrical impedance machines such as body fat analyzers (Tanita, Inc., Arlington Heights, VA, USA) are becoming common household items and give rough estimates of the percentage of fat in the body. The most common way to measure visceral fat in clinical practice is the waist circumference, but measurements of waist circumference vary with the examiner and are frequently inaccurate. According to expert guidelines, a waist circumference of at least 35 in (88 cm) in women and 40 in (102 cm) in men is associated with increased cardiovascular risk.[8]

Assessment for Cause of Overweight and Obesity

The causes of obesity are multifactorial, and some have not yet been identified. A careful history of lifestyle is necessary, but genetics (family history), laboratory values, and medication regimen of the patient should be assessed in conjunction to lifestyle factors.

Genetics/Family History

Genetics is a significant contributing factor to obesity and may account for almost half of the cases of obesity.[12,13] The most commonly associated gene is the FTO gene,[12–14] and its identification led the way to further study of many other obesity-associated genes.[14] Much less common (almost never identified) are mutations of the leptin gene or its receptor, but very-young-onset obesity (usually less than 2 years old) involving the MC4R gene is investigated by obesity specialists, particularly if the youngster has a voracious appetite.[13] Less rare is Prader-Willi syndrome, which presents at a young age, also characterized by the inability for satiation.[13]

The genetic contributions to obesity are extremely complex and beyond the scope of this chapter, but nonetheless worth mentioning, as healthy lifestyle habits should still be encouraged to minimize the weight gain and escalating weight trajectory that transpires. In fact, gene studies using twins have found that BMI differences were greater in adults than in children, indicating that adults may be making deliberate attempts at weight control, limiting the observed genetic effect.[15] Influence of the environment also had significant impact on body measures at all ages and in both sexes.[16]

Laboratory Values and Medication Regimen

In addition to genetics and the importance of family history, laboratory values and regular medication use ought to be considered. Thyroid indices should be obtained if there is no record of these values in the past year. These measurements include thyroid stimulating hormone, thyroxine, triiodothyronine, and thyroid antibody tests.[17] Such laboratory values can rule out the possibility of hypothyroidism, which may be a contributing factor to weight gain. Likewise, cortisol levels may identify the possibility of Cushing syndrome or hypercortisolism. The phenotype for this disease presents with weight gain in the midsection, fatty deposits around the face, a hallmark "fat hump" between the shoulders, dark pink or purple stretch marks, and fat loss in the legs.[18] Plasma cortisol levels, alone, are not enough to diagnosis this condition and other tests such as a 24-hour urinary free cortisol or a midnight plasma cortisol and late-night salivary cortisol measurement are needed.[18]

Medication use (i.e., glucocorticoid-steroid hormones) may be responsible for the development of Cushing syndrome, as these medications are chemically similar to naturally produced cortisol.[18] Other obesity-causing medications include antipsychotics, as they alter hunger signals, most likely owing to interaction with neurotransmitter systems (serotonergic, histaminergic, and dopaminergic).[19,20] A recent meta-analysis concluded that virtually all antipsychotics are associated with weight gain and the longer the duration of use the greater the weight gain.[21] A 1-unit BMI increase was noted after 4 to 8 weeks, whereas a 4-unit BMI increase resulted after 24 to 48 weeks.[21,22] More weight-neutral, effective antipsychotics are needed to minimize the weight gain side effect.[20]

Clearly, genetics, disease states, and pharmacologically induced obesity should be addressed before or concurrently with lifestyle assessment, such as food and beverage consumption, physical activity, sedentary behavior, and sleep patterns. However, lifestyle habits are common contributors of obesity and will be the focus of this chapter.

History of Weight Gain/Loss

Weight history of the patient is imperative, as it points to periods in the patient's life when a specific life event may have contributed to the weight gain. For example, pregnancy is a typical cause of obesity, as greater than 50% of women retain postpartum weight, particularly when excessive weight was gained during pregnancy.[23,24] Other typical life events that perpetuate weight gain include smoking cessation,[25] divorce, death of a loved one, or an injury.[26]

Along with weight gain history capturing previous weight loss attempts is important. This helps the clinician and patient determine a future direction for treatment. For example, if strict or fad dieting did not work long term (this is typically the case), it can be determined that a less rigid or more balanced approach is needed for long-term weight loss and its maintenance. In fact, overrestriction and yo-yo dieting can be considered causes of obesity in and of itself (see The Starvation Response and "Yo-Yo" Dieting section).

Caloric Intake

It is no secret that excessive calories contribute to obesity.[27] Assessing food and beverage consumption to determine a patient's typical caloric intake is challenging, particularly for the primary care clinician who has little time with the patient. Preferably a patient can be taught how to keep a food record for 3 days (2 weekdays and 1 weekend day) so that calories can be determined and patterns of eating triggers can be identified. Teaching the patient this task is also quite time consuming. In addition to time, accuracy is an issue because people typically tend to underreport for two reasons: they are embarrassed to be truthful to the clinician or they truly eat less than usual (which does not give the actual picture) simply because the very act of writing down one's food and beverage intake is a weight loss strategy (if you know you have to report it, you are more conscious with your food choices and amounts).

Although food records that collect dietary information for at least three consecutive days are most accurate,[28,29] a "usual daily intake" can be obtained in the clinic environment and may capture other aspects of a typical day for a patient. The clinician may ask what one eats and drinks from the time of waking up to the time of falling asleep. This "snap shot," ideally, can also include what one does in a typical day and lends clues to lack of activity, excessive sedentary behavior, poor sleep pattern, and emotional eating, all factors to be considered for lifestyle change to promote weight loss.

Physical Activity and Sedentary Behavior

Most adults do not meet the minimum physical activity (PA) guidelines for maintaining health (see Table 9.1).[30] However, these guidelines are intended to be *in addition* to activities of daily living (ADLs), but ADLs have decreased, primarily because of busy lifestyle and advances in technology, causing the increase in sedentary behavior, researched over the past few decades and the subsequent distinction made between PA and sedentary behavior.[31] In fact, some professionals have suggested that "sitting is the new smoking of the 21st century."[32]

When assessing for lack of activity, there are two types of physical activities clinicians can ask their patient about: structured activity and ADLs. Going to the gym or playing basketball for an hour is a planned activity, whereas grocery shopping or gardening is an ADL. Questions about a

TABLE 9.1 Physical Activity Recommendations by Health Goals	
Health Goal	Minutes/Week
Maintain/improve health	150
Prevent weight gain	150–250
Lose weight	225–420
Prevent weight gain after weight loss	200–300

Adapted from Swift DL, Johannsen NM, Lavie CJ, et al. The role of exercise and physical activity in weight loss and maintenance. *Prog Cardiovasc Dis.* 2014;56(4):441-447. Available at https://www.ncbi.nlm.nih.gov/pmc/articles/PMC3925973/.
Note: American College of Sports Medicine recommendations for amount of physical activity per week based on health goals.

usual day are important to assess how long the patient obtains activity. Equally important are the hours spent doing blatant sedentary activities (for example, watching television or using a computer), as these activities often displace PA because there are only so many hours in a day. If a "usual day" that includes food intake and activity cannot be captured because even this abbreviated method is too time consuming, the clinician may want to use a PA questionnaire. Such questionnaires can be found online (http://www.health.gov/PAGuidelines/), and the patient can be instructed to fill one out before the assessment visit.

Emotional Eating

Many overweight and obese patients eat for reasons other than hunger. It is estimated that about 40% of the U.S. population eats in response to emotions or maladaptive coping.[33] Chronic stress is a common problem in busy U.S. lifestyles and has been associated with obesity,[34,35,36] even in youth.[37,38] Stress can produce changes of hormones in the brain, causing a maladaptive pattern[36]; in fact, there is a significant overlap of brain neural action with substance addictions and overeating.[39] Hyperpalatable food, such as high-fat and sugar choices, activate areas of the brain, as drugs do, and animal studies have shown the display of withdrawal symptoms when these foods are taken away.[39]

The Perceived Stress Scale is a popular, self-reported tool for measuring psychological stress and captures the degree to which individuals appraise their life situations as stressful.[40,41] Although there are different versions, ranging from 4 (PSS-4) to 14 items (PSS-14), the 10-item questionnaire (PSS-10) appears to have the most validity while being easy to understand and quick for the clinician to score.[41] A more comprehensive measure of emotions, from boredom to stress, can be captured using the Emotional Eater Questionnaire (EEQ), which is also relatively short (10 questions) and easy to apply in clinical practice.[42]

Sleep Deprivation

Along with stress, lack of sleep can increase caloric intake for various reasons. One obvious reason sleep deprivation increases calories is that one is tired and is looking for energy. When we are sleep deprived, we often make overall bad choices, including poor food choices. This is problematic because more than one-third of U.S. adults sleep less than 6 hours per night.[43] There is an association between short sleep duration and increased prevalence of obesity in both adults and children.[44] In fact, when shift workers (evening workers) were compared with nonshift workers, less than 5 hours of sleep resulted in greater onset of obesity than those with 5 to 7 hours of sleep.[45] The effects of shift work on sleep has received increased attention because it accounts for 20% of the entire workforce in developed countries.[44]

Most patients know approximately how many hours of sleep they obtain per night, although this likely varies on weekdays and weekends. Sleep questionnaires are available for clinicians to use with patients,[46] and commercial wrist sleep trackers are also available that measure sleep patterns (www.sleephealthfoundation.org). If lack of sleep due to obstructive sleep apnea is suspected, a formal sleep study should be prescribed.[47]

METABOLISM OF WEIGHT GAIN AND LOSS

Mechanisms for Saving Energy

When individuals consume food energy (calories) beyond their immediate needs, the body stores much of the excess as body fat. Body fat, other than that which plays a protective, cushioning function, serves mainly to store potential energy. A certain level of stored energy is healthy. But for many people, the storage capacity and the amount stored are both well above any potential need other than in the case of famine.

Contrary to famine-like conditions, we live in an obesogenic environment today, with fast foods and other convenience foods at our disposal.[48] Moreover, high-fat and sugar foods are cheaper than fruits and vegetables, making better food choices less desirable.

The Starvation Response and "Yo-Yo" Dieting

A critical metabolic factor in weight gain, especially relevant to our weight reduction, diet-conscious culture, is a phenomenon called the *starvation response*. Like the fat energy storage system, it is a mechanism to enhance the survival of the individual and species.[49] If a person experiences a sudden decrease in caloric intake, the resting metabolic rate (RMR, the measure of energy required to maintain organ system function) will start to decrease, probably within 24 to 36 hours. During species development, this process was originally designed to conserve energy. The RMR, which is normally approximately 75 cal/hr, can in the first instance drop to 60 cal/

hr. A second exposure to sudden caloric deficit can lower the RMR further to approximately 50 cal/hr. In some people, the RMR may drop to as low as 35 to 40 cal/hr.[49]

The starvation response can be elicited by sudden calorie restriction (i.e., dieting). Unfortunately, the metabolic system responds the same way to intentional caloric deficit as it does to externally induced deficits. The metabolic system cannot recognize that the immediate caloric deficit in this instance does *not* indicate that food might be in short supply for quite some time. Therefore, when the person finishes with a diet designed for short-term weight loss with no long-term healthy eating component and returns to his or her prediet eating pattern (as often happens), there is no available built-in "second signal" to stimulate an immediate return to normal RMR.[49]

Usually, the sudden calorie restriction diets described in the lay literature contain little information about lifelong healthy eating and how to go about establishing that pattern. Many dieters using these methods lose some weight and then return to their normal eating pattern. If a person with a lowered RMR resumes normal eating without increasing energy expenditure, they will consume calories in excess of metabolic need. Most of the excess calories will be stored as body fat, and body weight will increase again. That outcome may well induce the person to try losing weight once more.[49]

If the same sudden calorie restriction dieting approach is followed, perhaps just formulated differently, the RMR may be further depressed. And again, even if some weight is lost on subsequent tries, unless the person has managed to change his or her regular eating pattern, the diet often produces immediate, sometimes significant, weight loss, followed by slow, but steady weight regain. This dieting-induced pattern is called *yo-yo dieting*. (After several such cycles, the RMR may be depressed to the point that the next episode of calorie restriction dieting has no effect on body weight at all, as well as having no further effect on an already greatly depressed RMR.)[49]

There is one known mechanism by which a depressed RMR can be raised, however: engaging in regular exercise.[49,50] Muscle requires more energy for maintenance of its basal functions than does fat. Regular exercise raises the RMR by gradually creating new muscle mass. For patients averse to regular exercise, this will be a "good news/bad news" message, but they should be encouraged to use this method to raise their RMR, if they feel that they can manage it[49] (see Activity Modification).

TREATMENT GOALS

Modest weight loss, between 5% and 10% of initial body weight, can significantly improve many comorbid conditions.[3] In fact, a weight loss of only 3% to 5% that is maintained can produce clinically relevant health improvements (e.g., reductions in triglycerides, blood glucose, and risk of developing type 2 diabetes).[51] Clinicians need to work on developing realistic weight loss goals with their obese patients so that they are not disillusioned and are more successful in maintaining the weight loss. Often it is better to set a short- and long-term weight loss goal so that the clinician and patient can interpret any changes in health with a modest weight loss. They then can decide if more loss is necessary or desired. A healthful, sustainable weight should be emphasized over a cosmetic goal.

Although the obese patient is attempting to lose weight, the goal(s) should be specific to the cause of obesity (yo-yo dieting, poor eating pattern, lack of activity, emotional eating, sleep deprivation, or a combination of any of these). Stating behavioral goals rather than numbers of pounds to be lost is preferred during the actual process because it is the behavior change of the individual that will result in the weight loss (see Setting Goals and Follow-up Care for practical ways to set goals with patients).

TREATMENT APPROACHES

Traditional weight loss approaches involve lifestyle modification. Most obese individuals know that, to lose weight, one must eat less and exercise more. In fact, many obese individuals are "experienced" and can identify which foods are healthy choices (perhaps even know appropriate portion sizes) and likewise can tell their clinician how many minutes of activity they should be engaging in per day. The challenge of the obese patient lies in *making the actual behavior change happen* and continuing with positive, healthy habits. That is, usually, it is *not* a knowledge problem, it is a behavior problem.

Although diet, activity, and behavior modifications often work simultaneously during weight loss, each component is described separately in the following text.

Diet Modification

The goal of diet modification for weight loss is to decrease energy intake enough so that a significant deficit of calories occurs over time to promote weight loss. The theoretical rule of a 3500-calorie deficit equating to a 1-lb weight loss[52] has recently been disputed.[53,54] First, the simplified rule does not take dynamic physiologic adaption into account during weight loss efforts,[53] and second, individual weight loss is dependent on baseline body composition, age, height, and gender.[54] The rule may be better utilized as a teaching tool to convey how excess calories add up to surplus weight, but clinicians should refrain from projecting a weight loss based upon the rule, as done in the past (e.g., 1–2-lb weight loss per week with a 500–1000-calorie deficit). Such overestimated projections can lead to a discouraged patient who has worked hard at compliance.

Indirect calorimetry is perhaps the most accurate method for determining a patient's RMR so that a deficit could be calculated (calorie level). This method, however, like other assessment methods described earlier, is reserved for the research environment. The use of the 3-day food record or "usual intake" can be used as a baseline to help the clinician determine the prescriptive calorie level for weight loss. An alternate method to estimate energy needs (instead of considering usual intake) of overweight and obese individuals is the Mifflin-St Jeor equation, which approximates RMR as follows[51]:

Man: (10 × weight in kilograms) + (6.25 × height in centimeters) − (5 × age in years) + 5.

Woman: (10 × weight in kilograms) + (6.25 × height in centimeters) − (5 × age in years) − 161.

After determining the patient's usual caloric intake or RMR, the clinician may prescribe a 500 to 1000-calorie deficit per day as a starting point to bring about weight loss over time.[51]

In addition to the caloric level of the diet, the quality of the diet must be considered. Nutritional balance and adequacy are important, and a meal plan that omits entire food groups will leave out the corresponding vitamins and minerals. For example, if a meal plan touts avoidance of dairy products, vitamin D and calcium needs will not be met. Also, because comorbidities often exist with obesity, effects of manipulating macronutrients need to be considered. For example, if a low-glycemic diet or low-carbohydrate diet does not reduce low-density lipoprotein (LDL)-cholesterol (or increases it) and an obese individual has hyperlipidemia at the start of a weight loss journey, these regimens may not be the best choice. Approaches to several diet modifications will be discussed along with reported pros and cons of each.

Low-Calorie Diets and Very-Low-Calorie Diets

Typically, a low-calorie diet (LCD) ranges from 1200 to 1600 calories per day.[51] The goal of the LCD is to induce an energy deficit of approximately 500 to 1000 calories per day.[51] The American Academy of Nutrition and Dietetics in conjunction with the American Diabetes Association publishes *Choose Your Foods: Food List for Weight Management* (2014). Many dietitians use this resource as the basis of meal planning with calorie restriction because it provides nutritional balance with the representation of all food groups. Each food group—Starch, Fruits, Milk and Milk Substitutes, Nonstarchy vegetables, Protein, Fats—is assigned a specific macronutrient and calorie level. There is also a Free Foods group with foods less than 20 cal. See Table 9.2 for an example of a 1500 cal/d meal plan using this method.

Very-low-calorie diets (VLCD), on the other hand, are much more aggressive with calorie restriction than the LCD because it only provides <800 calories per day.[51] A VLCD may also be known as a protein-sparing

TABLE 9.2 The 1500-Calorie Meal Plan

Exchange	Amount	Food Idea	Food Amount
Breakfast			
Starch	2	Shredded wheat cereal	1 cup
Milk	1	1% milk	8 oz
Fruit	1	Medium banana	1/2
Free		Coffee, black	1 cup
Snack:			
Fat	2	Almonds	12
Lunch			
Starch	2	Wheat bread	2 slices
Meat/meat alternative	2 low fat	Turkey	2 oz
	1 high fat	Cheese	1 oz
Vegetable	1	Lettuce and tomato	2 leaves and 2 slices
Fat	1	Mayonnaise	1 tbsp
Fruit	1	Grapes	17, small
Free		Iced tea, unsweetened	12 oz
Snack:			
Milk	1	Yogurt, plain or sweetened with artificial sweetener	6 oz container
Dinner			
Meat/meat alternative	3	Salmon, grilled	3 oz
Starch	1	Baked potato	Small (3 oz)
Vegetable	2	Green beans	1 cup, steamed
Free		Salad greens	
Fat	2	Butter or sour cream Olive oil Vinegar (free)	1 tbsp 2 tbsp 1 tsp To taste
Free		Seltzer	12 oz
Snack/dessert:			
Fruit	1	Cantaloupe	1 cup, diced

Adapted from American Diabetes Association & Academy of Nutrition and Dietetics. *Choose Your Foods: Food Lists for Weight Management*; 2014.
Note: A sample 1500-calorie meal plan.

modified fast when protein contents reach 1.2 to 1.5 g of protein per kg of ideal body weight.[55] The protein-sparing modified fast type of VLCD is intended to preserve muscle mass, so much of its source consists of protein, which is anabolic. This diet should be medically supervised, as in addition to a multivitamin, additional potassium is generally prescribed.[52,55,56]

Pros of the VLCD includes greater short-term weight loss than LCD, but long-term outcomes have been reported to be similar between the two diets,[56] and some studies report much greater weight regain in the VLCD group.[56] This modified fast might be indicated before bariatric surgery to drop weight quickly and prove compliance in the obese patient.[55] The LCD is perhaps a better choice for the obese individual who is not seeking a quick weight loss or bariatric surgery. In fact, a moderate calorie restriction may be more tolerable in the long term.[57]

Low-Carbohydrate Diet

A low-carbohydrate diet, with or without calorie restriction, generally consists of 20 g or less of carbohydrate intake per day.[58] The goal of this diet is to produce ketosis in the obese individual. Ketosis allows fat to be used as energy while sustaining fuel utilization in the brain.[59] Ketosis decreases hunger and consequently increases dietary compliance. Some research, however, has shown that the unintended decrease in energy intake may be the true mechanism behind weight loss rather than the ketosis.[59] An additional reason for weight loss in a low-carbohydrate diet is related to the depletion of glycogen stores, resulting in diuresis and an initial striking weight loss. Once a healthier weight or short-term weight loss goal is achieved, carbohydrate intake generally increases to 50 g/d.[51] This may still be difficult to sustain in the long term.

It should be noted that low-carbohydrate diets have shown more weight loss in the short term (3–6 months) than more traditional low-fat diets,[60] but several long-term (1–2 year) randomized control trials found no difference between weight loss using either a low-carbohydrate or low-fat, energy-restricted diet.[58,61,62]

As with any meal plan, high-quality carbohydrates (fruits, vegetables, legumes, and other high-fiber, nutrient-dense carbohydrates) should be consumed. However, with low-carbohydrate diets, there is no place for added sugars because milk and vegetables are also accounted for as carbohydrates along with typical carbohydrate foods such as potato or rice.

Low–Glycemic Index Diet

Glycemic index (GI) is based on the blood glucose response of a specific carbohydrate (expressed as a percentage) when compared with a reference food such as 50 g of glucose or slice of white bread of equal carbohydrate value.[63] Foods are typically categorized as low (<55), medium,[56–69] or high (>70) in GI, with a higher-GI food thought to raise blood sugar more than a lower-GI food.[64] Most lay persons do not know there is a difference between the GI of food and the glycemic load (GL) of food, as the GL is the product of the GI of the food and grams of available carbohydrate in food divided by 100.[65] That is, the GL takes the *total amount* of food one is consuming into account, whereas the GI does not (its ranking is based on 50 g of carbohydrate). For example, the GI of carrots is high, whereas the load is very low. Most people avoid carrots because of their high GI, but the reality is one would have to eat a lot of carrots (about 10 cups raw) to see the effect of the GI ranking. Outside of the research laboratory, where this food ranking was originally used, this meal planning method can be complex.

A meta-analysis of clinical trials studying the effects of low GI on insulin sensitivity and cardiovascular disease risk factors reports mixed results when low- and high-glycemic diets were compared.[64] This may be due to the complexity of studying different carbohydrates (total carbohydrate, ripeness, cooking duration, and fiber content) or different methods between studies.[64] However, when a clinical trial was carried out using four different diets (high GI, high carbohydrate; low GI, high carbohydrate; high GI, low carbohydrate; low GI, low carbohydrate) in the same institution, there were limited data to support a health benefit of low-GI diet, except when coupled with a low-carbohydrate diet as well[66]; this health benefit was a decrease in triglyceride levels.[66] Conversely, when a low-GI diet was used with a high-carbohydrate diet, metabolic outcomes worsened as insulin sensitivity decreased and LDL-cholesterol increased.[66] In addition to minimal cardiovascular risk effects, there also seems to be no difference between a high-GI diet and low-GI diet from a weight loss standpoint when caloric intake between diets are similar.[67]

Low-Fat Diet

Perhaps the most highly prescribed type of diet is the low-fat diet because it carries health benefits (CVD and diabetes risk reduction) and promotes weight loss.[52] More recently, the type of fat verses the amount of fat (within the total daily caloric goal) seems to be more important from a health stance. Because diabetes and CVD are common comorbidities of obesity, reducing the amount of saturated fat and trans-fatty acid content of the diet is recommended.[52] Randomized control trials that lowered the intake of dietary saturated fat and replaced it with polyunsaturated vegetable oil reduced CVD by approximately 30%, similar to reductions observed in statin regimens.[66] Both polyunsaturated and monounsaturated fats are suggested to replace saturated fats; however, studies consistently find polyunsaturated fats to reduce CVD risk more so than monounsaturated fats.[68]

The "take home" message for patients is to replace saturated fats with unsaturated fats. Table 9.3 identifies the primary type of fat found in several fats and oils. The Mediterranean dietary pattern in which unsaturated fats (high in olive oil) predominates repeatedly has been shown to lower the

TABLE 9.3 Primary Fats in Oils and Food Products		
Saturated Fat	**Monounsaturated Fat**	**Polyunsaturated Fat**
Butter	Olive oil	Soybean oil
Lard/Crisco	Canola oil	Sunflower oil
Coconut oil	Sesame oil	Corn oil
Palm oil	Peanut oil	Cottonseed oil
Palm kernel oil	Safflower oil	Flaxseed oil
Whole milk	Seeds (pumpkin and sesame seeds)	Seeds (flax, pumpkin, sesame, sunflower)
Dairy products made with whole milk (cheese, yogurt, cream cheese)	Nuts/nut butter (macadamia, hazelnuts, pecans, almonds, cashews)	Nuts (walnuts and pine nuts)
Cream	Peanuts/peanut butter	Fish (salmon, tuna, sardines, mackerel)
Processed meat (hot dogs, sausage, salami)	Avocados	Tofu
Baked goods (cinnamon rolls, donuts, some cookies)	Olives	Mayonnaise

Adapted from https://healthyforgood.heart.org/eat-smart/articles/saturated-fats; https://healthy-forgood.heart.org/eat-smart/articles/monounsaturated-fats; and https://healthyforgood.heart.org/eat-smart/articles/polyunsaturated-fats.

incidence of CVD.[69,70,71] However, in addition to the common use of olive oil, this diet emphasizes the consumption of fruits, vegetables, legumes, and nuts; moderate amounts of fish and dairy; and low amounts of meat.

In addition to replacing saturated fats with unsaturated fats, patients should be educated about the avoidance of trans-fatty acids. It should be noted that there are two types of trans-fatty acid—one that occurs naturally in meat and milk called ruminant trans-fatty acids and another that is produced by chemical and enzymatic action called industrial trans-fatty acids.[72] The latter type of trans-fatty acids typically found with other fats in margarines, baked foods, and commercial deep-fried foods are slowly coming off the market because of the adverse effects of health.[72]

Low-Carbohydrate Versus Low-Fat Diet—Overall Recommendation

As stated earlier, there have been no differences in weight loss between a low-carbohydrate and a low-fat diet long-term using a low-calorie approach; however, research does suggest that these two diets may produce differences in cardiometabolic outcomes.[51] For example, a low-fat LCD approach has shown a greater reduction in LDL cholesterol than a low-carbohydrate LCD diet, whereas a low-carbohydrate LCD approach has shown more reduction in triglyceride levels and larger increases in high-density lipoprotein cholesterol (these two have an inverse relationship).[51] Interestingly, there is no long-term (1 yr) difference in glycemic control between these two diets either.[73]

In either case, the author recommends healthier fats and high-quality carbohydrates discussed earlier. Severe calorie restriction is not advisable. In fact, a nondiet approach to avoid yo-yo dieting and to build a healthy relationship with food is advisable, particularly with children and teenagers who are still learning food habits.

Nondiet Approach or Intuitive Eating

Often used in conjunction with a low-fat approach is a nondiet approach that emphasizes healthy food choices of moderate portion sizes. In this approach, one does not count calories or grams of macronutrients but eats nutrient-dense/low-fat foods in moderation and tries to cook in a low-fat manner as well (grilling or baking verses frying, for example). Small, gradual changes are recommended for this approach for long-term success.[74]

When a group of dieters were compared with a group using the nondiet approach, both participating in a weight management program including nutrition education, behavior modification, and exercise, the dieters fared better at 1 year, but by 2 years, the dieters weight bounced back to baseline (the hallmark of dieting), whereas the nondiet approach group continued to decrease their BMI.[75] Dieting has been associated with weight regain and poor body image and eating disorders.[76] Dieters are eight times more likely than nondieters to develop an eating disorder. White females have the highest prevalence of this condition.[76] This, however, has been disputed by some researchers owing to possible clinician bias toward non-white ethnicities and those of male gender when assessing for symptoms.[77]

Dieting may predispose an individual to binge eating by increasing a desire for the "forbidden" food and terminating meals because of a regimen or self-imposed limit rather than satiation.[78] The latter interferes with self-regulation and satiation cues.[79] The practice of dieting has been reported in 46% of U.S. high school students.[80] Early behaviors set the stage for later behaviors[81]; this is important to consider because multiple attempts at dieting are often unsuccessful and may not predict weight loss or maintenance, but weight regain,[78,82] as mentioned earlier.

Intuitive eating is a nondieting approach. It teaches one to enjoy eating, reject the dieting mentality, and use nutrition information without judgment, while respecting one's body regardless of its shape.[83] The overall goal is to normalize one's relationship with food. Principles of this innate approach include both honoring hunger and the feeling of fullness.[84] Intuitive eating is inversely associated with BMI and disordered eating in both males and females.[84]

Nondieting approaches are a combination of nutrition and behavior modification, with attention to moderate exercise as well. The goal is to move away from deprivation and work associated with dieting and think of weight loss as a gradual process or journey while regaining self-regulation or intuition of hunger and satiety for long-term weight management.

Activity Modification

PA is a vital component for treating overweight and obesity. PA alone without reduction in energy intake through a nondieting or dieting approach results in minimal weight loss.[30] PA is associated with better weight loss maintenance. This may be due to increased muscle mass and decreased fat mass, which increase RMR as discussed earlier.[30,50] Clinicians should educate their patients on realistic weight loss expectation from PA and emphasize other benefits beyond weight loss.

Moderate to vigorous PA (the equivalence of brisk walking) is often recommended for weight loss.[85] Elevation of RMR has two phases: a short-term response to the exercise event and then an ongoing one lasting up to 48 hours later.[50] PA guidelines to promote a clinically significant weight loss is >225 min/wk (see Table 9.1)[30]; to maintain weight loss, these recommendations are almost as high (which contributes to the difficulty of maintaining a weight loss). When energy restriction is coupled with moderate to vigorous PA, 30% or more weight loss can occur.[30] It should be noted that no additional protein intake is suggested for the average individual engaging in PA, as these increased recommendations are intended for athletes in training.[86]

Besides weight loss and maintenance, however, benefits of exercise include improved cardiorespiratory fitness, increase in high-density lipoprotein cholesterol, decrease in LDL cholesterol, increase in glucose control, and the prevention of type 2 diabetes, osteoporosis, and certain cancers.[30,85,87] There is also evidence that exercise improves mood and promotes better sleep patterns.[88]

Busy adults find professional PA recommendations challenging, and the clinician should be cognizant that some exercise is better than no exercise, which comes from the feeling of being defeated by the recommended duration. Many obese adults are quite sedentary, and a 10- or 15-minute walk can be a realistic start to a more active lifestyle. Moreover, gradual addition of activity may lead to less soreness and more continued compliance. The obese patient should engage in activities that put minimal stress on joints, such as walking, swimming, water exercises, and cycling.[89] Although evidence supports high amounts of activity for long-term weight loss maintenance, the sedentary individual needs to start slowly and find a type of exercise that is not only tolerable but also enjoyable.

Integrating PA into daily activity is a reasonable first step with a sedentary obese patient. Taking the stairs instead of the elevator or taking a short walk at lunch verses sitting in the lunch room are examples. Sedentary behavior not only displaces more physically active behavior but can also result in increased caloric intake (such as snacking while watching television). Recent attempts to decrease sedentary behavior include the use of standing desks, pedometers, FitBits, and apps on smart phones to count steps.

Reducing sedentary behavior and increasing PA are critical steps in weight loss and better health and also help maintain weight loss. Once PA has been modified, it needs to be a regular component of a healthy lifestyle.

Behavior Modification

Behavioral approaches to weight loss generally encompass diet and activity modification. As stated earlier, obese patients generally know healthy food choices and how long they should exercise. Practicing and sustaining these healthy lifestyle behaviors are the challenges. Weight loss interventions using behavior modification components or individual weight loss counseling should teach individuals strategies for addressing unhealthy behavior patterns that lead to overeating or lack of activity.

If a patient is drinking six cans of soda a day, behavior modification is necessary, but a diet is not. This is an example of how a nondiet approach can be very successful. Whether it is going to bed earlier or switching from regular soda to a calorie-free drink, often one or two behavior changes is all one needs to initiate a weight loss.[74]

Whether in a group setting or individually, the clinician can use various behavioral strategies to increase awareness of eating triggers or problematic behavior patterns. Once the patient is aware of the problematic behavior, problem solving it, goal setting, and follow-up care are needed.

1. Identifying the problem

A clinician can obtain a "snap shot" of the patient's typical day as discussed previously. Together, the clinician and patient can identify challenging times of the day or situations, problem solve, and develop goals to try to promote change. Using the previous example of a patient drinking excessive soda, the clinician's obtained snap shot would reveal this poor dietary behavior. Another way to help patients identify obesity-contributing lifestyle behaviors is by teaching them to self-monitor. As discussed earlier, a 3-day food record that includes the time of day, food eaten, quantity, hunger level, mood of the patient, and type and duration of activity is the most comprehensive type of recording system. This allows the clinician and patient to look back and try to decipher patterns of overeating and lost opportunities for PA.

This same food and activity tool to help identify problematic areas can also serve as a tool to decrease food intake and increase PA as self-monitoring increases adherence to healthier lifestyle.[90] There are several smart phone apps available to track food and activity. These may be more convenient for the patient to use and may provide calorie intake and output with daily goals (e.g., My fitness pal; Lose it); however, there is no app, to date, that also includes the mood of the patient, which is an important element of overeating.[91] Helping a patient work through emotional eating involves basic counseling skills and is more involved than suggesting a food alternative or finding a window of opportunity for PA (see Emotional Eating at the end of Behavior Modification section).

2. Problem solving

Once a problematic behavior has been identified, both the patient and clinician try to develop strategies to overcome the behavior. The clinician should take the "back seat" on this process and allow the patient to develop his or her own strategy, if possible.[92] This patient-centered approach puts the patient in the expert position of their own life. After all, a patient can better assess how realistic a plan is for his or her own lifestyle. Moreover, ownership to a solution creates more "buy in" and desire to carry out the plan.[92] If the patient is having difficulty proposing a solution, the clinician may want to help with the development of the plan. Every effort should be made, including the use of silence, to give patients a chance to think to allow the opportunity for them to propose a solution.

3. Setting goal(s)

Although traditionally setting goals for weight management often has included the number of pounds per week or month one hopes to lose, the goal should, instead, be behavior based. For example, if skipping lunch is the problem that was identified that triggers overeating at 5:00 PM, a goal should include eating lunch each day. This goal is Specific, Measurable, Achievable, Rewarding, and Time specific. The acronym SMART is widely used for goal setting, both clinically and in corporate situations.[93,94]Table 9.4 outlines SMART goals useful for lifestyle modification. For the best outcome, each component is necessary when setting a goal. This is where the clinician may have to assist the patient with his or her proposed solution and tweak it to a concrete goal (for e.g., "That is great that you will go to the gym, but how many times, realistically, can you plan to go each week and for how long each time?" would be typical assistance to help patients better clarify their PA goal).

The importance of including the patient in the identification of the problem, problem solving, and goal setting (all steps) cannot be overemphasized. Not only is the clinician showing respect for the capability of the patient, but the clinician is also exhibiting cultural competence by ensuring that the patient's cultural and, perhaps, religious values are taken into consideration in the treatment plan.[95]

4. Follow-up

See Follow-up Care section later in the chapter.

TABLE 9.4   Setting SMART Goals With Your Patients

S.M.A.R.T.	Meaning	Example
Use the S.M.A.R.T. acronym to help patients set achievable goals. Be sure goals are as follows:		
Specific	The goal should be clear and focused on a particular behavior	"I will not drink beverages with sugar unless there is no other alternative"
Measurable	Quantifying the goal makes it clearer	"I will exercise for 20 minutes 6 days per week"
Achievable	Goal should be realistic for the patient's circumstance	"I will eat out no more than 2 times per week"
Rewarding and **R**elevant	Patient should perceive a benefit from meeting the goal set	"To feel and look better at my high school reunion in 3 mo, I will go to the gym and workout for 1 hr 3 times per week"
Timely	Goals should be trackable and have a timeline to encourage patients to work steadily on their goals	"For the next 6 wk, I will try one new vegetable each week"

Adapted from National Lipid Association. Setting SMART Goals With Your Patients. Clinicians Lifestyle Modification Toolbox. https://www.lipid.org/sites/default/files/clmt. goal_setting. final_o.pdf. Accessed 2 January 2018.

Emotional Eating

Emotional eating is a complex problem associated with obesity.[91] Eating has been described as a convenient way to "self-medicate" whether it is a serious trigger such as stress or depression or an emotional trigger as simple as boredom. These emotions are commonly identified as catalysts to overeating and all involve maladaptive coping behaviors to alleviate the unpleasant feeling.

Reward and gratification associated with eating eventually leads to dopamine production, which activates reward and pleasure centers in the brain similar to drugs.[91] Therefore, an individual will repeatedly eat a particular food (usually high in fat or sugar) to experience this positive feeling of gratification or satisfaction.[35,39]

Self-defeating thoughts can lead to the cycle of overeating. Cognitive behavior therapy is used to restructure maladaptive self-talk and to break the pattern of negative emotions cascading into overconsumption. Mental health counselors often use a form of cognitive behavior therapy called rational emotive behavior therapy that encompasses an A-B-C framework as follows[96]:

A (activating event) > B (belief) > C (emotional and behavioral consequence).

The activating event (A) does not directly cause the consequence (C). It is the belief (B) that interferes and brings about the consequence. Using this model, counselors attempt to dispute (D) the belief, which is usually irrational, and to bring on a different effect (E) or feeling (F). For example, if an overweight person is at a party (activating event) and eventually finds himself or herself eating cookies from a cookie platter (consequence), further inquiry might show that the person felt badly about himself or herself during the party. Perhaps the person was thinking that no one was paying attention to him or her because no one liked him or her (belief). Indeed, this inadequate, irrational belief could be disputed (for many reasons, including the fact that the person was invited to the party!). It is the counselor's job to ask the patient what proof he or she has to back up the irrational belief. Usually the patient can find no reasoning behind this thought and a new feeling would prevail. Counselors can teach patients to do this cognitive reframing if their thought process continually gets in the way of lifestyle goals.

When stress has been identified as an overeating trigger, stress reduction techniques or programs can be suggested as goals to help cope with the underlying problem. Deep breathing exercises, yoga classes, or more individual coping methods such as an aromatic bubble bath are all methods to decrease stress in one's daily life.

Mindfulness meditation, defined as a nonjudgmental attention and acceptance to the immediate experience,[97] is increasingly being used to address eating-related issues, including obesity caused primarily from emotional eating.[98,99] Awareness and acceptance of stressful moments allow one to replace automatic thoughts and reactions to adverse situations with more conscious and healthier responses.[99] Although this appears to be a promising coping mechanism, limited research is available to suggest that mindfulness, without other behavioral weight management strategies, produces a significant weight loss.[98]

Starkly different from stress is the emotion of boredom that often contributes to overeating simply to distract from the unpleasant experience.[100] Boredom not only has been associated with overeating but also increases the desire to eat unhealthy food choices.[100] Moreover, the consumption of food may take the place of social interaction for some.[101] The obvious solution to eating because of boredom is to suggest the patient to engage in a hobby, go for an outing, visit friends or family, or engage in PA. The last suggestion is the most ideal solution as it would burn the most calories, but the other suggestions, if enjoyable to the patient, can be effective ways to alleviate excessive calorie intake.

A less obvious and more complex emotion to deal with is depression. As a comorbidity to obesity, depression is associated with abdominal obesity and poor diet.[91,102] Interestingly, a reciprocal link exists between depression and obesity as obesity increases the risk for depression, whereas depression is found to be predictive of developing obesity.[103]

Patients who eat in response to depression should be referred to a mental health provider to help them work on the underlying reason(s) for depression.[103,104] The mental health provider can follow the patient regularly and utilize aggressive cognitive processes to treat the depression. Often a medication can be prescribed to alleviate symptoms of depression and, consequently, aid in the process of making healthier lifestyle choices.[103]

Sleep Deprivation

Some changes in behavior, such as increased sleep, may or may not involve changes in food intake and consequent weight loss. However, if a patient is going to bed very late each night and eating in the wee hours, suggesting an earlier bedtime will cut down on calorie intake. On the other hand, if the patient is sleep deprived and does not necessarily snack at night, getting to bed earlier may still promote weight loss. The added sleep allows the patient to feel better the next day, eat less, and feel rested enough to exercise.

Although there are several suggestions clinicians can make to help their patient obtain more sleep, the patient should be part of the problem-solving approach as stated earlier so that the solution or suggestion fits his or her lifestyle. See Table 9.5 for practical considerations to help a patient develop healthy sleep pattern goals.

Surgical and Pharmacologic Approaches

Lifestyle modification, including dietary intervention, exercise, and behavioral change, are the cornerstone of obesity and overweight management. However, like other chronic diseases, obesity can require multiple modalities for effective treatment. In addition to traditional approaches, surgical and pharmacologic approaches might also be used, particularly for the patient with higher BMIs. Surgical approaches are potentially indicated with severe obesity, BMI >40 kg/m^2, or those with BMI >35 kg/m^2 with significant comorbidities,[57] whereas pharmacologic agents demand a BMI >30 or 27 kg/m^2 with at least one comorbity.[105]

There are currently four types of bariatric surgical procedures, including gastric banding, sleeve gastrectomy, Roux-en-Y gastric bypass, and biliopancreatic diversion with or without duodenal switch.[106] Each procedure has its pros and cons with consideration patient specific.

Like surgical procedures, there are many pharmacologic agents on the market today, including orlistat, phentermine, topiramate, phentermine/topiramate, and lorcaserin hydrochloride.[51] There are specific mechanisms of action and side effects to each, and the use of one over the other should be carefully planned based on the health profile of the obese patient. As with the consideration of surgery, the use of anti-obesity medication should be prescribed and managed by an obesity specialist.

TABLE 9.5 Practical Suggestions for Patients to Develop Healthy Sleep Patterns	
1.	Refrain from caffeine-containing beverages or foods after 1:00 PM (or earlier if very sensitive)
2.	Do not eat high-sodium foods as a late dinner or evening snack as the sensation of thirst may hinder sleep
3.	Avoid strenuous exercise before bedtime. Exercise can decrease the production of melatonin, a natural tranquilizer made in the body
4.	Avoid deep or critical thinking before bedtime. Such issues may affect sleep due to anxiety. If worrying or trying to remember something, write it down and refer to this note the next day
5.	Take a warm shower or bath to relax muscles. Aromatherapy in the bath adds to the feeling of relaxation
6.	Turn off all electronics. A glaring computer light or television can easily keep one from sleeping. Even the vibration of the cell phone can interfere with sleep. For best sleep, these devices should not even be in the bedroom
7.	Set a comfortable temperature for the room (slightly cooler to allow for warmth from blanket)
8.	Develop a bedtime routine. Establish a pattern of doing the same thing before bed each evening (e.g., read, meditate, pray)
9.	Have a regular bedtime each evening, keeping weekends fairly close to weekdays

Adapted from Savoye-DeSanti M. *1 Thing "diet": It Doesn't Get Any Simpler.* Denver: Outskirts Press; 2012.

It should be noted that, although the clinician should start with a referral to the specialist to determine if the patient is a viable candidate for either surgery or pharmacologic treatment, in either case, traditional approaches would have to have been attempted to be considered for these more aggressive treatments. Diet, activity, and behavior modification will have to be maintained even with or after surgical and pharmacologic agents have been used. Most currently available pharmaceutical agents prescribed without an accompanying program of behavior modification achieve no more than a 5% to 10% long-term weight loss. Furthermore, weight regain is likely if the medication is discontinued or when health-promoting behaviors are not maintained.[107]

FOLLOW-UP CARE

Regular follow-up is associated with improved outcomes in weight management.[51] Dose responses have shown the more often a patient is seen in follow-up visits that review goals and reassess progress, the more successful the outcome is regardless of the delivery method.[86,108,109] Many overweight patients are seeking accountability for their behavior. A short follow-up visit provides this, whether one-on-one or a group setting, face-to-face or technology driven. If in-person, group follow-up may be more cost-effective (weight checks and group counseling), allowing for more patients to be seen in a specified time frame.

Whichever mode of follow-up is used, the patient should be encouraged to continue with the healthy lifestyle change, and in some cases, the clinician might encourage the patient to add an additional goal if more than one behavior change is needed (for example, activity increase in addition to a diet modification).

CONCLUSION

Although obesity is often viewed as preventable, its causes are multifactorial and complex. When assessing and treating an overweight or obese patient, there are several factors to consider. A comprehensive assessment should include genetics/family history, potential comorbidities or undiagnosed concurrent conditions, history of weight gain/loss (yo-yo dieting), caloric intake, activity level, emotional state and coping mechanisms employed, and sleep pattern.

Lifestyle treatment for obesity should include both diet and activity changes with the use of behavior modification to ensure solid behavior change verses short-term fixes. The clinician should be aware of pros and cons of different dietary approaches and consider comorbidities, if any already exists. A nondiet approach should be considered, particularly if there is room for lifestyle change in the patient's typical day. Small, gradual behavior changes can lead to significant weight loss, and the changes are more likely to be long term. Activity should be a regular part of the patient's plan for long-term success. Poor sleep patterns and coping mechanisms should not be overlooked. These, too, may be appropriate behavior changes to promote weight loss.

Clinicians should remind their patients that even modest weight losses of 5% to 10% are sufficient to improve physical health and prevent comorbid diseases from developing. The goals set for weight loss should be behavior oriented, realistic, and, most importantly, patient centered (developed with the input of the patient). Regular follow-up increases patient accountability of goals and improves outcomes.

A surgical or pharmacologic approach might be indicated for patients with higher BMIs who require multiple modalities. However, lifestyle modification needs to be at the forefront of these nontraditional approaches to ensure optimal effectiveness and weight loss maintenance.

ACKNOWLEDGMENTS:

I would like to thank Sonia Caprio, MD, for her careful review of this chapter and Jennifer Chick, BS, for her skillful formatting of the tables. I am greatly appreciative of these dear colleagues and friends.

SUGGESTED RESOURCES AND MATERIALS

An important role of a clinician is to link patients with other weight management resources outside of the clinic setting that may enhance patients' chances for success. Recommended programs should promote the diet and exercise principles outlined in this chapter and should teach the behavioral and cognitive skills that are essential if weight loss is to be achieved and then maintained.

Some commercial weight loss programs and peer-led support groups such as Weight Watchers and Take Off Pounds Sensibly (TOPS) Club, Inc., are widely available and can help patients achieve significant reductions in weight.[110] These organizations also have interactive online programs and resources that may be a more attractive option for busy lifestyles today. There are other Web-based programs available such as WebMD. Although technology-based weight-loss interventions are still in their infancy, important components, including regular monitoring, counselor feedback, social support, and use of structured program with ability to individualize, have been identified as effective for the facilitation of weight loss.[109] Although promising, more long-term research is needed. Clinicians should advise their patients that many commercial programs advertising quick weight loss are associated with high costs, high attrition rates, and the regain of 50% or more of lost weight in 1 to 2 years.[110]

The Centers for Disease Control and Prevention Task Force on Community Preventive Services found sufficient evidence that worksite programs can produce significant weight loss, particularly if staffed by appropriately credentialed individuals.[111] Multidisciplinary programs may also be offered through local health care facilities, health departments, fitness centers, and parks and recreation centers. These programs frequently offer professional guidance by dietitians, physical therapists, exercise physiologists, or other counselors and health educators. These may be found by contacting local dietitians and public health agencies.[49]

Online Resources

Academy of Nutrition and Dietetics
www.eatright.org (patient information and referral information to registered dietitian nutritionist)

American Academy of Family Physicians:
www.aafp.org or https://familydoctor.org/condition/obesity

American Heart Association
Re: Weight Management
http://www.heart.org/HEARTORG/HealthyLiving/WeightManagement/Weight-Management_UCM_001081_SubhomePage.jsp

Re: Mediterranean Diet
http://www.heart.org/HEARTORG/HealthyLiving/HealthyEating/Mediterranean-Diet_UCM_306004_Article.jsp#W092Vkjwauk

American Diabetes Association:
http://www.diabetes.org/

Re: weight loss
http://www.diabetes.org/food-and-fitness/weight-loss/getting-started/weight-loss-the-basics.html?referrer=https://www.google.com/

National Institute for Diabetes, Digestive, and Kidney Diseases
http://win.niddk.nih.gov/

Take off Pounds Sensibly (TOPS)
https://www.tops.org

WebMD
http://www.webmd.com

Weight Watchers
http://www.weightwatchers.com

Print Resources

MEAL PLANNING

American Diabetes Association & Academy of Nutrition and Dietetics. *Choose Your Foods: Food Lists for Weight Management;* 2014.

Duffy RL. *Complete Food and Nutrition Guide.* American Academy of Nutrition; 2017.

Easy Food Tips for Heart Healthy Eating. American Heart Association [brochure].

MEAL PLANNING & BEHAVIOR MODIFICATION

Brownell K. *The LEARN Program for Weight Management.* Dallas, TX: American Health Publishing; 2000.

Piechota T. *Real Solutions Weight Loss Workbook.* American Academy of Nutrition; 2015.

NON-DIETING APPROACH

Savoye-DeSanti M. *1 Thing "Diet": Doesn't Get Any Simpler.* Denver: Outskirts Press; 2012.

Tribole E, Resch E. *Intuitive Eating Workbook: Principles for Nourishing a Healthy Relationship With Food.* Oakland: Harbinger Publications; 2017.

Jonas S, Konner L. *Just the Weigh You Are: How to Be Fit and Healthy Whatever Your Size.* Shelburne: Chapters Publishing; 1997.

REFERENCES

1. Fryar CD, Carroll MD, Ogden CL. *Prevalence of Overweight, Obesity, and Extreme Obesity Among Adults Aged 20 and over: United States, 1960–1962 through 2011–2014.* National Center for Health Statistical Data, Health E-stats; July, 2016. Available at https://www.cdc.gov/nchs/data/hestat/obesity_child_13_14/obesity_child_13_14.htm. Retrieved on 25 January 2018.
2. Hales CM, Carroll MD, Frayar CD, et al. *Prevalence of Obesity Among Adults and Youth: United States, 2015–2016. NCHS Data Brief, No 288.* Hyattsville, MD: National Center for Health Statistics; 2017.
3. Pi-Sunyer X, Blackburn G, Brancati FL, et al. Reduction in weight and cardiovascular disease risk factors in individuals with type 2 diabetes: one-year results of the look AHEAD trial. *Diabetes Care.* 2007;30:1374-1383.
4. Bray GA, Kim KK, Wilding JPH. Obesity: a chronic relapsing progressive disease process. A position statement of the world obesity federation. *Obe Rev.* 2017;18(7):715-723. doi:10.1111/obr.12551.
5. Geloneze B, Mancini MC, Coutinho W. Obesity: knowledge, care, and commitment, but not yet cure. *Arq Bras Endocrinol Metabol.* 2009;53(2):117-119.
6. Flegal KM, Graubard BI, Williamson DF, et al. Excess deaths associated with underweight, overweight, and obesity. *JAMA.* 2005;293(15):1861-1867.
7. World Health Organization. *Preventing and Managing the Global Epidemic of Obesity. Report of the World Health Organization Consultation of Obesity.* Geneva: WHO; 1997.
8. NHLBI Obesity Education Initiative Expert Panel on the Identification, Evaluation and Treatment of Overweight in Adults. Clinical guidelines on the identification, evaluation, and treatment of overweight and obesity in adults: executive summary. *Am J Clin Nutr.* 1998;68:899-917.

9. Gasteyger C, Tremblay A. Metabolic impact of body fat distribution. *J Endocrinol Invest.* 2002;25(10):876-883.

10. Deurenberg P. Limitations of the bioelectrical impedance method for the assessment of body fat in severe obesity. *Am J Clin Nutr.* 1996;64(suppl 3):449S-452S.

11. Coppini LZ, Waitzberg DL, Campos AC. Limitations and validation of bioelectrical impedance analysis in morbidly obese patients. *Curr Opin Clin Nutr Metab Care.* 2005;8(3):329-332.

12. Ramachandrappa S, Farooqi IS. Genetic approaches to understanding human obesity. *J Clin Invest.* 2011;121(6):2080-2086.

13. Xia Q, Grant SFA. The genetics of human obesity. *Ann N Y Acad Sci.* 2013;1281(1):178-190. doi:10.1111/nyas.12020.

14. Fawcett KA, Barroso I. The genetics of obesity: FTO leads the way. *Trends Genet.* 2010;26(6):266-274. doi:10.1016/j.tig.2010.02.006.

15. Llewellyn CH, Trzaskowski M, Plomin R, et al. Finding the missing heritability in pediatric obesity: the contribution of genome-wide complex trait analysis. *Int J Obes.* 2013;37:1506-1509. doi:10.1038/ijo.2013.30.

16. Dubois L, Kyvik KO, Girard M, et al. Genetic and environmental contributions to weight, height, and BMI from birth to 19 years of age: an international study of over 12,000 twin pairs. *PLoS One.* 2012;7(2):e30153. doi:10.1371/jounrla.pone.0030153.

17. Garber JR, Cobin RH, Garib H, et al. Clinical practical guidelines for hypothyroidism in adults: cosponsored by the American association of clinical endocrinologists and the American thyroid association. *Endo Practice.* 2012;18(6):988-1028.

18. Nieman LK, Ilias I. Evaluation and treatment of cushing syndrome. *JAMA.* 2005;188(12):1340-1346.

19. Gentile S. Contributing factors to weight gain during long-term treatment with second-generation antipsychotics. A systematic appraisal and clinical implications. *Obes Rev.* 2009;10(5):527-542. doi:10.111/j.1467-789X.2009.00589.x.

20. Kim DH, Maneen MJ, Stahl SM. Building a better antipsychotic: receptor targets for the treatment of multiple symptom dimensions of schizophrenia. *Neurotherapeutics.* 2009;6(1):78-85. doi:10.1016/j.nurt.2008.10.020.

21. Bak M, Fransen A, Janssen J, et al. Almost all antipsychotics results in weight gain: a meta-analysis. *PLoS One.* 2014;9(4):e94112. doi:10.1371/journal.pone.0094112.

22. Tarricone I, Ferrari Gozzi B, Serretti A, et al. Weight gain in antipsychotic-naïve patients: a review and meta-analysis. *Psychol Med.* 2010;40:187-200.

23. Rooney BL, Schauberger CW. Excess pregnancy weight gain and long-term obesity: one decade later. *Obstet Gynecol.* 2002;100(2):245-252.

24. Linne Y, Dye L, Barkeling B, et al. Weight development over time in parous women—the SPAWN study—15 years follow-up. *Intl J Obes Rel Met Dis.* 2003;27(12):1516-1522.

25. Filozof C, Fernandez Pinilla MC, Fernandez-Cruz A. Smoking cessation and weight gain. *Obes Rev.* 2004;5(2):95-103. doi:10.1111/j.1467-789X.2004.00131.x.

26. Ogden J, Stavrinaki M, Stubbs J. Understanding the role of life events in weight loss and weight gain. *Psychol Health Med.* 2009;14(2):239-249. doi:10.1080/13548500802512302.

27. Food and Drug Administration. *Obesity Working Group Report. Calories Count: Report of the Working Group on Obesity;* 2012. https://www.fda.gov/Food/FoodScienceResearch/ConsumerBehaviorResearch/ucm081696.htm. Accessed 21 January 2018.

28. Shim JS, Oh K, Kim HC. Dietary assessment methods in epidemiologic studies. *Epidemiol Health.* 2014;36:e2014009.

29. Yang YJ, Kim MK, Hwang SH, et al. Relative validities of 3-day food records and the food frequency questionnaire. *Nutr Res Pract.* 2010;4(2):142-148.

30. Swift DL, Johannsen NM, Lavie CJ, et al. The role of exercise and physical activity in weight loss and maintenance. *Prog Cardiovasc Dis.* 2014;56(4):441-447. doi:10.1016/j.pcad.2013.09.012.

31. Owen N, Health GN, Matthews CE, et al. Too much sitting: the population-health science of sedentary behavior. *Exerc Sport Sci Rev.* 2010;38(3):105-113. doi:10.1097/JES.0b013e3181e373a2.

32. Egger G, Dixon J. Beyond obesity and lifestyle: a review of 21st century chronic disease determinants. *Biomed Res Int.* 2014. doi:10.1155/2014/731685.

33. American Psychological Association. *Stress Eating,* 2013. Retrieved from www.apa.org/news/press/releases/stress/2013/eating.aspx.

34. Block JP, He Y, Zaslavsky AM, et al. Psychosocial stress and change in weight among U.S. adults. *Am J Epidemiol.* 2009;170(2):181-192.

35. Epel E, Lapidus R, McEwen B, et al. Stress may add bite to appetite in women: a laboratory study of stress-induced cortisol and eating behavior. *Psychoneuroendocrinology.* 2001;26(1):37-49.

36. Sinha R, Jastreboff AM. Stress as a common risk factor for obesity and addiction. *Biol Psychiatry.* 2013;73:827-835. doi:10.1016/j.biopsych.2013.01.032.

37. Sato AF, Fahrenkamp AJ. From bench to bedside: understanding stress-obesity research within the context of translation to improve pediatric behavioral weight management. *Pediatr Clin North Am.* 2016;63:401-423.

38. Koch FS, Sepa A, Ludvigsson J. Psychological stress and obesity. *J Pediatr.* 2008;153(6):839-844.

39. Volkow ND, Wang GJ, Folwler JS, et al. Food and drug reward: overlapping circuits in human obesity and addiction. *Curr Top Behav Neurosci.* 2012;11:1-24. doi:10.1007/7854_2011_169.

40. Cohen S, Kamarch T, Mermelstein R. A global measure of perceived stress. *J Health Soc Behavior.* 1983;24:385-396.

41. Lee E. Review of the psychometric evidence of the perceived stress scale. *Asian Nurs Res.* 2012;6:121-127.

42. Garaulet M, Canteras M, Morales E, et al. Validation of a questionnaire on emotional eating for use in cases of obesity; the Emotional Eater Questionnaire (EEQ). *Nutr Hosp.* 2012;27(2):645-651. doi:10.3305/nh.2012.27.2.5649.

43. Center for Disease Control and Prevention (CDC). QuickStats: Sleep Duration Among Adults Aged > 20 years, by Race/Ethnicity – National Health and Nutrition Examination Survey, US, 2007–2010. Available at https://www.cdc.gov/mmwr/preview/mmwrhtml/mm6236a9.htm. Accessed 28 January 2018.

44. Gangwisch JE, Malaspina D, Boden-Albala B, et al. Inadequate sleep as a risk factor for obesity: analyses of NHANES 1. *Sleep.* 2005;10:1289-1296.

45. Itani O, Kaneita Y, Murata A, et al. Association of onset of obesity with sleep duration and shift work among Japanese adults. *Sleep Med.* 2011;12(4):341-345.

46. Grandner MA, Jackson N, Gooneratne NS, et al. The development of a questionnaire to assess sleep-related practices, beliefs, and attitudes. *Behav Sleep Med.* 2014;12(2):123-142.

47. Motamedi KK, McClary AC, Amedee RG. Obstructive sleep apnea: a growing problem. *Ochsner J.* 2009;9(3):149-153.

48. Cummins S, Macintyre S. Food environment and obesity: neighborhood or nation? *Int J Epidemiology.* 2006;35(1):100-104. doi:10.1093/ije/dyi276.

49. Jonas S, Schelbert KB. Weight management. In: Woolf SH, Jonas S, Kaplan-Liss E, eds. *Health Promotion and Disease Prevention in Clinical Practice.* 2nd ed. Philadelphia: Wolters Kluwer Health/Lippincott Williams & Wilkins; 2008.

50. Speakman JR, Selman C. Physical activity and resting metabolic rate. *Proc Nutr Soc.* 2003;62(3):621-634.

51. American Academy of Nutrition and Dietetics. Position of the academy of nutrition and dietetics: interventions for the treatment of overweight and obesity in adults. *J Acad Nutr Diet.* 2016;116:129-147. doi:10.1016/j.jand.2015.10.031.

52. American Dietetic Association. Position of the American dietetic association: weight management. *J Am Diet Assoc.* 2009;109:330-346. doi:10.1016/j.ada.2008.11.041.

53. Hall KD, Chow CC. Why is the 3500 kcal per pound weight loss rule wrong? *Int J Obes (Lond).* 2013;37(12):1614.

54. Thomas DM, Martin CK, Lettieri S, et al. Can a weight loss of one pound a week be achieved with a 3500-kcal deficit? Commentary on a commonly accepted rule. *Int J Obes (Lond).* 2013;37(12):1611-1613.

55. Bakhach M, Shah V, Harwood T, et al. The protein-sparing modified fast diet: an effective and safe approach to induce rapid weight loss in severely obese adolescents. *Glob Pediatr Health.* 2016;3:1-6. doi:10.1177/2333794X15623245.

56. Tsai AG, Wadden TA. The evolution of very-low-calorie diets: an update and meta-analysis. *Obesity.* 2006;14:1283-1293.

57. Jensen MD, Ryan DH, Apovian CM, et al. 2013 AHA/ACC/TOS guideline for the management of overweight and obesity in adults: a report of the American College of Cardiology/American heart association task force on practice guidelines for the obesity society. *Circulation.* 2014;129(suppl 2):S102-S38. doi:10.1161/01.cir.000437739.71477.ee.

58. Foster GD, Wyatt HR, Hill JO, et al. Weight and metabolic outcomes after 2 years on a low-carbohydrate versus low-fat diet: a randomized trial. *Ann Intern Med.* 2010;153:147-157.

59. Bravata D, Sanders L, Huang L, et al. Efficacy and safety of low-carbohydrate diets: a systematic review. *JAMA.* 2003;289:1837-1850.

60. Nordman AJ, Nordmann A, Briel M, et al. Effects of low-carbohydrate vs low-fat diets on weight loss and cardiovascular risk factors: a meta-analysis of randomized controlled trials. *Arch Intern Med.* 2006;166(3):285-293.

61. Yancy WS, Olsen MK, Guyton JR, et al. A low-carbohydrate, ketogenic diet versus a low-fat diet to treat obesity and hyperlipidemia: follow up of a randomized, controlled trial. *Ann Intern Med.* 2004;140:769-777.

62. Stern L, Iqbal N, Seshadri P, et al. The effects of low carbohydrate versus conventional weight loss diets in severely obese adults: one-year follow up of a randomized trial. *Ann Intern Med.* 2004;140:778-785.

63. Jenkins D, Wolever T, Taylor R, et al. Glycemic index of foods: a physiological basis for carbohydrate exchange. *Am J Clin Nutr.* 1981;34:362-366.

64. Livesey G, Taylor R, Hulshof T, et al. Glycemic response and health—a systematic review and meta-analysis: relations between dietary glycemic properties and health outcomes. *Am J Clin Nutr.* 2008;87(1):258S-268S.

65. Barclay AW, Brand-Miller JC, Wolever T. Glycemic index, glycemic load, and glycemic response are not the same. *Diabetes Care.* 2005;28(7):1839-3840. doi:10.2337/diacare.28.7.1839.

66. Sacks FM, Carey VJ, Anderson C, et al. Effects of high vs low glycemic index of dietary carbohydrate on cardiovascular disease risk factors and insulin sensitivity. *JAMA.* 2014;312(23):2531-2541.

67. Das S, Gilhooly C, Golden J, et al. Long-term effects of 2 energy-restricted diets differing in glycemic load on dietary adherence, body composition, and metabolism in CALERIE: a 1-y randomized controlled trial. *Am J Clin Nutr.* 2007;85:1023-1030.

68. Mozaffarian D, Micha R, Wallace S. Effects on coronary heart disease of increasing polyunsaturated fat in place of saturated fat: a systematic review and meta-analysis of randomized controlled trials. *PLoS Med.* 2010;7:e1000252. doi:10.1371/journal.pmed.1000252.

69. Serra-Majem L, Roman B, Estruch R. Scientific evidence of interventions using the mediterranean diet: a systematic review. *Nutr Rev.* 2006;64:S27-S47.

70. Trichopoulou A, Costacou T, Bamia C, et al. Adherence to a mediterranean diet and survival in a Greek population. *N Engl J Med.* 2003;348:2599-2608. doi:10.1056/NEJMoa025039.

71. De Lorgeril M, Salen P, Martin JL, et al. Mediterranean diet, traditional risk factors, and the rate of cardiovascular complications after myocardial infarction: final report of the lyon diet heart study. *Circulation.* 1999;99:779-785.

72. Food and Drug Administration. *FDA News Release: The FDA Takes Step to Remove Artificial Trans Fats in Processed Foods*; June 16, 2016. http://www.fda.gov/newsevents/newsroom/pressannouncements/ucm451237.htm. Accessed 27 January 2018.

73. Davis NJ, Tomuta N, Schechter C, et al. Comparative study of the effects of a 1-year dietary intervention of a low-carbohydrate diet versus a low-fat diet on weight and glycemic control in type 2 diabetes. *Diabetes Care.* 2009;32(7):1147-1152.

74. Savoye-DeSanti M. *1 Thing "diet": It Doesn't Get Any Simpler.* Denver: Outskirts Press; 2012.

75. Savoye M, Berry D, Dziura J, et al. Anthropometric and psychosocial changes in obese adolescents enrolled in a weight management program. *J Am Diet Assoc.* 2005;105:364-370.

76. Brownell KB, Fairburn CG, eds. *Eating Disorders and Obesity: A Comprehensive Handbook.* New York: The Guilford Press; 1995.

77. Becker AE, Franko DL, Speck A, et al. Ethnicity and differential access to care for eating disorder symptoms. *Int J Eat Disord.* 2003;33(2):205-212.

78. Neumark-Sztainer D, Wall M, Story M, et al. Dieting and unhealthy weight control behaviors during adolescence: do they predict changes in weight ten years later? *J Adol Health.* 2012;50:80-86.

79. Birch LL, Fisher JO, Davison KK. Learning to overeat: maternal use of restrictive feeding practices promotes girls' eating in the absence of hunger. *A J Clin Nutr.* 2003;78:215-220.

80. Centers for Disease Control. Youth risk behavior surveillance – United States, 2011. *MMWR.* 2012;61(SS-4):1-162.

81. Birch LL, Fisher JO. Development of eating behaviors among children and adolescents. *Pediatrics.* 1998;101(S2):539-550.

82. Field AE, Haines J, Rosner B, et al. Weight-control behaviors and subsequent weight change among adolescents and young adult females. *Amer J Clin Nutr.* 2010;69:1264-1272.

83. Cole RE, Horacek T. Effectiveness of the my body knows when intuitive eating pilot program. *Am J Health Behav.* 2010;34:286-297.

84. Denny KN, Loth K, Eisenberg ME, et al. Intuitive eating in young adults: who is doing it, and how is it related to disordered eating behaviors? *Appetite.* 2013;60(1):13-19. doi:10.1016/j.appet.2012.09.029.

85. LaMonte MJ, Lewis CE, Buchner DM, et al. Both light intensity and moderate-to-vigorous physical activity measured by accelerometry are favorably associated with cardiometabolic risk factors in older women: the objective physical activity and cardiovascular health (OPACH) study. *J Am Heart Assoc.* 2017;6:e007064. doi:10.1161/JAHA.117.007064.

86. Phillips K, Wood F, Kinnersely P. Tackling obesity: the challenge of obesity management for practice nurses in primary care. *Fam Pract.* 2014;31(1):51-59.

87. Wing RR, Lang W, Wadden TA, et al. Benefits of modest weight loss in improving cardiovascular risk factors in overweight and obese individuals with type 2 diabetes. *Diabetes Care.* 2011;34(7):1481-1486. doi:10.2337/dc10-2415.

88. Gebhart C, Erlacher D, Schredl M. Moderate exercise plus sleep education improves self-reported sleep quality, daytime mood, and vitality in adults with chronic sleep complaints: a waiting list-controlled trial. *Sleep Disord.* 2011. doi:10.1155/2011/809312.
89. Schmidt S. Obesity and exercise. ACSM. Retrieved from www.acsm.org/public-information/articles/2016/10/07/obesity-and-exercise.
90. Burke LE, Wang J, Sevick MA. Self-monitoring in weight loss: a systematic review of the literature. *J Am Diet Assoc.* 2011;111:92-102.
91. Singh M. Mood, food, and obesity. *Front Psychol.* 2014;5:925. doi:10.3389/fpsyg.2014.00925.
92. Elwyn G, Dehlendorf C, Epstein RM, et al. Shared decision making and motivational interviewing: achieving patient-centered care across the spectrum of health care problems. *Ann Fam Med.* 2014;12(3):270-275. doi:10.1370/afm.1615.
93. National Lipid Association. Setting SMART Goals With Your Patients. Clinicians Lifestyle Modification Toolbox. https://www.lipid.org/sites/default/files/clmt.goal_setting.final_o.pdf. Accessed 2 January 2018.
94. Doran GT. There's a SMART way to write management's goals and objectives. *Manage Rev.* 1981;70(11):35-36.
95. Saha S, Beach MC, Cooper LA. Patient centeredness, cultural competence and healthcare quality. *J Natl Med Assoc.* 2008;100(11):1275-1285.
96. Corey G, ed. *Theory and Practice of Counseling and Psychotherapy.* 8th ed. Belmont: Thompson Brooks/Cole; 2009.
97. Kabat-Zinn J. *Coming to Our Senses: Healing Ourselves and the World Through Mindfulness.* New York: Hachette Books; 2005.
98. Dalen J, Smith BW, Shelley BM, et al. Pilot study: mindful eating and living (MEAL): weight, eating behavior, and psychological outcomes associated with a mindfulness-based intervention for people with obesity. *Compl Ther Med.* 2010;18:260-264.
99. Katterman SN, Kleinman BM, Hood MM, et al. Mindfulness meditation as an intervention for binge eating, emotional eating, and weight loss: a systematic review. *Eat Behav.* 2014;15:197-204.
100. Moynihan AB, van Tilburg WAP, Igou ER, et al. Eaten up by boredom: consuming food to escape awareness of the bored self. *Front Psychol.* 2015;6:369. doi:10.3389/fpsyg.2015.00369.
101. Baumeister RF, deWall CN, Ciarocco NJ, et al. Social exclusion impairs self-regulation. *J Pers Soc Psychol.* 2005;88:589-604.
102. Roberts RE, Deleger S, Strawbridge WJ, et al. Prospective association between obesity and depression: evidence from the Alameda county study. *Int J Obes Relat Metab Disord.* 2003;27:514-521.
103. Luppino FS, deWit LM, Bouvy PF, et al. Overweight, obesity, and depression: a systematic review and meta-analysis of longitudinal studies. *Arch Gen Psychiatry.* 2010;67(3):220-229. doi:10.1001/archgenpsychiatry.2010.2.
104. Talen MR, Mann MM. Obesity and mental health. *Primary Care.* 2009;36(2):287-305.
105. Apovian CM, Aronne LJ, Bessesen DH, et al. Pharmacological management of obesity: an endocrine society clinical practice guideline. *J Clin Endocrinol Metab.* 2015;100(2):342-362.
106. Colquitt JL, Pickett K, Loveman E, et al. Surgery for weight loss in adults. *Cochrane Database Syst Rev.* 2014;(8):CD00364. doi:10.1002/14651858.CD00364.pub 4.
107. Li Z, Maglione M, Tu W, et al. Meta-analysis: pharmacologic treatment of obesity. *Ann Intern Med.* 2005;142(7):532-546.

108. Wadden TA, Volger S, Tsai AG, et al. Managing obesity in primary care practice: an overview and perspective from the POWER-UP study. *Int J Obes (Lond).* 2013;37(01):S3-S11. doi:10.1038/ijo.2013.90.
109. Khaylis A, Yiaslas T, Bergstrom J, et al. A review of efficacious technology-based weight-loss interventions: five key components. *Telemed J E Health.* 2010;16(9):931-938. doi:10.1089/tmj.2010.0065.
110. Tsai AG, Wadden TA. Systematic review: an evaluation of major commercial weight loss programs in the United States. *Ann Intern Med.* 2005;142(1):56-66.
111. Katz DL, O'Connell M, Yeh MC, et al. Public health strategies for preventing and controlling overweight and obesity in school and worksite settings: a report on recommendations of the task force on community preventive services. *MMWR.* 2005;54(RR-10):1-12.

Please see Online Appendix: Apps and Digital Resources for additional information.

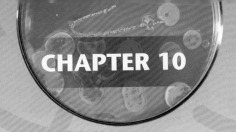

CHAPTER 10

Tobacco Use

LISA M. FUCITO

BACKGROUND

Tobacco use is the leading preventable cause of morbidity and mortality worldwide, accounting for an estimated 6 million deaths annually.[1] In the United States, tobacco use and secondhand tobacco smoke exposure account for more than 480,000 deaths and $170 billion in health care costs for smoking-related illness each year.[1,2]

The health consequences known to be causally related to tobacco use and secondhand exposure continue to increase with new research.[1] Tobacco use damages nearly every organ, causes numerous diseases and negative health effects (see Table 10.1), and lowers the overall health status.[1,3] Moreover, many of these consequences occur in children and adults who do not smoke because of secondhand tobacco smoke exposure.[1] Cigarette smoking accounts for the majority of tobacco-related harm.[1] However, smokeless tobacco and other combustible forms of tobacco (e.g., cigars, cigarillos, pipe tobacco, hookah) pose similar health risks.[1,4–6]

Tobacco cessation clearly and unequivocally reduces tobacco-related health consequences and improves overall health and life expectancy for individuals of all ages.[7,8] The National Commission on Prevention Priorities ranks tobacco-use screening and cessation support among the top three most effective and cost-effective clinical preventive services that clinicians can offer patients.[9]

In 2016, an estimated 15.1% of adults in the United Stated smoked cigarettes,[10] which represents the majority of tobacco use (~69%) among adults 25 years and older.[11] The highest smoking rates are among men (17.5%), people aged 25 to 44 (17.6%) and 45 to 64 years (18%), non-Hispanic American Indians and Alaskan Natives (31.8%) and people who identify as multiple races (25.2%), people who identify as lesbian/gay/bisexual/transgender (20.5%), people with a General Educational Development certificate but not a standard high-school diploma (40.6%), and people living below the poverty level (25.3%).[10] Noncigarette tobacco use is less common among adults but accounts for approximately 50% of tobacco use among

TABLE 10.1   Health Effects Causally Related to Tobacco Use and Secondhand Tobacco Smoke Exposure

Cancer

Bladder

Cervical
Colorectal

Esophageal

Kidney

Laryngeal

Leukemia
Liver

Lung[a]

Oral

Pancreatic

Stomach

Respiratory

Asthma[a]

Chronic obstructive pulmonary disease

Tuberculosis

Pneumonia[a]

Respiratory symptoms (coughing, phlegm, wheezing, dyspnea)[a]
Lung function decline[a]
Impaired lung growth

Cardiovascular

Aortic aneurysm
Abdominal aortic aneurysm

Atherosclerosis

Cerebrovascular disease

Coronary heart disease[a]
Stroke

Reproductive

Reduced fertility
Ectopic pregnancy
Male sexual function—erectile dysfunction
Low birth weight[a]

Placental abruption

TABLE 10.1   Health Effects Causally Related to Tobacco Use and Secondhand Tobacco Smoke Exposure   (Continued)

Placenta previa

Preterm birth

Sudden infant death syndrome[a]

Congenital
Orofacial cleft

Metabolic
Diabetes

Other Effects

Blindness, cataracts, age-related macular degeneration
Periodontitis
Middle ear disease in children (secondhand exposure only)[a]

Hip fractures

Low bone density

Rheumatoid arthritis
Immune function
Peptic ulcer disease (*Helicobacter pylori* positive)

Poor surgical outcomes

Poor wound healing

Adapted from U.S. Department of Health and Human Services. *The Health Consequences of Smoking-50 Years of Progress: A Report of the Surgeon General.* Atlanta, GA: U.S. Department of Health and Human Services, National Centers for Disease Control and Prevention, National Center for Chronic Disease Prevention And Health Promotion, Office on Smoking and Health; 2014.
[a]Health effects also linked to secondhand tobacco smoke exposure.

youth (under 18 years of age) and young adults (18–25 years old).[11] Outside of the United States, tobacco use prevalence is comparable in countries with strong tobacco control policies, which are typically high-income countries.[12] Conversely, prevalence rates in low- to middle-income countries are two to three times higher than that of the United States.[12]

The U.S. Department of Health and Human Services Office of Disease Prevention and Health Promotion set a national goal in *Healthy People 2020* to reduce cigarette smoking rates in adults and adolescents to 12% and 16%, respectively.[13] This target was achieved for adolescents in 2013; however, new benchmarks were set to reduce the increasing rates of other tobacco use in this cohort.[13] Among adults, the national smoking rate is slowly declining, but more work is needed to achieve the 2020 goal.[13]

This chapter provides clinicians and their associates with an evidence-based approach to address their patients' tobacco use based on the U.S. Public Health Services (PHS) *Guidelines for Treating Tobacco Use and Dependence.*[14] The emphasis is smoking cessation, but the interventions can also help patients change to other forms of tobacco use. Clinicians have the option to either offer comprehensive tobacco treatment through a series of clinic visits or brief cessation advice coupled with a referral to an external tobacco treatment resource. The latter option may be more feasible for some clinicians to incorporate into their daily practice.

Although most clinicians recognize that tobacco use poses a major threat to a patient's health, many do not feel confident intervening for several reasons: (1) lack of formal training in evidence-based tobacco treatment, (2) limited infrastructure and/or organizational support to deliver interventions, and (3) a history of unsuccessful attempts to help patients with significant tobacco-related diseases quit. The evidence is clear, however, that brief advice (~3 min) to quit tobacco use from a health care provider is a proven effective and efficient intervention technique that significantly increases long-term quit rates.[14,15] In addition, tobacco use disorder should be conceptualized as a chronic disease in which most individuals will undergo multiple cycles of remission and relapse and require repeated quit attempts to eventually achieve permanent tobacco abstinence.[14] It is important for clinicians and patients to expect this likely pattern, so that initial failed attempts do not discourage future cessation efforts. Only a small percentage of individuals successfully maintain abstinence after an initial quit attempt.[14] The methods outlined here are consistent with a chronic disease framework and demonstrate how best to use the limited time available to impact tobacco use among patients.

METHODS

Treating Tobacco Use and Dependence, which is available online,[14] details the PHS clinical practice guidelines for promoting tobacco cessation among patients.

Clinician Intervention

The PHS guideline comprises five activities, each beginning with the letter "A" (often referred to as the *5 A's*):

- *Ask* all patients about tobacco use
- *Advise* patients to quit tobacco use
- *Assess* patients' motivation to quit tobacco use
- *Assist* patients who are motivated to quit with evidence-based behavioral and pharmacologic interventions either directly or via referral
- *Arrange* for follow-up contacts

This intervention plan describes a general approach for patients who use tobacco and can be used in almost any outpatient encounter, whether the clinician and patient have 30 seconds or 30 minutes for the discussion.[16]

Ask *all patients about tobacco use at every opportunity.* All patients should be asked about their tobacco use (i.e., cigarette smoking, other combustible tobacco use, smokeless tobacco, electronic cigarettes) at their initial visit. The tobacco assessment should evaluate (1) lifetime use of any of these products and (2) current use defined as any use within the past 30 days.[14] For example, a nurse or other staff member should routinely ask patients "*Have you ever smoked or used other forms of tobacco?*" or "*Are you still using?*" at each visit. Tobacco use status should be documented in the patient's health record to remind the clinician and staff to discuss tobacco use at all subsequent visits. Each health system will need to determine the optimal model for identifying patients' tobacco use status. One possible method is to add tobacco use status as a *vital sign.*[17] Patients who report former tobacco use should be congratulated for achieving abstinence.

Advise *all patients who report tobacco use to stop.* A clear statement of advice (e.g., "*As your physician, I am concerned about your tobacco use. Quitting is the most important step you can take to improve your health.*") is essential. The best advice is short, clear, and personalized to the patient's clinical condition and/or other relevant information such as family history. The factors that motivate tobacco cessation will likely differ from patient to patient. It is helpful to listen to what patients value and personalize tobacco messages accordingly. Although almost any clinical encounter provides an opportunity to discuss smoking, the timing of advice can also be very important. Changes in health status often represent teachable moment opportunities in which patients may be more receptive to advice and more motivated to change their tobacco use. Clinicians and their associates should take advantage of these opportunities to provide clear advice about the benefits of tobacco cessation for health outcomes. This advice from a health care provider is a proven effective and efficient strategy that significantly increases long-term quit rates and can be as brief as 3 minutes.[14,15]

Assess *patients' motivation to quit tobacco use.* Patients' level of interest in stopping smoking is usually evident in discussions with the clinician. If it is not, ask patients if they want to stop. Patients who are motivated to quit should immediately receive behavioral and pharmacologic interventions and the development of a treatment plan either directly or via a referral to an external tobacco treatment resource. For patients who are not willing to quit, clinicians should utilize evidence-based motivational techniques to enhance tobacco cessation motivation, a model known as the *5 R's,* which is effective in increasing future quit attempts compared with no motivational advice.[14]

- *Relevance*—engage the patient in a discussion of why quitting is personally relevant
- *Risks*—ask the patient to identify potential negative consequences of tobacco use

- *Rewards*—ask the patient to identify potential benefits of stopping tobacco use
- *Roadblocks*—ask the patient to identify barriers or impediments to quitting and brainstorm how to address these, if relevant
- *Repetition*—repeat motivational steps at subsequent clinic visits

The recommendation to triage tobacco treatment based on patients' motivation to quit has received criticism. For example, only 12% to 20% of individuals who smoke cigarettes report willingness to quit smoking in the next month and motivation to quit fluctuates often.[18] Thus, requiring motivation to quit as a necessary condition to treat (i.e., an *opt-in* model) means that most patients will not receive tobacco cessation treatment. In comparison, the default treatment approach for other chronic diseases (e.g., hypertension, diabetes) is an *opt-out* model in which treatment is offered on detection with the option to decline. An alternative approach to the 5 R's for unmotivated patients would be to offer treatment and advise that patients use treatment to at least help them reduce their tobacco use.[18] Providing tobacco pharmacotherapies to smokers who are not ready to quit can significantly increase quit rates.[19-21] This treatment approach may promote cessation by increasing unmotivated smokers' motivation to quit and abstinence self-efficacy.[19] Furthermore, abrupt cessation (i.e., setting a quit date and attempting to stop altogether) is not the only successful pathway to achieve long-term tobacco abstinence. A gradual approach in which patients reduce tobacco use before complete cessation can also be effective.[22-25] Patients who express willingness to reduce tobacco use but are not motivated to quit entirely should be managed similarly to those who are willing to quit completely, and tobacco treatment should be offered.

Assist *patients in stopping.* Patients who are motivated to quit should be provided with evidence-based behavioral and pharmacologic tobacco interventions. **Combined behavioral and pharmacologic tobacco interventions are superior to either individual treatment** and are recommended in most cases.[14] A member of the care team can provide these interventions or patients can be referred to an external tobacco treatment resource such as a tobacco quit line, Web-based or text-based interventions for tobacco cessation (e.g., SmokefreeTxt.gov), and/or a service/provider with expertise in treating tobacco use disorder. One example is simply to provide the national toll-free number (1-800-QUIT-NOW) that automatically routes callers to their state's quit line and to recommend that patients call (reactive telephone counseling). This can be done in 30 seconds. This alternative care model is *Ask, Advise,* and *Refer.*[14] In this model, the initial clinician would still remain responsible for ensuring that the patient receives appropriate treatment and subsequent follow-up.[14] Care models that include all 5 steps may be more effective for tobacco cessation than the alternative three-step model.[14]

Arrange follow-up visits. Last, clinicians should *arrange* for follow-up contacts with patients by telephone or in person soon after patients initiate tobacco treatment, regardless of whether they provided tobacco treatment directly or referred patients to external tobacco resources.[14] When patients know that their progress will be reviewed, their chances of stopping successfully improve. Nurses or other clinicians as well as the physician may conduct this follow-up in the office or by telephone. It should consist of an assessment of the patient's progress, reinforcing the decision to stop, troubleshooting for any problems encountered or anticipated, and discussion of the effectiveness or side effects of cessation medications. Most relapses occur within the first weeks of initiating abstinence. Patients who are followed by a health care provider during this early phase have a greater chance of remaining abstinent than those without follow-up.[26] Although follow-up visits are critical during the first 2 weeks after cessation, clinic staff should remain in contact with patients and schedule formal follow-up visits in 1 to 2 months. For patients who cannot return for an appointment, contact by telephone or by mail may be helpful.

Pharmacologic Interventions

Pharmacotherapy is the standard of care for tobacco use disorder in addition to counseling and should be offered to all patients regardless of their motivation level. There are currently seven U.S. Food and Drug Administration (FDA)-approved pharmacologic treatments for tobacco use disorder: (1) nicotine replacement therapy (i.e., patch, gum, lozenge, inhaler, nasal spray), (2) varenicline, and (3) bupropion (see Table 10.2).[14] These treatments have minimal contraindications and are generally well tolerated. Nevertheless, all patients should be monitored for adverse events, the most common of which may be neuropsychiatric symptoms, regardless of which treatment is selected.

Selection of an appropriate agent should be based on any treatment contraindications, tobacco use disorder severity, patient preference, and cost/coverage issues. It is also important to assess patients' nicotine withdrawal symptoms and craving at treatment initiation to determine the optimal pharmacologic dose and which intervention strategies (i.e., pharmacologic and behavioral) may be beneficial. These symptoms should then be monitored throughout treatment to determine if any modifications are needed. Validated scales are available to easily quantify withdrawal symptoms,[27,28] including free Web-based versions that provide instant feedback.[29] Common withdrawal symptoms include craving, negative affect (e.g., anger, sadness, anxiety, irritability), fatigue, restlessness, difficulty concentrating, insomnia, increased appetite, or weight gain.[30] These symptoms can predict treatment failure or relapse. Thus, withdrawal symptoms should be monitored at follow-up to determine if more intensive or alternative treatment (i.e., higher nicotine replacement dose, additional pharmacologic treatment, and/or alternative behavioral strategies) is needed.

TABLE 10.2 Tobacco Cessation Pharmacotherapy

Medication	Dosing	Advantages	Disadvantages	Contraindications
Nicotine transder-mal patch	• 21 mg if >10 cig/d • 14 mg if ≤10 cig/d	• OTC • Single application daily • Different strengths available • Safe for longer-term use • Safe to combine with short-acting NRT, varenicline, and bupropion • Overnight use may reduce early morning cravings	• Slow nicotine delivery • Less flexible dosing • Side effects: skin irritation, sleep disturbance, vivid dreams	• Severe skin conditions
Nicotine gum	• 2 mg if smoke 1st cig >30 min after waking • 4 mg if smoke 1st cig ≤30 min after waking • Use every 1–2 hr	• OTC • Flexible dosing • Fast nicotine delivery • Safe for longer-term use • Safe to combine with nicotine patch, varenicline, and bupropion	• Frequent dosing required • No food or drink 15 min before use • Side effects: jaw pain, mouth soreness, dyspepsia, hiccups	• Conditions that limit saliva production; dental problems; temporomandibular joint syndrome
Nicotine lozenge	• 2 mg if smoke 1st cig >30 min after waking • 4 mg if smoke 1st cig ≤30 min after waking • Use every 1–2 hr	• OTC • Flexible dosing • Fast nicotine delivery • Safe for longer-term use • Safe to combine with nicotine patch, varenicline, and bupropion	• Frequent dosing required • No food or drink 15 min before use • Side effects: nausea, hiccups, heartburn, headache, cough	• Conditions that limit saliva production

Medication	Dosing	Advantages	Considerations/Side effects	Contraindications/Cautions
Nicotine nasal spray	0.5 mg/inhalation/nostril, 1–2 times/hr or PRN dosing	• Flexible dosing • Fastest nicotine delivery • Reduces cravings in minutes • Safe to combine with nicotine patch, varenicline, and bupropion	• Frequent dosing required • Most addictive nicotine replacement therapy • Side effects: nasal irritation, nasal congestion, change in sense of smell and taste	• Severe nasal disease; severe reactive airways disease; patients with high bleeding risk
Nicotine inhaler	6–16 cartridges/d	• Flexible dosing • Faster nicotine delivery • Mimics hand-to-mouth routine of smoking • Safe to combine with nicotine patch, varenicline, bupropion	• Frequent dosing required • Considerable effort required to achieve nicotine levels of other short-acting NRT • Side effects: mouth and throat irritation, cough, rhinitis	• Severe reactive airways disease
Bupropion SR	Titrate: 150 mg/d × 3 d, then 150 mg BID	• Non-nicotine medication • Safe for longer-term use • Safe to combine with NRT and varenicline • May delay weight gain • May be effective for comorbid depression	• Side effects: decreased seizure threshold, insomnia, dry mouth	• Seizure disorders; eating disorders; use of monoamine oxidase inhibitor in past 14 d; history of adverse reactions to stimulants and/or antidepressants; pregnant/breast-feeding
Varenicline tartrate	Titrate: 0.5 mg/d × 3 d, then 0.5 mg BID × 4 d, then 1 mg BID	• Most effective monotherapy • Non-nicotine medication • Safe for longer-term use • Safe to combine with NRT and bupropion	• Side effects: nausea, sleep disturbance, vivid dreams	• History of renal disease/decreased kidney function; pregnant/breast-feeding

NRT, nicotine replacement therapy; OTC, over the counter.

Nicotine Replacement Therapy

Nicotine is the primary addictive component of tobacco products.[31,32] Cigarettes have been engineered to deliver high levels of nicotine very quickly (~10–20 s), making them highly addictive.[33] Compared with cigarettes, nicotine replacement therapy (NRT) delivers lower nicotine levels to the brain more slowly through alternative routes (see Table 10.2), reducing the addiction potential but potentially limiting craving relief if underdosed.[33] Clinicians should advise patients about these nicotine delivery differences because it may affect satisfaction with NRT.

The nicotine patch delivers nicotine transdermally over the course of a 24-hour period; nicotine peak levels occur within 3 to 8 hours.[33] Dosing is based on number of cigarettes smoked per day. All other forms of NRT are short acting and used to relieve tobacco cravings as needed.[33] Nicotine gum and lozenges deliver nicotine through the buccal mucosa; nicotine peak levels occur within approximately 30 minutes.[33] Dosing is based on time to first cigarette of the day.[33] Patients are advised to take a gum/lozenge every 1 to 2 hours as needed, but actual nicotine delivery is far lower than the amount contained in each piece because 50% to 60% is ingested and subjected to first pass metabolism.[34,35] The nicotine inhaler delivers an aerosol to the buccal mucosa and airway,[36] and nicotine nasal spray delivers nicotine through the nasal mucosa within 5 to 10 minutes.[33]

All forms of NRT are efficacious for smoking cessation, nearly doubling the odds of quitting, and may also be helpful for treating other forms of tobacco use.[14,37–40] As monotherapy, the nicotine patch is less effective than other tobacco pharmacologic interventions such as varenicline.[41] The nicotine patch used in combination with shorter-acting NRT (i.e., nicotine gum, lozenge, inhaler, or nasal spray), however, is safe and more effective than NRT monotherapy.[41] Dual NRT may be more effective than NRT monotherapy because it delivers a higher total nicotine dose that may better approximate dose levels achieved from cigarette smoking.[33]

NRT is safe and generally well tolerated, including in patients with acute and chronic cardiovascular disease.[42,43] The long-term use of NRT does not pose a known health risk and may be helpful for patients vulnerable to relapse following cessation. NRT side effects typically reflect the route of administration: (1) oral forms can cause gastrointestinal symptoms, hiccups, mouth soreness, and jaw ache; (2) transdermal nicotine patch can cause skin irritation; (3) intranasal and inhaled forms can cause local irritation to the nose and throat, respectively. Fatal nicotine overdose from NRT is extremely rare (even when used concurrently with tobacco use) because users typically titrate their nicotine levels to the desired physiologic effect.[31] Patients may need to titrate NRT if they experience symptoms of nicotine intoxication, which include stimulatory gastrointestinal and cardiovascular symptoms such as nausea, vomiting, abdominal pain, heart palpitations, dizziness, and anxiety.[33] The FDA has revised the NRT label warnings against the use of NRT in the setting of concurrent smoking. Importantly, patients who report concurrent smoking with NRT may have inadequate control of withdrawal symptoms or cravings and require more aggressive treatment.

Varenicline

Varenicline, a partial agonist of the alpha4-beta2 nicotinic acetylcholine receptor, is more efficacious for smoking cessation than bupropion and NRT monotherapy.[44,45] Varenicline reduces the rewarding effects of smoking (i.e., inhibits dopaminergic activation) and attenuates the withdrawal syndrome in individuals who stop smoking.[46] Varenicline is also effective for other forms of tobacco use.[40] Varenicline is the most effective *monotherapy* for tobacco cessation[44] and is equivalent to dual NRT (e.g., nicotine patch plus gum or lozenge).[41]

The standard dosing guide is to initiate varenicline while patients are still using tobacco, titrating up gradually to 1 mg twice a day for a minimum duration of 12 weeks.[14] The medication is also safe and efficacious when used for up to a year.[47,48] A longer treatment duration should be strongly considered, as it is more consistent with a chronic disease model for tobacco use disorder.

The most common side effects of varenicline are nausea, sleep disturbance, and vivid dreams.[44] Early studies suggested that varenicline could cause severe neuropsychiatric symptoms in rare cases; however, subsequent meta-analyses showed that there was no greater incidence of neuropsychiatric symptoms among patients treated with varenicline compared with usual care controls.[44,49,50] A recent large-scale, placebo-controlled, double-blind trial evaluating the safety and efficacy of NRT, varenicline, and bupropion for smoking cessation in patients with and without a history of psychiatric disorders (i.e., EAGLES study) commissioned by the FDA showed no significant increase in neuropsychiatric symptoms from varenicline or bupropion relative to placebo or the nicotine patch.[51] As a result of this study, the FDA removed the warning on varenicline and bupropion regarding severe neuropsychiatric side effects in 2016.

Bupropion SR

Bupropion SR is a medication used to treat depression that has also been shown to be effective for tobacco cessation as monotherapy or in combination with other tobacco pharmacologic interventions.[52] Bupropion inhibits the reuptake of dopamine and norepinephrine.[53] The standard dosing guide is to initiate bupropion while patients are still using tobacco, titrating up gradually to 150 mg twice a day, and continued for at least 7 to 12 weeks.[14] Bupropion is also safe to use beyond 12 weeks for patients for long-term maintenance.[14] Because bupropion is less effective than varenicline as monotherapy,[54] it should be used as part of a combination therapy regimen with NRT or in patients who are unable to tolerate varenicline. Bupropion may delay weight gain associated with tobacco cessation and therefore may be preferred among obese individuals or those concerned about weight gain.[55,56] Common side effects include sleep disturbance and dry mouth. There is a small risk of seizure associated with use,[52] so bupropion should be avoided in patients with seizure disorders or at increased seizure risk. Following the recent EAGLES study noted earlier, the FDA has removed the boxed warning language regarding the potential for severe neuropsychiatric adverse events associated with bupropion.[51]

Combination Therapy

For patients highly dependent on tobacco, multiple medications may be required to control withdrawal symptoms and relieve cravings. The specific combination will likely be based on the patient's comorbidities and preference. Dual NRT typically combines the nicotine patch (long-acting drug) with a shorter-acting form of nicotine replacement (i.e., gum, lozenge).[57,58] Other studies have shown the effectiveness and safety of using two or more long-acting drugs (i.e., combinations of nicotine patch, varenicline, and bupropion).[57,59]

Behavioral Interventions

Behavioral interventions are effective for tobacco cessation either alone or in combination with pharmacotherapies.[14,37] In fact, the *combination* of behavioral and pharmacologic interventions is superior to either individual modality and is recommended in most cases.[14] Behavioral interventions increase in effectiveness with greater intensity and multiple format delivery (i.e., individual/group counseling, phone-based counseling, self-help).[14] Clinicians can provide these interventions directly or refer patients to external tobacco cessation programs/resources such as telephone-based tobacco cessation services, commonly known as quit lines.[60] Quit lines are accessible and eliminate many barriers associated with traditional tobacco cessation classes or support groups (e.g., transportation, wait times, childcare). Patients underrepresented in traditional cessation services, such as individuals who identify as members of racial or ethnic minorities, actively seek help from quit lines.[61] Depending on the state, clinicians can send referrals directly to the quit line for patients who are ready to quit within the next 30 days or are willing to reduce, whose counselors will then contact the patient directly (i.e., proactive counseling). Proactive counseling eliminates the need for the patient to call, is more effective than reactive counseling,[60] and is usually arranged by completing a referral form (often signed by both patient and clinician), which is then faxed to the service.[62]

Practical counseling and supportive treatment are the two behavioral interventions that are effective for tobacco cessation.[14] Practical counseling helps patients recognize and cope with internal (e.g., negative emotional states) and external tobacco use triggers (e.g., alcohol use, being around others who use tobacco).[14] Practical counseling also focuses on helping patients cope with tobacco cravings and learn how to change the habit of tobacco use.[14] Supportive treatment focuses on encouraging patients to stop by identifying personal cessation benefits, emphasizing the effectiveness of tobacco treatment, communicating confidence in patients' ability to stop, and conveying empathy.[14] Supportive interventions also address patients' concerns about quitting (e.g., weight gain, withdrawal symptoms/cravings, failing) and prior difficulties with initiating and/or maintaining tobacco abstinence.[14]

To address patients' weight concerns, advise them of the following: (1) small weight gain is common (~5–10 lb) and self-limited with lifestyle changes, (2) use low-calorie substitutes for tobacco use (e.g., vegetables, mints) and start/increase physical activity, (3) the risks from tobacco use far exceed the risks from small weight gain, and (4) maintain pharmacotherapy use to limit weight gain (e.g., bupropion, 4 mg nicotine gum/lozenge).[63] With respect to patients' concerns about withdrawal symptoms/cravings, it is helpful to inform patients of the nature and course of these symptoms (i.e., common symptoms, normal part of tobacco recovery process, time limited) and to advise them of the benefits of pharmacotherapy and behavioral techniques for managing them.[14] For patients who are discouraged by prior failed attempts at quitting, clinicians should educate patients that tobacco cessation often requires multiple attempts to achieve permanent abstinence. A clinician can help patients benefit from past relapses rather than view them as personal failures by helping patients to identify the circumstances that led to past relapses and to develop strategies for either avoiding those circumstances or responding to them in a different manner. Several common relapse risk factors include withdrawal symptoms, weight gain, stress, alcohol use, and social pressure.[14]

Last, it is important for patients to have positive social support to help them quit. All patients should be encouraged to tell their family, friends, and coworkers of their decision to stop tobacco use and to seek their support and encouragement. Patients with significant others who also use tobacco can have particular difficulty quitting. Spouses/partners should also be encouraged to stop. If they are unwilling to stop, they should at least be encouraged to use tobacco only outside of the home to support their partners' cessation efforts.

Tobacco Harm Reduction

Tobacco cessation remains the primary goal for all patients because there is no safe level of tobacco use. For patients who are unwilling or unable to quit tobacco, however, a secondary goal is to lower tobacco harm by either reducing tobacco use and/or switching to less toxic products.[64–66] There is limited evidence to support the use of behavioral interventions and/or standard tobacco pharmacotherapies (i.e., NRT, varenicline, bupropion) for helping patients successfully reduce tobacco use.[64] Recently, two other options, switching from cigarette smoking to electronic nicotine delivery systems and/or snus, a form of smokeless tobacco, have been investigated as potential tobacco harm reduction strategies. We briefly review these two common product groups.

Electronic Nicotine Delivery Systems/Electronic Cigarettes

Electronic nicotine delivery systems or electronic cigarettes (ECs) are battery-operated vaporizing devices that heat a liquid solution, typically propylene glycol or glycerin, which may also contain nicotine and flavorings.[65] The liquid solution, stored in disposable or refillable cartridges or a reservoir, converts into an aerosol for inhalation when heated.[65] ECs better approximate the sensory experience of cigarette smoking than the nicotine inhaler and are marketed as harm reduction products because they do not contain tobacco and are not combustible.[65] Since ECs first became available in 2006, their use has increased rapidly and created controversy within the public health community.[67] Proponents of ECs believe that they expose individuals to less harm than smoking cigarettes and may facilitate smoking cessation.[65,68] Conversely, critics contend that ECs could maintain tobacco addiction and prevent the transition to less harmful forms of nicotine replacement among individuals who currently smoke cigarettes and could increase the risk of subsequent cigarette initiation among young people.[68–70]

The rapidly changing EC industry makes the products difficult to study. There are a wide range of devices and liquids with different toxicity profiles.[71,72] Recent studies of currently available products suggest that ECs likely have adverse health effects[73,74] but are less harmful than tobacco smoking.[75,76] The long-term health effects of ECs, however, remain unknown. Large-scale clinical trials of ECs for tobacco cessation are limited.[77,78] The two trials to date did not show conclusive benefit of ECs, but the products are currently obsolete and may not have delivered adequate nicotine to users.

The FDA Center for Tobacco Products recently requested that the National Academies of Science, Engineering, and Medicine convene a panel of experts to conduct a review of the available evidence of EC health effects.[79] Among the findings, there is *conclusive evidence* that most ECs contain and emit numerous potentially toxic substances but the type and level of toxicant exposure varies by device and completely substituting ECs for combustible tobacco cigarettes reduces exposure to numerous toxicants and carcinogens founds in combustible cigarettes. Furthermore, there is *substantial evidence* that use of ECs increases the risk of ever using combustible tobacco cigarettes among young people and completely switching to ECs from combustible tobacco cigarettes results in short-term adverse health outcomes in several organ systems. Last, there is *limited evidence* that e-cigarettes are effective for smoking cessation. In light of these findings, what should we advise our patients who are interested in ECs?

Consistent with the statements of major medical associations, smokers should be encouraged to use FDA-approved tobacco pharmacotherapies in conjunction with counseling in lieu of using ECs for smoking cessation.[80,81]

Snus

"Snus" is a Swedish oral smokeless tobacco product that delivers nicotine and other chemicals through the oral mucosa. Snus may have lower levels of toxicants than other forms of smokeless tobacco. It contains carcinogens such as heavy metals and tobacco-specific nitrosamines and is associated with increased risk for pancreatic cancer but not for lung or head and neck cancers.[82] Snus has gained a lot of attention for its potential role in the reduction of cigarette smoking prevalence in Sweden. Swedish men had the largest reduction in smoking prevalence and tobacco-related diseases between 1976 and 2002, and this reduction is linked to snus use.[83,84] Similar to ECs, however, there is insufficient evidence to conclude that snus is effective for smoking cessation or for the purpose of harm reduction in the general population. Individual smokers who use snus for harm reduction should be advised that it is not harmless or without risk. Patients should still be advised to quit all forms of tobacco and use approved tobacco pharmacotherapies.

SPECIAL POPULATIONS

The tobacco cessation advice and assistance a clinician provides should reflect an understanding of the patient's medical, social, and cultural background. By discussing with patients anticipated tobacco cessation problems and potential solutions, clinicians can help patients construct solutions that are relevant to their social and cultural setting. Clinicians should be prepared to provide factual medical information that is personalized for their patients. For example, the older smoker who believes it is too late to stop and that cessation would be of limited benefit, should be reminded that quitting at any age decreases the risk of future smoking-related illness and can increase both the length and quality of life.[85-87]

Clinicians also need to recognize that smoking and tobacco use are viewed differently by various cultural groups, and that these views may influence how and why patients stop. The Centers for Disease Control and Prevention Tips from Former Smokers® Web-based program has culturally tailored information about tobacco use and tobacco cessation tips as well as links to cessation resources.

Young people comprise another group that can benefit from the advice and assistance of clinicians because most adult smokers first become addicted to nicotine during childhood and adolescence. Although cigarette smoking may be declining among young people, use of other tobacco products, including ECs, is rapidly increasing in this group.[88,89] Clinicians should review the full report by the National Academies of Science, Engineering, and Medicine to advise young people about the acute health risks of ECs (e.g., ingestion of EC liquids containing nicotine can cause acute toxicity and possibly death; batteries of ECs can explode).[79] (http://nationalacademies.org/hmd/reports/2018/public-health-consequences-of-e-cigarettes.aspx) and the negative effects of nicotine exposure on the developing brain (e.g., deficits in attention and cognition, reduced impulse control).[90] Clinicians can provide reasons for avoiding tobacco use that are relevant to adolescents and help them practice refusal skills. Adolescents who are already regular smokers should be advised and assisted in the same manner as an adult patient. However, adolescents may be more concerned about the immediate effects of cigarette smoking, such as "smokers' breath and smell" and diminished athletic performance, than information about long-term risks such as cancer and other tobacco-related diseases.

Finally, clinicians should routinely ask about vulnerable household members who might be exposed to secondhand smoke. Children of any age should be protected from exposure to environmental tobacco smoke. Parents who smoke should be advised to stop and to keep their children in smoke-free environments at home, at day care, and in other settings. Similar precautions must be taken when older adults are receiving care in the home. Even brief exposure to secondhand smoke could pose significant acute risks to ill older adults or to anyone at high risk for cardiovascular or respiratory disease. Those caring for relatives with heart or lung disease should be advised not to smoke in the presence of the sick relative. Some clinicians systematically identify passive smokers (including children) in their practices and routinely provide recommendations to reduce their exposure.

OFFICE AND CLINIC ORGANIZATION

Tobacco cessation interventions cannot be delivered to patients routinely and systematically without a supportive office organization. The goal is to ensure that all patients who use tobacco are routinely and efficiently identified, consistently monitored, and appropriately treated. Evidence-based office practices that reduce tobacco use among patients include the following[91]:

- Implementing a tobacco-user identification system in every clinic (e.g., expand vital signs to include an assessment of tobacco use)
- Providing education, resources, and feedback to promote interventions by clinicians
- Dedicating staff to provide tobacco dependence treatment and then assessing delivery of these interventions in staff performance evaluations

To act as a coordinated team, all office staff members must understand that tobacco cessation is an important task for the practice and they must know their roles. The team approach is facilitated by designating a tobacco cessation coordinator, usually a nurse. With the help of the other staff members, the coordinator incorporates the various components of the planned intervention program into the day-to-day activities of the practice (i.e., ensuring that all patients are identified, facilitating access to treatment, and scheduling follow-up visits). The tobacco cessation coordinator also helps maintain the staff members' commitment to the program and ensures that the system operates smoothly. Both the system itself and staff fulfillment of their roles should be reviewed periodically and adjustments made as necessary.

The team approach emphasizes staff identification of each patient who uses tobacco. When patients are identified as current tobacco users, their charts should be marked in a prominent manner. For paper records, a typical identifier could be a brightly colored permanent sticker or stamp or a removable sticker that is put on the chart at each visit. Practices with paper records can revise their forms to include tobacco use as a vital sign, and those with electronic health records can go one step further and display screen prompts to staff to obtain this information. The regular use of these chart reminders, which facilitates the provision of brief cessation advice as a routine part of every office visit for patients who smoke, has been shown to significantly increase cessation rates in office practices.[91] It is important that all staff members understand and use this kind of charting system.

CONCLUSION

Clinician assistance for tobacco cessation can have an enormous public health impact as well as benefit each individual patient who quits. In conjunction with other tobacco-control efforts in communities, practice-based cessation intervention can lead to a marked reduction in the morbidity and mortality caused by smoking.

SUGGESTED RESOURCES AND MATERIALS

American Academy of Family Physicians
Links to AAFP and National Resources for Patients and Clinicians, Including Patient Education Materials, Information About the "Ask and Act" Tobacco Cessation Program, Quit Lines, Pharmacotherapy, and Tips on Reimbursement.
https://www.aafp.org/patient-care/public-health/tobacco-nicotine/ask-act.html.

American Cancer Society
Online Cessation Guide, Tools for Clinicians, and Information on the Great American Smokeout.
https://www.cancer.org/cancer/cancer-causes/tobacco-and-cancer.html.

Centers for Disease Control and Prevention
Tobacco Information and Prevention Source (TIPS) With Links to Free How to Quit Guides, Education Materials, TIPS for Youth. Much of the Information and Materials are Also Available There in Spanish.

Quitline: 1-800-QUIT-NOW
http://www.cdc.gov/tobacco.

National Cancer Institute
Links to Tobacco Information, Statistics, Research, and Other Resources
NCI Quitline: 1-877-448-7848
http://www.cancer.gov/cancertopics/tobacco.

Smoke Free
NCI's Free Online Smoking Cessation Program
http://www.smokefree.gov.

Clinical Practice Guideline
Fiore MC, Jaen CR, Baker TB, et al. *Treating Tobacco Use and Dependence: 2008 Update. Clinical Practice Guideline*. Rockville, MD: Department of Health and Human Services. Public Health Service; 2008.

REFERENCES

1. U.S. Department of Health and Human Services. *The Health Consequences of Smoking-50 Years of Progress: A Report of the Surgeon General*. Atlanta, GA: U.S. Department of Health and Human Services, National Centers for Disease Control and Prevention, National Center for Chronic Disease Prevention And Health Promotion, Office on Smoking and Health; 2014.
2. Xu X, Bishop EE, Kennedy SM, Simpson SA, Pechacek TF. Annual healthcare spending attributable to cigarette smoking: an update. *Am J Prev Med.* 2015;48(3):326-333.
3. U.S. Department of Health and Human Services. *A Report of the Surgeon General: How Tobacco Smoke Causes Disease: What It Means to You*. Atlanta, GA: U.S. Department of Health and Human Services, Centers for Disease Control and Prevention, National Center for Chronic Disease Prevention and Health Promotion, Office on Smoking and Health; 2010.
4. Chang CM, Corey CG, Rostron BL, Apelberg BJ. Systematic review of cigar smoking and all cause and smoking related mortality. *BMC Public Health.* 2015;15:390.
5. Andreotti G, Freedman ND, Silverman DT, et al, Tobacco use and cancer risk in the agricultural health study. *Cancer Epidemiol Biomarkers Prev.* 2016:390.
6. Montazeri Z, Nyiraneza C, El-Katerji H, Little J. Waterpipe smoking and cancer: systematic review and meta-analysis. *Tob Control.* 2017;26(1):92-97.
7. Brawley OW, Glynn TJ, Khuri FR, Wender RC, Seffrin JR. The first surgeon general's report on smoking and health: the 50th anniversary. *CA Cancer J Clin.* 2014;64(1):5-8.
8. Samet JM. The 1990 report of the surgeon general: the health benefits of smoking cessation. *Am Rev Respir Dis.* 1990;142(5):993-994.
9. Maciosek MV, LaFrance AB, Dehmer SP, et al. Updated priorities among effective clinical preventive services. *Ann Fam Med.* 2017;15(1):14-22.
10. Prevention C.f.D.C.a. Current cigarette smoking among adults—United States, 2016. *Morb Mortal Wkly Rep.* 2018;67(2):6.
11. Kasza KA, Ambrose BK, Conway KP, et al. Tobacco-product use by adults and youths in the United States in 2013 and 2014. *N Engl J Med.* 2017;376(4):342-353.
12. Bilano V, Gilmour S, Moffiet T, et al. Global trends and projections for tobacco use, 1990–2025: an analysis of smoking indicators from the WHO comprehensive information systems for tobacco control. *Lancet.* 2015;385(9972):966-976.
13. Healthy People 2020 [Internet]. Washington, DC: U.S. Department of Health and Human Services, Office of Disease Prevention and Health Promotion. Available from https://www.healthypeople.gov/. Accessed March 6, 2018.

14. Fiore MC, Jaén CR, Baker TB, et al. *Treating Tobacco Use and Dependence: 2008 Update. Clinical Practice Guideline.* Rockville, MD: U.S. Department of Health and Human Services. Public Health Service; 2008.

15. Hughes JR. Motivating and helping smokers to stop smoking. *J Gen Intern Med.* 2003;18(12):1053-1057.

16. Okuyemi KS, Nollen NL, Ahluwalia JS. Interventions to facilitate smoking cessation. *Am Fam Physician.* 2006;74(2):262-271.

17. Fiore MC, Jorenby DE, Schensky AE, Smith SS, Bauer RR, Baker TB. Smoking status as the new vital sign: effect on assessment and intervention in patients who smoke. *Mayo Clin Proc.* 1995;70(3):209-213.

18. Richter KP, Ellerbeck EF. It's time to change the default for tobacco treatment. *Addiction.* 2015;110(3):381-386.

19. Burris JL, Heckman BW, Mathew AR, Carpenter MJ. A mechanistic test of nicotine replacement therapy sampling for smoking cessation induction. *Psychol Addict Behav.* 2015;29(2):392-399.

20. Jardin BF, Cropsey KL, Wahlquist AE, et al. Evaluating the effect of access to free medication to quit smoking: a clinical trial testing the role of motivation. *Nicotine Tob Res.* 2014;16(7):992-999.

21. Carpenter MJ, Hughes JR, Gray KM, Wahlquist AE, Saladin ME, Alberg AJ. Nicotine therapy sampling to induce quit attempts among smokers unmotivated to quit: a randomized clinical trial. *Arch Intern Med.* 2011;171(21):1901-1907.

22. Wang D, Connock M, Barton P, Fry-Smith A, Aveyard P, Moore D. 'Cut down to quit' with nicotine replacement therapies in smoking cessation: a systematic review of effectiveness and economic analysis. *Health Technol Assess.* 2008;12(2):iii-iv, ix-xi, 1-135.

23. Ebbert JO, Hughes JR, West RJ, et al. Effect of varenicline on smoking cessation through smoking reduction: a randomized clinical trial. *JAMA.* 2015;313(7):687-694.

24. Lindson-Hawley N, Aveyard P, Hughes JR. Reduction versus abrupt cessation in smokers who want to quit. *Cochrane Database Syst Rev.* 2012;11:CD008033.

25. Hughes JR, Carpenter MJ. Does smoking reduction increase future cessation and decrease disease risk? A qualitative review. *Nicotine Tob Res.* 2006;8(6):739-749.

26. Kenford SL, Fiore MC, Jorenby DE, Smith SS, Wetter D, Baker TB. Predicting smoking cessation. Who will quit with and without the nicotine patch. *JAMA.* 1994;271(8):589-594.

27. Welsch SK, Smith SS, Wetter DW, Jorenby DE, Fiore MC, Baker TB. Development and validation of the Wisconsin smoking withdrawal scale. *Exp Clin Psychopharmacol.* 1999;7(4):354.

28. Etter JF. A self-administered questionnaire to measure cigarette withdrawal symptoms: the cigarette withdrawal scale. *Nicotine Tob Res.* 2005;7(1):47-57.

29. U.S. Department of Health and Human Services. Quiz: What Are Your Withdrawal Symptoms? Available at https://smokefree.gov/challenges-when-quitting/managing-withdrawal/quiz-withdrawal [cited 2017 August 7].

30. Hughes JR, Hatsukami D. Signs and symptoms of tobacco withdrawal. *Arch Gen Psychiatry.* 1986;43(3):289-294.

31. Benowitz NL. Nicotine addiction. *N Engl J Med.* 2010;362(24):2295-2303.

32. Henningfield JE, Stapleton JM, Benowitz NL, Grayson RF, London ED. Higher levels of nicotine in arterial than in venous blood after cigarette smoking. *Drug Alcohol Depend.* 1993;33(1):23-29.

33. Le Houezec J. Role of nicotine pharmacokinetics in nicotine addiction and nicotine replacement therapy: a review. *Int J Tuberc Lung Dis.* 2003;7(9):811-819.

34. Russell MA, Feyerabend C, Cole P. Plasma nicotine levels after cigarette smoking and chewing nicotine gum. *Br Med J.* 1976;1(6017):1043-1046.

35. Lunell E, Curvall M. Nicotine delivery and subjective effects of Swedish portion snus compared with 4 mg nicotine polacrilex chewing gum. *Nicotine Tob Res.* 2011;13(7):573-578.

36. Schneider NG, Olmstead RE, Franzon MA, Lunell E. The nicotine inhaler. *Clin Pharmacokinet.* 2001;40(9):661-684.

37. Lancaster T, Stead LF. Individual behavioural counselling for smoking cessation. *Cochrane Database Syst Rev.* 2005;(2):CD001292.

38. Stead LF, Perera R, Bullen C, et al. Nicotine replacement therapy for smoking cessation. *Cochrane Database Syst Rev.* 2012;11:CD000146.

39. Cahill K, Stead LF, Lancaster T. Nicotine receptor partial agonists for smoking cessation. *Cochrane Database Syst Rev.* 2012;4:CD006103.

40. Ebbert JO, Elrashidi MY, Stead LF. Interventions for smokeless tobacco use cessation. *Cochrane Database Syst Rev.* 2015;(10):CD004306.

41. Cahill K, Stevens S, Lancaster T. Pharmacological treatments for smoking cessation. *JAMA.* 2014;311(2):193-194.

42. Woolf KJ, Zabad MN, Post JM, McNitt S, Williams GC, Bisognano JD. Effect of nicotine replacement therapy on cardiovascular outcomes after acute coronary syndromes. *Am J Cardiol.* 2012;110(7):968-970.

43. Critchley J, Capewell S. Smoking cessation for the secondary prevention of coronary heart disease. *Cochrane Database Syst Rev.* 2004;(1):CD003041.

44. Cahill K, Lindson-Hawley N, Thomas KH, Fanshawe TR, Lancaster T. Nicotine receptor partial agonists for smoking cessation. *Cochrane Database Syst Rev.* 2016;(5).

45. Jorenby DE, Hays JT, Rigotti NA, et al. Efficacy of varenicline, an alpha4beta2 nicotinic acetylcholine receptor partial agonist, vs placebo or sustained-release bupropion for smoking cessation: a randomized controlled trial. *JAMA.* 2006;296(1):56-63.

46. Coe JW, Brooks PR, Vetelino MG, et al. Varenicline: an α4β2 nicotinic receptor partial agonist for smoking cessationVarenicline: an α4β2 nicotinic receptor partial agonist for smoking cessationVarenicline: an α4β2 nicotinic receptor partial agonist for smoking cessation. *J Med Chem.* 2005;48(10):3474-3477.

47. Tonstad S, Tønnesen P, Hajek P, et al. Effect of maintenance therapy with varenicline on smoking cessation: a randomized controlled trial. *JAMA.* 2006;296(1):64-71.

48. Williams KE, Reeves KR, Billing CB, Pennington AM, Gong J. A double-blind study evaluating the long-term safety of varenicline for smoking cessation. *Curr Med Res Opin.* 2007;23(4):793-801.

49. Kishi T, Iwata N. Varenicline for smoking cessation in people with schizophrenia: systematic review and meta-analysis. *Eur Arch Psychiatry Clin Neurosci.* 2014.

50. Tonstad S, Davies S, Flammer M, Russ C, Hughes J. Psychiatric adverse events in randomized, double-blind, placebo-controlled clinical trials of varenicline: a pooled analysis. *Drug Saf.* 2010;33(4):289-301.

51. Anthenelli RM, Benowitz NL, West R, et al. Neuropsychiatric safety and efficacy of varenicline, bupropion, and nicotine patch in smokers with and without psychiatric disorders (EAGLES): a double-blind, randomised, placebo-controlled clinical trial. *Lancet.* 2016;387(10037):2507-2520.

52. Hughes JR, Stead LF, Lancaster T. Antidepressants for smoking cessation. *Cochrane Database Syst Rev.* 2007;(1):CD000031.

53. Ascher JA, Cole JO, Colin JN, et al. Bupropion: a review of its mechanism of antidepressant activity. *J Clin Psychiatry.* 1995.

54. Gonzales D, Rennard SI, Nides M, et al. Varenicline, an alpha4beta2 nicotinic acetylcholine receptor partial agonist, vs sustained-release bupropion and placebo for smoking cessation: a randomized controlled trial. *JAMA.* 2006;296(1):47-55.

55. Croft H, Houser TL, Jamerson BD, et al. Effect on body weight of bupropion sustained-release in patients with major depression treated for 52 weeks. *Clin Ther.* 2002;24(4):662-672.
56. Filozof C, Fernández Pinilla MC, Fernández-Cruz A. Smoking cessation and weight gain. *Obes Rev.* 2004;5(2):95-103.
57. Piper ME, Smith SS, Schlam TR, et al. A randomized placebo-controlled clinical trial of 5 smoking cessation pharmacotherapies. *Arch Gen Psychiatry.* 2009;66(11):1253-1262.
58. Cahill K, Stevens S, Perera R, Lancaster T. Pharmacological interventions for smoking cessation: an overview and network meta-analysis. *Cochrane Database Syst Rev.* 2013;5:CD009329.
59. Koegelenberg CF, Noor F, Bateman ED, et al. Efficacy of varenicline combined with nicotine replacement therapy vs varenicline alone for smoking cessation: a randomized clinical trial. *JAMA.* 2014;312(2):155-161.
60. Stead LF, Perera R, Lancaster T. Telephone counselling for smoking cessation. *Cochrane Database Syst Rev.* 2006(3):CD002850.
61. Schroeder SA. What to do with a patient who smokes. *JAMA.* 2005;294(4):482-487.
62. Perry RJ, Keller PA, Fraser D, Fiore MC. Fax to quit: a model for delivery of tobacco cessation services to Wisconsin residents. *WMJ.* 2005;104(4):37-40, 44.
63. Bush T, Lovejoy JC, Deprey M, Carpenter KM. The effect of tobacco cessation on weight gain, obesity, and diabetes risk. *Obesity (Silver Spring).* 2016;24(9):1834-1841.
64. Lindson-Hawley N, Hartmann-Boyce J, Fanshawe TR, Begh R, Farley A, Lancaster T. Interventions to reduce harm from continued tobacco use. *Cochrane Database Syst Rev.* 2016;10:CD005231.
65. Hartmann-Boyce J, Begh R, Aveyard P. Electronic cigarettes for smoking cessation. *Cochrane Database Syst Rev.* 2016;9:CD010216.
66. McRobbie H, Bullen C, Hartmann-Boyce J, Hajek P. Electronic cigarettes for smoking cessation and reduction. *Cochrane Database Syst Rev.* 2014;12:CD010216.
67. Drummond MB, Upson D, Electronic cigarettes. Potential harms and benefits. *Ann Am Thorac Soc.* 2014;11(2):236-242.
68. Britton J, Arnott D, McNeill A, et al. Nicotine without smoke-putting electronic cigarettes in context. *BMJ.* 2016;353:i1745.
69. Schraufnagel DE, Blasi F, Drummond MB, et al. Electronic cigarettes. A position statement of the forum of international respiratory societies. *Am J Respir Crit Care Med.* 2014;190(6):611-618.
70. Leventhal AM, Strong DR, Kirkpatrick MG, et al. Association of electronic cigarette use with initiation of combustible tobacco product smoking in early adolescence. *JAMA.* 2015;314(7):700-707.
71. Kosmider L, Sobczak A, Fik M, et al. Carbonyl compounds in electronic cigarette vapors: effects of nicotine solvent and battery output voltage. *Nicotine Tob Res.* 2014;16(10):1319-1326.
72. Goniewicz ML, Knysak J, Gawron M, et al. Levels of selected carcinogens and toxicants in vapour from electronic cigarettes. *Tob Control.* 2014; 23(2):133-139.
73. Hutzler C, Paschke M, Kruschinski S, Henkler F, Hahn J, Luch A. Chemical hazards present in liquids and vapors of electronic cigarettes. *Arch Toxicol.* 2014;88(7):1295-1308.
74. Farsalinos KE, Kistler KA, Gillman G, Voudris V. Evaluation of electronic cigarette liquids and aerosol for the presence of selected inhalation toxins. *Nicotine Tob Res.* 2015;17(2):168-174.
75. Hecht SS, Carmella SG, Kotandeniya D. Evaluation of toxicant and carcinogen metabolites in the urine of E-cigarette users versus cigarette smokers. *Nicotine Tob Res.* 2015;17(6):704-709.

76. Goniewicz ML, Gawron M, Smith DM, Peng M, Jacob P, Benowitz NL. Exposure to nicotine and selected toxicants in cigarette smokers who switched to electronic cigarettes: a longitudinal within-subjects observational study. *Nicotine Tob Res.* 2016.
77. Bullen C, Howe C, Laugesen M, et al. Electronic cigarettes for smoking cessation: a randomised controlled trial. *Lancet.* 2013;382(9905):1629-1637.
78. Caponnetto P, Campagna D, Cibella F, et al. EffiCiency and safety of an eLectronic cigAreTte (ECLAT) as tobacco cigarettes substitute: a prospective 12-month randomized control design study. *PLoS One.* 2013;8(6):e66317.
79. National Academies of Sciences Engineering, and Medicine. *Public Health Consequences of E-Cigarettes.* Washington, DC: The National Academies Press; 2018.
80. Brandon TH, Goniewicz ML, Hanna NH, et al. Electronic nicotine delivery systems: a policy statement from the American association for cancer research and the American society of clinical oncology. *J Clin Oncol.* 2015; 33(8):952-963.
81. Cummings KM, Dresler CM, Field JK, et al. E-cigarettes and cancer patients. *J Thorac Oncol.* 2014;9(4):438-441.
82. Luo J, Ye W, Zendehdel K, et al. Oral use of Swedish moist snuff (snus) and risk for cancer of the mouth, lung, and pancreas in male construction workers: a retrospective cohort study. *Lancet.* 2007;369(9578):2015-2020.
83. Lund KE, Scheffels J, McNeill A. The association between use of snus and quit rates for smoking: results from seven Norwegian cross-sectional studies. *Addiction.* 2011;106(1):162-167.
84. Foulds J, Ramstrom L, Burke M, Fagerström K. Effect of smokeless tobacco (snus) on smoking and public health in Sweden. *Tob Control.* 2003;12(4):349-359.
85. Gellert C, Schottker B, Brenner H. Smoking and all-cause mortality in older people: systematic review and meta-analysis. *Arch Intern Med.* 2012;172(11):837-844.
86. Jha P, Ramasundarahettige C, Landsman V, et al. 21st-century hazards of smoking and benefits of cessation in the United States. *N Engl J Med.* 2013;368(4):341-350.
87. Takashima N, Miura K, Hozawa A, et al. Cigarette smoking in middle age and a long-term risk of impaired activities of daily living: NIPPON DATA80. *Nicotine Tob Res.* 2010;12(9):944-949.
88. Centers for Disease Control and Prevention. Tobacco use among middle and high school students—United States, 2011–2017. *Morb Mortal Wkly Rep.* 2018;67(22):629-633. Accessed June 8, 2018.
89. Centers for Disease Control and Prevention. Tobacco product use among middle and high school students—United States, 2011 and 2012. *Morb Mortal Wkly Rep.* 2013;62(45):893-897. Accessed June 15, 2018.
90. U.S. Department of Health and Human Services. *E-Cigarette Use Among Youth and Young People: A Report of the Surgeon General.* Atlanta, GA: U.S. Department of Health and Human Services, Centers for Disease Control and Prevention, National Center for Chronic Disease Prevention and Health Promotion, Office on Smoking and Health; 2016.
91. Agency for Healthcare Research and Quality. *Systems Change: Treating Tobacco Use and Dependence. Content Last Reviewed*; December 2012. Available at http://www.ahrq.gov/professionals/clinicians-providers/guidelines-recommendations/tobacco/decisionmakers/systems/index.html.

Please see Online Appendix: Apps and Digital Resources for additional information.

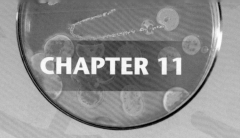

CHAPTER 11

Substance Use

ROBERT M. WEINRIEB

BACKGROUND

In 2014, an estimated 21.5 million Americans (8.1%) over the age of 12 had a substance use disorder (SUD)[1] the yearly economic impact of substance misuse is enormous, and estimates indicate costs of $740 billion for alcohol, tobacco and illicit drugs.[2] This includes costs related to crime, work productivity and healthcare. One measure of clinical impact is emergency department (ED) visits, and in 2011, the most recent data available, there were more than 1.5 million ED visits related to illicit drug and alcohol use.[1] Currently, a significant proportion of visits to emergency departments in the United States are due to an epidemic of opioid overdoses and deaths. The Vital Signs report from the Centers for Disease Control and Prevention (CDC) estimated an average 30% increase in ED visits for opioid overdoses in the US from July 2016 through September 2017, but these increases varied according to geographic location.[3] In 2017, it was estimated that there were over 64,000 opioid overdose deaths, or one death every 20 minutes. Although prescription opioids have previously accounted for the majority of fatal overdoses, increasingly greater numbers of people injecting opioids are dying compared to those who die from oral opioid overdoses because of the addition of the synthetic opiate Fentanyl (Table 11.1).[4]

Substance use disorders span a continuum starting with abstinence and continuing through at-risk use to what was previously referred to as Substance Abuse and Dependence in the Diagnostic and Statistical Manual of Mental Disorders, Fourth Edition (DSM-IV).[5] In the current edition of the DSM (DSM V), Substance Abuse and Dependence are combined into a single diagnostic category called Substance Use Disorders[6] which is further differentiated from mild to severe. For the diagnosis of a mild substance use disorder, individuals must have two to three criteria from a list of 11 (see Table 11.2), and at least seven criteria are needed for a Severe Substance Use Disorder diagnosis.

TABLE 11.1   Criteria for Substance Use Disorder

According to the DSM-5, a "substance use disorder describes a problematic pattern of using alcohol or another substance that results in impairment in daily life or noticeable distress." They must display 2 of the following 11 symptoms within 12-mo:

1. Consuming more alcohol or other substance than originally planned
2. Worrying about stopping or consistently failed efforts to control one's use
3. Spending a large amount of time using drugs/alcohol, or doing whatever is needed to obtain them
4. Use of the substance results in failure to "fulfill major role obligations" such as at home, work, or school.
5. "Craving" the substance (alcohol or drug)
6. Continuing the use of a substance despite health problems caused or worsened by it. This can be in the domain of mental health (psychological problems may include depressed mood, sleep disturbance, anxiety, or "blackouts") or physical health.
7. Continuing the use of a substance despite its having negative effects on relationships with others (for example, using even though it leads to fights or despite people's objecting to it).
8. Repeated use of the substance in a dangerous situation (for example, when having to operate heavy machinery or when driving a car)
9. Giving up or reducing activities in a person's life because of the drug/alcohol use
10. Building up a tolerance to the alcohol or drug. Tolerance is defined by the DSM-5 as "either needing to use noticeably larger amounts over time to get the desired effect or noticing less of an effect over time after repeated use of the same amount."
11. Experiencing withdrawal symptoms after stopping use. Withdrawal symptoms typically include, according to the DSM-5: "anxiety, irritability, fatigue, nausea/vomiting, hand tremor or seizure in the case of alcohol."

The DSM V also has a new diagnostic category of behavioral addictions that includes Gambling Disorder. This new term and its location in the new manual reflect research findings that a gambling disorder is similar to substance-related disorders in clinical expression, brain origin, comorbidity, physiology, and treatment.[6]

Adverse effects due to SUDs are numerous and can affect every organ system. The nature of the adverse effects that may be experienced by one individual depends on the type of substance, the route of use, and an individual's predisposition to such harm(s). Common complications of substance use and SUDs appear in Tables 11.2A and B.

For many individuals with substance use disorders, primary care clinicians are their first point of contact with the health care system. The primary care clinician can play a critical role in the assessment and treatment

TABLE 11.2A Medical Complications Associated With Alcohol and/ or Drug Use and Use Disorders

Alcohol

Trauma

Hypertension

Depression

Suicide

Ischemic heart disease

Stroke

Throat and esophageal cancer

Breast and colon cancer

Hepatitis

Hepatic cirrhosis

Hepatocellular carcinoma

Gastritis/gastric ulceration

Encephalopathy

Peripheral neuropathy

Myopathy

Cerebellar ataxia

Anemia

Thrombocytopenia

Withdrawal syndromes and sequellae

Injection Drug Use Complications

Blood-borne viruses

Hepatitis B/hepatitis C

Human immunodeficiency virus infection

Cutaneous infections

Endocarditis

Cardiomyopathy

Nephropathy

Restrictive pulmonary disease

(Continued)

TABLE 11.2A   Medical Complications Associated With Alcohol and/or Drug Use and Use Disorders   (Continued)
Stimulant Use Complications
Stroke
Myocardial infarction
Acute liver failure from hepatic artery thrombosis
Cardiac arrhythmia
Seizure
Mood disorders
Psychosis

TABLE 11.2B   Common Social Complications of Substance Use and Substance Use Disorders (SUDs)
Job loss
Criminal behavior
Domestic violence
Assault (victim or perpetrator)
Social isolation

of substance-related disorders and in so doing, prevent some of the devestating individual and societal sequelae of SUDs. Primary care clinicians are ideally situated to provide initial assessment, brief counseling, pharmacotherapy, and referrals to appropriate specialists and psychosocial rehabilitation. This chapter serves as a review of the risk factors, screening instruments, assessment, diagnosis, and treatment of SUDs in the primary care setting. (See Chapter 3 for screening and exploratory questions about substance use to include in the periodic health examination [PHE] and for guidance on discussing this topic with adolescents.)

WHO SHOULD BE SCREENED?

As noted in Chapter 3, according to the U.S. Preventive Services Task Force, the Institute of Medicine, the American Academy of Family Physicians, and the National Institute on Alcohol Abuse and Alcoholism, routine screening for alcohol use disorders is recommend for adults, including pregnant women. Screening of adolescents and the elderly is also encouraged. Screening for illicit drug use and drug-related problems in PHEs is recommended by the American Academy of Pediatrics and the American Medical Association. "Illicit drugs" are virtually all of the psychoactive drugs that federal law deems illegal to sell, possess, or use (e.g., marijuana, heroin, and cocaine) and include prescription pharmaceuticals that are used on a nonprescription basis.

SCREENING INSTRUMENTS

Screening instruments for at-risk alcohol use and alcohol use disorders are much more varied and well-studied than instruments for illicit drug use. Similar to screens for other clinical conditions, the clinician should keep in mind that these instruments are not diagnostic for substance use disorders. A positive finding upon screening mandates further evaluation through detailed interviews and/or specialist consultation.

Screening for Alcohol

Several instruments have been developed and studied as screens for at-risk alcohol use and/or alcohol use disorders. Each has its advantages and disadvantages in terms of testing characteristics and convenience of administration. Because the diagnosis of SUDs is based on historical factors related to substance use, the gold standard used to determine the performance of screening instruments for SUDs is most frequently a clinical interview based on the DSM-V, such as the Structured Clinical Interview for DSM-V.[7]

This section focuses on those screens found to be most practical for use in the primary care setting. Such sophisticated screening instruments as the Michigan Alcoholism Screening Test (MAST) or the Substance Abuse Subtle Screening Inventory (SASSI) are very detailed and therefore impractical for use in a busy primary care setting. They involve complicated weighted scoring systems, are time consuming to administer, and do not provide substantially greater sensitivity, specificity, or predictive value than do instruments reviewed in this chapter. Test performance characteristics of several of the most common alcohol screening instruments targeting the general adult population are provided in Table 11.3, however they are based upon the DSM-IV diagnoses of Alcohol Abuse and Dependence.

An instrument familiar to most providers is the CAGE questionnaire (see Table 11.4).[8] It should be noted that the CAGE questions are time insensitive; therefore, they do not distinguish a past from a current problem. Two positive responses are most generally considered criteria for a positive screen. Reducing the cutoff for a positive screen to one positive response improves test sensitivity (from approximately 76%–88%) but reduces test specificity (from approximately 86%–74%).

A more detailed screening instrument, the Alcohol Use Disorders Identification Test (AUDIT, see Table 11.5), was developed by the World Health Organization as a screen for current at-risk drinking and alcohol

TABLE 11.3 Test Characteristics of Common Screening Instruments for At-Risk Alcohol Use and Alcohol Use Disorders in the General Clinic Population

Instrument and Cutoff Point	Diagnosis	Sensitivity (%)	Specificity (%)	PPV (%)	NPV (%)
CAGE score ≥2 positive responses	Abuse or dependence	74–78	76–96	32–75	95–97
CAGE score ≥1 positive response	Abuse or dependence	86–90	52–93	21–66	96–98
AUDIT score ≥8	At-risk use, abuse, or dependence	38–63	95–96	68–82	84–94
MAST score ≥5	Abuse or dependence	80	70	29	96
BMAST score ≥5	Abuse or dependence	30–78	80–99	19–92	88–97
Single quantity/frequency question (yes)[a]	Abuse or dependence	62	93	74	88

Adapted from Magruder-Habib K, Stevens HA, Alling WC. Relative performance of the MAST, VAST, and CAGE versus DSM-III-R criteria for alcohol dependence. *J Clin Epidemiol.* 1993;46:435-441; and Mayfield D, McLeod G, Hall P. The CAGE questionnaire: validation of a new alcoholism screening instrument. *Am J Psychiatry.* 1974;131:1121-1123.[5-7]

[a]"On any single occasion during the last 3 mo, have you had more than five drinks containing alcohol?"[11]

AUDIT, Alcohol Use Disorders Identification Test; BMAST, Brief Michigan Alcohol Screening Test; MAST, Michigan Alcoholism Screening test; NPV, negative predictive value; PPV, positive predictive value.

TABLE 11.4 CAGE Questionnaire
Have you ever felt you should **C**ut down on your drinking?
Have people **A**nnoyed you by criticizing your drinking?
Have you ever felt **G**uilty about drinking?
Have you ever had a drink in the morning (**E**ye-Opener) to steady your nerves or relieve a hangover?

Adapted from Ewing JA. Detecting alcoholism. The CAGE questionnaire. *JAMA.* 1984;252:
1905-1907 and Mayfield DG, McLeod G, Hall P. The CAGE questionnaire: validation of a new
alcoholism screening instrument. *Am J Psychiatry.* 1974;131:1121-1123.

use disorders.[9] The AUDIT consists of ten questions, each scored on a five-point Likert scale (0–4) yielding a possible range of 0 to 40. A score of eight or greater indicates the need for further evaluation. In the outpatient clinic population, the AUDIT exhibits improved specificity (95%–96%) over the CAGE at traditional cutoffs, but at the expense of sensitivity (38%–63%).[10]

A single quantity question (e.g., "On any single occasion during the last 3 months, have you had more than five drinks containing alcohol?") has also been evaluated as a screen for at-risk drinking and alcohol use disorders in the outpatient clinical setting and for binge drinking. Its performance compares favorably to that of the other short screening instruments for problematic alcohol use.[11]

The application and utility of the widely used screening instruments, such as CAGE, AUDIT, and variations of the MAST, have primarily been studied among men, using cutoff values and diagnostic criteria more appropriate for men. Therefore, test characteristics and the goals for alcohol screening tools may differ significantly when applied to groups other than adult males.

Among pregnant women, for instance, dependent drinking is less common than in men and cutoffs for potentially harmful drinking patterns are lower than that for men. Studies also indicate that traditional screening instruments may not provide accurate results in the general female population and among adolescents.

Pregnancy

The CAGE has been modified to yield screening questionnaires more appropriate for pregnant women. Screening in the population of pregnant women is designed to detect at-risk drinking and more severe alcohol-related behaviors. At-risk drinking for a pregnant woman has been defined as consuming 1 oz or more of alcohol daily.[12] Screening instruments are therefore designed for the detection of this lower volume of consumption. Epidemiologic studies, however, indicate that fetal harm may be associated with even lower levels of consumption: three drinks per week or 0.5 oz

TABLE 11.5   Alcohol Use Disorders Identification Test (AUDIT)[a]

	0	1	2	3	4
How often do you have a drink containing alcohol?	Never	Monthly	Two to four times a mo	Two to three times a wk	Four or more times a wk
How many drinks containing alcohol do you have on a typical day when you are drinking?	One or two	Three or four	Five or six	Seven to nine	Ten or more
How often do you have six or more drinks on one occasion?	Never	Less than monthly	Monthly	Weekly	Daily or almost daily
How often during the last year have you found that you were not able to stop drinking once you had started?	Never	Less than monthly	Monthly	Weekly	Daily or almost daily
How often during the last year have you failed to do what was normally expected of you because of drinking?	Never	Less than monthly	Monthly	Weekly	Daily or almost daily
How often during the last year have you needed a first drink in the morning to get yourself going after a heavy drinking session?	Never	Less than monthly	Monthly	Weekly	Daily or almost daily
How often during the last year have you had a feeling of guilt or remorse after drinking?	Never	Less than monthly	Monthly	Weekly	Daily or almost daily
How often during the last year have you been unable to remember what happened the night before because of your drinking?	Never	Less than monthly	Monthly	Weekly	Daily or almost daily
Have you or someone else been injured because of your drinking?	No	—	Yes, but not in the last year	—	Yes, during the last year
Has a relative, friend, doctor, or other health care worker been concerned about your drinking or suggested you cut down?	No	—	Yes, but not in the last year	—	Yes, during the last year

Adapted from Saunders JB, Aasland OG, Babor TF, et al. Development of the alcohol use disorders identification test (AUDIT): WHO collaborative project on early detection of persons with harmful alcohol consumption-II. *Addiction.* 1993;88:791-804.

[a]Each response is scored using the numbers at the top of each response column. Add all numbers in that column to obtain the total score. A total score of eight or more indicates the need for further evaluation.

of alcohol daily.[13] Due in part to this lack of clarity in the literature, women should be counseled that no level of alcohol consumption is known to be safe during pregnancy.

T-ACE (see Table 11.6) and TWEAK (see Table 11.7) are examples of screening instruments modified for the purposes of evaluating risky drinking by pregnant women. The T-ACE replaces the "guilt" question of CAGE with a tolerance question (Table 11.6). The T-ACE was further revised to yield the TWEAK (Table 11.7).[14] The comparative performance of the more commonly used screens for risky drinking during pregnancy (1 oz or more daily) is summarized in Table 11.8.

Among non-pregnant women, asking about tolerance using the T-ACE or TWEAK may be a more effective method to ascertain an alcohol use disorder or at-risk drinking. Since many healthier, or younger drinkers may not experience a need to ameliorate withdrawal symptoms, they will not

---

TABLE 11.6 T-ACE Questions

1. Tolerance: "How many drinks does it take to make you feel high?" (a quantity of >2 is considered a positive response.)

2. Have people **A**nnoyed you by criticizing your drinking?

3. Have you ever felt you should **C**ut down on your drinking?

4. Have you ever had a drink in the morning (**E**ye-Opener) to steady your nerves or relieve a hangover?

Adapted from Sokol RJ, Martier SS, Ager JW. The T-ACE questions: practical prenatal detection of risk-drinking. *Am J Obstet Gynecol.* 1989;160:863-868; discussion 868-870.

TABLE 11.7 TWEAK Questions

1. How many drinks can you hold before falling asleep or passing out? (Tolerance: score >5 is a positive response)

2. Have close friends or relatives **W**orried or complained about your drinking in the past yr?

3. Have you ever taken a drink in the morning (**E**ye-Opener) to steady your nerves or relieve a hangover?

4. Has a friend or family member ever told you about things you said or did while you were drinking that you could not remember? (**A**mnesia)

5. Have you ever felt you should "**K**ut" [sic] down on your drinking?

Derived from Russell M, Martier SS, Sokol RJ, et al. Detecting risk drinking during pregnancy: a comparison of four screening questionnaires. *Am J Public Health.* 1996;86:1435-1439.

TABLE 11.8 Test Performance of Screening Instruments for At-Risk Drinking During Pregnancy

Instrument	Sensitivity (%)	Specificity (%)	PPV (%)	NPV (%)
CAGE score ≥2 positive responses	38	92	5–22	96–99
T-ACE score ≥2 positive responses	60–69	66–89	2–27	96–99
TWEAK score ≥2	79	85	5–24	99
AUDIT score ≥8	15	94	3–13	95–99
MAST score ≥5	36	96	9–35	96–99
SMAST ≥2	11	96	3–14	95–99

Adapted from Sokol RJ, Martier SS, Ager JW. The T-ACE questions: practical prenatal detection of risk-drinking. *Am J Obstet Gynecol.* 1989;160:863-868; discussion 868-870 and Windham GC, Von Behren J, Fenster L, et al. Moderate maternal alcohol consumption and risk of spontaneous abortion. *Epidemiology.* 1997;8:509-514.

AUDIT, Alcohol Use Disorders Identification Test; MAST, Michigan Alcoholism Screening Test; NPV, negative predictive value; PPV, positive predictive value; SMAST, Short Michigan Alcoholism Screening Test.

endorse the need for an "eye opener". Furthermore, many patients are reluctant or embarrassed to disclose how much they are drinking to their health care provider, so how the clinician asks about their patient's alcohol consumption can significantly influence how comfortable and honest a patient will be answering the questions. For example, if a clinician starts their inquiry about the quantity and frequency of their patient's drinking by asking "how many drinks do you drink each day". This can seem judgmental to a some patients even if the clinician was not trying to be critical. Motivational Interviewing (MI) is based upon the premise that patients can be at different stages of their awareness, acceptance and readiness to to make changes toward making healthier choices about their drinking or drug use.[15] One such approach derived from Motivational Interviewing that can help patients feel less reluctant to discuss their drinking or drug use begins with the clinician asking permission to ask about it. Rather than switching from questions about medication adherence, diet and exercise by abruptly asking about alcohol or drug use, the clinician can say "now I'd like to ask you some lifestyle questions I ask all my patients. "Would it be OK with you if I ask some questions about alcohol and drug use?" If your patient agrees, begin by asking the screening questions that get at the psychosocial consequences of drinking before asking questions about quantity and frequency of drinking. This can improve rapport with your patient because it conveys that their clinician is interested in the problems they are facing in their lives that may be related to alcohol and drug use. Initiating the interview by asking patients about the quantity and frequency of their drinking can put them on the defensive by conveying that the clinician is less interested in them as a whole person. Once the clinician is ready to ask about how much and how often their patient is drinking, the patient may be more honest if they are not asked "how many drinks do you drink each day". Instead, ask whether they mostly drink at home or in bars. If they drink at home, ask if they buy their own beer, wine or liquor? If so, then what quantity do they buy, ie. for beer, "how many cases (24, 12 oz. beers) do you go through in a typical week?"; for wine, "what size do you buy, a standard size bottle (750 mL); a big bottle (1.5 L), or a box (3,4 or 5 L), and how many they go through in a week; for liquor, a pint, a fifth or 1.75 L ("a handle"). The clinician can then extrapolate how many drinks that translates to, for example, in a fifth of vodka, there is about 25 oz, which is likely to be about 10 to 12 slightly larger drinks.

Screening for Other Drug Use

Far fewer instruments have been investigated for screening of SUDs other than alcohol-related disorders. The evaluation of screens for which there are published results has focused on conjoint screening, or screening simultaneously for alcohol and other drug use disorders. Two such instruments are the CAGE-AID[16] (see Table 11.9) and the two-item conjoint screen (TICS).[17] The two-item conjoint screen asks the following two questions:

- In the last year, have you ever drunk or used drugs more than you meant to?
- Have you felt that you wanted or needed to cut down on your drinking or drug use in the last year?

Test performance characteristics of these instruments appear in Table 11.10.

TABLE 11.9 CAGE-AID Questions[a]
Have you felt you ought to **C**ut down on your drinking or drug use?
Have people **A**nnoyed you by criticizing your drinking or drug use?
Have you felt bad or **G**uilty about your drinking or drug use?
Have you ever had a drink or used drugs first thing in the morning to steady your nerves or to get rid of a hangover (**E**ye-Opener)?

Adapted from Brown RL, Rounds LA. Conjoint screening questionnaires for alcohol and other drug abuse: criterion validity in a primary care practice. *Wis Med J.* 1995;94:135-140 and Muntaner C, Eaton WW, Diala C, et al. Social class, assets, organizational control and the prevalence of common groups of psychiatric disorders. *Soc Sci Med.* 1998;47:2043-2053.
[a]Greater than or equal to two positive responses is considered a positive screen warranting further evaluation.

TABLE 11.10 Testing Characteristics of Conjoint Screens for Alcohol and Other Drug Use Disorders

Instrument/Cutoff	Sensitivity (%)	Specificity (%)	PPV (%)	NPV (%)
CAGE-AID (score ≥2 positive responses)	70	85	52	92
TICS (1 positive response)	78	84	69	93

Adapted from Brown RL, Rounds LA. Conjoint screening questionnaires for alcohol and other drug abuse: criterion validity in a primary care practice. *Wis Med J*. 1995;94:135-140 and Brown RL, Leonard T, Saunders LA, et al. A two-item screening test for alcohol and other drug problems. *J Fam Pract*. 1997;44:151-160.
NPV, negative predictive value; PPV, positive predictive value; TICS, two-item conjoint screen.

ADOLESCENCE

The adolescent population presents unique challenges to screening and deserves dedicated instruments for the detection of alcohol and other SUDs. Refer to Chapter 18 for a discussion of how to ask adolescents about drug and alcohol use and the sensitivities that surround these issues in this age group.

As mentioned above, the "Eye-Opener" question of the CAGE questionnaire, is unlikely to be appropriately targeted to the typical substance use pattern among adolescents. Factors such as self-esteem, peer acceptance, and family influence serve to predict substance use among adolescents to a greater degree than among adults.

The literature characterizing the performance of substance misuse screening instruments among adolescents, particularly adolescents not attending university, is scant. Short substance-use screening tests for adolescent populations include the RAFFT[18] (see Table 11.11), CRAFFT (see Table 11.12), CAGE-AA (CAGE questions adapted for adolescents), the

TABLE 11.11 RAFFT Questionnaire[a]

Do you drink/drug to **R**elax, feel better about yourself, or fit in?

Do you ever drink/drug while you are **A**lone?

Do any of your closest **F**riends drink/drug?

Does a close **F**amily member have a problem with alcohol/drugs?

Have you ever gotten into **T**rouble from drinking/drugging?

Adapted from Bastiaens L, Francis G, Lewis K. The RAFFT as a screening tool for adolescent substance use disorders. *Am J Addict*. 2000;9:10-16.
[a]Two or more positive responses is considered a positive screen warranting further evaluation.

TABLE 11.12   CRAFFT Questions[a]

Have you ever ridden in a **C**ar driven by someone (including yourself) who was "high" or had been using alcohol or drugs?

Do you ever use alcohol or drugs to **R**elax, feel better about yourself, or fit in?

Do you ever use alcohol/drugs while you are **A**lone?

Do your family or **F**riends ever tell you that you should cut down on your drinking or drug use?

Do you ever **F**orget things you did while using alcohol or drugs?

Have you gotten into **T**rouble while you were using alcohol or drugs?

Adapted from Knight JR, Sherritt L, Shrier LA, et al. Validity of the CRAFFT substance abuse screening test among adolescent clinic patients. *Arch Pediatr Adolesc Med.* 2002;156:607-614.
[a]Two or more positive responses is considered a positive screen warranting further evaluation. Instruments screening for substance misuse other than alcohol have not been studied in samples of pregnant women.

TABLE 11.13   Test Performance of Alcohol/Drug Screens for Adolescents

Instrument/Cutoff	Sensitivity (%)	Specificity (%)	PPV (%)	NPV (%)
RAFFT score ≥2 positive responses	89	69	89	79
CRAFFT score ≥2 positive responses	80	86	53	96

Adapted from Bastiaens L, Francis G, Lewis K. The RAFFT as a screening tool for adolescent substance use disorders. *Am J Addict.* 2000;9:10-16 and Knight JR, Sherritt L, Shrier LA, et al. Validity of the CRAFFT substance abuse screening test among adolescent clinic patients. *Arch Pediatr Adolesc Med.* 2002;156:607-614.
NPV, negative predictive value; PPV, positive predictive value.

Simple Screening Instrument for Alcohol and Other Drug Abuse, and questions from the Drug and Alcohol Problem QuickScreen. Test performance characteristics of the RAFFT and CRAFFT are presented in Table 11.13.

RISK FACTORS

Knowledge of the factors associated with the development of SUDs may help the clinician overcome some of the shortcomings of traditional screening tests. SUDs are multifactorial in their etiology. For any individual, risk is determined by an array of biological, behavioral, and environmental factors, such as family history, sex, age, ethnicity, employment status, education, and psychiatric history. The existence of such risk factors may well be revealed in the course of a general medical or social history, indicating that further evaluation for the presence of SUDs is indicated.

Family history is the most powerful and consistent risk factor for the development of SUDs. Alcohol and drug use disorders are generally more common among men than women. However, among those who consume drugs, the likelihood of developing a SUD is similar for men and women. The prevalence of alcoholism declines with age. The prevalence of the SUDs associated with the use of drugs (other than prescription drugs used on a nonprescription basis) peaks in adolescence and young adulthood (age 21–35 yr) and declines thereafter. Alcohol use disorders tend to develop at a later age among African Americans than other ethnicities, and a greater proportion of African Americans tend to abstain from alcohol use. When alcohol or drug dependence develops among African American men, their substance use disorders are less persistent than in whites, and Hispanic females with alcohol use disorders also have less persistence than white females. Hispanic males with drug use disorders are less persistent than white males, and in general, polysubstance users were consistently higher in persistence than people with either drug or alcohol use disorders.[19] Unemployment has been linked to alcohol use disorders. Longer work hours and dropping out of high school are each associated with a greater risk of drug and alcohol use among adolescents,[20] although excessive alcohol use can be a cause of these circumstances as well as a consequence.

The prevalence of alcohol and drug disorders has been estimated to be 20% to 50% respectively among individuals reporting a history of a psychiatric disorder.[21] The nature of the link between specific psychiatric syndromes and SUDs is complex and beyond the scope of this chapter.[22]

TREATMENT

There are a number of evidence-based methods available to treat alcohol and drug use disorders. These include brief primary care office-based interventions, motivational interviewing therapy, pharmacotherapy, cognitive behavioral therapy (CBT), Mindfulness Meditation? Alcoholics Anonymous (AA)-based self-help groups, and traditional alcohol and drug group therapy. There is sufficient evidence to recommend each of these methods for the treatment of alcohol and drug use disorders. Other methods such as acupuncture, herbal medication, and massage therapy have insufficient evidence to recommend implementation and therefore will not be reviewed in this chapter.

Primary Care Office-Based Interventions

"Brief intervention" is a technique widely utilized by clinicians to help patients change behaviors, increase medication adherence, and improve follow-through with clinic appointments. There is compelling evidence that brief intervention can change behavior in patients who drink more than the recommended amounts.[23–25] In a randomized clinical trial of patients in primary care clinics, however, brief intervention was not shown to have efficacy for decreasing unhealthy drug use in primary care patients who were identified by screening.[27]

There are six basic steps in the "brief intervention." The first step is for the clinician to express concern that the patient is drinking above recommended levels, or concern about the patient's drug use. The second step is to connect the patient's drinking or drug use to health, social, or family concerns of importance to that patient. Providing this objective, concrete feedback may be particularly useful in patients who are resistant to changing their alcohol or drug use behavior. The third step is to ask the patient if they have any concerns about their alcohol or drug use. The fourth step is to make a specific recommendation for the patient to reduce use or become abstinent in an effort to reduce the potential for drug-related harm. The fifth step is to negotiate with the patient a realistic change in alcohol or drug use in the next 30 days. The sixth step is to provide a self-help booklet, online references, or a list of community resources for follow-up appointments. Follow-up telephone calls and visits over the next 6 to 12 months can reinforce face-to-face visits. The National Council for Behavioral Health recently released a guide to assist primary care providers implement substance abuse services with an emphasis on SBIRT (Screening Brief Intervention and Referral to Treatment). It can be found at https://www.thenationalcouncil.org/press-releases/national-council-releases-guide-assist-primary-care-providers-implement-substance-use-disorder-services/.

Client-Centered Counseling

There are a number of client-centered counseling therapies available for clinician referral that are effective in helping patients reduce their substance use or to become abstinent[27]: *Client-centered therapy* allows the clinician and the client to establish and prioritize a limited number of goals during a series of short counseling sessions. Included among them are Motivational Enhancement Therapy (MET), cognitive behavioral therapy (CBT), 12-step facilitation therapy, and peer self-help groups.[26]

MET is a technique that can be learned by primary care clinicians to help patients move along in the readiness-to-change paradigm (see pages 133–134). Techniques utilized in MET include rolling with patient resistance, dealing with patient ambivalence, setting up cognitive dissonance, which is the emotional distress a patient feels when they hold two opposing viewpoints about their substance use, and using behavioral change contracts. This technique can move patients from contemplating reducing their drinking or drug use to actual behavior change.

CBT provides patients with specific skills designed to deal with triggers, craving, and high-risk situations. Relapse prevention programs are based on CBT counseling strategies, which are primarily used by counselors in 1-hour sessions lasting 10 to 16 weeks. Clinicians can use CBT to role-play with patients on how to deal with high-risk social situations that often lead to relapse. CBT therapy is used to change a variety of behaviors and/or their results including tobacco use disorders, alcohol use disorders, and obesity.

The 12-step facilitation method is another technique that can be learned by clinicians to help patients improve the ability to become abstinent. This includes having patients keep a weekly diary of their alcohol use and relapse events, read AA materials or other self-help books, and work through the 12 steps of the AA program. These techniques can be combined with pharmacotherapy. Of the AA 12 steps, completion of steps 4 and 5 is predictive of recovery and long-term abstinence. Step 4 focuses on recording how alcohol and/or drugs have damaged patients' lives and those around them. Step 5 involves sharing these events with another person. Clinicians can ask patients to complete step 4 on their own and then use a regular clinician visit to go over the items.

Self-help peer groups remain the main source of help for patients trying to deal with their alcohol and drug use. As part of the information on community resources that practices should keep on hand for patients, clinicians may want to have a list of local AA chapters and Al-Anon meetings available in the waiting room or as a handout. This list can be obtained from the local AA chapter, which is often listed in telephone directories or on websites. There is an increasing number of self-help organizations designed to address the needs of diverse groups of people trying to deal with their alcohol or drug problems. These include groups for women, gay men and women, underage drinkers, older adults, nonreligious persons, people with cocaine addiction, people with prescription drug addictions, nonsmokers, and professionals. AA meetings remain one of the most widely used options for the treatment of alcohol and drug dependence throughout the world. Unlike a patient's primary care clinician, AA is free and available after 5 PM, on weekends, and during the holidays. Patients should be encouraged to work with a sponsor in their journey through the 12-steps. When your patient is ready, they should seek out AA sponsors who are stably sober alcoholics. They must be willing and able to be available to the patient (within reason) when they need additional support to stay sober.

Counseling Patients About Drinking and Driving

Alcohol use is a major cause of motor vehicle crashes. When counseling patients regarding drinking and driving and the risk for motor vehicle accidents and injury, it should be emphasized that, although legal blood alcohol limits promote safety to some degree, evidence indicates that impairment occurs within legal blood alcohol concentration limits. In addition to increasing the risk of injury, recent alcohol consumption also increases the probability of sustaining more severe injury with poorer clinical outcome.[27] Patients should be made aware of local safe ride programs (transportation alternatives for intoxicated drivers) as a preventive measure.

PHARMACOTHERAPY

Alcohol Dependence

There are two groups of medications that can be helpful in the primary treatment of alcohol dependence: aversive agents and anticraving agents (see Table 11.14). These medications are not recommended for the treatment of patients engaged in at-risk or problem drinking, pregnant women, or patients younger than 16 years.

The first class consists of aversive agents such as disulfiram and metronidazole. Patients who take the medication at least 5 days a week are likely to remain sober. Supervised medication dosing by a partner or close personal contact may facilitate compliance. Liver function tests should be monitored at baseline, 2 months after initiation, and every 6 months thereafter. Placebo controlled studies show that most patients who are prescribed disulfiram are not compliant with taking it. Furthermore, results from a large, multi-center randomized, controlled study found that in patients who were compliant with the study drug, rates of abstinence for those randomized to disulfiram were no better than patients randomized to the placebo.[30]

The second class of medications is the anticraving drugs. Two are currently approved by the U.S. Food and Drug Administration (FDA): naltrexone and acamprosate. An injectable formulation of naltrexone has received FDA approval for monthly administration for alcohol dependence (Vivitrex), and results from the studies are positive Also, Vivitrex was not found to adversely affect liver chemistries.[31,32] Acamprosate has been widely used in Europe for some years. Anticraving drugs are most effective when administered for 3 to 12 months. They are meant to be used in patients who whose goal is abstinence, and they are therefore less effective in patients who continue to drink intermittently while taking the medication. Liver and renal function should be checked at baseline and 2 months after initiation.

If your practice is located near a university based outpatient substance abuse treatment center, a research study evaluating novel medications for alcohol use disorders may be available for eligible patients.

Drug Dependence

Available pharmacotherapy for drug dependence is limited primarily to the treatment of opioid dependence. Developing effective pharmacotherapy for the treatment of cocaine, amphetamine, marijuana, and other illicit drug use is an active area of research.

With regards to the current opioid overdose epidemic, it is well known that among injection heroin users, the illicitly manufactured synthetic opiate. Fontanel is one of the major reasons for the increase in heroin overdose deaths. Fontanel is dangerously potent, and most opioid dependent people simply do not possess the pharmacological tolerance to survive it.

TABLE 11.14 Pharmacotherapy for Dependence

Diagnosis	Medication	Mechanism	Dosing	Contraindications/Cautions
Alcohol dependence	Disulfiram Aversive agent[a]	250 mg p.o. QD	Age >65 yr Liver disease[b]	Can cause severe hypotension, neurological complications
	Naltrexone	Anticraving	25–100 mg p.o. QD 380 mg i.m. monthly	Liver disease[b] Active opioid dependence on opioid analgesics
	Acamprosate	Anticraving	666 mg p.o. TID	Severe renal disease[c]
Opioid dependence	Methadone[d]	Anticraving prevents withdrawal	60–150 mg p.o. QD	Severe liver disease (cirrhosis)
	Buprenorphine/ Naloxone	Anticraving prevents withdrawal	8–32 mg p.o. or s.l. QD	Initiation <24 hr after other opioid use (<48 hr after last methadone dose)

[a]Produces reaction when alcohol used concomitantly characterized by nausea, vomiting, flushing, and anxiety.
[b]Gamma–glutamyl transferees (GGT) or transaminase levels greater than three times upper limit of normal. Although there is a black box warning in the labeling for using naltrexone in people with elevated liver chemistries, if the elevations were due to alcohol misuse, studies have shown subsequent reductions in liver chemistries due to reduced alcohol consumption associated with naltrexone.
[c]Creatinine clearance less than or equal to 30 mol/min.
[d]only legally prescribed for dependence through appropriately licensed treatment facilities.

People who were recently detoxified from opiates in a hospital setting or in the community are especially vulnerable due to the rapid loss of tolerance they experience. That is why it is critical for individuals who are newly abstinent from opiates to seek medication assisted therapies (MAT). There are currently three FDA approved medications for the treatment of opioid dependence; naltrexone, methadone and suboxone. Naltrexone can be self-administered daily in an oral pill form, or monthly from a health care provider as an extended release injectable intramuscular suspension (Vivitrex).

Methadone and buprenorphine remain the primary treatments for opioid dependence and are currently approved by the FDA for medication assisted treatment (MAT). These medications reduce craving, prevent withdrawal, and when combined with counseling, often lead to abstinence from opioids and other illicit drugs, thereby preventing related complications, such as blood-borne virus transmission and cutaneous infections. In a special report published by the New England Journal of Medicine, May 2017 edition, the National Institute of Drug Abuse (NIDA) director Dr. Nora Volker and NIH Director Dr. Francis Collins eloquently described ways in which science can provide solutions to the opioid crisis.[33]

Methadone can only be prescribed for the treatment of opioid dependence at an approved methadone maintenance clinic, although any clinician with a Drug Enforcement Administration license can prescribe methadone for pain. Some states will grant clinicians who practice in rural communities permission to prescribe methadone to addicted patients living more than 50 miles from a methadone maintenance program. The effective methadone dose is 60 to 150 mg/d dispensed as a single morning dose. Most patients who are successfully treated receive methadone for a minimum of 5 years. Each state has different rules that govern the dispensing of methadone for opioid dependence.

Suboxone (Buprenorphine/Naloxone) can be prescribed for outpatient use by any physician with a DEA license who has taken an 8-hour training course. Suboxone must be combined with psychosocial counseling and regular drug testing. Suboxone is a partial agonist of the Mu-opioid receptor that is combined with naloxone to prevent diversion by injection of the medication. Unlike methadone which is a full agonist of the opiate receptor, it is very difficult for patients to overdose on Suboxone. Suboxone is meant to be prescribed in doctors' offices (Office Based Opioid Treatment or OBOT) and is dispensed monthly by pharmacists as a pill or dissolvable film Studies have found that Suboxone is effective in reducing injection opioid use and the frequency of hepatitis C and human immunodeficiency virus (HIV) transmission.

Treatment of Comorbid Mental Health Disorders

Comorbidity is a common problem seen in patients with alcohol and drug use disorders. Many patients with SUDs often have mental health disorders such as unipolar depression, anxiety, panic attacks, bipolar disorders, and post-traumatic stress disorder (PTSD). Primary care clinicians need to identify these comorbidities before developing a SUD treatment plan. It's useful to remember that substance use is sometimes related to a patient "self-medicating" an underlying anxiety disorder, PTSD, insomnia or untreated chronic pain. Patients are not likely to become abstinent from alcohol and drugs if these comorbidities are not treated. In contradistinction, many people with an alcohol use disorder present as depressed or with panic disorder when they are still drinking or newly abstinent, but in the majority of patients who maintain abstinence for a few weeks or more, their psychiatric symptoms will resolve without medication. These patients usually have no history of psychiatric problems when they are sober, and therefore, they may not need medications for their transient symptoms of depression or anxiety.

Treatment of Tobacco and Marijuana Use and Dependence

Tobacco and marijuana use are the cause of the two most common SUDs in the United States and throughout the world. The number of persons using these two substances on a regular basis far exceeds those using alcohol and all other illicit drugs combined. Continued use of these substances not only has adverse health and societal effects but these substances also interact with treatments for alcohol and other drug problems. Tobacco use is the leading cause of death in the United States and deserves special emphasis. Chapter 10 discusses the public health significance of tobacco and the important steps clinicians should take to facilitate smoking cessation. In general, however, clinicians should recommend cessation of all mood-altering drugs and then negotiate with patients as to how to proceed. Some patients will agree to try cessation of multiple drugs while others prefer to start with one at a time. The key is to develop a partnership with the patient to successfully address these very challenging problems (see Chapter 6).

CHRONIC PAIN AND SUBSTANCE USE DISORDERS

Professional guidelines have advocated the use of opioid analgesics for chronic nonmalignant pain, but because of the emergence of the opioid epidemic, clinicians have reevaluated this guideline and now do their best to manage chronic, nonmalignant pain by using the lowest effective doses of opiates, rotating different opiate analgesics or supplementing opiates in other ways. According to figures outlined in the National Institute on Drug Abuse's website, last updated in March, 2018, between 21% and 29% of people using opiates for chronic pain misuse them[34] and between 8% and 12% develop an opioid use disorder.[35] Strikingly, about 80% of people using heroin started by misusing prescription opioids.[36]

Clinicians and patients often misinterpret physical dependence on opioids, an expected consequence of long-term opioid use, as opioid dependence or addiction. Withdrawal and tolerance, the manifestations of physical dependence, constitute two of the 11 DSM-V criteria, which qualifies for a diagnosis of a substance use disorder if it has lasted at least 12 months and causes "impairment in daily life or noticeable distress."

Pseudoaddiction was a term coined in 1989. It has been widely accepted to describe the seeking of additional medications, appropriately or inappropriately, due to undertreatment of pain. Thus, when the pain is adequately treated, the aberrant behaviors ceased. However, the term is controversial and the authors of one literature review concluded that there is insufficient empirical evidence to support pseudoaddiction as a diagnosis distinct from addiction.[28]

Clinicians treating chronic pain should assess and monitor for signs and symptoms of substance dependence, such as aberrant behaviors surrounding medication use that might indicate a loss of control over opioid use. Clinicians should monitor the manner in which the patient is taking the medication and whether the patient complies with the recommendations of the prescribing provider. Clinicians should also determine whether the patient is taking opioid analgesics for reasons other than pain relief, such as craving, anxiety relief, insomnia, or depression.

OFFICE AND CLINIC ORGANIZATION

The development of office-based programs to deal with substance use and dependence are modeled after programs developed over the last 20 years for tobacco prevention and treatment. The model developed for tobacco use is discussed in Chapter 10, and a general systems approach for delivering preventive care in practices is discussed in Chapter 21. When applied to alcohol and drug use, the first step in such an approach is to establish a system for routinely screening for these behaviors on a regular basis. This can be accomplished by asking all new patients to complete a short set of questions on alcohol and drug use. Computer prompts can be set to remind clinicians and nurses to query all patients at some predetermined frequency and to be sure to target high-risk patients: pregnant women, patients with uncontrolled hypertension, and tobacco users. Some clinics assess alcohol use as a "vital sign," the process for identifying tobacco users discussed in Chapter 10.

Toxicology screens are helpful in high-risk patients such as those receiving pain medication or sedative drugs. Examples of newer tests of alcohol consumption are Carbohydrate Deficient Transferrin (CDT), Ethyl Glucuronide (EtG) and Phosphatidyl Ethanol (P-Eth).[29] Of the three biomarkers, P-Eth is probably the most useful as it has no known false positive sources, and is not affected by sex or age. P-Eth is a serum derived measure of longer-term drinking that detects drinking in patients consuming four or more drinks per day for two-three weeks. The relationship between P-Eth levels and alcohol intake is linear, and results are not affected by hypertension or liver disease. Patients can be advised that this lab test can help them stay sober by allowing their doctors a more precise tool to assess their progress. Traditional serum ethanol tests only measure the presence of alcohol for a period of 12 hours or less.

SUGGESTED RESOURCES AND MATERIALS

Substance Abuse and Mental Health Services Administration (SAMHSA)
National Helpline 1-800-662-HELP (4357). Open 24/7/365
www.SAMHSA.gov. Accessed 2018.

National Institute on Drug Abuse
Drug Facts Plain Language Research Summaries are available on substances of abuse, treatment, and prevention topics among many other clinical references
http://www.nida.nih.gov/Infofacts/Infofaxindex.html. Accessed 2018.

Alcoholics Anonymous
The Big Book of AA, AA brochures, and AA meeting times and locations are available online through the AA website
www.alcoholics-anonymous.org. Accessed 2018.

FamilyDoctor.org resources
Substance Abuse
https://familydoctor.org/condition/substance-abuse/. Accessed 2018.

How to Support an Addict
https://familydoctor.org/how-to-support-an-addict/. Accessed 2018.

Alcohol Abuse
https://familydoctor.org/condition/alcohol-abuse/. Accessed 2018.

Opioid Addiction
https://familydoctor.org/condition/opioid-addiction/. Accessed 2018.

Finding the Right Addiction Treatment Program
https://familydoctor.org/finding-right-addiction-treatment-program/. Accessed 2018.

Taking Medicines Safely After Alcohol or Drug Abuse Recovery
https://familydoctor.org/taking-medicines-safely-after-alcohol-or-drug-abuse-recovery/. Accessed 2018.

Teens and Alcohol
https://familydoctor.org/teens-and-alcohol/. Accessed 2018.

Resources for Family Practitioners

American Academy of Family Physicians (Search "Addiction" for Multiple Topics). www.aafp.org. Accessed 2018.
American Academy of Pediatrics (Search "Addiction" for Multiple Topics). www.aap.org. Accessed 2018.
Ways that primary care settings can improve access to addiction treatment. The Annals of Family Medicine. http://www.annfammed.org/content/15/4/306.long. Accessed 2018.

8 *Things Every Primary Care Physician Should Know About Addiction.* https://www.rehabs.com/author/anne-fletcher/. Accessed 2018.

National Institute on Alcohol Abuse and Alcoholism (NIAAA). *Helping Patients Who Drink too Much: A Clinicians Guide.* NIH Pub. No. 07-3769. http://pubs.niaaa.nih.gov/publications/Practitioner/CliniciansGuide2005/guide.pdf. Accessed 2018.

Websites for Specific Screening Instruments

https://www.integration.samhsa.gov/clinical-practice/screening-tools#drugs. Accessed 2018.

Additional Reading for Clinicians

Ait-Daoud N, Blevins D, Khanna S, Sharma S, Holstege CP. Women and addiction. *Psychiatr Clin North Am.* 2017;40(2):285-297. UI: 28477653.

Babor TF, Del Boca F, Bray JW. Screening, brief intervention and referral to treatment: implications of SAMHSA's SBIRT initiative for substance abuse policy and practice. *Addiction.* 2017;112(suppl 2):110-117. UI: 28074569.

Dackis C, O'Brien C. Neurobiology of addiction: treatment and public policy ramifications. *Nat Neurosci.* 2005;8(11):1431-1436.

Franck J, Jayaram-Lindstrom N. Pharmacotherapy for alcohol dependence: status of current treatments. [Review]. *Curr Opin Neurobiol.* 2013;23(4):692-699. UI: 23810221.

Kaye DL. Office recognition and management of adolescent substance abuse. *Curr Opin Pediatr.* 2004;16(5):532-541.

Saitz R. Clinical practice. Unhealthy alcohol use. *N Engl J Med.* 2005;352(6):596-607.

U.S. Department of Health and Human Services. *The Surgeon General's Call to Action to Prevent and Reduce Underage Drinking*U.S. Department of Health and Human Services, Office of the Surgeon General; 2007. https://www.ncbi.nlm.nih.gov/books/NBK44360/. Accessed 2018.

Velleman RD, Templeton LJ, Copello AG. The role of the family in preventing and intervening with substance use and misuse: a comprehensive review of family interventions, with a focus on young people. *Drug Alcohol Rev.* 2005;24(2):93-109.

Volkow ND, Li TK. Drugs and alcohol: treating and preventing abuse, addiction and their medical consequences. *Pharmacol Ther.* 2005;108(1):3-17.

Williams SH. Medications for treating alcohol dependence. *Am Fam Physician.* 2005;72(9):1775-1780.

REFERENCES

1. Center for Behavioral Health Statistics and Quality. *Behavioral Health Trends in the United States: Results From the 2014 National Survey on Drug Use and Health.* (HHS Publication No. SMA 15-4927, NSDUH Series H-50); 2015. Retrieved at http://www.samhsa.gov/data/.
2. NIDA. *Trends & Statistics*; April 24, 2017. Retrieved at https://www.drugabuse.gov/related-topics/trends-statistics on 2018, March 29.
3. Centers for Disease Control and Prevention. DC Newsroom "Emergency Department Data Show Rapid Increases in Opioid Overdoses". https://www.cdc.gov/media/releases/2018/p0306-vs-opioids-overdoses.html. Page last updated: March 6, 2018.
4. Rudd RA, Seth P, David F, Scholl L. Increases in drug and opioid-involved overdose deaths — United States, 2010–2015. *MMWR Morb Mortal Wkly Rep.* 2016;65:1445-1452. doi:10.15585/mmwr.mm655051e1.
5. Buchsbaum DG, Buchanan RG, Welsh J, et al. Screening for drinking disorders in the elderly using the CAGE questionnaire. *J Am Geriatr Soc.* 1992;40:662-665.
6. *Diagnostic and Statistical Manual of Mental Disorders.* 5th ed. Arlington, VA: American Psychiatric Publishing. American Psychiatric Association; 2013.

7. First MB, Williams JBW, Kart RS, Spitzer RL. *Structured Clinical Interview for DSM-5 Disorders, Clinician Version (SCID-5-CV)*. Arlington, VA: American Psychiatric Association; 2015.

8. Ewing JA. Detecting alcoholism. The CAGE questionnaire. *JAMA*. 1984;252: 1905-1907.

9. Saunders JB, Aasland OG, Babor TF, et al. Development of the alcohol use disorders identification test (AUDIT): WHO collaborative project on early detection of persons with harmful alcohol consumption-II. *Addiction*. 1993;88:791-804.

10. Isaacson JH, Butler R, Zacharek M, et al. Screening with the alcohol use disorders identification test (AUDIT) in an inner-city population. *J Gen Intern Med*. 1994;9:550-553.

11. Canagasaby A, Vinson DC. Screening for hazardous or harmful drinking using one or two quantity-frequency questions. *Alcohol Alcohol*. 2005;40:208-213.

12. Sokol RJ, Martier SS, Ager JW. The T-ACE questions: practical prenatal detection of risk-drinking. *Am J Obstet Gynecol*. 1989;160:863-868; discussion 868-870.

13. Windham GC, Von Behren J, Fenster L, et al. Moderate maternal alcohol consumption and risk of spontaneous abortion. *Epidemiology*. 1997;8:509-514.

14. Russell M, Martier SS, Sokol RJ, et al. Detecting risk drinking during pregnancy: a comparison of four screening questionnaires. *Am J Public Health*. 1996;86:1435-1439.

15. DiClemente CC, Corno CM, Grayson MM, Wiprovnick AE, Knoblach DJ. Motivational interviewing, enhancement, and brief interventions over the last decade: a review of reviews of efficacy and effectiveness. *Psychol Addict Behav*. 2017;31(8):862-887. doi:10.1037/adb0000318.

16. Brown RL, Rounds LA. Conjoint screening questionnaires for alcohol and other drug abuse: criterion validity in a primary care practice. *Wis Med J*. 1995;94:135-140.

17. Brown RL, Leonard T, Saunders LA, et al. A two-item screening test for alcohol and other drug problems. *J Fam Pract*. 1997;44:151-160.

18. Bastiaens L, Francis G, Lewis K. The RAFFT as a screening tool for adolescent substance use disorders. *Am J Addict*. 2000;9:10-16.

19. Knight JR, Sherritt L, Shrier LA, et al. Validity of the CRAFFT substance abuse screening test among adolescent clinic patients. *Arch Pediatr Adolesc Med*. 2002;156:607-614.

20. Evans EA, Grella CE, Washington DL, Upchurch DM Gender and race/ethnic differences in the persistence of alcohol, drug, and poly-substance use disorders. *Drug Alcohol Depend*. 2017;174:128-136. doi:10.1016/j.drugalcdep.2017.01.021. Epub 2017 Mar 7.

21. Muntaner C, Eaton WW, Diala C, et al. Social class, assets, organizational control and the prevalence of common groups of psychiatric disorders. *Soc Sci Med*. 1998;47:2043-2053.

22. Armstrong TD, Costello EJ. Community studies on adolescent substance use, abuse, or dependence and psychiatric comorbidity. *J Consult Clin Psychol*. 2002;70:1224-1239.

23. Brady KT, Myrick H, Sonne SC. Co-occurring addictive and affective disorders. In: Graham A, Schultz T, Mayo-Smith M, et al. eds. *Principles of Addiction Medicine*. 3rd ed. Chevy Chase: American Society of Addiction Medicine; 2003.

24. Whitlock EP, Polen MR, Green CA, et al. Behavioral counseling interventions in primary care to reduce risky/harmful alcohol use by adults: a summary of the evidence for the U.S. Preventive Services Task Force. *Ann Intern Med*. 2004;140:557-568.

25. Cuijpers P, Riper H, Lemmers L. The effects on mortality of brief interventions for problem drinking: a meta-analysis. *Addiction*. 2004;99:839-845.

26. Fleming M, Mundt M, French M, et al. Brief physician advice for problem drinkers: long-term efficacy and benefit-cost analysis. *Alcohol Clin Exp Res*. 2002;26:36-43.

27. Seitz R, Palfai TPA, Cheng DA, et al. Screening and brief intervention for drug use in primary care-the ASPIRE randomized clinical trial. *JAMA*. 2014;312(5):502-513. doi:10.1001/jama.2014.7862.

28. Anonymous. Matching alcoholism treatments to client heterogeneity: project MATCH posttreatment drinking outcomes. *J Stud Alcohol*. 1997;58:7-29.

29. Ogden EJ, Moskowitz H. Effects of alcohol and other drugs on driver performance. *Traffic Inj Prev*. 2004;5:185-198.

30. Fuller RK, Branchey L, Brightwell DR, et al. Disulfiram treatment of alcoholism. A veterans administration cooperative study. *JAMA*. 1986;256(11):1449-1455.

31. Gastfriend DR. Intramuscular extended-release naltrexone: current evidence. *Ann N Y Accad Sci*. 2011;1224(1):207. [Erratum appears in *Ann N Y Accad Sci*. 2011;1224(1):207; PMID: 28605079].

32. Lucey MR, Silverman BL, Illeperuma A, O'Brien CP. Hepatic safety of once-monthly injectable extended-release naltrexone administered to actively drinking alcoholics. *Alcohol Clin Exp Res*. 2008;32(3):498-504. Comparative Study. Journal Article. Randomized Controlled Trial. Research Support, Non-U.S. Gov't UI: 18241321

33. Volkow ND, Collins FS. The role of science in addressing the opioid crisis. *N Engl J Med*. 2017;377(4):391-394. [Special Report]. AN: 00006024-201707270-00018.

34. Vowels KE, Mentee ML, Jules PS, Froe T, Ney JP, van der Goes DN. Rates of opioid misuse, abuse, and addiction in chronic pain: a systematic review and data synthesis. *Pain*. 2015;156(4):569-576. doi:10.1097/01.j.pain.0000460357.01998.f1.

35. Muhuri PK, Gfroerer JC, Davies MC. Associations of nonmedical pain reliever use and initiation of heroin use in the United States. *CBHSQ Data Rev*, 2013. https://www.samhsa.gov/data/sites/default/files/DR006/DR006/nonmedical-pain-reliever use-2013.htm.

36. Carlson RG, Nahhas RW, Martins SS, Daniulaityte R. Predictors of transition to heroin use among initially non-opioid dependent illicit pharmaceutical opioid users: a natural history study. *Drug Alcohol Depend*. 2016;160:127-134. doi:10.1016/j.drugalcdep.2015.12.026.

37. Greene M, Chambers R. Pseudoaddiction: fact or fiction? An investigation of the medical literature. *Curr Addict Rep*. 2015. doi:10.1007/s40429-015-0074-7.

38. Allen JP, Worst FM, Thon N, Latten RZ. Assessing the drinking status of liver transplant patients with alcoholic liver disease. *Liver Transpl*. 2013;19:369-376.

Please see Online Appendix: Apps and Digital Resources for additional information.

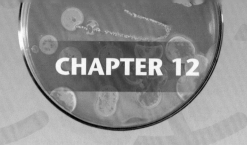

CHAPTER 12

Contraception

ALISON MORIARTY DALEY

BACKGROUND

In the United States, there are 61 million women between the ages of 15 and 44 years.[1] Most sexually active women report that they have used at least one method of contraception.[1] Reversible hormonal contraceptive methods (pill, patch, injection, implant, intrauterine contraceptive [IUC]) and condoms are the most commonly used methods by women (67%) with fewer opting for female (25%) or male (8%) sterilization.[1] The oral contraceptive pill (OCP) is the most commonly used method, although the use of other hormonal contraceptive methods has increased in recent years.[1]

Women are sometimes reluctant to use contraceptives because of perceived side effects or potential health risks, but most women are unaware that pregnancy often carries far greater risks. The latter is especially true for women with coexisting medical problems that can complicate a pregnancy. Highly effective contraception is essential for those women who are using teratogenic medications.

Nearly half (47%) of all pregnancies in the United States are reported by women to be unintended.[1-4] The rate of unintended pregnancy is higher, 75%, among adolescents 15 to 19 years old.[5] Contraceptive access and long-active contraceptive methods have been credited with decreasing the teen birth rate steadily since the early 1990s from 77.1 per 1000 to 20.3 per 1000 among 15- to 19-year-olds.[6] Unintended pregnancies are a concern for all women, not just adolescents, because of the potential for adverse outcomes for both the mother and child.[7]

Maternal deaths are all too common in developing countries, with maternal mortality rates nearly 20 times higher in developing (239/100,000 live births) versus developed countries (12/100,000 live births).[8] The largest health impact of family planning in such settings is the reduction of maternal mortality through a decrease in unwanted and potentially dangerous pregnancies. Contraceptive use also leads to a decrease in infant mortality through increased spacing between pregnancies.[9] Spacing pregnancies more than 2 years apart decreases infant mortality by 50%.[9] In addition to these health benefits, allowing women to control their fertility can give them opportunities to pursue education and employment outside the home.[10]

In addition to pregnancy prevention, hormonal contraception provides additional health-related benefits to women, including the decrease in dysmenorrhea, decreased risk of ovarian and endometrial cancer, menstrual regularity, improvement of acne, and decreased premenstrual symptoms.[11] Condoms reduce the risk of the transmission of human immunodeficiency virus (HIV) and other sexually transmitted infections (STIs) between partners. Suppression of menses for transgender male patients either before or with testosterone therapy can also be achieved through hormonal contraception.[12,13]

CONTRACEPTIVE COUNSELING

The choice of a contraceptive method is highly personal. Female and male patients need to be educated about all available contraceptive methods, the efficacy of each method (Table 12.1), how to properly use the chosen method(s), and possible side effects. Patients also need education and written instructions on what to do if they take their contraceptive method off schedule or have an unintended event (e.g., lose a pill, patch comes off, IUC expelled). Clinicians need to consider first what their patient feels will work best and if this method is safe for the patient to use within the context of a comprehensive medical history and physical examination. A complete list of contraindications for each contraceptive method and guidance for the clinician to contraceptive use can be found in the *U.S. Medical Eligibility Criteria for Contraceptive Use, 2016.*[14]

The need for protection from STIs also needs to be considered. Patients can make this decision only with excellent access to information and timely access to the full spectrum of methods. The primary care clinician can help reduce unintended pregnancy by proactively asking each patient about her contraceptive needs and experience at each encounter (see Chapter 3). The discussion should both elicit the patient's concerns and address any misinformation about contraception (e.g., hormonal contraceptives cause infertility). Many women avoid using effective methods because they, their partners, family members, or friends hold mistaken beliefs. Clinicians who effectively address these concerns and beliefs can improve the initiation of a method, continuation, and contraceptive adherence.[14] Clinicians can also refer patients to online (e.g., www.bedsider.com) or community resources, such as Planned Parenthood (www.plannedparenthood.org), for further counseling about family planning options.

TABLE 12.1   Contraceptive Methods by Effectiveness

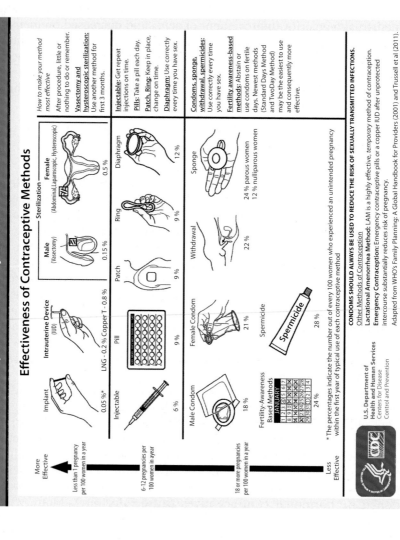

Effectiveness of Contraceptive Methods

Adolescents

Contraceptive counseling is especially important for adolescents because most teen pregnancies are unintended (75%).[4] The United States has had a steady decline in teen birth rates since 1991 from a rate of 61.8 births per 1000 to the current rate of 20.3 per 1000 in 15- to 19-year-olds.[6] In 2015, 229,715 babies were born to women aged 15 to 19 years. Much of this decline has been credited to increased access to contraception for adolescents.[4,15] Despite these declines, the rate of teen pregnancy is higher than many other similar countries, including the United Kingdom and Canada.[16] Most teens report contraceptive use at sexual initiation or within the same month.[5] Younger teens are less likely to be using contraception at the time they initiate sex.[5]

Clinicians should counsel adolescents in private, with the assurance that all discussions will remain confidential (see Chapter 18).[17] Many adolescents will not raise the issue of contraception, so a clinician needs to start this discussion on a routine basis, perhaps by inquiring what the patient has heard from her friends. Early puberty is a good time to begin to discuss, with teens and parents, the availability of contraception.[18] Although the advantages of abstinence merit discussion, as discussed in Chapter 13, clinicians should also discuss contraception because most adolescents become sexually active at some point. The discussion can occur during any visit and should start with the most effective methods and need for consistent condom use for the prevention of STIs.[19,20] Adolescents benefit from clinical services that protect their confidentiality, can be easily accessed, and are available either in school (e.g., through a school-based health center) or outside school hours.[21] Ideally, contraceptive services are best integrated into primary care services for adolescents because it removes a significant barrier to care and avoids unnecessary delay in accessing contraception.

All adolescents starting a contraceptive method need to be encouraged to call or return to discuss perceived side effects, concerns, or ask questions.[19,21] Frequent follow-up visits for adolescents, especially after the initiation of a method are important to enhance continuation of contraception use. Many teens are unsure of their reproductive physiology and also likely to be unsure of how contraception will prevent pregnancy or how condoms provide STI prevention. Providing oral and written instructions and providing condoms and a contraceptive method within the same visit facilitates timely use of contraception.[20]

A pelvic examination is not required before the initiation of a hormonal contraceptive method, with the exception of a diaphragm, cervical cap, or IUC.[2] Requiring a pelvic examination introduces a barrier to the initiation of hormonal contraception especially for adolescents. Regular Pap smear screening, being at age 21 years, is encouraged for all female-bodied individuals.[22] Pelvic examinations for adolescents are indicated for several

---

Box 12.1   Criteria for Reasonable Certainty That a Woman is Not Pregnant

No symptoms/signs of pregnancy and (one of the following)
Last menstrual cycle began ≤7 days ago
No sexual intercourse since first day of last menstrual period
Using a method of contraception correctly and consistently
Less than or equal to 7 days since spontaneous or induced abortion
Within 4 weeks postpartum
Fully/nearly fully breastfeeding (≥85% of feeds are breastfeeds) and amenorrheic and <6 months postpartum

CDC. U.S. selected practice recommendations for contraceptive use. Adapted from the World Health Organization selected practice recommendations for contraceptive use, 2nd edition. *MMWR Recomm Rep.* 2013;62(No. RR-2).

---

reasons including symptoms of a vaginal or upper reproductive tract infection, pelvic pain, menstrual irregularities, or after a sexual assault.[23,24] Most contraceptive methods can be started at any time as long as the clinician is reasonably certain that the woman is not pregnant (Box 12.1; Fig. 12.1).

As compared with "no method," use of contraception by adolescents or adults leads to medical care cost savings.[1,3] Male condom use along with a female-based method, and advance provision of emergency contraception (EC), provide additional savings.[26]

CONTRACEPTIVE METHODS

Highly Effective Reversible Methods: Injectable Contraceptives, Intrauterine Devices, and Implants

Long-acting reversible methods are highly effective and provide continuous contraception that either cannot be passively discontinued (IUCs and implants) or are only slowly reversible (depot medroxyprogesterone acetate). None of these methods contain estrogen, and they are generally the first choice for women who cannot take estrogen and for those women in whom pregnancy is medically contraindicated. All of these methods are discrete, enhance patient privacy, and forgettable.

Injectable Contraceptive

Depot medroxyprogesterone acetate (DMPA), or Depo Provera, is an injectable contraceptive consisting of microcrystals suspended in an aqueous solution.[27,28] It is available as a deep intramuscular injection of 150 mg every 3 months (13 weeks) or as a subcutaneous injection of 104 mg every 3 months (13 weeks). The efficacy rate with perfect use is >99% and 94% with typical use.[29] Failure rates quoted with perfect use are achieved when the method is used exactly as directed. DMPA works by blocking the mid-cycle

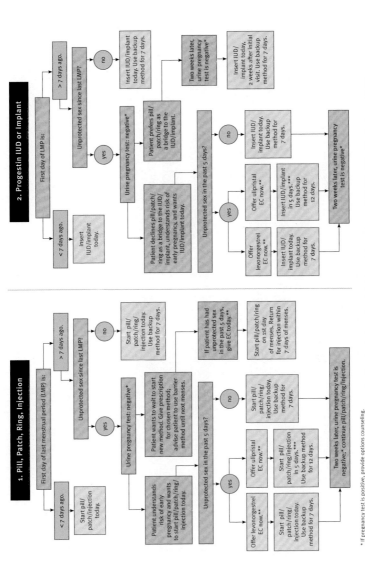

Figure 12.1 Quick start algorithm. Reproduced with permission from https://www.reproductiveaccess.org/wp-content/uploads/2014/12/QuickstartAlgorithm.pdf.

Quick Start Algorithm — Patient requests a new birth control method:

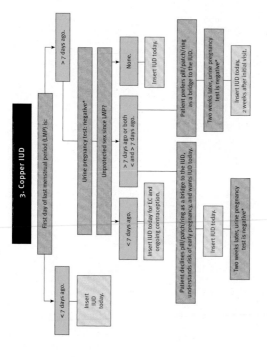

3. Copper IUD

First day of last menstrual period (LMP) is:

< 7 days ago.
> Insert IUD today.

> 7 days ago.
> Urine pregnancy test: negative*

Unprotected sex since LMP?

< 7 days ago.
> Insert IUD today for EC and ongoing contraception.

> 7 days ago or both < and > 7 days ago.

None.
> Insert IUD today.

Patient declines pill/patch/ring as a bridge to the IUD, understands risk of early pregnancy, and wants IUD today.
> Insert IUD today.
> Two weeks later, urine pregnancy test is negative*

Patient prefers pill/patch/ring as a bridge to the IUD.
> Two weeks later, urine pregnancy test is negative*
> Insert IUD today, 2 weeks after initial visit.

* If pregnancy test is positive, provide options counseling.

Citation: Curtis KM, Jatlaoui TC, Tepper NK, et al. U.S. Selected Practice Recommendations for Contraceptive Use, 2016. MMWR Recomm Rep 2016;65(No. RR-4):1–66. DOI: https://dx.doi.org/10.15585/mmwr.rr6504a1.

October 2016 / Reproductive Health Access Project / www.reproductiveaccess.org

reproductive
health
access
project

Figure 12.1 *(Continued)*

luteinizing hormone surge, thickening cervical mucus, and causing atrophy of the endometrium. The only absolute medical contraindication to use is active breast cancer.[25] Noncontraceptive benefits of DMPA include diminished menstrual bleeding and dysmenorrhea, decreased risk of pelvic inflammatory disease and of endometrial and ovarian cancers, and fewer sickle cell crises.[12] After their third injection, almost half of DMPA users become amenorrheic. Amenorrhea occurs in 70% of women after 2 years of use and 80% of women after 5 years. Data from prospective studies of DMPA do not support a causal relationship between its use and either depression or marked weight gain.[30–35]

Bone density loss during use is comparable with that seen during breastfeeding, and studies indicate that bone density is regained after discontinuing this method.[36,37] DMPA is contraindicated in women who may be pregnant because it would offer no benefit and because its use may delay the diagnosis of pregnancy. The contraceptive effect of DMPA is slowly reversible. Although continued reliable contraceptive protection requires a reinjection every 3 months, the average time for return to ovulation ranges between 15 and 49 weeks.[25] Therefore, DMPA may not be an ideal method for women who are planning pregnancy in the near future.

Intrauterine Devices

The ParaGard Copper T 380A IUC is a highly effective low-maintenance method. It has greater than 99% efficacy,[29] which is comparable with sterilization, and it may remain in place for 10+ years.[38,39] The mechanism of action of the Copper T is impairment of sperm function, rendering sperm unable to fertilize ova. It is recommended for women who desire long-term contraception. Owing to the immediate return of fertility after removal, it is also suitable for women who are spacing pregnancies. The clinician can easily insert the IUC during an office visit at any time during the menstrual cycle (see Fig. 12.2). The copper IUC typically causes longer or heavier menstrual bleeding, especially in the first few months after insertion.[20,39] The risk of involuntary expulsion is approximately 5% in the first year after insertion. To ensure that the device is still in place, women should be advised to feel the strings of the IUC after every menses.[2]

The initial cost of the IUC is higher than that of many other contraceptives, but IUCs become the most cost-effective method when utilized for 2 years or longer.[40] The copper IUC can also be used for EC (see section on "Emergency Contraception," page 291) as well as immediately postpartum[2] (see section on "Contraception after Pregnancy").

Currently four levonorgestrel intrauterine systems (LNG IUSs) are available in the United States: Mirena (52 mg), Kayleena (19.5 mg), Liletta (52 mg), and Skyla (13.5 mg).[41–45] Each is a T-shaped device inserted into the uterus. Mirena and Kayleena provide up to 5 years of contraception,[41,42] Liletta 4 years,[43,44] and Skyla 3 years.[45] Levonorgestrel

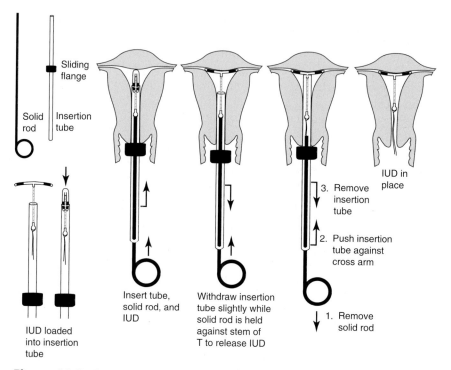

Solid rod

Insertion tube

Sliding flange

IUD loaded into insertion tube

Insert tube, solid rod, and IUD

Withdraw insertion tube slightly while solid rod is held against stem of T to release IUD

3. Remove insertion tube

2. Push insertion tube against cross arm

1. Remove solid rod

IUD in place

Figure 12.2   Insertion technique for Copper T380A intrauterine device. High fundal placement is achieved by using a withdrawal technique. *IUD*, intrauterine device. Reproduced with permission from Beckmann CRB, Ling FW, Laube DW, et al. *Obstetrics and Gynecology*. 4th ed. Baltimore: Lippincott Williams & Wilkins; 2002.

is released from the device into the uterus. Efficacy rates for perfect and typical use are >99%.[29] The mechanisms of action for the LNG-IUS are thickening of the cervical mucus, which impairs sperm motility, reduces survival, and the suppression of the endometrium.[14,41] In some women, the systemic absorption of levonorgestrel may suppress ovulation. The LNG-IUS has major noncontraceptive benefits, including improving dysmenorrhea, reducing menorrhagia with a 90% decrease in blood loss compared with a typical menstrual cycle, and the development of amenorrhea in approximately 20% of women.[46] For women with menorrhagia, use of the LNG-IUS provides an alternative to endometrial ablation and hysterectomy.[41,46] Women using the LNG-IUS experience a gradual decrease in menstrual duration, blood loss, and spotting during the first 6 months after insertion. Most women experience light bleeding or amenorrhea over time.[2] The LNG-IUS is also acceptable for use to protect the endometrium in menopausal women using estrogen therapy.[46]

Contraindications to IUC insertion are current pelvic infection and anomalies of the uterine cavity, as these might increase the risk of expulsion of the device.[2] Insertion should not occur in the presence of active cervical or pelvic infection, but it can occur after treatment of both partners. IUCs do not increase the risk of pelvic inflammatory disease.[2] If, while an IUC is being used, an asymptomatic cervical infection is detected by screening, the woman can be treated with the device in place and reassessed in 24 to 48 hours.[2] If a woman develops symptomatic upper genital tract infection during IUC use, she should be tested for STIs, treated with the appropriate antibiotic regimen, and followed per current guidelines.[17] IUCs can be used in nulliparous women, in adolescents, in women with a past ectopic pregnancy, in women infected with HIV, and in women with past pelvic infection.[14,47]

Subdermal Progestin Implant

Nexplanon is a reversible single-rod implant, measuring 40 by 2 mm, that is impregnated with 68 mg of etonogestrel, a progestin.[48] The implant releases approximately 40 µg of etonogestrel daily, providing continuous contraception for up to 3 years.[48] Efficacy for perfect and typical use is also >99%.[29] The implant is inserted subcutaneously in the upper arm during an office procedure performed by a trained clinician. Noncontraceptive benefits include a decrease in dysmenorrhea and endometriosis and the improvement of acne.[20] The main side effect of this implant is irregular bleeding throughout use; however, the bleeding pattern for most women is established by 3 months post insertion.[49] Nexplanon does not adversely affect bone mineral density.[48,50] Removal of the implant is accomplished via a quick and simple office procedure. Fertility returns immediately following removal.[48]

Effective Reversible Methods: Pills, Patch, and Vaginal Ring

Combined ethinyl estradiol and progestin methods (OCPs, transdermal patch, and vaginal ring) and the progestin-only pills (POPs) have perfect-use efficacy rates of >99%; however, the typical use efficacy is 91%.[29] These hormonal methods all require active decision making and a regular routine for successful use. These are generally cyclic methods designed to produce a regular withdrawal bleeding episode but can be used continuously.

Oral Contraceptives

OCPs are the most popular reversible method of contraception in the United States.[1] There are combined estrogen and progestin formulations (COCs) and POPs. The estrogen in COCs in the United States is ethinyl estradiol.[20] To decrease the risk of thromboembolic events, the estrogen dose has been steadily reduced since the first introduction of the pill in the 1960s. Currently, low-dose contain 10 to 35 μg of ethinyl estradiol per tablet, compared with 100 to 150 μg of ethinyl estradiol in the 1960s. The amount of progestin in the pill has been lowered even more than the amount of estrogen. There are eight different progestins in current pills. Many believe that the choice of progestin can influence the tolerability of the pill, with different women preferring different products. Efficacy rates of both COCs and POPs is >99% and 91% with typical use.[29]

Traditional cyclic use of COCs involves following the routine prescribed by the monthly pill pack for 28 days, taking 21 active pills followed by 7 placebo pills. The predictable withdrawal bleeding occurs during the week in which the placebo pills are taken. A new pill pack is started the day after finishing the placebo pills regardless of the bleeding pattern. The most recently approved 28-day COC regimens typically contain more days of active pills[24] and fewer days of placebo[51]; the rationale is to minimize cyclic symptoms that may be related to fluctuations in hormone levels. These regimens may also yield fewer days of withdrawal bleeding.

Continuous use of COCs is achieved in three U.S. Food and Drug Administration–approved products (Seasonale, Seasonique, Loseasonique) by daily use of active pills for 84 consecutive days followed by 7 days of placebo (or low-estrogen-dose) tablets.[52–54] The benefit of this approach is less frequent withdrawal bleeding.[51] Comparison of continuous and cyclic use of COCs demonstrates that continuous use is safe, effective, and well tolerated.[55] Breakthrough bleeding and spotting decrease with successive cycles.[56]

Conventional approaches to the initiation of oral contraception require waiting until the next menstrual period to take the first pill either on the first day of menses or as a Sunday start. Newer alternative approach encourages patients to take the first tablet on the same day as it was prescribed regardless of menstrual cycle day as long as the clinician is reasonably certain the women is not pregnant (see Box 12.1 for these criteria). This approach, called *Quick Start,* has been shown to increase OCP use initially among adolescents; however, frequent follow-up enhances continuation of OCP.[51] The World Health Organization recommends prescribing 1 year of OCPs at the annual visit and access to refills should be flexible.[57] Condoms should be used for 7 days after starting OCP via Quick Start. This approach is safe, acceptable, and useful for the initiation of OCPs as well as for all hormonal contraceptives.[58–60]Figure 12.1 provides the Quick Start Algorithm.

Despite dose reductions, potential risks exist to the use of OCPs. Some women should not take estrogen-containing contraception because of an increased risk of myocardial infarction or stroke.[20] A family history of adverse effects from OCPs does not raise the risk of most adverse events. Regardless of age, the use of an estrogen-containing OCP is contraindicated in the presence of known ischemic heart disease, a personal history of stoke, migraine headaches with aura, diabetes with vascular changes, or uncontrolled hypertension.[20] Such women need other forms of highly effective contraception because of the risks of major complications during pregnancy. A complete list of contraindications and guidance for the clinician to contraceptive use can be found in the *U.S. Medical Eligibility Criteria for Contraceptive Use, 2016.*[20]

The increased risk of venous thromboembolism (VTE) generally contraindicates the use of COCs (or patch or ring) in women with a personal history of VTE, those with a known high-risk thrombogenic mutation, and postpartum women within 21 days of giving birth. Most studies agree that the greatest risk of VTE occurs in the first 1 to 2 years of COC use.[2,20] The risk of VTE in young women is greatest during pregnancy, particularly during the puerperium; the risk of VTE associated with COC use is substantially lower than the VTE risk attributable to pregnancy itself.[62] Despite widely held beliefs that the use of COC leads to weight gain, a systematic review of 44 randomized controlled trials found no evidence of a causal relationship between combination contraceptives and weight gain.[61]

POPs (or "minipills") contain 0.35 mg of norethindrone, in Micronor (Camila and Errin).[63] The mechanisms of action for POPs are inhibition of ovulation, thickening of cervical mucus, decreasing activity of cilia in the fallopian tubes, and altering the endometrium.[20,63] They are to be taken every day with no hormone-free interval. POPs may be most appropriate in women who should not take estrogen-containing contraceptives. The only absolute contraindication to use is current breast cancer. Noncontraceptive benefits of POPs include reduced menstrual bleeding (and in some cases amenorrhea), anemia, dysmenorrhea, and premenstrual symptoms such as bloating and breast tenderness. As with COCs there is a decreased risk of endometrial and ovarian cancer. Like the COCs, the contraceptive effect of POPs is immediately reversible. Disadvantages of POPs include the need to take the pills on a very regular schedule. Missing pills or taking them at irregular intervals reduces effectiveness. Back-up methods such as condoms or other barrier methods (see "Barrier and Related Methods" section, pages 287-291) are generally recommended for 48 hours if a pill is taken more than 3 hours late.[20] Menstrual irregularities are a reason that many women discontinue use of this particular type of OCP; adequate counseling on this side effect may reduce discontinuation rates.[64]

Transdermal Contraceptive Patch

Xulane (generic of Ortho Evra available in the United States) is a combined hormonal contraceptive patch. Each patch measures 1.75 × 1.75 in and contains 0.75 mg ethinyl estradiol and 6.0 mg norelgestromin.[65] As with OCPs, the main mechanism of action is the prevention of ovulation. Each patch is worn for 7 days and replaced each week, for 3 weeks out of every four. A withdrawal bleed occurs during the fourth week, when no patch is worn. Once-a-week dosing is convenient and may enhance the chances of correct use, compared with OCPs. The benefits of the patch are similar to combined OCPs, including usefulness in the management of both menorrhagia and dysmenorrhea.[20,51] Disadvantages include lack of privacy when the patch is worn on a visible area and possible skin irritation and pigment change at the site of application.[20] Like the OCP, the patch does not protect against STIs. Women who have contraindications to using estrogen may not use the patch.[20]

Vaginal Ring

NuvaRing is a monthly vaginal contraceptive that is inserted by the patient and remains in place for 3 weeks.[66] It is a soft flexible ring made of ethylene vinyl acetate (see Fig. 12.3). Its outer diameter is 5.4 cm, and it is 4 mm thick. It contains ethinyl estradiol and etonogestrel, which is dispersed evenly throughout the ring. It releases 15 µg of ethinyl estradiol and 120 µg of etonogestrel each 24-hour period. The vaginal ring has the advantage of once-a-month dosing, and its use is completely discreet.[20,66]

The vaginal ring may be used in a cyclic or continuous manner, both of which are acceptable to patients and well tolerated.[27,67] If used in a cyclic manner, the ring is removed after the third week and there is a withdrawal bleed. A new ring is placed 1 week later. For continuous use, a new ring is inserted immediately after the ring that has been in place for 3 weeks is removed. Alternatively, each ring contains enough hormone for 28 to 35 days and therefore can be changed monthly (on the same day each month).[66,68] The continuous method may reduce cyclic symptoms such as premenstrual syndrome. It yields fewer total bleeding days but results in more spotting. Comparison of the pharmacokinetics of the vaginal ring, transdermal patch, and combined OCPs demonstrated significantly lower

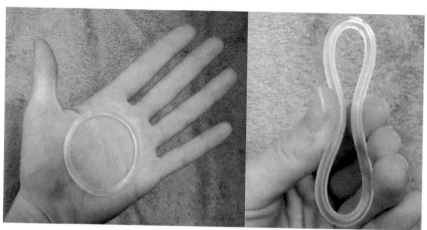

Figure 12.3 NuvaRing (Organon Pharmaceuticals USA Inc, Roseland, NJ, USA), a monthly vaginal contraceptive that is inserted by the patient and remains in place for 3 weeks.

and less varied ethinyl estradiol serum levels among ring users compared with women using the other methods.[69] A disadvantage of this method is that the individual must be comfortable inserting and removing it from the vagina; patient education with a pelvic model may be necessary.

Less Effective Methods: Condoms, Diaphragms, Sponges, and Spermicides

When less effective contraceptive methods are used, outcomes are widely variable with typical use. These methods must be in use at the time of coitus. Annual failure rates range from 10% to 25%. Parous women experience higher failure rates.[2,29]

Condoms

Condoms are widely available and are the method most frequently used at first intercourse.[1] Male condoms are available in latex; for latex-sensitive or allergic users, condoms manufactured with natural membrane from animal skin or with polyurethane and synthetic elastomers are available. The animal membrane material has a larger pore size that prevents transmission of sperm but may allow passage of infectious organisms. As noted in Chapter 13, this type of condom is not recommended for prevention of STIs, including HIV.[68]

A Cochrane review of all randomized controlled trials evaluated male nonlatex condoms made of polyurethane film or synthetic elastomers as compared with latex condoms. Nonlatex condoms had higher rates of breakage than latex condoms but are still an acceptable alternative.[70]

Typical efficacy of male condoms is 82% versus perfect use efficacy of 98%.[29] Actual per-use failure rates experienced by condom users vary greatly depending on the correctness and consistency of use. Unplanned pregnancy among condom users occur owing to numerous factors including slippage and breakage; failure to use condoms during an imperfectly calculated "safe period"; and nonuse of the condom during the early minutes of intercourse, leading to insemination by the pre-ejaculatory fluid.

The key noncontraceptive benefit of synthetic condoms is that they are the only contraceptive method proved to reduce the risk of STIs, including infection with HIV and human papillomavirus[20,23,71] (see Chapter 13). In addition, condoms are inexpensive, often free to patients, and easy to use. *Dual method use* refers to the simultaneous use of condoms and an additional effective or highly effective pharmaceutical contraceptive to provide optimal protection against both infection and pregnancy. Women who rely on effective hormonal contraceptives, but who do not use condoms consistently, have a higher risk of acquiring STIs. Consistent dual method use is uncommon, however.[23]

Female Condoms

The first-generation female condom (formerly called *Reality*) is made of polyurethane. Efficacy for the female condom for perfect use 95% and typical use 79% are lower than that of male condoms.[29] The female condom is inserted into the vagina before sexual intercourse. FC2 is a second-generation female condom made of synthetic latex, which is less expensive than polyurethane.[72] Female condoms are 17 cm long and contain two flexible polyurethane rings, one at each end. The ring at the closed end is inserted into the vagina, and the open ring remains outside the vagina after insertion. Female condoms provide protection against both pregnancy and STIs, and they can be inserted up to 8 hours before intercourse. Female and male condoms should not be used together; they can adhere to each other, causing breakage, slippage, or displacement of one or both devices.[51]

Diaphragm and Cervical Cap

The diaphragm is a dome-shaped latex rubber cup that was much more popular decades ago before the introduction of more highly effective methods. The diaphragm and cervical cap is used by less than 1% of contraceptive users in the United States.[1] Efficacy rates are 94% and 88% for perfect and typical use, respectively.[29] It has a flexible rim available with diameters from 60 to 100 mm. It is inserted into the vagina before intercourse, covering the cervix (see Fig. 12.4). The cervical cap fits more tightly over the cervix than does the diaphragm, with diameters of 18 to 25 mm.[14,51] Both the diaphragm and cap must be individually fitted. They are both designed for use with a spermicide. After intercourse, the diaphragm must remain in place for 6 hours to maximize spermicidal action. The spermicide must be reapplied with an applicator with the diaphragm in place before subsequent intercourse. The cap can provide continuous contraception for 48 hours without the need to reapply spermicide.[68]

Prolonged use of either device for greater than 24 consecutive hours is associated with an increased risk of toxic shock syndrome,[51] which is a systemic infection with *Staphylococcus aureus*. Both caps and diaphragms protect against upper genital tract infections that ordinarily gain entry through the cervical mucosa, including gonorrhea and chlamydia. Contraceptive failure rates with these devices are approximately 12% per year, with a wide range depending on the correctness and consistency of use.[1] Diaphragm use carries an increased risk of urinary tract infection. If a woman has prolapse of the uterus or relaxation of the introitus or is immediately postpartum, it may not be possible to fit a diaphragm or cap successfully. Users should be refitted after childbirth or substantial changes in weight.[51]

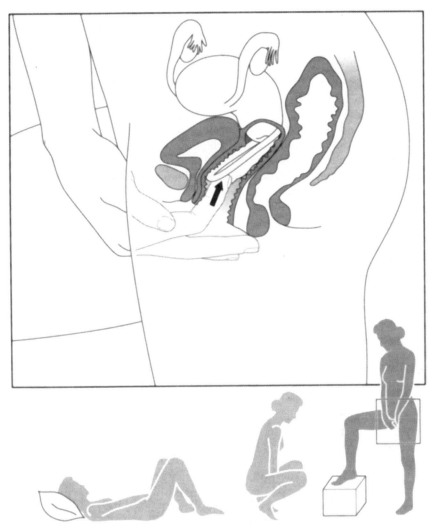

Figure 12.4   Insertion of the diaphragm. Proximal edge fits in posterior fornix and distal edge behind symphysis. Reproduced with permission from Speroff L, Darney PD. *A Clinical Guide for Contraception*. Baltimore: Williams & Wilkins; 1992.

Spermicides

Spermicides are reversible, temporary, nonprescription methods of contraception. They are available as foams, creams, jellies, film, and suppositories that melt after they are inserted into the vagina. The efficacy of these methods is 82% for perfect use and 72% for typical use.[29] All spermicide preparations are short acting, with the intent of providing protection for a single act of intercourse that takes place within minutes to a few hours following the application of the spermicide. Suppositories and films need to melt and disperse in the vagina, and they therefore may not be active until 20 minutes after application. Their efficacy in pregnancy prevention is 70% to 85%. Spermicides may be used alone or as adjuncts to barrier contraceptive methods. Nonoxynol-9 is a spermicide that may irritate vaginal and rectal mucosa and may therefore increase the risk of HIV and other STIs. Therefore, current recommendations are for nonoxynol-9 use only by couples at low risk of STIs.[73] Hypersensitivity is a common adverse reaction, either from nonoxynol-9 itself or from the vehicle. Spermicides are not recommended for use in women at risk for HIV infection.[23,68]

Sponge

The Today sponge is a polyurethane sperm barrier available over the counter.[74] It contains 1 g of nonoxynol-9 spermicide. Efficacy of this method is better, 88%, for nulliparous women than for parous women, 76%.[74] There is a dimple on one side that is designed to fit over the cervix and a loop on the other side for removal. The sponge provides continuous contraception for 24 hours and must be left in place for 6 hours after intercourse. Wearing the sponge for greater than 30 hours may increase the risk of toxic shock syndrome.[74–76]

Fertility Awareness Methods

Periodic abstinence techniques (rhythm method) are designed to work by avoiding coitus during the fertile days of the menstrual cycle. All variations of this method rely on assumptions about the timing of ovulation.[77] Examples of periodic abstinence techniques include the calendar method, which estimates fertile days based on cycle length; the temperature method, which relies on recording the basal body temperature to detect ovulation; and the symptothermal method, which relies on temperature and cervical mucous changes. Advantages of periodic abstinence methods include no cost and no direct medical risks. Disadvantages include long training periods, unreliability in predicting fertility, poor adherence and continuation rates, and resulting high failure rates. This method may be difficult to use for women who recently had menarche, are in the postpregnancy state, are currently breastfeeding, recently discontinued a contraceptive method, have irregular cycles, or are nearing menopause.[77]

Anovulation During Lactational Amenorrhea

Anovulation during lactational amenorrhea can be exploited as a contraceptive method. Natural postpartum infertility occurs when a woman is amenorrheic and fully breastfeeding. To rely on this method, women must be exclusively breastfeeding at least six times a day or 85% breastfeeding, have not had menses since delivery, and be less than 6 months postpartum.[2] Done correctly, this temporary method is highly effective (up to 98%). It does not provide protection from STIs.

EMERGENCY CONTRACEPTION

Emergency contraception (EC) is intended for use after unprotected intercourse, sexual assault, or contraceptive failure. Efficacy is estimated to be as high as 90% for emergency contraceptive pills and >99% for the copper IUC.[78]

EC pills work by inhibiting or delaying ovulation. *Plan B One-step (Teva)* and several generic brands *Take Action (Teva)*, Next Choice One Step (Actavis Pharma, Inc.), My Way (Gavis Pharmaceuticals), and AfterPill (Syzygy Healthcare Solution LLC) all are one tablet formulations containing 1.5 mg of levonorgestrel.[79] EC is more effective the sooner it is used, but it has been shown to decrease the incidence of pregnancy when taken up to 5 days after unprotected sex. It is available over the counter ($20–$50), mail order (add $5 shipping cost), and by prescription. In the United States, progestin-only EC is available to anyone over the counter.

Ella (Afaxys, Inc.) is another oral EC method that contains 30 mg of ulipristal acetate, a synthetic progesterone.[80] It is available by prescription through an online prescription service ($67 including shipping). Unlike levonorgestrel EC, Ella's efficacy is similar on day 1 and day 5 of use because it inhibits follicular rupture even after mid-cycle rise in luteinizing hormone.[81]

Screening for pregnancy is not required before taking EC.[2] All patients should be offered STI screening and asked to return for a pregnancy test if they have not had menses within 1 week of when their next period was due.[25] Patients should be instructed not to use levonorgestrel EC and Ella within 5 days of each other. EC will not interfere with an established pregnancy or cause teratogenic effects. Women using EC after unprotected intercourse should be counseled on available contraceptive options. Any method of contraception can be started immediately after EC.[25] Women who were the victim of a sexual assault should be offered EC and need information on their legal rights, referral to appropriate health services for evidence collection, and mental health services.

Paragard, a copper T-shaped intrauterine device, is the most efficacious EC method if placed within 5 days after unprotected intercourse in women who desire up to 12 years of hormone-free contraception.[2] The copper IUC prevents pregnancy by impairing sperm function and survival and may also prevent implantation.[78]

CONTRACEPTION AFTER PREGNANCY

Discussion of contraceptive methods with parturient patients should begin during prenatal care. Sterilization may be performed immediately after delivery and is the most common contraceptive method utilized by U.S. couples.[82] All progestin-only methods and the copper IUC can be used by women <21 days postpartum regardless of breastfeeding (all category 1–2).[2,14]

Combined methods should not be used until after 42 days postpartum.[2,14] IUCs can be inserted immediately post delivery in the absence of postpartum sepsis. Please consult *U.S. Medical Eligibility Criteria for Contraceptive Use, 2016* for additional guidance.[14]

CONTRACEPTION AFTER ABORTION

The unwanted pregnancies that lead to induced abortions often occur because women did not receive sufficient information about family planning before becoming pregnant. In a nationwide survey, 46% of women undergoing abortion had not used contraception in the month they conceived. The main reasons cited were the perceived low risk of pregnancy and concerns about contraception.[83] Women undergoing abortion should be counseled that pregnancy can occur again almost immediately. Delaying the initiation of contraception post abortion only increases the probability of a repeat unintended pregnancy. Patients interested in hormonal methods of contraception can initiate any of these methods on the same day or within 7 days of an abortion procedure.[14] If patients say that they will never be sexually active again and refuse contraception, they should nevertheless be provided with information on a variety of contraceptive methods and how to obtain them should circumstances change.

OFFICE AND CLINIC ORGANIZATION

Practices that care for women of childbearing age should maintain supplies of relevant patient education materials (or listings of pertinent websites), such as those listed in the subsequent text, to help women learn more about contraceptive options. As noted earlier, being able to provide contraception during an appointment can help women begin use immediately. If a chosen method cannot be provided at the same visit, consider providing another method as a bridge (e.g., OCPs until they can receive their IUC) and schedule an appointment as soon as possible for patients to receive their desired method of contraception. Adolescents benefit from providers who are aware of their unique developmental needs regarding contraception and health care services and clinicians who are willing to honor their confidentiality. It is also important for patients to understand that they can switch methods as desired and they are not "stuck" with a method if they are unhappy with it.

SUGGESTED RESOURCES AND MATERIALS
Bedsider. http://www.bedsider.org/

American College of Obstetricians and Gynecologists
http://www.acog.org/publications/patient_education/

Association of Reproductive Health Professionals
www.arhp.org

Planned Parenthood
http://www.plannedparenthood.org/learn/birth-control

not-2-late
http://www.not-2-late.com

The Emergency Contraception Website
http://ec.princeton.edu/

Go Ask Alice!
http://goaskalice.columbia.edu/new-qas

Center for Disease Control and Prevention
http://www.cdc.gov/reprodectivehealth/contraception/index.htm

Guttmacher Institute
http://www.guttmacher.org/united-states/contraception

SUGGESTED READINGS

American College of Obstetricians and Gynecologists. *ACOG Committee Opinion #337. Noncontraceptive Uses of the Levonorgestrel Intrauterine System.* Washington, DC: American College of Obstetricians and Gynecologists; June 2006.

American College of Obstetricians and Gynecologists. *ACOG Practice Bulletin #59. Intrauterine Device.* Washington, DC: American College of Obstetricians and Gynecologists; January 2005.

American College of Obstetricians and Gynecologists. *ACOG Practice Bulletin #69. Emergency Contraception.* Washington, DC: American College of Obstetricians and Gynecologists; December 2005.

American College of Obstetricians and Gynecologists. *ACOG Practice Bulletin #73. Use of Hormonal Contraception in Women with Coexisting Medical Conditions.* Washington, DC: American College of Obstetricians and Gynecologists; June 2006.

American College of Obstetricians and Gynecologists. *ACOG Committee Opinion #534, Well-Woman Visit.* Washington, DC: American College of Obstetricians and Gynecologists; August 2012. (Reaffirmed 2016).

Hatcher RA, Trussel J, Nelson AL, et al. *Contraceptive Technology.* 20th rev. ed. New York: Ardent Media Inc.; 2011.

World Health Organization. *Medical Eligibility Criteria for Contraceptive Use.* 3rd ed. 2004.

REFERENCES

1. Guttmacher Institute. *Fact Sheet: Contraceptive Use in the United States.* Guttmacher Institute; 2016. Retrieved from http://www.guttmacher.org/fact-sheet/contraceptive-use-united-states.
2. Curtis KM, Jataoui TC, Tepper NK, et al. U.S. selected practice recommendation for contraceptive use, 2016. *MMWR Recomm Rep.* 2016;65(No. RR-4):1-66.
3. Mosher WD, Jones J, Abma JC. Intended and unintended births in the United States: 1982–2010. *Natl Health Stat Rep.* 2012;55:1-16.
4. Finer LB, Zolna MR. Declines in unintended pregnancy in the United States, 2008–2011. *N Eng J Med.* 2016;374:843-852.
5. Finer LB, Philbin JM. Sexual initiation, contraceptive use, and pregnancy among young adolescents. *Pediatrics.* 2013;131:886-891.

6. Hamilton BE, Martin JA, Osterman MJK, et al. *Births: Provisional Data for 2016. Vital Statistics Rapid Release; No 2.* Hyattsville, MD: National Center for Health Statistics; June 2017. Available at https://www.cdc.gov/nchs/data/vsrr/report002.pdf.

7. Gipson JD, Koenig MA, Hindin MJ. The effects of unintended pregnancy on infant, child, and parental health: a review of the literature. *Stud Fam Plan.* 2008;39(1):18-38. doi:10.1111/j.1728-4465.2008.00148.x.

8. Moos MK, Bartholomew NE, Lohr KN. Counseling in a clinical setting to prevent unintended pregnancy: an evidence-based research agenda. *Contraception.* 2003;67:115-132.

9. World Health Organization. *Trends in Maternal Mortality: 1990 to 2015: Estimates by WHO, UNICEF, UNFPA, World Bank Group and the United Nations Population Division.* Geneva: World Health Organization; 2015.

10. U.S. Agency for International Development. *Healthy Timing and Spacing of Pregnancies: A Family Planning Investment Strategy for Accelerating the Pace of Improvements in Child Survival.* Washington, DC: U.S. Agency for International Development Bureau of Global Health, Office of Population and Reproductive Health; 2012.

11. Sedgh G, Ashford LS, Hussain R. *Unmet Need for Contraception in Developing Countries: Examining Women's Reasons for not Using a Method.* Guttmacher Institute; 2016. http://www.guttmacher.org/report/ unmet-need-for-contraception-in- developing-countries.

12. Armstrong C. ACOG guidelines on noncontraceptive uses of hormonal contraceptives. *Am Fam Physician.* 2010;82(3):294-295.

13. Deutsch MB. *Guidelines for the Primary and Gender-Affirming Care of Transgender and Gender Nonbinary People.* San Francisco, CA: Center of Excellence for Transgender Health; 2016:1-199.

14. CDC. U.S. Medical eligibility criteria for contraceptive use, 2016. *MMWR Recomm Rep.* 2016;65(No RR-3);1-106.

15. Santelli L, Dubersten L, Linberg D. Explaining recent declines in adolescent pregnancy in the United States: the contribution of abstinence and improved contraceptive use. *Am J Public Health.* 2007;97(1):150-156.

16. Sedgh G, Finer LB, Bankole A. Adolescent pregnancy, birth, and abortion rates across countries: levels and recent trends. *J Adolesc Health.* 2015;56(2):223-230.

17. American Academy of Pediatrics. Policy statement: contraception for adolescents. *Pediatrics.* 2014;134(4):e1244-1256.

18. American Academy of Pediatrics. *Bright Futures: Guidelines for Health Supervision of Infants, Children, and Adolescents.* 3rd ed. Elks Grove Village, IL: American Academy of Pediatrics; 2008.

19. American College of Obstetricians and Gynecologists. ACOG Committee Opinion #710. *Counseling Adolescents About Contraception.* Washington, DC: American College of Obstetricians and Gynecologists; August 2017.

20. Hartman LB, Monasterion E, Hwang LY. Adolescent contraception: review and guidance for pediatric clinicians. *Curr Probl Pediatr Adolesc Health Care.* 2012;42:221-263.

21. Moriarty Daley A, Sadler LS, Reynolds H. Tailoring clinical services to address the unique needs of adolescents from pregnancy test to parenthood. *Curr Probl Pediatr Adolesc Health Care.* 2013;43:71-95. doi:10.1016/j. cppeds.2013.01.001.

22. Moyer VA, U.S. Preventive Services Task Force. Screening for cervical cancer: U.S. Preventive Services Task Force recommendation statement. *Ann Intern Med.* 2012;156:880-891. Available at http://annals.org/article.aspx?articleid=1183214(annals.org). Accessed 21 November 2012.

23. Centers for Disease Control and Prevention. Sexually transmitted diseases treatment guidelines 2015. *MMWR.* 2015;64(3):1-137.

24. American College of Obstetricians and Gynecologists. ACOG Committee Opinion #534, *Well-Woman Visit.* Washington, DC: American College of Obstetricians and Gynecologists; August 2012. (Reaffirmed 2016).

25. CDC. U.S. selected practice recommendations for contraceptive use. Adapted from the World Health Organization selected practice recommendations for contraceptive use, 2nd edition. *MMWR Recomm Rep.* 2013;62(No. RR-2).

26. Trussell J, Koenig J, Stewart F, et al. Medical care cost savings for adolescent contraceptive use. *Fam Plann Perspect.* 1997;29:248-255, 295.

27. Depo-Provera Intramuscular Package. https://www.accessdata.fda.gov/drug-satfda_doc/label/2003/20246scs019_Depo-provera_lbl.pdf.

28. Depo-Provera Subcutaneous Package. https://www.accessdata.fda.gov/drug-satfda_doc/label/2017/021583s023_lbl.pdf.

29. Trussell J. Contraceptive failure in the United States. *Contraception.* 2011; 83(5):397404.

30. Westhoff C, Truman C, Kalmuss D, et al. Depressive symptoms and depo-provera. *Contraception.* 1998;57:237-240.

31. Westhoff C. Depot medroxyprogesterone acetate contraception: metabolic parameters and mood changes. *J Reprod Med.* 1996;41:401-406.

32. Pelkman C. Hormones and weight change. *J Reprod Med.* 2002;47:791-794.

33. Pelkman C, Chow M, Heinbach R, et al. Short-term effects of a progestational contraceptive drug on food intake, resting energy expenditure, and body weight in young women. *Am J Clin Nutr.* 2001;73:19-26.

34. Bonny AE, Ziegler J, Debanne SM, et al. Weight gain in obese and nonobese adolescent girls initiating depot medroxyprogesterone, oral contraceptive pills or no hormonal method. *Arch Pediatr Adolesc Med.* 2006;160(1):40-45.

35. Lopez LM, Ramesh S, Chen M, et al. Progestin-only contraceptives: effects on weight. *Cochrane Database Syst Rev.* 2018;(8):CD008815.

36. Scholes D, LaCroix AZ, Ichikawa LE, et al. Injectable hormone contraception and bone density: results from a prospective study. *Epidemiology.* 2002;13(5):581-587. Erratum in: *Epidemiology.* 2002;13(6):749.

37. American College of Obstetricians and Gynecologists. ACOG Committee Opinion #602. *Depot Medroxyprogesterone Acetate and Bone Effects.* Washington, DC: American College of Obstetricians and Gynecologists; June 2014.

38. Paragard. http://www.paragard.com/pdf/PARAGARD-PI.pdf.

39. Grimes D. Intrauterine devices (IUDs). In: Hatcher R, Trussell J, Nelson A, Cates W, Stewart F, Kowel D, eds. *Contraceptive Technology.* 19th ed. New York: Ardent Media; 2008.

40. Trussell J, Koenig J, Ellertson C, et al. Preventing unintended pregnancy: the cost-effectiveness of three methods of emergency contraception. *Am J Public Health.* 1997;87:932-937.

41. Mirena Package. http://labeling.bayerhealthcare.com/html/products/pi/Mirena_PI.pdf.

42. Kyleena Package. http://labeling.bayerhealthcare.com/html/products/pi/Kylena_PI/pdf.

43. Skyla Package. http://labeling.bayerhealthcare.com/html/products/pi/Skyla_PI/pdf.

44. Liletta Package. https;//www.allergan.com/assets/pdf/lilettashi_pi.

45. Liletta Package-2 Handed. https;//www.allergan.com/assets/pdf/liletta_pi.

46. American College of Obstetricians and Gynecologists. ACOG Committee Opinion #110. *Noncontraceptive Uses of the Levonorgestrel Intrauterine System.* Washington, DC: American College of Obstetricians and Gynecologists; January 2010.

47. American College of Obstetricians and Gynecologists. ACOG Committee Opinion #672. *Clinical Challenges of Long-Acting Reversible Contraceptive Methods.* Washington, DC: American College of Obstetricians and Gynecologists; September 2016.

48. Nexplanon Package. http://www.merck.com/product/usa/pi_circulars/n/nexplanon/nexplanon_pi.pdf.

49. Mansour D, Korver T, Marintcheva-Petrova M, et al. The effects on Impnaon on menstrual bleeding patterns. *Eur J Contracept Reprod Health Care.* 2008;13(suppl 13):13-28.

50. Beerthuizen R, van Beek A, Massai R, et al. Bone mineral density during long-term use of the progestagen contraceptive implant Implanon compared to a non-hormonal method of contraception. *Hum Reprod.* 2000;15:118-122.

51. Nelson AL, Cwiak C. Combined oral contraceptives (COCs). In: Hatcher RA, Trussel J, Nelson AL, et al, eds. *Contraceptive Technology.* 20th rev. ed. New York: Ardent Media Inc.; 2011:249-341.

52. Seasonale Package. https://www.accessdata.fda.gov/drugsatfda_docs/label/2017/021544s013lbl.pdf.

53. Seasonique Package. https://www.accessdata.fda.gov/drugsatfda_docs/label/2017/021840s011lbl.pdf.

54. Loseasonique Package. https://www.accessdata.fda.gov/drugsatfda_docs/label/2017/022262s002lbl.pdf.

55. Anderson FD, Hait H. A multicenter, randomized study of an extended cycle oral contraceptive. *Contraception.* 2003;68:89-96. Erratum in: *Bontraception.* 2004;69:175.

56. Anderson F, Hait H. Seasonale-301 Study Group. A multicenter, randomized study of an extended cycle oral contraceptive. *Contraception.* 2003;68:89-96.

57. World Health Organization. *Selected Practice Recommendations for Contraceptive Use.* 3rd ed. Geneva, Switzerland; 2016:1-66. Retrieved from http://apps.who.int/iris/bitstream/handle/10665/252267/9789241565400-eng.pdf; jsessionid=FC2D6F78C40A7A61F0F24DCEF5937E84?sequence=1.

58. Westhoff C, Kerns J, Morroni C, et al. Quick start: novel oral contraceptive initiation method. *Contraception.* 2002;66:141-145.

59. Brahni D, Curtis KM. When can women start combined hormonal contraceptives (CHCs)? A systematic review. *Contraception.* 2013;87:524-538.

60. Lopez LM, Newmann SJ, Grimes DA. Immediate start of hormonal contraceptives for contraception. *Conchrane Database Syst Rev.* 2012;12:CD0062.

61. Gallo MF, Lopez LM, Grimes DA, et al. Combination contraceptives. *Cochrane Database Syst Rev.* 2006;(1):CD003987.

62. van Hylckama VA, Helmerhorst FM, Vanderenbrouke JP, et al. The venous thrombotic risk of oral contraceptives, effects of oestrogen dose and progestogen type: results of the MEGA case-control study. *BMJ.* 2009;339:b2921.

63. Micronor Package. https://www.accessdata.fda.gov/drugsatfda_docs/label/2008/016954s101lbl.pdf.

64. Belsey EM. The association between vaginal bleeding patterns and reasons for discontinuation of contraceptive use. *Contraception.* 1998;38:207-225.

65. Xulane Package. https://dailymed.nlm.nih.gov/dailymed/fda/fdaDrugXsl.cfm?setid=f7848550-086a-43d8-8ae5-047f4b9e4382&type=display.

66. Nuvaring Package. http://merck.com/product/usa/pi_circulars/n/nuvaring/nuvaring_pi.pdf.

67. Miller L, Verhoeven CHJ. Results of a randomized, multicenter trial comparing extended contraceptive ring regimens. *Obstet Gynecol.* 2005;105:6S.

68. Ott MA, Sucato GA, Committee on adolescence. Contraception for adolescents. *Pediatrics.* 2014;134;e1257-1281.

69. van den Heuvel M, van Brigt A, Alnabawy A, et al. Comparison of ethinyl estradiol pharmacokinetics in three hormonal contraceptive formulations: the vaginal ring, the transdermal patch and an oral contraceptive. *Contraception.* 2005;72:168-174.

70. Gallo MF, Grimes DA, Lopez LM, et al. Non-latex versus latex condoms for contraception. *Cochrane Database Syst Rev.* 2006;(1).

71. Winer RL, Hughes JP, Feng Q, et al. Condom use and the risk of genital human papillomavirus infection in young women. *N Engl J Med.* 2006;354:2645-2654.

72. The Female Health Company. FC and FC2 Female Condom Website. http://www.femalehealth.com/theproduct.html.

73. Planned Parenthood. Nonoxynol-9: Benefits and Risks. http://www.planned-parenthood.org/news-articles-press/politics-policy-issues/birth-control-access-prevention/nonoxyonol-9-6546.htm.

74. Today Sponge. http://todaysponge.com/about.html.

75. McClure DA, Edelman DA. Worldwide method effectiveness of the today vaginal contraceptive sponge. *Adv Contracept.* 1985;1:305-311.

76. Cates W, Harwood B. Vaginal barriers and spermicides. In Hatcher RA, Trussel J, Nelson AL, et al, eds. *Contraceptive Technology.* 20th rev. ed. New York: Ardent Media Inc; 2011:391-408.

77. Jennings VH, Burke AE. Fertility awareness-based methods. In Hatcher RA, Trussel J, Nelson AL, et al, eds. *Contraceptive Technology.* 20th rev. ed. New York: Ardent Media Inc.; 2011:417-434.

78. Cleland K, Zhu H, Goldstuck N, Cheng L, Trussell J. (2012). The efficacy of intra-uterine devices for emergency contraception: a systematic review of 35 years of experience. *Hum Reprod.* 2012;27(7):1994-2000.

79. BPlan. One-Step Package. http://accessdata.fda.gov/drugsatfda_docs/label/2019/021998lbl.pdf.

80. Ella Package. http://accessdata.fda.gov/drugsatfda_docs/label/2015/022474s007lbl.pdf.

81. Trussell J, Schwarz EB. Emergency contraception. In: Hatcher RA, Trussel J, Nelson AL, et al, eds. *Contraceptive Technology.* 20th rev. ed. New York: Ardent Media Inc; 2011:121-136.

82. Bartz D, Greenberg JA. Sterilization in the United States. *Rev Obstet Gynecol.* 2008;1(1):23-32.

83. Jones RK, Darroch JE, Henshaw SK. Contraceptive use among US women having abortions in 2000–2001. *Perspect Sex Reprod Health.* 2002;34(6):294-303.

Please see Online Appendix: Apps and Digital Resources for additional information.

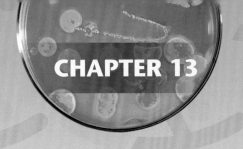

CHAPTER 13

Sexually Transmitted Infections

ALISON MORIARTY DALEY

BACKGROUND

More than two decades ago the Institute of Medicine (1997) described sexually transmitted infections (STIs) as the "hidden epidemic."[1] STIs remain a public health problem. Beyond the spectrum of clinically evident STIs that are encountered frequently in practice, the much larger burden of asymptomatic infection highlights the magnitude of the problem confronting both clinicians and health policy planners. The clinical outcomes of such infections include not only short-term symptomatic states but also pelvic inflammatory disease (PID), epididymitis, and proctitis. STIs also act as cofactors that increase the risk of human immunodeficiency virus (HIV) transmission.[2] They are a major cause of chronic pelvic pain, infertility, and adverse outcomes of pregnancy, such as ectopic pregnancy, low birthweight and fetal loss, prematurity, and vertically transmitted neonatal infections.[2] As noted in Chapter 4, persistent human papillomavirus (HPV) infection can cause cervical, genital, anal, and head and neck cancers.[3] Congenital Zika virus (ZIKV) infection can cause microcephaly and other congenital malformations.[4]

The prevention of STIs and their long-term consequences remains an important clinical and public health goal. According to Centers for Disease Control and Prevention (CDC) guidelines,[2] STI prevention and control are based on five key principles:

- accurate risk assessment and education and counseling of persons on ways to avoid sexually transmitted diseases (STDs), through changes in behavior and use of recommended prevention services;
- pre-exposure vaccination of persons at risk for vaccine-preventable STDs;
- identification of asymptomatically infected persons and persons with symptoms associated with STDs;
- effective diagnosis, treatment, counseling, and follow-up of infected persons; and
- evaluation, treatment, and counseling of sex partners of persons who are infected with an STD.

A number of factors must work in conjunction to achieve the best prevention outcomes based on these principles:

1. Clinicians should remain aware of current screening, diagnostic, and treatment protocols that most effectively prevent and identify STIs, and they should find practice opportunities for implementing them.
2. Clinical practice and counseling should respect individual needs as well as evolving societal norms for sexual and health behaviors.
3. Health systems should facilitate counseling, diagnosis, and treatment through appropriate office systems, health insurance coverage, and community resources.

The goals of this chapter are to describe effective strategies for clinicians to foster STI prevention and to review briefly current recommendations for STI screening, diagnosis, treatment, and reporting with a focus on prevention strategies. The emphasis is on STIs, resources, and clinical practice in the United States. The spectrum and severity of disease burden, as well as the range of available and effective management options, differ widely in other countries where STIs remain an overwhelming public health problem. Sexual practices to prevent unwanted pregnancy are discussed in Chapter 12.

Epidemiology

Chlamydia trachomatis infection is the most prevalent of all reportable STIs.[5] Approximately 70% of chlamydia infections are asymptomatic. In 2016, a total of 1,598,354 chlamydia cases were reported to the CDC in the United States.[5] This corresponds to a rate of 497.3 cases per 100,000 population, a 4.7% increase since 2015.[5] Rates increased among individuals in all regions of the United States.[5] The highest rates are among adolescent and young adult women (15–24 yr old).[5] The continued increase in the case rate reflects increased screening, the use of more sensitive diagnostic tests, and improved efforts to ensure case reporting, as well as a real increase in incidence.[2,5]

Neisseria gonorrhoeae is the second most commonly reported notifiable disease in the United States.[5] In 2016, there were 468,514 cases reported for a rate of 145.8 cases per 100,000.[5] This represents an increase of 18.5% from 2015.[5] This infection is more common among 15- to 24-year-old females and 20- to 29-year-old males.[5] Gonococcal antibiotic resistance to cephalosporin continues to be a public health concern.[2,5]

Untreated chlamydia and gonorrhea infections can result in PID and subsequently ectopic pregnancy, infertility, or chronic pelvic pain in women.[2] If not adequately treated, approximately 15% of women with chlamydia will develop PID; estimates of PID from untreated gonorrhea are even higher.[5–8] A perihepatitis (Fitz-Hugh-Curtis syndrome) can result from untreated PID.[9] Epididymitis can result from untreated gonorrhea or chlamydia infections in men.[2] Untreated gonorrhea infections can also cause a disseminated infection.[2]

The incidence of primary and secondary syphilis (caused by *Treponema pallidum*) has increased steadily since 2001, from a rate of 2.1 to 8.7 cases per 100,000.[5] Rates are highest among individuals 20 to 29 years old; however they increased in all age groups greater than 15 years old. The majority (90%) of cases of primary and secondary syphilis occurred in men particularly among men with male sexual partners (MSM).[2,5]

An estimated 1.1 million people in the United States are living with HIV; 15% are unaware they have HIV.[10] In 2015, 38,500 new infections were reported; the majority of these, 70%, were among MSM.[10] About 50% to 90% of individuals will experience acute retroviral syndrome (acute HIV infection) within the weeks following exposure to the virus.[2] Symptoms of acute HIV are similar to other viral illnesses and include fever, malaise, skin rash, and lymphadenopathy.[2] People are highly contagious during this time. Following the acute infection, a chronic infection follows that attacks CD4 cells and effects the individual's immune response to infection. If the condition is untreated, autoimmune deficiency syndrome can develop.[2] HIV is spread through unprotected sexual activity with an infected partner through exposure to blood, semen, and vaginal secretions.

HPV is the most common viral STI. Forty types of this virus are known to infect the genital tract. Most sexually active individuals in the United States are infected with at least one virus type.[5] Although the majority of those infected will clear the infection, some infected with high-risk HPV types will have a persistent infection resulting in precancer or cancer. Types 16 and 18 are responsible for the majority of cervical, vulvovaginal, anal, and head and neck cancers. Low-risk types, 6 and 11, can result in external or internal genital warts.[2,3,5] Vaccination is available to protect against 9 HPV types and is recommended for male and female adolescents at age 11 to 12 years[3] (refer to Table 13.1).

Herpes Simplex Virus (HSV) is also a very common STI and is often asymptomatic.[2,5] Genital infections caused by HSV type 2 are characterized by painful genital or anal vesicles that are recurrent. HSV type 1 is more commonly orolabial; however, it can cause anogenital infection.

Trichomoniasis is a protozoal STI and the most common nonviral STI.[11] The prevalence of trichomoniasis in a recent study was 0.5% among men and 1.8% among women 18 to 59 years old.[12] Most people are asymptomatic. This infection can cause vaginitis, PID, urethritis, epididymitis, and preterm birth. Trichomoniasis has also been linked to an increased risk of HIV acquisition and transmission.[13]

Hepatitis A virus (HAV) is a viral infection transmitted by the fecal-oral route from person to person through sex or more commonly contaminated water.[2] The incubation period from exposure to clinical symptoms is 5 to 50 days; however, the virus is shed through feces 2 to 3 weeks before and 1 week after the onset of symptoms.[5] Clinical symptoms include nausea, anorexia, fever, malaise, dark-colored urine, clay-colored stool, or

TABLE 13.1 Recommendations for Safer Sexual Practices to Reduce Transmission of Sexually Transmitted Infection/Human Immunodeficiency Virus (STI/HIV)

Measure	Information to Share With Patients
Pre-exposure vaccination	• HPV-9 vaccination is recommended for male and female adolescents aged 11–12 yr; catch-up vaccination for 13–26-yr-old females and 13–21-yr-old males is recommended. HPV vaccine recommended through age 26 yr for MSM and males with HIV. HPV-9 can be given as early as age 9 yr[3,23] • Hepatitis A and B vaccines are recommended for all uninfected and previously unvaccinated persons seeking STI testing. These vaccines are also recommended for previously unvaccinated and uninfected injection-drug users, MSM, and persons with chronic liver disease or HIV infection[14,15]
Abstinence and reduction of the number of partners	• Counsel patients that abstinence from all types of sexual activity or being in a long-term mutually monogamous relationship with an uninfected partner is the most reliable way to avoid transmission of STIs • Counsel patients to abstain from sexual activity until both (all) partners have completed STI treatment
Pre-exposure prophylaxis for HIV (PreP)	• Daily oral antiretroviral with Truvada (emtricitabine and tenofovir disproxil fumarate) reduces the rate of HIV acquisition among those at risk for HIV
Male condoms	• When used consistently and correctly, male latex condoms are highly effective at reducing the transmission of HIV and other STIs, including the Zika virus • Polyurethane condoms provide similar protection against STIs and unintended pregnancy as do latex condoms and can be used for patients with latex allergy • Natural membrane or "natural" condoms prevent passage of sperm, but they have pores that allow transmission of HIV and HBV and are not recommended for STI prevention
Female condoms	• When male condoms cannot be used properly, patients should be counseled to consider using female condoms (see page 288), which can substantially reduce the risk for STIs, including Zika virus • Male and female condoms should not be used together
Diaphragms and nonbarrier hormonal contraception	• Diaphragms do not provide adequate protection against STIs or HIV • Women using hormonal contraception should be advised to use condoms to prevent STDs and HIV
Male circumcision	• Reduces risk of HIV, HSV, and high-risk HPV infection

(Continued)

TABLE 13.1   Recommendations for Safer Sexual Practices to Reduce Transmission of Sexually Transmitted Infection/Human Immunodeficiency Virus (STI/HIV)   (Continued)

Measure	Information to Share With Patients
Retesting after treatment for repeat infection(s)	• Rescreen for gonorrhea and chlamydia 3 mo after treatment • Rescreen females for trichomonas 3 mo after treatment • Follow-up serologic testing for syphilis per recommendations
Expedited partner therapy	• Treatment of sexual partner(s) diagnosed with gonorrhea or chlamydia. Medications are provided to the patient for their partner(s) from the previous 60 d or more recent sex partner if last sex was >60 d
Mosquito bite prevention[18]	• Use insect repellent per package instructions containing DEET, Picaridin (KBR 3023 or icaridin), IR3535, Oil of Eucalyptus (OLE) or para-methane-diol (PMD) or 2-umdecanone • Permethrin Spray to clothing and gear • Bed nets, screens on doors/windows, long sleeves/pants, remove standing water from yard • Avoid travel to affected areas if pregnant or planning pregnancy

Adapted from Centers for Disease Control and Prevention. Sexually transmitted diseases treatment guidelines 2015. *MMWR*. 2015;64(3):4-9.

HBV, hepatitis B virus; HPV, human papillomavirus; HSV, herpes simplex virus; MSM, men having sex with men.

abdominal pain and either jaundice or elevated serum aminotransferase levels.[14] The incidence of hepatitis A has decreased since HAV vaccine became available in 1996. In 2010, the reported incidence of HAV infection was 0.5 cases/100,000.[14] Vaccination is available and recommended for all children at age 12 to 24 months (and those >2 yr old who desire vaccination). HAV can be sexually transmitted, and therefore vaccination is recommended also for MSM. Postexposure prophylaxis, for previously unimmunized individuals, is recommended as soon as possible, but within 2 weeks, following exposure to the virus.[5,14]

Hepatitis B virus (HBV), also a viral liver infection, is transmitted through sexual contact via percutaneous exposure to hepatitis B–infected blood or body fluids.[2,5,15] Risk factors for exposure to this virus include unprotected sex with an infected partner, history of other STDs, MSM, multiple sexual partners, and injection-drug use.[2,5] The incubation period from exposure to clinical symptoms is 6 weeks to 6 months. Affected individuals may have a short, mild illness or develop chronic infection.[2,15] Signs and symptoms, if present, include fever, fatigue, nausea/vomiting, abdominal pain, loss of appetite, joint pain, jaundice, clay-colored stools, and dark urine.[15] Approximately 1% of individuals with HBV will develop acute liver failure.[2] The incidence of new HBV infections decreased from 1990 to 2014; however, since 2014 there has been an increase in HBV infection owing to increased injection-drug use.[15] Vaccinations are available for the prevention for HBV and are recommended at birth, for previously unvaccinated children/adolescents through age 18 years, and for unvaccinated adults with risk for infection[2,15] (refer to Table 13.1).

ZIKV can be contracted through the bite of infected *Aedes* mosquitos or through unprotected sexual activity (vaginal, oral, anal sex and sharing of sex toys) with an infected partner or transmitted from mother to fetus prenatally.[4] ZIKV is a flavivirus and has been associated with microcephaly in infants exposed prenatally and Guillain-Barré syndrome in adults.[16] The ZIKV has been identified in mosquitos in Africa, Asia, the Caribbean, Central America, North America (Mexico, Puerto Rico, Cuba, Dominican Republic), the Pacific Islands, and South America (updates are available through the CDC website (http://www.cdc.gov/zika).

Most people infected with ZIKV are asymptomatic.[4,16] Others may experience a mild illness with symptoms that include fever, headache, rash, conjunctivitis, malaise, and joint and muscle pain for 2 to 7 days.[16] Time from exposure to clinical symptoms is estimated to be 3 to 14 days following exposure; however, prolonged shedding can occur for 8 weeks in vaginal fluids and 6 months in semen.[17] The World Health Organization and the CDC recommend consistent condom use (male or female) and dental dams for men and women for the 3 months following a potential exposure to ZIKV and for pregnant women, abstinence or consistent condom use throughout her entire pregnancy if her partner has traveled to an area of potential exposure to the virus.[4,18] There is currently no vaccine available to prevent ZIKV infection. Women who are pregnant or are planning on becoming pregnant are advised to avoid travel to endemic areas.[4,18] Those who either live in endemic areas or must travel are encouraged to use preventive measures that include insect repellent, permethrin spray to clothing and gear, wearing long sleeves and pants, using bed nets, using screens on doors and windows, and removing standing water sources from the yard.[18] If a woman is infected with ZIKV during pregnancy, her infant may develop congenital Zika syndrome.[4] Clinical features associated with this syndrome include microcephaly, seizures, irritability, craniofacial disproportion and cutis gyrata, hypertonicity and hyperreflexia, abnormal neuroradiology findings, dysphagia/feeding difficulties, ocular abnormalities, sensorineural hearing loss, and arthrogryposis.[4,16] Laboratory testing is available; however, results in pregnant women should be interpreted within the context of the timing of infection during pregnancy, clinical findings, and serological results.[4] Up-to-date guidance is available through the CDC.[18]

The rates of STIs, especially antibiotic-resistant gonorrhea and primary and secondary syphilis, are higher among MSM than the rates found in women or men.[2,5] Young age (younger than 25 yr) is an important risk factor for the acquisition of an STI[2] (see Chapter 5). Other demographic characteristics such as race and ethnicity, marital status, living in an urban location, and low income have been less consistently associated with infection.[2] Therefore, STI prevention and screening guidelines are aimed at reaching those individuals with risk factors for infection. STIs can also be transmitted following a sexual assault. The CDC provides clinicians with clinical guidance on testing and prophylactic treatment for victims of assault.[2]

STRATEGIES FOR THE PREVENTION OF SEXUALLY TRANSMITTED INFECTIONS

Education and Counseling

As discussed in Chapter 6, counseling for any behavioral change is challenging. Counseling people at risk for STIs to change their sexual behaviors is a special challenge for clinicians, who strive to communicate effectively with their patients. For many clinicians and patients, sexual activity is an especially difficult matter to discuss. Counseling to change sexual behaviors must be conducted with an extra measure of sensitivity, in a way that respects individuals' health needs, privacy, and motivation to prevent illness.

A number of techniques can be used to approach the general sexual history, as described elsewhere.[2,19] Assuring confidentiality is an important aspect of STI assessment. The key features include the following:

1. Approach the sexual history in a matter-of-fact yet sensitive manner.
2. Ask the patient's permission to discuss sexual behavior and health issues.
3. Acknowledge and provide support for positive steps already made; previous risk reduction attempts, whether successful or not, or even efforts to get tested for STIs or HIV, should be recognized.
4. Avoid assumptions about the patient's sexual orientation or activity—initially use the term *partner* rather than *boyfriend, girlfriend, husband, or wife.*
5. Communicate clearly and teach patients the correct terminology regarding sexual behaviors. Use appropriate language and terminology: avoid compromising professionalism by using slang terms.
6. Avoid moral or religious judgment of patients' behaviors. Provide information that is directed at emotional and psychological as well as physical health.
7. Correct misinformation and dispel myths, but provide factual information in limited amounts so that patients can ask for further details if desired. Clarify specific misconceptions rather than correcting "common" or general misinformation; focus on patients' personal risk factors and clarify misinformation about their own behaviors.

8. Keep the discussion focused on personal STI/HIV risk reduction.
   - Avoid emphasizing delivery of predetermined didactic information.
   - Use open-ended questions that keep the patient focused on personal STI/HIV risks.
   - Discuss specific STI/HIV risks and risk reduction in depth.
9. Negotiate a concrete, achievable behavioral change step that will reduce STI or HIV risk.
   - Small behavioral changes are significant, and counseling should emphasize realistic, specific, achievable steps, at the outset possibly targeted to just one of many high-risk behaviors (see Chapter 5).
   - Behavioral change steps should be acceptable to patients and relevant to their specific behaviors.
   - Identifying and resolving barriers to achieving this goal, possibly through role playing or discussion, can increase the likelihood of success.
   - Writing down the goal, for the patient and/or in the chart, may be helpful for later reinforcement.
   - Be flexible in the prevention approach and counseling process.
10. Provide skill-building opportunities.

The CDC (2016) recommends using an STD/HIV risk assessment focused on five areas: Partners, Practices, Prevention of Pregnancy, Protection from STDs, and Past History of STDs. Box 13.1 provides the clinician with questions related to each of these areas. Following the history, the clinician should offer STI screening and encourage risk reduction through prevention counseling. This counseling is most effective when it is patient centered and is presented in a sensitive, nonjudgmental manner. The counseling should be tailored to best address the specific needs of the person, with special attention to the individual's age, developmental level, beliefs, culture, language, gender identity, and sexual orientation.[2]

COUNSELING FOR SAFER SEXUAL PRACTICES

The CDC STD Treatment Guidelines (2016) provide specific information regarding the efficacy of various "safer" sexual practices. They include detailed instructions for male condom use that can be shared with patients. Table 13.1 summarizes these recommendations. Although these counseling guidelines apply to all patient populations, some specific recommendations for STI risk reduction counseling pertain to particular patient groups or situations.

Counseling Adolescents

Adolescent present with specific risk factors, barriers to effective treatment, and other issues that affect effective STI prevention.[2,19] In 2015, 41.2% of high school adolescents reported ever having sex.[20] The percentage of

---

Box 13.1   The 5 P's: Partners, Practices, Prevention of Pregnancy, Protection from STDs, and Past History of STDs.

1. Partners
   - "Do you have sex with men, women, or both?"
   - "In the past 2 months, how many partners have you had sex with?"
   - "In the past 12 months, how many partners have you had sex with?"
   - "Is it possible that any of your sex partners in the past 12 months had sex with someone else while they were still in a sexual relationship with you?"
2. Practices
   - "To understand your risks for STDs, I need to understand the kind of sex you have had recently."
   - "Have you had vaginal sex, meaning 'penis in vagina sex'?" If yes, "Do you use condoms: never, sometimes, or always?"
   - "Have you had anal sex, meaning 'penis in rectum/anus sex'?" If yes, "Do you use condoms: never, sometimes, or always?"
   - "Have you had oral sex, meaning 'mouth on penis/vagina'?"
   - For condom answers:
   - If "never": "Why don't you use condoms?"
   - If "sometimes": "In what situations (or with whom) do you use condoms?"
3. Prevention of pregnancy
   - "What are you doing to prevent pregnancy?"
4. Protection from STDs
   - "What do you do to protect yourself from STDs and HIV?"
5. Past history of STDs
   - "Have you ever had an STD?"
   - "Have any of your partners had an STD?"

Additional questions to identify HIV and viral hepatitis risk include:
   - "Have you or any of your partners ever injected drugs?"
   - "Have your or any of your partners exchanged money or drugs for sex?"
   - "Is there anything else about your sexual practices that I need to know about?"

From Centers for Disease Control and Prevention. Sexually transmitted diseases treatment guidelines 2015. *MMWR.* 2015;64(3):3. https://www.cdc.gov/std/tg2015/tg-2015-print.pdf.
STD, sexually transmitted disease.

---

sexually active teens increases throughout high school, with 24.1% 9th graders and 58.1% of 12th graders reporting ever having sexual intercourse.[20] Few report first sex before age 13 years (3.9%) or four or more sexual partners (11.5%).[20] Among currently sexually active high school students (30.1%), 56.9% (52% females, 61.5% males) report use of a condom before last sexual intercourse.[20] Rates of condom use decreased throughout high school, from 60.5% among 9th graders to 52.9% among sexually active 12th graders.[20] See Chapter 3 for suggestions on how to approach the discussion of sexual practices with teenage patients. Lack of correct and consistent condom use, older sexual partners, use of alcohol and/or drugs at the time of sex, barriers to health care services for education and screening for STIs, and confidentiality concerns are additional factors that place adolescents at risk for STI acquisition and delayed testing and treatment.[2,21]

Despite statutes in all states allowing minors to receive STI testing and treatment without parental consent, concerns about confidentiality and fears of parental discovery limit the willingness of many adolescents to seek effective health care for STIs.[2,21,22] Although discussions with adolescent patients can emphasize the parameters for confidentiality, it is also important that clinicians encourage and possibly facilitate open communication of sexual health matters between minors and their parents. This is especially important if insurance billing for these services may come to parental attention despite the best efforts of the clinician to prevent disclosure. Out-of-pocket expenditures for office visits, testing, and treatment may be prohibitive for adolescents. Clinicians should be flexible about providing effective and affordable care while maintaining adolescents' confidentiality. Referral to a publicly funded clinic may be appropriate in some cases.

Many teens report that sex was not planned rather it "just happened." Clinicians should encourage abstinence and safer sex.[2] Other potential barriers that are more pronounced among adolescents include lack of awareness of what constitutes abnormal physical symptoms of STIs, fears of physical examination or embarrassment about pelvic examination, concerns about the discovery of sexual activity or sexual abuse by others, or reluctance to confront the reality of an STI that may raise questions about the fidelity or stability of their relationship with their partner.[21] Patient education regarding abstinence, safer sexual practices, and health beliefs and behaviors is especially important for adolescent patients. These topics are difficult for many clinicians to discuss with teenagers. Such discussions are also limited by the misconception of clinicians that their patients are not sexually active or that the prevalence of STIs is low in their patient population.

It is important to help teens to identify factors that would place the patient at risk for unsafe sexual activity and subsequent STIs. These factors include lack of consistent condom use, alcohol or substance use, social settings that would create pressure for unwanted sexual activity, or a new partner who might apply pressure to become sexually active. Reminders about the benefits of abstinence may be helpful, especially for adolescents who are ambivalent about whether to become sexually active. Secondary prevention in patients who already have STIs should emphasize behaviors that can be modified to reduce the risk of STIs.

Screening for Sexually Transmitted Infections

Screening patients for early detection of asymptomatic STIs remains one of the most important measures to reduce disease transmission, prevent the development of symptoms or complications in the individual patient, and reduce the overall prevalence of common STIs. See Chapter 5 and Appendix A to this book for details on screening guidelines issued by clinical and professional organizations for various patient groups. Clinicians should be aware of local STI rates, which are available from the local or state public health department. Current screening recommendations are provided in Table 13.2.

Identification of asymptomatic HPV infection in women through routine Pap testing may help prevent HPV-related illness, including genital cancers, but such screening is not universally recommended.[2,24] CDC

TABLE 13.2 STI Screening Recommendations	
Patient Population	**Screening**
Sexually active adolescents	• Annual chlamydia and gonorrhea screening females <25 yr • Consider chlamydia and gonorrhea screening for males in settings with high prevalence of infection • Offer chlamydia and gonorrhea screening to young MSM • HIV screening for all adolescents, repeat based on risk • Screening for asymptomatic adolescents for syphilis, trichomoniasis, HSV, HBV, HAV, and HPV not generally recommended • Screen young MSM and pregnant adolescents for syphilis • Cervical cancer screening beginning at age 21 yr[24]
Pregnant women	• Chlamydia screening for women <25 yr old and older women with risk factors at first prenatal visit • Retest for cure 3–4 wk after diagnosis • Retest in 3 mo after treatment • Gonorrhea screening for women <25 yr old and older women with risk factors at first prenatal visit • Retest in 3 mo after treatment if positive • Retest in third trimester if high risk • Screen for HIV and syphilis at first prenatal visit regardless of previous testing • Retest for HIV at 36 wk gestation for those considered high risk • Retest for syphilis around 28 wk gestation and at delivery for those considered high risk or living in areas of high syphilis morbidity • Rapid HIV test for those women in labor who have not been screened for HIV • Hepatitis B surface antigen first prenatal visit even if received the vaccination or tested • Retest at time of delivery for those considered high risk for HBV infection • Screen for HCV infection at first prenatal visit • Papanicolaou screening at recommended intervals • Test pregnant women for Zika virus if symptomatic *and* possible exposure • Offer screening to asymptomatic women with ongoing Zika virus exposure (consult CDC and local health department for up-to-date guidance)[18]

TABLE 13.2   STI Screening Recommendations   (Continued)

Patient Population	Screening
Men <30 yr and women ≤35 yr in correctional facilities	• Screen for gonorrhea and chlamydia at intake • Screen for syphilis based on prevalence in community
Men having sex with men (MSM)	At least annually, • HIV • Syphilis • Urethral gonorrhea and chlamydia for those with a history of insertive sex in past year • Rectal gonorrhea and chlamydia for those with history of receptive anal sex in past year • Pharyngeal screening for gonorrhea for those with a history of receptive oral sex in past year
Women having sex with women	• Routine cervical cancer screening[24]
Transgender men and women	• Assess risk for STIs and HIV based on current anatomy and sexual history

Adapted from Centers for Disease Control and Prevention. Sexually transmitted diseases treatment guidelines 2015. *MMWR.* 2015;64(3):9-19.
CDC, Centers for Disease Control and Prevention; HAV, hepatitis A virus; HBV, hepatitis B virus; HCV, hepatitis C virus; HIV, human immunodeficiency virus; HPV, human papillomavirus; HSV, herpes simplex virus; STI, sexually transmitted infection.

guidelines recommend testing patients with genital ulcers for herpes and syphilis and possibly for *Haemophilus ducreyi* in settings in which chancroid is prevalent to help reduce the transmission of HIV.[2]

Effective Diagnosis and Treatment of Sexually Transmitted Infections

The diagnosis and treatment of symptomatic STIs in community clinics, primary care offices, school-based health centers, emergency rooms, and other settings are generally straightforward. In addition to improving short-term STI-related symptoms, prompt diagnosis and treatment of STIs play a key role in preventing coinfection, complications, and transmission of STIs to others. Recommended treatment regimens for genital STIs are provided in Table 13.3. Guidance on alternative regimens for STIs are available in the *STD Treatment Guidelines 2015*[2] and should be used only if a recommended regimen cannot be used for treatment. Clinicians should also consult the aforementioned guidelines for treatment regimens for infections not listed in Table 13.3, special populations (pregnant women, HIV-positive individuals, infants, children), nongenital infections (rectal, pharyngeal, ocular, disseminated), recurrent infections, PID, epididymitis, victims of sexual assault, acute HIV, neurosyphilis, and tertiary syphilis.

TABLE 13.3   Signs and Symptoms of STIs and Recommended Treatment Regimens

STI	Signs/Symptoms	Recommended Treatment Regimen(s)*
Chlamydia	Often asymptomatic Vaginal or urethral discharge Dysuria Rectal pain, discharge, or bleeding	Azithromycin 1 g orally one dose *or* doxycycline 100 mg orally twice a day for 7 d
Gonorrhea (uncomplicated infection of cervix, urethra, rectum, and pharynx)	Dysuria White, yellow, or green discharge Increased vaginal discharge Vaginal bleeding between menses Rectal discharge, anal pruritis, soreness, bleeding, or pain with bowel movement Sore throat	Ceftriaxone 250 mg IM in a single dose *and* azithromycin 1 g orally in a single dose
Trichomoniasis	Frothy, malodorous vaginal discharge, genital itching/irritation, dysuria, discomfort with sex Males often asymptomatic; urethral discharge and/or irritation/burning	Metronidazole 2 g orally in a single dose *or* Tinidazole 2 g orally in a single dose
Genital herpes simplex	May be asymptomatic to mild Pinpoint vesicles on an erythematous based any-where in genital area Initial outbreak: longer and more severe and may include fever, body aches, lymphadenopathy, or headache Subsequent outbreak: prodromal symptoms may include genital pain or tingling or shooting pain in legs, hips, or buttock before the appearance of lesions; shorter duration and less severe lesions/symptoms	First episode: Acyclovir 400 mg orally 3 times a day for 7–10 d or Acyclovir 200 mg orally 5 times a day for 7–10 d or Valacyclovir 1 g orally 2 times a day for 7–10 d or Famciclovir 250 mg orally 3 times a day for 7–10 d Episodic, recurrent: Acyclovir 400 mg orally 3 times a day for 5 d or Acyclovir 800 mg orally 2 times a day for 5 d or Acyclovir 800 mg orally 3 times a day for 2 d or Valacyclovir 500 mg orally 2 times a day for 3 d or Valacyclovir 1 g orally 1 time a day for 5 d or Famciclovir 125 mg orally 2 times a day for 5 d or Famciclovir 1000 mg orally 2 times a day for 1 d or Famciclovir 500 mg orally once, followed by 250 mg 2 times a day for 2 d

Genital warts, external anogenital (penis, groin, scrotum, vulva, perineum, external anus, and perianus)	Anogenital warts are typically asymptomatic, may be painful or pruritic. Flesh-colored rough lesions that are papular, flat, or pedunculated	Patient applied: Imiquimod 3.75% or 5% cream may weaken latex condoms/diaphragms *or* Podofilox 0.5% solution or gel *or* Sinecatechins 15% ointment may weaken latex condoms/diaphragms Provider applied: Cryotherapy *or* Surgical removal *or* Trichloroacetic acid or bichloroacetic acid 80%–90%, apply small amount weekly if necessary
Syphilis	Primary: Chancre or chancres (painless ulcer) on genitals, rectum, or mouth Secondary: Rash, lymphadenopathy, fever Latent: Asymptomatic	Primary, secondary, or early latent <1 yr: Benzathine penicillin G 2.4 million units IM in a single dose Latent >1 yr or unknown duration: Benzathine penicillin G 2.4 million units IM in 3 doses at 1-wk intervals (7.2 million units total)

Adapted from Centers for Disease Control and Prevention. Sexually transmitted diseases treatment guidelines 2015. *MMWR.* 2015;64(3):1-137. https://www.cdc.gov/std/general/default.htm. Consult guidelines for additional information and guidance on regimens.
IM, intramuscular; STI, sexually transmitted infection.

Preventing Transmission of Sexually Transmitted Infections

An important way to prevent transmission of STIs from the patient to sexual contacts is through required reporting of selected illnesses to local and/or state public health departments with subsequent contact tracing. The list of reportable STIs varies somewhat from state to state, and different infections have different reporting requirements in terms of the time permitted between patient diagnosis and the reporting of the infection.

All persons diagnosed with STIs should be counseled to notify all of their sex partners within the past 60 days or last partner if sex occurred more than 60 days ago.[2] Patient-provided partner therapy also called expedited partner therapy is legal in most states (check http://www.cdc.gov/std/ept) and should be offered to heterosexual partners for the treatment of gonorrhea or chlamydia. Many states have partner letters available on their Department of Public Health website. The medication or prescription and written information that includes treatment instructions, medication warnings, and a statement to seek medical evaluation for symptoms of STIs are given to the patient to be delivered to their partner(s). The CDC (2016) does not recommend routine use of patient-provided partner therapy in MSM because of concerns regarding HIV infection. All persons diagnosed with an STI should be encouraged to have HIV testing.[2]

Vaccinations to Prevent Sexually Transmitted Infections

Vaccination is an important prevention strategy. Currently, vaccinations are available for HPV, hepatitis A, and hepatitis B. The Advisory Committee on Immunization Practices recommends routine vaccination with HPV-9 at age 11 to 12 years for male and female adolescents and catch-up vaccination for females 13 to 26 and males 13 to 21 years old.[3,14,15,23] Hepatitis A vaccine and hepatitis B vaccine are recommended for all individuals who have not been previously immunized[14,15,23] (refer to Chapter 17).

OFFICE AND CLINIC ORGANIZATION

At the level of the individual practice, a number of systems interventions can help expand effective provision of services for preventing STIs:

- Offer condoms, male and/or female, to all adolescents and adults at every visit. Provide education on the proper use and storage of condoms.
- On the basis of local STI rates, determine which subset of patients should be screened for STIs during routine health maintenance examinations. The practice should adopt a protocol as discussed in Chapter 21.

- Incorporate reminder systems through the use of electronic health records that will prompt clinicians when STI screening is indicated.
- Consider dedicating physical space and/or personnel to providing behavioral counseling focused on STI prevention.
- Consider posting flyers or handouts with STI prevention information, and listings of helpful websites, in places where patients can access this information privately and discreetly.

STI screening, counseling, and other prevention measures have not been implemented with the frequency and effectiveness that are warranted by the high prevalence of STIs in many communities. This occurs because effective STI prevention involves the larger health care system, including not only the individual practice but also community-based and national resources and a policy environment involving insurers and local, regional, and national institutions. Each of these entities influences the effectiveness with which clinicians can prevent the transmission of STIs and HIV infection. With STI prevention as with other aspects of medical care, a systems approach is as important as individual patient management. Community resources and community-based STI prevention measures are therefore increasingly important to address these widespread diseases.

SUGGESTED RESOURCES AND MATERIALS

Centers for Disease Control and Prevention Sexually Transmitted Diseases
https://www.cdc.gov/std/default.htm

HPV (Human Papillomavirus) Vaccine: What You Need to Know
https://www.cdc.gov/vaccines/hcp/vis/vis-statements/hpv.pdf

Hepatitis A Vaccine: What You Need to Know
http://www.immunize.org/VIS/hepatitis_a.pdf

Hepatitis B Vaccine: What You Need to Know
https://www.cdc.gov/vaccines/hcp/vis/vis-statements/hep-b.pdf

Zika Virus Prevention and Transmission
https://www.cdc.gov/zika/prevention/index.html
https://www.cdc.gov/zika/prevention/protect-yourself-and-others.html
https://www.cdc.gov/zika/prevention/sexual-transmission-prevention.html
https://www.cdc.gov/zika/prevention/plan-for-travel.html
https://www.cdc.gov/zika/pdfs/fs-Zika-Sex-PartnerTravel.pdf (English)
https://www.cdc.gov/zika/pdfs/spanish/fs-zika-sex-partnertravel-sp.pdf(Spanish)
https://www.cdc.gov/zika/pdfs/MosqPrevInUS.pdf (English)
https://www.cdc.gov/zika/pdfs/spanish/mosqprevinus-sp.pdf (Spanish)
https://www.cdc.gov/pregnancy/zika/pregnancy/documents/ZIKA-PregnancyTravel.pdf (English)
https://www.cdc.gov/pregnancy/zika/pregnancy/documents/ZIKA-PregnancyTravel-SP.pdf (Spanish)

Zika Virus Travel Information
https://wwwnc.cdc.gov/travel/page/zika-information

SUGGESTED TRAINING/READINGS

Centers for Disease Control and Prevention STD Training. https://www.cdc.gov/std/training/onlinetraining.htm.

ACOG Committee on Adolescent Health Care. Sexually transmitted diseases in adolescents. *ACOG Comm Opin No. 301.* 2004;104(4):891-898.

Centers for Disease Control and Prevention. Sexually transmitted diseases treatment guidelines 2015. *MMWR.* 2015;64(3):1-137. (app available through iTunes or Google Play).

Golden MR, Whittington WL, Handsfield HH, et al. Effect of expedited treatment of sex partners on recurrent or persistent gonorrhea or chlamydia infection. *New Engl J Med.* 2005;352(7):676-685.

Centers for Disease Control and Prevention. *Epidemiology and Prevention of Vaccine-Preventable Diseases.* In: Hamborsky J, Kroger A, Wolfe S, eds. 13th ed. Washington, DC: Public Health Foundation; 2015.

Centers for Disease Control and Prevention. *CDC Yellow Book 2018: Health Information for International Travel.* Atlanta, GA: Centers for Disease Control and Prevention. (app available through iTunes or Google Play).

Deutsch MB. *Guidelines for the Primary and Gender-Affirming Care of Transgender and Gender Nonbinary People.* San Francisco, CA: Center of Excellence for Transgender Health; 2016:1-199.

REFERENCES

1. Eng TR, Butler WT, eds. *The Hidden Epidemic: Confronting Sexually Transmitted Diseases. Institute of Medicine. Committee on Prevention and Control of Sexually Transmitted Diseases.* Washington, DC: National Academy Press; 1997:1-432.
2. Centers for Disease Control and Prevention. Sexually transmitted diseases treatment guidelines 2015. *MMWR.* 2015;64(3):1-137.
3. Centers for Disease Control and Prevention. *Epidemiology and Prevention of Vaccine-Preventable Diseases. Human Papillomavirus.* In: Hamborsky J, Kroger A, Wolfe S, eds. 13th ed. Washington, DC: Public Health Foundation; 2015:175-186.
4. Shirley DT, Nataro JP. Zika virus infection. *Pediatr Clin of North Am.* 2017;64:937-951. doi:10.1016/j.pcl.2017.03.012.
5. Centers for Disease Control and Prevention. *Sexually Transmitted Disease Surveillance 2016.* Atlanta: U.S. Department of Health and Human Services; 2017.
6. Haggerty CL, Gottlieb SL, Taylor BD, et al. Risk of sequelae after *Chlamydia trachomatis* genital infection in women. *J Infect Dis.* 2010;201:S134-S155.
7. Oakeschott P, Kerry S, Aghaizu A, et al. Randomised controlled trial of screening for Chlamydia trachomatis to prevent pelvic inflammatory disease: the POPI (prevention of pelvic infection) trial. *BMJ.* 2010;340:c1642.
8. Price MJ, Ades AE, De Angelis D, et al. Risk of pelvic inflammatory following Chlamydia trachomatis infection: analysis of prospective studies with a multistate model. *Am J Epidemiol.* 2013;178(3):484-492.
9. Marrazzo J, Hynes NA, Bloom A. *Pelvic Inflammatory Disease: Clinical Manifestations and Diagnosis.* UpToDate; 2018. https://www.uptodate.com/contents/pelvic-inflammatory-disease-clinical-manifestations-and-diagnosis?-search=fitz%20hugh%E2%80%93curtis%20syndrome&source=search_result&selectedTitle=1~36&usage_type=default&display_rank=1.
10. Centers for Disease Control and Prevention. *HIV in the United States: At a Glance.* Altlanta, GA: National Center for HIV/AIDS, Viral Hepatitis, and TB Prevention, Division of HIV/AIDS Prevention; 2018. https://www.cdc.gov/hiv/pdf/statistics/overview/cdc-hiv-us-ataglance.pdf.
11. World Health Organization. Sexually Transmitted Infections. http://www.who.int/mediacentre/factsheets/fs110/en/.

12. Patel EU, Gaydos CA, Packman ZR, et al. Prevalence and correlates of *Trichomonas vaginalis* infection among men and women in the United States. *Clin Infect Dis.* 2018;67(2):211-212. (published ahead of print).
13. Kissinger P, Adamski,A. Trichomoniasis and HIV interactions: a review. *Sex Transm Infect.* 2013;89:426-433.
14. Centers for Disease Control and Prevention. *Epidemiology and Prevention of Vaccine-Preventable Diseases. Hepatitis A.* In: Hamborsky J, Kroger A, Wolfe S, eds. 13th ed. Washington, DC: Public Health Foundation; 2015:135-148.
15. Centers for Disease Control and Prevention. *Epidemiology and Prevention of Vaccine-preventable Diseases. Hepatitis B.* In: Hamborsky J, Kroger A, Wolfe S, eds. 13th ed. Washington, DC: Public Health Foundation; 2015:149-174.
16. World Health Organization. Zika Virus. http://www.who.int/news-room/fact-sheets/detail/zika-virus.
17. Stassen L, Armitage CW, van der Heide D, Beagley KW, Frentiu FD. Zika virus in the male reproductive tract. *Viruses.* 2018;10:1-15. doi:10.3390/v10040198.
18. Centers for Disease Control and Prevention. Zika Virus. https://www.cdc.gov/zika/index.html.
19. Nusbaum MRH. The proactive sexual health history. *Am Fam Physician.* 2002;66(9):1705-1712.
20. Frieden TR, Jaffe W, Cono H, et al. Youth risk behavior surveillance—United States 2015. *MMWR.* 2016;65(6):1-180.
21. Leichliter JS, Copen C, Dittus PJ. Confidentiality issues and use of sexually transmitted disease services among sexually experienced persons aged 15–25 years — United States, 2013–2015. *MMWR.* 2017;66:237-241. doi:10.15585/mmwr.mm6609a1.
22. Guttmacher Institute. *Minors' Access to STI Services.* Guttmacher Institute; 2018. https://www.guttmacher.org/print/state-policy/explore/minors-access-sti-services.
23. Kroger AT, Duchin J, Vázquez M. General Best Practice Guidelines for Immunization. Best Practices Guidance of the Advisory Committee on Immunization Practices (ACIP). https://www.cdc.gov/vaccines/hcp/acip-recs/general-recs/index.html. Accessed 13 April 2018.
24. American Cancer Society. *Cervical Cancer Prevention and Early Detection;* 2014. http://www.cancer.org/acs/groups/cid/documents/webcontent/003167-pdf.pdf.

Please see Online Appendix: Apps and Digital Resources for additional information.

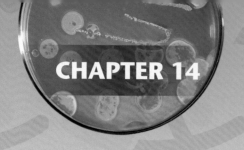

CHAPTER 14

Depression, Mood Disorders, and Cognitive Impairment

LINDA TRINH

BACKGROUND

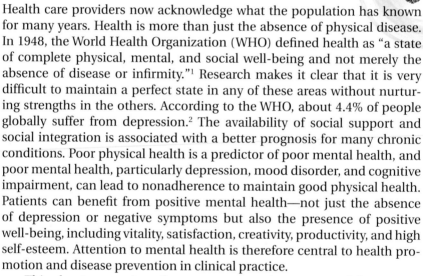

Health care providers now acknowledge what the population has known for many years. Health is more than just the absence of physical disease. In 1948, the World Health Organization (WHO) defined health as "a state of complete physical, mental, and social well-being and not merely the absence of disease or infirmity."[1] Research makes it clear that it is very difficult to maintain a perfect state in any of these areas without nurturing strengths in the others. According to the WHO, about 4.4% of people globally suffer from depression.[2] The availability of social support and social integration is associated with a better prognosis for many chronic conditions. Poor physical health is a predictor of poor mental health, and poor mental health, particularly depression, mood disorder, and cognitive impairment, can lead to nonadherence to maintain good physical health. Patients can benefit from positive mental health—not just the absence of depression or negative symptoms but also the presence of positive well-being, including vitality, satisfaction, creativity, productivity, and high self-esteem. Attention to mental health is therefore central to health promotion and disease prevention in clinical practice.

This chapter examines the assessment and treatment of depression, mood disorders, and cognitive impairment. It predominantly focuses on depression, the treatment of which shows the strongest evidence of benefit. The presentation and treatment of depression in the clinical setting are the subject of an extensive literature. This chapter does not discuss the assessment and treatment of patients with other mental or behavioral concerns (e.g., autism, bipolar mood disorder, schizophrenia, borderline personality disorder, or obsessive compulsive disorder). For depression, outcomes can be greatly improved by closing the gap between the ideal and current treatment practices. Managing depression should be a priority for all clinicians, as good management can lead to improved adherence in improving physical health. Studies have shown that, in the elderly, medication management, psychotherapy, socializing with family and friends, and regular exercise were all preferred treatment options.[3]

Mental health relates to many of the topics discussed in this book. Depression is a risk factor for many of the conditions that are targeted by clinical preventive services. For example, depression approximately doubles the risk of a new myocardial infarction or an ischemic stroke. A study shows that patients with acute myocardial infarction with untreated depression had higher 1-year mortality when compared with patients without depression.[4] Individuals with depression are less likely to be adherent to taking medications, such as aspirin chemoprophylaxis for heart disease or to successfully adopt new health behaviors. Patients with depression are more likely to smoke cigarettes, less likely to try quitting, and less successful at quitting than those without depression. Current evidence supports that depression actually primes smoking behaviors.[5] Adolescents with depression are more likely to start smoking than are their peers. Alcohol and substance abuse are also more common among those with depression. Individuals with depression may be more likely to be sedentary and obese.[6] Given the low levels of self-efficacy and the undervaluing of the future that characterize depression, it is not surprising that behavior change is particularly difficult for this group of patients. Anxiety and cognitive impairment also affect the ability of patients to pursue health-promoting behavior change, to obtain recommended clinical preventive services, and to adhere to follow-up regimens.

DEPRESSION

Screening and Clinical Assessment

The first step in the appropriate management of depression is accurate detection. Depression screenings should include a plan for identifying patients with possible depression. If a patient screens positive, further appropriate referrals or diagnostic testing should be done to confirm the condition. The patient should then be offered effective options for treatment or management. Depression is present in approximately 5% to 15% of patients who present in primary care, with higher prevalence rates observed among postpartum women, elders, and young adults. The diagnosis of *major depressive disorder* requires the presence of at least five symptoms, with one being depressed mood or lack of pleasure for a duration of at least 2 weeks. *Dysthymia* requires depressed mood or lack of pleasure lasting at least 2 years with fewer depression symptoms than are required for major depressive disorder.

A variety of questionnaire instruments are available to screen for depression. Instruments that have been used for many years include the Zung Self-Rating Depression Scale, the Center for Epidemiological Studies Depression Scale, and the Beck Depression Inventory. In its 2002 review of depression screening, the U.S. Preventive Services Task Force provided details about instruments available at the time.[3] It concluded that the accuracy of most depression questionnaires for the primary care setting was comparable. The decision about which depression instrument to use in practice is guided less by the accuracy of the questionnaire and more by the number of questions, the ease of formatting, the associated costs, and the symptom domains the questionnaire covers.

The Patient Health Questionnaire (PHQ-9) is a recently developed depression assessment instrument that is becoming the most commonly

PATIENT HEALTH QUESTIONNAIRE-9 (PHQ-9)

Over the last 2 weeks, how often have you been bothered by any of the following problems? (Use "✔" to indicate your answer)	Not at all	Several days	More than half the days	Nearly every day
1. Little interest or pleasure in doing things	0	1	2	3
2. Feeling down, depressed, or hopeless	0	1	2	3
3. Trouble falling or staying asleep, or sleeping too much	0	1	2	3
4. Feeling tired or having little energy	0	1	2	3
5. Poor appetite or overeating	0	1	2	3
6. Feeling bad about yourself — or that you are a failure or have let yourself or your family down	0	1	2	3
7. Trouble concentrating on things, such as reading the newspaper or watching television	0	1	2	3
8. Moving or speaking so slowly that other people could have noticed? Or the opposite — being so fidgety or restless that you have been moving around a lot more than usual	0	1	2	3
9. Thoughts that you would be better off dead or of hurting yourself in some way	0	1	2	3

FOR OFFICE CODING   _0_ + _____ + _____ + _____

=Total Score: _____

If you checked off any problems, how difficult have these problems made it for you to do your work, take care of things at home, or get along with other people?

Not difficult at all	Somewhat difficult	Very difficult	Extremely difficult
☐	☐	☐	☐

Figure 14.1 Patient Health Questionnaire. Courtesy of Pfizer. Developed by Drs. Robert L. Spitzer, Janet B.W. Williams, Kurt Kroenke and colleagues, with an educational grant from Pfizer Inc.

Fold back this page before administering this questionnaire

INSTRUCTIONS FOR USE

for doctor or healthcare professional use only

PHQ-9 QUICK DEPRESSION ASSESSMENT

For initial diagnosis:

1. Patient completes PHQ-9 Quick Depression Assessment on accompanying tear-off pad.
2. If there are at least 4✓s in the shaded section (including Questions #1 and #2), consider a depressive disorder. Add score to determine severity.
3. *Consider Major Depressive Disorder*
   –if there are at least 5✓s in the shaded section (one of which corresponds to Question #1 or #2)
   Consider Other Depressive Disorder
   –if there are 2 to 4✓ s in the shaded section (one of which corresponds to Question #1 or #2)

Note: Since the questionnaire relies on patient self-report, all responses should be verified by the clinician and a definitive diagnosis made on clinical grounds, taking into account how well the patient understood the questionnaire, as well as other relevant information from the patient. Diagnoses of Major Depressive Disorder or Other Depressive Disorder also require impairment of social,occupational, or other important areas of functioning (Question #10) and ruling out normal bereavement, a history of a Manic Episode (Bipolar Disorder), and a physical disorder, medication, or other drug as the biological cause of the depressive symptoms.

To monitor severity over time for newly diagnosed patients or patients in current treatment for depression:

1. Patients may complete questionnaires at baseline and at regular intervals (eg, every 2 weeks) at home and bring them in at their next appointment for scoring or they may complete the questionnaire during each scheduled appointment.
2. Add up ✓s by column. For every✓: Several days = 1   More than half the days = 2   Nearly every day = 3
3. Add together column scores to get a TOTAL score.
4. Refer to the subsequent PHQ-9 Scoring Card to interpret the TOTAL score.
5. Results may be included in patients' files to assist you in setting up a treatment goal, determining degree of response, as well as guiding treatment intervention.

PHQ-9 SCORING CARD FOR SEVERITY DETERMINATION

for healthcare professional use only

Scoring–add up all checked boxes on PHQ-9

For every ✓ : Not at all = 0; Several days = 1;
More than half the days = 2; Nearly every day = 3

Interpretation of Total Score

Total Score Depression Severity

      0-4 None
      5-9 Mild depression
    10-14 Moderate depression
    15-19 Moderately severe depression
    20-27 Severe depression

Figure 14.1 *(Continued)*

used standard.[4,5] Its advantages include its relative brevity—it has only nine questions (see Fig. 14.1)—and its sensitivity (85%) and specificity (75%) compared with structured clinical interviews by mental health specialists. The questions in the PHQ-9 are very similar to those used in the most common psychiatric diagnostic interviews and reflect the criteria for major depression presented in the Diagnostic and Statistical Manual of Mental Disorders, fourth edition. Perhaps the most important advantage of the PHQ-9 is that it can serve to help the clinician not only to make the diagnosis but also to follow the course and severity of the depression. A PHQ-9 score of below 5 indicates resolution of depression, 10 to 14 indicates moderate depression, and 15 or more indicates severe depression. A five-point reduction in the PHQ-9 score is considered a significant clinical improvement in depression even if complete resolution is not achieved.

The PHQ-9, like other depression questionnaires, has its limitations. For example, the PHQ-9 score does not by itself establish the primary diagnosis. When patients present with both a high PHQ-9 score and substantial medical comorbidity, substance abuse, or severe mental illness, clinicians must use their clinical judgment to identify the primary treatment target. Furthermore, the PHQ-9 does not measure anxiety, pain, hopelessness, or loneliness. Functional status, a very important factor in assessing the need for treatment, is addressed by only one question (question 10) appended to the PHQ-9. The PHQ-9 does include a question on suicidal ideation (question 9); clinicians who use the instrument must therefore institute a plan to examine the patient's response in a timely manner.

Awareness to identify depression in primary care has improved in recent years. Clinicians understand depression more than they formerly did, rates of detection have increased, and treatment has increased. Yet there is still a substantial gap between patients with depression and patients whose depression is being managed or treated. Closing the gap requires not only greater diligence in detecting the disease and assessing its severity but also the adoption of a system to ensure that those identified with the disease receive proper care. In its last review of the topic, the U.S. Preventive Services Task Force in 2016 recommends screening the general adult population, pregnant women, and postpartum women for depression. Screenings should include systems in which, after identification, patients will have access to treatment and management.[7] Studies that have evaluated isolated depression screening without standardized follow-up have not reported improved outcomes. Effective management and follow-up in the treatment of depression should include antidepressants, psychotherapy, and lifestyle changes, alone or in combination.[7] Greater resources are required to improve outcomes for screen-detected cases not previously recognized by the patient or clinician, because these individuals are less likely to accept usual forms of depression treatment and may have more associated comorbidities.

Treatment

Treatment of depression should be multifactorial and include addressing biological, psychological, and social needs, particularly in postpartum women.[8] Addressing the biological factors usually includes medication management to address neurotransmitter imbalance; psychosocial factors can be addressed with psychotherapy, lifestyle changes, and having strong social support systems. Lifestyle changes that have proven to decrease symptom of depression include daily exercise, good sleep hygiene, avoiding alcohol consumption, and meditation. Exercise is known to improve both physical and mental health in patients with depression.[9] Successful treatment addresses all three factors, and like any physical chronic conditions, regular follow-up is a necessity. All patients who appear to have acute symptoms of depression need to be screened for suicidal or homicidal ideation. If suicidal plans are evident, the patient needs to be hospitalized to ensure 24/7 supervision. In patients presenting with signs of depression and who do not require urgent treatment, clinicians can reasonably initiate a "watchful waiting" protocol. This protocol involves a brief diagnostic assessment, including a determination of the level of functioning, risk factors, education about the natural history and consequences of depression, presentation of depression treatment options, and agreement on the criteria for initiating treatment. With any treatment plan that involves medication management, psychotherapy is always recommended in conjunction. Healthy lifestyle changes continue to supplement treatment plans as well.

COUNSELING/PSYCHOTHERAPY

At least 50% of patients diagnosed with depression prefer to begin with the counseling/psychotherapy approach. Patients should be informed that counseling/psychotherapy is generally effective only if they complete six to eight sessions at a periodicity of every 1 to 2 weeks under the care of a competent therapist. Cognitive-behavioral, interpersonal, and problem-solving therapy have all been demonstrated to be more effective than unfocused talk therapy. Access to competent therapists who do not charge high out-of-pocket copayments is limited under many health plans, but locating such therapists to whom their patients can be referred should be a priority for primary care clinicians. This is particularly true for those practices serving a large number of African American and Hispanic patients, who tend to prefer counseling over pharmacotherapy.[6]

In general, licensed professionals such as psychologists, marriage family therapists, social workers, or Master's-level prepared counselors are thought to consistently provide the highest level of quality care in psychotherapy. Although primary care physicians can provide supplemental counseling that may increase the effectiveness of pharmacotherapy, most do not have the allotted time or therapeutic skills to provide intensive counseling for those patients who elect a counseling-only approach. Increasingly, psychiatrists, psychiatric mental health nurse practitioners, and psychiatric physician assistants are focusing on diagnostics and medication management while deferring psychotherapy to licensed psychologists, marriage family therapists, social workers, or Master's-level prepared counselors.[10]

PHARMACOTHERAPY

Currently available antidepressant medications are listed in Table 14.1. The foundation for successful pharmacotherapy involves creating a trusting, therapeutic relationship with the patient so that the prescriber and patient

TABLE 14.1 Commonly Used Antidepressant Medications				
Antidepressant[a]	Daily Therapeutic Dose Range	Initial Suggested Dose	Advantages	Disadvantages
Serotonin Reuptake Inhibitors (SSRIs)[b]				
Citalopram (Celexa)	20–40 mg	20 mg in morning with food (10 mg in elderly or those with panic disorder)	Possibly fewer cytochrome P-450 interactions; generic available	May cause Q-T prolongation, caution in patients with cardiac conditions
Escitalopram (Lexapro)	10–20 mg	10 mg	S-enantiomer more potent than racemic; 10 mg dose usually effective for most patients	—
Fluoxetine (Prozac)	10–80 mg	20 mg in morning with food (10 mg in elderly or children)	Indicated for obsessive compulsive disorder; long half-life good for poor medication adherence and missed doses; generic available; less frequent discontinuation symptoms	Slower to reach steady state; sometimes too stimulating thus should be taken in the morning; possibly more cytochrome P-450 interactions
Paroxetine (Paxil)	10–50 mg (40 mg in elderly)	20 mg once daily, usually in morning with food (10 mg in elderly and those with comorbid panic disorder)	FDA approved for most anxiety disorders; generic available	Sometimes sedating; occasionally more anticholinergic-like effects; possibly more cytochrome P-450 interactions); may have more frequent discontinuation symptoms
(Paxil CR)	25–62.5 mg (50 mg in elderly)	25 mg daily (12.5 mg in elderly and those with panic disorder)	May cause less nausea and GI distress	May have greater risk of major congenital malformations than other SSRIs

(Continued)

Sertraline (Zoloft)	25–200 mg	50 mg once daily, usually in morning with food (25 mg for elderly)	FDA approved for anxiety disorders; safety shown post myocardial infarction; generic available; most widely studied SSRI in pregnancy and breast-feeding women	GI side effects; may increase risk of pulmonary hypertension in third-trimester pregnant patients
Mirtazapine (Remeron)	15–45 mg	15 mg at bedtime (7.5 mg to start in frail elder patients)	Few drug interactions; less or no adverse effects on sexual function; may stimulate appetite	Sedation at low dose only; may stimulate appetite and weight gain
Norepinephrine and Dopamine-Reuptake Inhibitors (NDRI)				
Bupropion^c (Wellbutrin, Wellbutrin SR, Wellbutrin XL)	100–400 mg	XL 150 mg in morning or SR 100 mg in the morning	Stimulating; less or no adverse effects on sexual function; also used in smoking cessation and off-label for treatment of ADHD	At higher dose, may induce seizures in persons with seizure disorder; no effect on anxiety disorders; headaches, weight loss, decreased appetite
Serotonin and Norepinephrine-Reuptake Inhibitor (SNRIs)				
Venlafaxine (Effexor, Effexor XR)	75–375 mg	75 mg with food; if anxious or debilitated, 37.5 mg	XR version can be taken QD; helpful for anxiety disorders; not affiliated with weight gain or sexual side effects	May cause tachycardia, increase blood pressure, increase heart rate
Duloxetine (Cymbalta)	30–120 mg	20–30 mg	Seen helpful in neuropathic pain; not affiliated with weight gain or sexual side effects	May cause tachycardia, increase blood pressure, increase heart rate

TABLE 14.1   Commonly Used Antidepressant Medications   (Continued)

Antidepressant[a]	Daily Therapeutic Dose Range	Initial Suggested Dose	Advantages	Disadvantages
Tricyclic Antidepressants (TCA)				
Desipramine[d] (Norpramin, Pertofrane)	100–300 mg (25–100 mg in elderly)	50 mg in the morning	More effect on norepinephrine than serotonin; less sedating; generic available	Anticholinergic effects of TCAs; caution with BPH; can exacerbate cardiac conduction problems or CHF
Nortriptyline[d] (Aventyl, Pamelor)	25–150 mg	25 mg (10 mg in frail elderly) in the evening	Availability of reliable, valid blood levels; less likely than other TCAs to induce orthostatic hypotension; generic available	Anticholinergic effects of TCAs; caution with BPH; can exacerbate cardiac conduction problems or CHF
Serotonin Modulators				
Vortioxetine (Trintellix)	5–20 mg	5 mg daily	Works on multiple serotonin receptors to increase efficacy while decreasing side effects; very potent	Newer medication in the market, thus more expensive

[a]There are more antidepressants than those listed in this table; however, this list provides a reasonable variety of drugs that have different side effects and act by different neurotransmitter mechanisms. Monoamine oxidase inhibitors are not included.

[b]For SSRIs, generally start at the beginning of the therapeutic range. If side effects are bothersome, reduce the dose and increase more slowly. In debilitated patients or those sensitive to medications, start at a lower dose. For all antidepressants, allow 4 wk at a therapeutic dose and assess for a response. If the response is only partially effective, then increase the dose. If there is no response or symptoms worsen, then consider switching drugs.

[c]Generally avoid bupropion in patients with a history of seizures or anorexia nervosa.

[d]TCAs have lower costs but somewhat higher discontinuation rates compared with SSRIs due to side effects, and they are more lethal in an overdose.

ADHD, attention deficit hyperactivity disorder; BPH, benign prostatic hyperplasia; CHF, congestive heart failure; FDA, U.S. Food and Drug Administration; GI, gastrointestinal; QD, once a day.

can discuss medication options and potential side effects openly. There is no medication that is free of side effects; thus, it is important to find a medication that manages the patient's depression adequately while minimizing the patient's risk of side effects. Genetic testing is now available to test how well a patient can metabolize a medication. The ability to metabolize a medication is different from the efficacy of the medication, but the testing can provide insights on which medication can lead to higher chances of side effects. Because parents have half the identical genes of their children, it is helpful to take a thorough family history as well as successful treatment of anyone in the family who also suffers from depression. If a medication was successful in managing a parent's depression, there is a higher chance it would be helpful in treating the child's depression.[11]

Selective serotonin reuptake inhibitors (SSRIs) remain the first choice for antidepressant pharmacotherapy because of their effectiveness, once-a-day dosing, and relatively low incidence of side effects. Depending on the patient's demographic, comorbidity, and age, certain SSRIs are more favorable than others. For example, the most widely studied SSRI in children is Prozac because it has the longest half-life of all SSRIs. Zoloft, on the other hand, is most widely used in pregnant or breast-feeding mothers with depression, as it is also the most widely studied, although pregnant women also need to understand the increased risk of pulmonary hypertension in third-trimester pregnancies before starting or continuing treatment.[12]

Starting treatment with bupropion is also a reasonable choice as long as the patient does not also have a comorbidity of anxiety disorder, particularly because approximately 50% of patients with depression may be current smokers.[5] Buproprion has also been used successfully in smoking cessation with a 33.3% success rate and a 54.1% success rate when used with naltrexone.[13] Bupropion is more likely than SSRI medications to increase motivation and physical activity, but this may be difficult for patients who have had high levels of anxiety and insomnia before starting treatment, as the medication may worsen anxiety and insomnia.

Effective management of antidepressant medications extends beyond the initial prescription, as patients usually require subsequent medication adjustments. Initial rates of adherence to antidepressants are relatively low. Many patients require an adjustment in the medication dosing to address either the occurrence of side effects or an inadequate therapeutic response. Patients prescribed an antidepressant should be given a return appointment in 4 to 8 weeks, as the medication does take time to work. If this is not possible, they should be contacted by telephone during this time. Clinicians should be prepared to increase the dose of the medication to the accepted limit in an effort to achieve remission, and they should not be satisfied with partial treatment of the depression, assuming there are little or no side effects.

By 6 weeks of treatment, if there has not been at least some improvement in the level of clinical depression, a change in medication may be recommended with possible genetic testing warranted. More than half of patients with depression will require either a switch from or augmentation of their first antidepressant medication. If a patient does not respond to one SSRI and experiences minimal or no side effects, switching to a second SSRI is a reasonable choice. Switching to a serotonin and norepinephrine dual agent, such as venlafaxine or duloxetine, is also a possible option as long as patient's blood pressure is controlled.[14] Clinicians should be aware that venlafaxine can raise blood pressure, a potential concern for patients at high risk of cardiovascular disease.

Tricyclic antidepressants are also effective, but they carry a higher risk of anticholinergic side effects (e.g., orthostatic hypotension, dry mouth, urinary retention). Managing these side effects is particularly challenging with older adults. Tricyclic antidepressants with fewer anticholinergic effects, such as nortriptyline or desipramine, are preferred over amitriptyline.

Serotonin modulator is a newer class of antidepressants that have multimodal action specific to serotonin receptors.[15] On some serotonin receptors, the medication will inhibit reuptake, whereas on other receptors, it will modulate serotonin. Because of this multimodal action, the medication is able to increase efficacy and decrease the risk of side effects associated with SSRIs that can only inhibit reuptake.[16] Cost appears to be an obstacle to access of serotonin modulators as generic forms are not yet available, most notably Trintellix.[17]

As with hypertension, treatment of depression frequently requires the use of multiple medications to reach target goals. The key to multiple medication management is to use medications that have different modes of action. It is not recommended to use multiple medications with the same mode of action, as this will increase chances and severity of side effects. Both the clinician and the patient must be prepared for multiple assessments and have patience until goals are reached. When augmenting with a second agent, such as adding bupropion to an SSRI, the clinician should first prescribe a low dose to check for tolerability.

It is important to regularly monitor patients on antidepressant medication. The primary care clinician must be conscientious about intervening when therapy is proving to be unsatisfactory (i.e., inadequate resolution of the depression). Most primary care clinicians are capable of managing basic antidepressant medication schedules. However, if the clinician feels that referral to a psychiatric provider is necessary, it is better to make such a referral sooner rather than later.

COMPREHENSIVE PROGRAMS

The elements of a comprehensive approach to the care of depression in primary care are captured in the chronic care model synthesized by Edward Wagner et al.[8] This model emphasizes six elements that are necessary for a prepared patient and health care delivery system: (1) organizational support, (2) enhancing self-management, (3) decision support, (4) practice design, (5) information technology, and (6) community linkages. These elements are reviewed further in the subsequent text. Furthermore, studies of depression care indicate that successful comprehensive depression programs apply more than one practice intervention (including more than one clinician in the team) and are supported by a long-term commitment by the practice.[14]

Organizational Support

The extensive changes required to support the chronic care model in primary care call upon practices and systems of care to provide organizational support to provide the necessary resources and to keep the staff engaged when the inevitable bumps in the road arise. Leaders need to communicate their vision for the new program, invest the resources for requisite information technology, provide time off for staff to plan and be trained, and be willing to reward those staff who adopt the new model of care. Although the requisite organizational leadership is most easily identified in larger practices, even smaller practices can ensure that the senior management will support implementation of the new model of care. High quality care for depression will often require practices to consider new relationships with behavioral health organizations. Practice managers and health systems need to provide support and take initiative in working through the funding and care coordination issues that are part of forging new relationships between primary care and behavioral health providers.

Enhancing Self-management

Patients with depression spend a tiny portion of their lives with clinicians. Each day, patients with depression and other chronic diseases must decide whether and how to manage their conditions and respond to symptoms. The goal of each patient visit should be to prepare patients for this work. The support of self-management can begin by asking patients exactly what they do when they have a bad day and feel depressed or how they typically respond when someone invites them to go shopping or see a movie. Knowing this, the clinician can discuss constructive alternatives that are more likely to mitigate their depression.

The objective during the patient visit should be to identify a specific measurable self-management goal that the patient feels can be successfully achieved. For example, a patient might respond that she tends to stay home and eat more when she feels blue. A constructive goal to be achieved before the next visit might be to not eat and instead walk to her sister's house at least half the days she feels depressed. Other self-management goals might include taking antidepressant medication 6 of 7 days, making an appointment at an employment agency, reading a book on depression, visiting a depression Internet support group, or leaving the house every day for at least 1 hour.[18] By having this discussion, clinicians acknowledge the day-to-day struggles of their patients, help their patients identify specific problems, assess potential coping strategies, deconstruct problems into smaller pieces, respect patients' choices, and ultimately enhance their self-efficacy.

Decision Support

Primary care clinicians should have ready access to treatment protocols for patients with depression. Most primary care practices will benefit from developing a close working relationship with a mental health specialist who can provide overall decision support for a comprehensive depression detection and treatment program. The mental health specialist can help the practice develop strategies/protocols for diagnosing and monitoring depression, assessing psychiatric comorbidity, developing complex psychopharmacology protocols, and establishing criteria for referral to mental health specialists. This consultant may also be able to outline clearer pathways for referring patients to specialty mental health providers as well.

Aside from this general consultative role, clinicians should also engage mental health specialists for consultations concerning difficult cases, patients who will not accept referrals to mental health specialists, or those lacking insurance coverage. Some practices hire part-time mental health specialists or forge new relationships with behavioral health centers to enhance this level of decision support. Mental health specialists are often identified to supervise and provide decision support to the depression care coordinators of a practice (see subsequent text). Decision support for patients is also important. Clinicians should provide patients with information about best practices for treatment of depression and how depression is treated at the practice. See "Suggested Readings: "Clinical practice guidelines for the management of depression" at the end of the chapter.

Practice Design

Several elements of practice design are necessary for quality depression care. The first is to utilize a standard for both diagnosing and monitoring depression treatment within the practice. A depression assessment instrument, such as the PHQ-9 discussed earlier, should be adopted. If optimal outcomes are to be achieved for patients with depression, in most primary care practices it will be necessary to utilize the services of a mental health care manager. The care manager may have several roles, including performing the follow-up for patients who do not return for their appointments, assessing the severity of depression symptoms, educating patients about depression treatment options, reinforcing treatment plans, monitoring self-management goals and patients' efforts to achieve them, and providing emotional support.

If resources are available to support a dedicated individual to work exclusively as a depression care manager, there is a high probability that depression outcomes will improve. If such resources are lacking, quite often the best alternative is to divide the work of the care manager among multiple personnel in the office, such as the primary care clinicians, nurses, or extant behavioral health specialists. Personnel with limited professional education can undergo training to provide a limited but very useful service of following up and monitoring patients with depression.

Although it is ideal to have the care manager based within the primary care practice, this is often not feasible or financially viable. Telephone-based care management from a central location, such as that offered through health plans and employers, has been shown to be effective.[19] When the care management services are not based within the practice, however, clinicians may take longer to acquire confidence in the care managers and the depression protocols.

Clinical Information Systems

Effective monitoring of depression to establish whether remission is partial or complete is best accomplished by using some type of clinical information system. The optimal clinical information should include some form of electronic medical record. In one study, electronic medical record was successfully used to screen and identify a stepped-care approach in the management of depression.[20] Although direct entry of data by patients is ideal, the most common systems require data entry by staff. Finding an efficient way to accomplish data entry is essential to the long-term success of a comprehensive depression treatment program.

The clinical information system should also provide prompts for staff when processes of care and outcomes are not reaching goals. In the trials that demonstrated the effectiveness of multicomponent collaborative care, an essential element was the existence of procedures to make certain that clinicians received reminders when a patient had not undergone a reassessment of their depression within 4 weeks of starting treatment.[21] Finally, a clinical information system can help measure overall performance in relation to depression care. Performance measures might include the proportion of patients with depression who make contact with the health care system 1 to 3 weeks after starting treatment, who are adherent to the depression treatment plan, and who meet criteria for resolution of depression by 6 months.

Measuring these process and outcome measures serves several purposes. First, performance is usually less than what the practice might predict, and documenting the discrepancy can act as a catalyst for change. Primary care practices with established systems for quality improvement and "benchmarking" can motivate individual clinicians to improve the quality of their care by demonstrating how their performance compares with that of their peers.[22] Second, tracking the process and outcome measures over time can guide strategic planning on where to most efficiently target resources to improve outcomes. For example, performance data might persuade a practice that its depression care manager should emphasize recontact with patients for the first depression reassessment (1–3 weeks after initiating treatment) and that additional follow-up will not be cost-effective.

Third, performance data are increasingly being requested from quality assessment organizations as a measure of the quality of care in a practice. With these data a practice can negotiate with funders for additional resources, and performance data are essential for "pay-for-performance" arrangements.[23] Primary care practices are better positioned to obtain payment for additional resources when they can provide data to substantiate a need and underscore the potential improvement in outcomes that would be achieved by more rational funding of depression care.

Linkages With Community Resources

Primary care clinicians sometimes believe that they must provide all of the services required by patients in their care. Patients with depression, however, often face a complex array of challenges, including financial difficulties, inadequate housing, lack of health insurance, unstable employment, disrupted relationships and living arrangements, and lack of social support. For women presenting with depression in primary care, the exposure to interpersonal violence is substantial. Primary care clinicians should engage community resource support organizations informally, and, when possible, under more formal arrangements. These organizations commonly include community mental health centers, domestic violence shelters, the local Young Men's Christian Association, and vocational rehabilitation centers. Community resource organizations may be willing to trade easier access to their services in exchange for primary care for their clients. Through these partnerships, clinicians can help ensure that their patients receive the highest quality of care and level of support for their depression.

SCREENING AND MANAGEMENT OF OTHER MENTAL DISORDERS

There is limited evidence that screening for other mental disorders, such as anxiety and cognitive impairment, is effective in improving patient outcomes even when accompanied by a comprehensive treatment program. However, many primary care practices find it inefficient to implement a new program for mental disorders that only addresses depression. Expanding the focus to include screening for anxiety and cognitive disorders in certain circumstances may be more efficient and more consistent with the comprehensive philosophy of primary care.

Anxiety Disorders

Common anxiety disorders in the primary care population include generalized anxiety disorder, panic disorder, phobias, and posttraumatic stress disorder. An evidence-based argument to support screening for these conditions would require evidence that screening methods (beyond the usual clinical interview) would identify individuals with previously undetected anxiety disorders and that treatment at this earlier stage would produce better outcomes than usual care. For several reasons, this is a difficult threshold to meet.

First, there is wide variation in usual care. Some clinicians are much better at detection and treatment of anxiety disorders than others. The best performing clinicians would have the least to gain from new screening programs. Second, there are multiple anxiety disorders and specific questions that are required to screen for each disorder. Third, failure to recognize a mental disorder is less common with anxiety disorders than with depression, creating less of a need for screening. Fourth, there is a large overlap between depression and the more severe anxiety disorders. Screening programs for depression can also detect a large percentage of patients with severe anxiety disorders.[24]

The generalized anxiety disorder 7-item (GAD-7) scale has been successfully used to screen for anxiety disorders. Treatment of anxiety with medication management is usually started when the patient exhibits loss of daily function whether in the work place, at home, or at school. Psychotherapy has also shown to improve symptoms. Randomized clinical trials have demonstrated improved outcomes and reasonable costs when primary care practices adopt comprehensive treatment programs for anxiety disorders that come to clinical attention under usual care.[25] For example, in one trial the comprehensive intervention consisted of cognitive behavioral therapy and pharmacotherapy, delivered by a mental health therapist and primary care physician over six sessions with up to six follow-up telephone calls for 1 year.[26] In another trial, the practices adopted a telephone-based care management program for patients with panic and generalized anxiety disorder.[27]

With a comprehensive treatment program in place, a primary care practice might find it reasonable to look for anxiety disorders in patients with atypical presentations or anxiety symptoms that are too subtle to normally trigger treatment. Validated screening instruments for anxiety disorders are limited, but another option is the generalized anxiety disorder severity scale.[28]

Cognitive Impairment or Dementia

Dementia is defined as an acquired syndrome of decline in memory and at least one other cognitive domain such as language, visual-spatial, or executive function sufficient to interfere with social and occupational functioning in an alert person.[2] Dementia is most frequently due to Alzheimer disease or multiple infarcts from cerebrovascular disease also known as vascular dementia. Other types of less common dementia exist, including Lewy bodies dementia, Parkinson dementia, mixed dementia, frontotemporal dementia, Huntington disease dementia, or Wernicke-Korsakoff syndrome.

Interest in cognitive impairment has heightened in recent years with the growth in the number of seniors and of patients with dementia and the availability of new medications that have at least a modest impact on the decline of cognitive function. Currently all medications are geared at preventing further decline in memory and function, and up to date, no medication has been approved for improving memory in dementia. Pharmacotherapy is focused on prevention rather than curing, as there is no cure for dementia as yet.[29]

SCREENING

Screening for cognitive impairment could be considered for patients 65 years and older, especially those with a family history of dementia or with a high risk of cardiovascular disease. Potential approaches include directly testing cognitive function, assessing functional deficits, or asking for reports of cognition and function from proxy informants.

The U.S. Preventive Services Task Force concluded that evidence is lacking to recommend routine screening for dementia because of poor outcomes regardless of screening. At the same time, many experts in the field, including Mitchell Clionsky and Emily Clionsky, who are codevelopers of the Memory Orientation Screening Test, continue to recommend brief routine cognitive evaluation for early identification of cognitive imparement.[30] The U.S. Preventive Services Task Force states that available data do not permit the magnitude of benefit from early detection and treatment to be accurately gauged. Screening could be of potential benefit by finding a reversible cause of dementia (e.g., hypothyroidism, vitamin B_{12} deficiency), but such causes explain only 1% to 2% of cases and are often detected in other ways. Cognitive function screening could identify individuals who cannot safely drive a motor vehicle, but evidence that such screening is of practical utility is limited.[30] Nor has control of cardiovascular risk factors (e.g., with blood pressure control or aspirin chemoprophylaxis) been shown to reduce the progression of dementia due to cerebrovascular disease.[31]

Standardized instruments for evaluating cognitive function are available but unfortunately have limited diagnostic precision. The Mini-Mental Status Examination (MMSE, see Table 14.2) has been studied the most.[32] The MMSE takes approximately 7 minutes to administer. Its scores are affected by the patient's level of educational attainment. Depending on the cutoff utilized for scoring, the MMSE has a sensitivity of 70% to 92% and a specificity of 56% to 96%. The poor specificity leads to a relatively low positive predictive value and the need for clinicians to sort out positive screening results. Rather than reflecting a deterioration in cognition, the MMSE score may be falsely low because of other medical conditions, such as hearing impairment or failure to complete the questions.

TABLE 14.2   **Mini-Mental Status Examination**

Orientation

1. What is the

   Year? (1 point)

   Season? (1 point)

   Date? (1 point)

   Day? (1 point)

   Month? (1 point)

2. Where are we?

   State? (1 point)

   County? (1 point)

   Town/city? (1 point)

   Floor? (1 point)

   Address/name of building? (1 point)

Registration

3. Name three objects, taking 1 s to say each. Then ask the patient all three after you have said them. Repeat the answers until the patient learns all three. (3 points)

Attention and Calculation

4. Serial sevens: give one point for each correct answer. Stop after five answers.

   (Alternative: spell *world* backward.) (5 points)

Recall

5. Ask for names of three objects learned in question 3. Give one point for each correct answer. (3 points)

Language

6. Point to a pencil and a watch. Have the patient name them as you point. (2 points)

7. Have the patient repeat "No ifs, ands, or buts." (1 point)

8. Have the patient follow a three-stage command: "Take the paper in your right hand. Fold the paper in half. Put the paper on the floor." (3 points)

9. Have the patient read and obey the following: "Close your eyes." (1 point)

TABLE 14.2 Mini-Mental Status Examination   (Continued)
10. Have the patient write a sentence of his or her own choice. (The sentence should contain a subject and an object and should make sense. Ignore spelling errors when scoring.) (1 point)
11. Show the patient a picture of two overlapping pentagrams. Ask the patient to copy it. (Give one point if all the sides and angles are preserved and if the intersecting sides form a quadrangle.) (1 point)

Adapted from Crum RM, Anthony JC, Bassett SS, et al. Population-based norms for the mini-mental state examination by age and educational level. *JAMA*. 1993;269:2386-2391. A total score of less than 24 of 30 points is generally considered abnormal.

There are other tests that show promise. They include the Modified MMSE, Short Portable Mental Status Questionnaire, and the Mini-Cog.[33] The Mini-Cog consists of a clock drawing task and the recall of three unrelated words.[34] Some questionnaires ask the patient to rate their problems with memory across a range of activities. Finding more severe cases of cognitive impairment is possible by administering informant-based functional tests (completed by relatives or caregivers) such as the Functional Activities Questionnaire, the Informant Questionnaire on Cognitive Decline in the Elderly, and the Instrumental Activities of Daily Living questionnaire.

TREATMENT

If cognitive impairment is detected, use of cholinesterase inhibitors (see Table 14.3) has been shown to reduce progression of dementia, but their benefits are modest and not curative. Randomized controlled trials indicate that the medication effect is equivalent to delaying progression by up to 7 months in those with mild dementia and 2 to 5 months in those with moderate dementia. Cholinesterase inhibitors have had no demonstrable effect on maintaining function. Memantine, an N-methyl D-aspartate receptor antagonist, may be neuroprotective. It is generally well tolerated and appears to modestly reduce progression of dementia. It has also not been demonstrated to preserve function. These medications are often used together as they have different modes of action. Consistent evidence of effectiveness is also lacking for supplements to improve cognition, such as *Ginkgo biloba*, selegiline, and vitamin E.

Nonpharmacologic interventions such as mental exercises, behavioral training, and caregiver education have been proposed, but in rigorous trials, no improvements in functional status have been demonstrated. Observational studies suggest that integrated social networks, physical activity, and nonphysical activities that require mental work may reduce the risk of dementia.[35]

TABLE 14.3 Medications for Dementia

Drug	Therapeutic Dose Range	Starting Dose	Advantages	Disadvantages
Acetylcholinesterase Inhibitors				
Tacrine (Cogrex)	20–40 mg QID	10 mg QID	First in class	Rarely used; needs frequent dosing; must be avoided in the presence of liver disease; substantial GI side effects
Donepezil (Aricept)	5–10 mg QD	5 mg QD	Once-a-day dosing	Abnormal dreams; insomnia possible; avoid if a history of arrhythmia is present
Galantamine (Razadyne)	BID 8–12 mg	4 mg BID	Cognitive benefits sustained for 3 yr	Avoid if history of seizures; may have more GI side effects than donepezil
Rivastigmine (Exelon)	4–6 mg BID	1.5 mg BID	Useful for Parkinson-associated dementia	Slow titration recommended; possibly more GI side effects than donepezil; avoid if a history of arrhythmias is present
N-methyl-D-aspartate (NMDA) Blockers				
Memantine (Namenda)	10 mg BID	5 mg QD	Very low side effect rate	Dizziness; do not use with sodium bicarbonate or acetazolamide (Diamox)

BID, twice a day; GI, gastrointestinal; QD, once a day; QID, four times a day.

CONCLUSION

Although further research will be required to establish supporting evidence to justify routine screening for mental disorders other than depression—dementia, anxiety, and other conditions—clinicians should remain alert for these disorders as they interview patients, family members, and caregivers. Concerns raised by relatives and friends and subtle clues in the behavior and comments of patients can help the astute clinician recognize findings that require further diagnostic evaluation. Depression and other conditions often coexist with substance abuse. It is equally important to provide assessment of alcohol and drug use in the primary care setting.

Although clinicians do need to improve their assessment skills, more complete detection and treatment of depression and other mental disorders will most likely also require greater public education. Patient attitudes regarding the need for depression treatment play an important role in their acceptance of and adherence to treatment.

As noted at the outset of this chapter, mental health involves more than the absence of pathology. The mental well-being of patients often suffers because of emotional difficulties, stress-related illness, personality disorders, and dysfunctional relationships. Such patients often benefit from individual counseling and/or family therapy. The amelioration of these conditions can play an important preventive role in averting secondary health and social consequences.

Finally, clinicians caring for children and adolescents should be conscientious about recognizing the presenting features of depression and other mental illnesses at these life stages. They should also recognize parents in need of emotional support, training in parenting skills, or reporting to protective service agencies for investigation of potential child abuse or neglect.

SUGGESTED RESOURCES AND MATERIALS

National Institute of Mental Health
Depression
https://www.nimh.nih.gov/health/publications/depression/index.shtml. Accessed 2018.

Psych Central Telephone Hotlines and Helplines
https://psychcentral.com/lib/telephone-hotlines-and-help-lines/. Accessed 2018.

American Psychiatric Association. *Diagnostic and Statistical Manual of Mental Disorders.* 5th ed. Arlington, VA: American Psychiatric Publishing; 2013.

Gautam S., Jain A, Gautam M, Vahia VN, Grover S. Clinical practice guidelines for the management of depression. *Indian J Psychiatry.* 2017;59(suppl 1):S34.

REFERENCES

1. World Health Organization Constitution. *Basic Documents.* Geneva: World Health Organization; 1948.
2. World Health Organization. *Depression and Other Common Mental Disorders: Global Health Estimates*; 2017.

3. Luck-Sikorski C, Stein J, Heilmann K, et al. Treatment preferences for depression in the elderly. *Int Psychogeriatr.* 2017;29(3):389-398.
4. Smolderen KG, Buchanan DM, Gosch K, et al. Depression treatment and 1-year mortality following acute myocardial infarction: insights from the TRIUMPH registry. *Circulation.* 2017;135(18):1681-1689.
5. Mathew AR, Hogarth L, Leventhal AM, Cook JW, Hitsman B. Cigarette smoking and depression comorbidity: systematic review and proposed theoretical model. *Addiction.* 2017;112(3):401-412.
6. Quek Y-H, Tam WWS, Zhang MWB, Ho RCM. Exploring the association between childhood and adolescent obesity and depression: a meta-analysis. *Obesity Rev.* 2017;18(7):742-754.
7. Siu AL, U.S. Preventive Services Task Force (USPSTF), , Bibbins-Domingo K, et al. Screening for depression in adults: US preventive services task force recommendation statement. *JAMA.* 2016;315(4):380-387.
8. Abdollahi F, Rohani S, Sazlina GS, et al. Bio-psycho-socio-demographic and obstetric predictors of postpartum depression in pregnancy: a prospective cohort study. *Iran J Psychiatry Behav Sci.* 2014;8(2):11.
9. Knapen J, Vancampfort D, Moriën Y, Marchal Y. Exercise therapy improves both mental and physical health in patients with major depression. *Disabil Rehabil.* 2015;37(16):1490-1495.
10. DeRubeis RJ, Hollon SD, Amsterdam JD, et al. Cognitive therapy vs medications in the treatment of moderate to severe depression. *Arch Gen Psychiatry.* 2005;62(4):409-416.
11. McGrane IR, Mertens S. Depression and pharmacogenetics: a psychiatric pharmacist's perspective. *Arch Psychiatr Nurs.* 2018;32(3):329-330.
12. Bérard A, Sheehy O, Zhao JP, Vinet É, Bernatsky S, Abrahamowicz M. SSRI and SNRI use during pregnancy and the risk of persistent pulmonary hypertension of the newborn. *Br J Clin Pharmacol.* 2017;83(5):1126-1133.
13. Mooney ME, Schmitz JM, Allen S, et al. Bupropion and naltrexone for smoking cessation: a double-blind randomized placebo-controlled clinical trial. *Clin Pharmacol Ther.* 2016;100(4):344-352.
14. Rush AJ, Trivedi MH, Wisniewski SR, et al. Bupropion-SR, sertraline, or venlafaxine-XR after failure of SSRIs for depression. *N Engl J Med.* 2006;354(12):1231-1242.
15. Hirsch M, Birnbaum RJ. *Serotonin Modulators; Pharmacology, Administration, and Side Effects.* UptoDate; 2016.
16. Frampton JE. Vortioxetine: a review in cognitive dysfunction in depression. *Drugs.* 2016;76(17):1675-1682.
17. Antonio S, Valley S, Florida S. *Lundbeck Canada Inc. Announces Health Canada Approval of Trintellix™ (vortioxetine Hydrobromide) for Treatment of Adults with Major Depressive Disorder;* 2016.
18. Kleiboer A, Donker T, Seekles W, van Straten A, Riper H, Cuijpers P. A randomized controlled trial on the role of support in Internet-based problem solving therapy for depression and anxiety. *Behav Res Ther.* 2015;72:63-71.
19. Saeed SA, Johnson TL, Bagga M, Glass O. Training residents in the use of telepsychiatry: review of the literature and a proposed elective. *Psychiatr Q.* 2017;88(2):271-283.
20. Loeb D, Sieja A, Corral J, Zehnder NG, Guiton G, Nease DE. Evaluation of the role of training in the implementation of a depression screening and treatment protocol in 2 academic outpatient internal medicine clinics utilizing the electronic medical record. *Am J Med Qual.* 2015;30(4):359-366.
21. Lanata A, Valenza G, Nardelli M, Gentili C, Scilingo EP. Complexity index from a personalized wearable monitoring system for assessing remission in mental health. *IEEE J Biomed Health Inform.* 2015;19(1):132-139.

22. Jakobsen H, Andersson G, Havik OE, Nordgreen T. Guided internet-based cognitive behavioral therapy for mild and moderate depression: a benchmarking study. *Internet Interv.* 2017;7:1-8.
23. Mendelson A, Kondo K, Damberg C, et al. The effects of pay-for-performance programs on health, health care use, and processes of care: a systematic review. *Ann Intern Med.* 2017;166(5):341-353.
24. Kent P, Mirkhil S, Keating J, Buchbinder R, Manniche C, Albert HB. The concurrent validity of brief screening questions for anxiety, depression, social isolation, catastrophization, and fear of movement in people with low back pain. *Clin J Pain.* 2014;30(6):479-489.
25. Scaini S, Belotti R, Ogliari A, Battaglia M. A comprehensive meta-analysis of cognitive-behavioral interventions for social anxiety disorder in children and adolescents. *J Anxiety Disord.* 2016;42:105-112.
26. Katon W, Russo J, Sherbourne C, et al. Incremental cost-effectiveness of a collaborative care intervention for panic disorder. *Psychol Med.* 2006;36(3):353-363.
27. Rollman BL, Belnap BH, Mazumdar S, et al. A randomized trial to improve the quality of treatment for panic and generalized anxiety disorders in primary care. *Arch Gen Psychiatry.* 2005;62:1332-1341.
28. Shear K, Belnap BH, Mazumdar S, et al. Generalized anxiety disorder severity scale (GADSS): a preliminary validation study. *Depress Anxiety.* 2006;23:77-82.
29. Ulrike D, Meyer ET, Schroeder R. *Big Data for Advancing Dementia Research: An Evaluation of Data Sharing Practices in Research on Age-related Neurodegenerative Diseases. No. 246.* OECD Publishing; 2015.
30. Moyer VA. Screening for cognitive impairment in older adults: US preventive services task force recommendation statement. *Ann Intern Med.* 2014;160(11):791-797.
31. O'Brien JT, Thomas A. Vascular dementia. *Lancet.* 2015;386(10004):1698-1706.
32. McDowell I, Kristjansson B, Hill GB, et al. Community screening for dementia: the mini mental state exam (MMSE) and modified mini-mental state exam (3 MS) compared. *J Clin Epidemiol.* 1997;50:377-383.
33. Borson S, Scanlon JM, Watanabe J, et al. Improving identification of cognitive impairment in primary care. *Int J Geriatr Psychiatry.* 2006;21:349-355.
34. Borson S, Scanlan JM, Chen P, et al. The mini-cog: a cognitive 'vital signs' measure for dementia screening in multi-lingual elderly. *Int J Geriatr Psychiatry.* 2000;15:1021-1024.
35. Fratiglioni L, Paillard-Borg S, Winblad B. An active and socially integrated lifestyle in late life might protect against dementia. *Lancet Neurol.* 2004;3:343-353.

Please see Online Appendix: Apps and Digital Resources for additional information.

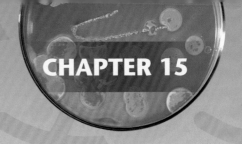

CHAPTER 15

Self-Examination of the Breasts, Testes, and Skin

GERALDINE F. MARROCCO

INTRODUCTION

The chapter focuses on the examination of three organs—breasts, testes, and skin—for which self-examination is most commonly recommended. Self-examination of the oral cavity, eyes, and other parts of the body is recommended less frequently, is supported by even weaker scientific evidence, and is therefore not discussed in this chapter. Screening for cancer through clinical examinations and laboratory screening tests (e.g., mammography) is discussed in Chapters 4 and 5.

When diagnosed at an early stage, cancers of the breast, skin (e.g., malignant melanoma), and testes have relatively good prognoses. In addition to obtaining periodic cancer screening by clinicians, which is discussed in Chapters 4 and 5, the public has been advised for many years to perform monthly self-examinations at home to help detect malignant or premalignant conditions at a curable stage. Clinicians have been encouraged to devote time during clinical encounters to train and remind patients how to correctly perform self-examination.

Over the last decade these recommendations have changed and are not universally accepted based on the clinical evidence and the appropriateness of these recommendations. For example, it has been determined that women of average risk should not perform the breast self-examination (BSE). Therefore, performing and teaching (BSE) has continued to lack any benefit and often leads to higher unnecessary invasive breast procedures. These procedures often show benign disease with the BSE, coupled with unnecessary anxiety during the time the patient needs to wait for results. However, women are encouraged to have an "awareness" of their breast tissue and bring any concerns of changes to their primary care provider. This self-awareness empowers women to know their body, yet, it is critical that they know self-awareness is no substitute for mammography.[1,2]

The U.S. Preventative Service Task Force review of skin cancer screening found "little evidence to determine the effects of counseling on other preventive behaviors ... such as practicing skin self-examination."[3] Its 2013 review of screening for testicular cancer recommended against routine screening and reported that there was "no new evidence that screening with clinical examination or testicular self-examination is effective in reducing mortality from testicular cancer."[4] The American Academy of Family Physicians has adopted similar positions.[5] All of these positions have remained the same as of 2018.

Recognizing this weak supporting evidence for self-examinations, the American Cancer Society, which for two decades had recommended that all women older than 20 years and all postpubertal males should perform monthly breast or testicular self-examinations, respectively, has softened its position on the topic.[6] In 2015, the American Cancer Society reclassified BSE as optional and advised clinicians to educate women about the benefits and limitations of the practice.[7] It now no longer recommends taking time during the periodic health examination to systematically teach patients how to perform self-examination of the breast, skin, or testicles. Its 2006 guidelines for clinicians state only that, "self-examination techniques or increased awareness about signs and symptoms of skin cancer, breast cancer, or testicular cancer can be discussed."[6] Data from a large randomized trial of BSE screening have shown that instruction in BSE has no effect on reducing breast cancer mortality. In one study, 266,064 women were randomly assigned to either receive instruction in BSE or not. Compliance was encouraged through feedback and reinforcement sessions. "After 10 to 11 years of follow-up, 135 breast cancer deaths in the instruction group and 131 in the control group occurred and the cumulative breast cancer mortality rates were not significantly different between the arms. The number of benign breast lesions detected in the BSE instruction group was higher than that detected in the control group. Nevertheless, women should be encouraged to be aware of their breasts because this may facilitate detection of interval cancers between routine screenings."[1]

Other groups have also revisited their view on self-examination practices. For example, in 2017, the American College of Obstetricians and Gynecologists stated that "breast self-examination is not recommended in average-risk women because there is a risk of harm from false-positive test results and a lack of evidence of benefit."[8]

This chapter examines both sides of the controversy. For those clinicians interested in teaching self-examination to their patients, the chapter discusses current methods for teaching and for promoting adherence among patients who have been taught the techniques. The inclusion of these sections by the editors, however, is offered as an information resource for readers but does not necessarily imply an endorsement of self-examination.

THE CONTROVERSY OVER SELF-EXAMINATION

The primary debate over self-examination concerns the question of whether it reduces morbidity or mortality. There is currently no direct evidence from controlled prospective studies that persons who practice self-examination have longer survival from cancer than those who do not. There is some indirect supporting evidence for that outcome, however, primarily related to self-detection of breast cancer. Most breast cancers are first discovered by patients, not by their clinicians.[9] Observational studies suggest that breast cancers detected through self-examination are likely to be smaller and less advanced than those first discovered by clinicians, to have less axillary node involvement, and to be associated with higher survival rates than cancers detected by other means. Another view is when considering health disparities, access to care issues, and no mammograms, detection of a breast mass may indicate there is an advanced malignancy.[10] Similarly, a thin malignant melanoma (less than 0.76 mm thickness) carries little risk of metastatic spread to other sites. Five-year survival for patients with melanomas between 1.5 and 4 mm is approximately 70%, and survival for those with melanomas thicker than 4 mm is approximately 45%.[11]

Skeptics cite several problems with this evidence. First, some observational studies found no benefit from self-examination (although many of these studies suffered from design limitations themselves). Second, although some observational studies have reported a benefit, for example, a case-control study reporting lower incidence and mortality associated with self-examination of melanomas,[12] the higher survival rates may reflect statistical artifacts (e.g., lead-time, length, or selection biases) rather than an actual reduction in mortality. In *lead-time bias,* survival appears to be longer simply because the cancer was diagnosed at an earlier age and not because death was postponed. In *length bias,* self-examination preferentially detects slowly growing tumors rather than aggressive malignancies, producing an artificially higher estimate of survival rates. *Selection bias* reflects the tendency of persons who practice self-examination to come from a more health-conscious population than the general public, making it unclear whether health-promoting practices other than self-examination (e.g., low dietary fat or alcohol intake) are more directly responsible for the observed benefits.

A third limitation relating to BSE data is that many, if not most, women engaging in this practice also undergo screening by clinicians and routine mammography, making it difficult to isolate the benefits attributable to self-examination. Fourth, in the case of testicular cancer, survival is good even without screening. Approximately 60% of testicular seminomas are diagnosed at stage I without screening, and current survival rates approach 100% for early-stage disease.[13] According to the National Cancer Institute, "[t]esticular cancer is so curable even at advanced stages and there are so few cases that it would be virtually impossible to document a decrease in mortality associated with screening."[14] Given these potential biases, the only type of study that can convincingly demonstrate the effectiveness of self-examination is one that is both controlled and prospective, comparing morbidity and mortality rates in persons who do and do not perform self-examination.

Such studies, conducted in China,[15] Russia,[16] and the United Kingdom,[17] did evaluate the effect of teaching BSE on mortality and other outcomes. The three trials, which involved a total of approximately 400,000 women, each demonstrated that self-examination produced no reduction in breast cancer mortality or significant improvements in the number or stage of cancers detected. The Chinese trial, which involved 266,064 female textile workers, concluded that intensive instruction in BSE not only had no effect on mortality but also increased the chances of having a benign breast biopsy, because of the high proportion of false-positive results. In a good-quality nested case-control analysis from a Canadian screening study, the overall practice of BSE was not associated with a reduction in mortality.[18] Meta-analyses and systematic reviews by the Cochrane Collaboration also reported no benefit from BSE in terms of mortality and near doubling in the performance of biopsies.[19] Although none of these studies provides support for BSE, these studies do not entirely exclude the possibility of benefit owing to their limited duration of follow-up and questions about whether results from other countries are generalizable to women in North America.[20]

Proponents of self-examination cite other benefits of the practice beyond lowering mortality. Introducing self-examination at an early age may make patients more familiar with the appearance and texture of their breasts, skin, and testes, thereby enabling more accurate and prompt detection of malignant changes later in life. Self-examination is inexpensive and empowers patients to take a more active role in the care of their body. In rural areas or other regions of the country with limited access to clinicians or imaging centers (e.g., facilities for mammography or scrotal ultrasonography), self-examination may provide the only available means of early cancer detection. However, these potential benefits have remained unproven.

The seeming harmlessness and low cost of self-examination are also debated. The examination skills of patients are often less sensitive and specific than those of clinicians trained in physical examination techniques and familiar with the physical characteristics of suspicious lesions. For example, although breast examination by physicians has a reported sensitivity of 40% to 69%, the reported sensitivity of BSE is only 26% to 41%.[21] The sensitivity of skin and testicular self-examination in detecting cancer is unknown. Reports indicate that the sensitivity of skin self-examination in detecting large nevi or those with new changes is approximately 70%,[22] suggesting that there is an even lower sensitivity in detecting more subtle, malignant lesions.

Self-examination is thought to have a low positive predictive value: a large proportion of abnormalities found by the patient are likely to be benign conditions or normal tissue. For statistical reasons outlined in Chapter 5, the chances of false-positive results are even greater when the target condition is rare. For example, the incidence of testicular cancer is extremely low (less than 3:100,000).[23] Therefore, it is far more likely that abnormal findings on testicular self-examination will be for benign conditions (e.g., epididymitis, spermatocele, and hydrocele) than cancer. The low positive predictive value of self-examination has led some to worry that it may lead to an overdetection of harmless findings and to the unnecessary anxiety, discomfort, and cost of follow-up office visits and biopsies for benign lesions. A Dutch study reported that women who were at increased risk of breast cancer and examined their breasts twice a week had higher scores for psychological distress.[24] As noted earlier, BSE is also associated with an increased risk of breast biopsies generated by false-positive results.

Other potential harms of self-examination have also been discussed. For example, it has been proposed that persons who perform self-examination may mistakenly conclude that, if they do not find an abnormality, routine examinations by clinicians are unnecessary. A particular concern for women is that this misunderstanding about BSE might lead to poorer adherence in obtaining routine examinations by clinicians and mammography screening. Another concern is that a negative workup for an abnormality detected through self-examination might be misjudged by the patient as a reason to discontinue further screening. However, there is little evidence to support these concerns or to suggest that they could not be remedied by proper patient education. In fact, some studies suggest that women who perform BSE are more health conscious and therefore more likely than other women to comply with screening examinations by clinicians.

Another focus of controversy is whether standardized self-examination is more sensitive or specific than incidental detection. Many lesions detected by patients are discovered during bathing, dressing, and other routine activities. It is unclear whether the detection rate that occurs with these normal activities differs appreciably from that of self-examination performed according to a schedule (e.g., monthly) or to the step-by-step techniques recommended by experts.

Recommendations that clinicians incorporate self-examination instructions into routine visits have also drawn criticism. Many practitioners lack enthusiasm for teaching self-examination. In one survey, for example, 82% of physicians were unfamiliar with how to teach testicular self-examination or had not thought about it.[25] A national survey of family physicians in 2002 found that only 24% recommended skin self-examinations in average-risk patients. Lack of time and training and patient reluctance to engage in the practice were cited as the most significant barriers to teaching skin self-examination.[26]

There are several key objections to teaching self-examination. First, a thorough demonstration of self-examination technique is time consuming; busy clinicians often lack the time for such counseling or do so at the expense of other forms of health education. A second concern is the lack of evidence that teaching is effective. Although some studies suggest that teaching self-examination improves patient knowledge levels and self-reported performance of self-examination, other studies have shown no effect. There is evidence that certain techniques do improve the accuracy of skin self-examination. For example, partner interventions and mole-mapping diagrams show promise. Third, self-reports of performance may not correlate with either actual performance or improved detection; knowing how to perform the examination does not necessarily mean that the patient will adhere to the technique.

In a national survey, 88% of women 18 years or older reported that they knew how to perform BSE, but only 43% of the same sample reported performing the procedure at least 12 times each year.[27] Among respondents to the Women Physicians' Health Study, only 21% reported performing monthly BSE[28] (and the patients in that study were *physicians*). A fourth concern, as discussed on page 341, is recidivism: patients who begin practicing self-examination on the advice of their clinician often abandon the practice over time or perform the technique incorrectly.

Nevertheless, these concerns aside, self-examination clearly has the *potential* to reduce morbidity and mortality through early detection. In the case of breast cancer, for example, between 50% and 90% of tumors are first detected by patients and not clinicians. Studies of women undergoing regular breast cancer screening with clinical breast examinations and mammography report that 13% to 17% of cancers are detected by patients, between screenings. Some evidence suggests that breast cancers detected on self-examination are more virulent than those detected on mammography.[29] Although, as noted earlier, theoretic harms from self-examination have been raised, the risks and costs of this simple practice are certainly far less than those of expensive or invasive clinical procedures that are routinely used in patient care despite similarly inadequate supporting evidence. Whether the benefits of self-examination outweigh its harms therefore remains uncertain.

PROPER TECHNIQUE

Clinicians should consider these issues in deciding whether to devote time to teaching patients how to perform self-examination. For those interested in doing so, Tables 15.1–15.3 summarize the key instructions that patients are generally given. **The editors of this book include this information for clinicians who wish to teach self-examination, but the inclusion does not necessarily indicate an endorsement of the practice.**

TABLE 15.1 Instructions for Breast Self-Examination*

Do not check your breasts during your period. The best time is 3–7 d after your period ends.

How to Examine Your Breasts

- Lie down and place your right arm behind your head. The examination is done while lying down, and not standing up. This is because when lying down the breast tissue spreads evenly over the chest wall and it is as thin as possible, making it much easier to feel all the breast tissue.

- Use the finger pads of the three middle fingers on your left hand to feel for lumps in the right breast. Use overlapping dime-sized circular motions of the finger pads to feel the breast tissue.

- Use three different levels of pressure to feel all the breast tissue. Light pressure is needed to feel the tissue closest to the skin; medium pressure to feel a little deeper; and firm pressure to feel the tissue closest to the chest and ribs. A firm ridge in the lower curve of each breast is normal. If you are not sure how hard to press, talk with your doctor or nurse. Use each pressure level to feel the breast tissue before moving on to the next spot.

- Move around the breast in an up and down pattern starting at an imaginary line drawn straight down your side from the underarm and moving across the breast to the middle of the chest bone (sternum or breastbone). Be sure to check the entire breast area going down until you feel only ribs and up to the neck or collarbone (clavicle).

- There is some evidence to suggest that the up and down pattern (sometimes called the *vertical pattern*) is the most effective pattern for covering the entire breast without missing any breast tissue.

- Repeat the examination on your left breast, using the finger pads of the right hand.

- While standing in front of a mirror with your hands pressing firmly down on your hips, look at your breasts for any changes of size, shape, contour, dimpling, pulling, or redness or scaliness of the nipple or breast skin. (The pressing down on the hips position contracts the chest wall muscles and enhances any breast changes.) Continue to look for changes with your arms down at your sides and then with your arms raised up over your head with your palms pressed together.

- Examine each underarm while sitting up or standing and with your arm only slightly raised so you can easily feel in this area. Raising your arm straight up tightens the tissue in this area and makes it difficult to examine.

If there are lumps, knots, nipple discharge, or other suspicious changes, contact your provider.

*The American Cancer Society (ACS) Recommendations for the Early Detection of Breast Cancer do not include breast self-exam. For current ACS breast cancer screening guidelines and statement related to breast self-exam please visit: https://www.cancer.org/cancer/breast-cancer/screening-tests-and-early-detection/american-cancer-society-recommendations-for-the-early-detection-of-breast-cancer.html

TABLE 15.2   Instructions for Skin Self-Examination

Your doctor or nurse may suggest that you do a regular skin self-examination to check for skin cancer, including *melanoma*.

The best time to do this examination is after a shower or bath. You should check your skin in a room with plenty of light. You should use a full-length mirror and a handheld mirror. It is best to begin by learning where your birthmarks, moles, and other marks are and their usual look and feel.

Check for anything new:

- New mole (that looks different from your other moles)
- New red or darker color flaky patch that may be a little raised
- New flesh-colored firm bump
- Change in the size, shape, color, or feel of a mole
- Sore that does not heal

Check yourself from head to toe. Do not forget to check your back, scalp, genital area, and between your buttocks.

- Look at your face, neck, ears, and scalp. You may want to use a comb or a blow dryer to move your hair so that you can see better. You also may want to have a relative or friend check through your hair. It may be hard to check your scalp by yourself.
- Look at the front and back of your body in the mirror. Then, raise your arms and look at your left and right sides.
- Bend your elbows. Look carefully at your fingernails, palms, forearms (including the undersides), and upper arms.

Contact your provider if you notice a change in a mole or other skin marking or if you have a new unexplained mole, skin lump, ulcer, or unhealed sore that has appeared since your last examination.

Adapted from National Cancer Institute. Skin Cancer Treatment - Patient Version. https://www.cancer.gov/types/skin/patient/skin-treatment-pdq. Accessed January 25, 2019.

Unfortunately, the absence of conclusive scientific evidence makes it difficult to know whether each of the steps outlined in Tables 15.1–15.3 is necessary. Few self-examination protocols have been validated in studies that measured clinical outcomes. Studies using intermediate outcomes have often produced conflicting results regarding the importance of specific self-examination procedures.

The lack of evidence of an optimal self-examination protocol should be kept in mind in interpreting the recommendations of some experts that patients perform a series of specific self-examination procedures in special positions, using certain equipment, and sometimes with the assistance of spouses or friends. For example, some instructions for skin

TABLE 15.3 Instructions for Testicular Self-Examination
• Perform the examination after a warm bath or shower, while your hands are still warm.
• Examine each testicle gently with both hands. The index and middle fingers should be placed underneath the testicle, whereas the thumbs are placed on top. Roll the testicle gently between the thumbs and fingers.
• Your testicles should feel smooth, rubbery, and slightly tender. Surfaces should be smooth and without lumps. It is common for one testicle to be larger than the other.
• Feel for any abnormal hard lumps, nodules, or swelling on the front or side of the testicle.
• The epididymis is a cordlike structure on the top and back of the testicle. Do not confuse the epididymis with an abnormal lump.
If you find a lump, nodule, swelling, or dull ache, or if you notice another change, contact your provider.

Adapted from National Cancer Institute. *Testicular Self-Examination NIH Publication No. 94-2636.* Bethesda: National Cancer Institute; 1994.

self-examination specify multiple examination positions and the need for a full-length or hand-held mirror, blow dryer, two chairs, or an examination partner. Although common sense suggests that following these instructions would help patients examine themselves more carefully, there is no evidence that they achieve higher detection rates than more limited self-examinations. Quite the contrary, routines that are so complex may discourage patients from performing self-examination. Finally, there is no evidence to support the common advice to perform self-examination every month; no studies have determined whether monthly self-checks achieve higher detection rates than less frequent examinations.

ADHERENCE

Most persons who are advised to perform monthly self-examinations do not do so, and a large proportion of persons who receive counseling or training to perform self-examination do not maintain the habit over time. Persons are more likely to perform self-examination if they fear cancer and believe that they are susceptible, believe that self-examination is an effective screening tool, understand how to perform the procedure, and have confidence in their examination skills (self-efficacy).

The principal barriers to performance include the absence of these beliefs, as well as fears of finding an abnormality, embarrassment, lack of time, and forgetting to do so. Poor adherence is also sometimes due to misconceptions, such as believing that cancer can be detected early by simply paying attention to symptoms or that a healthy lifestyle is fully protective against cancer. Some barriers are related to age. BSE and the recognition of suspicious lesions by older women can be impaired by poor visual acuity, tactile sensation, and range of motion. Testicular examination and BSE by adolescent boys and girls, respectively, can be influenced by embarrassment and uncomfortable feelings about body image.

Teaching patients how to perform self-examination, by itself, is unlikely to be effective if the clinician does not also address these concerns. Therefore, clinicians who have decided, despite the caveats mentioned earlier, to teach self-examination must do more than teach the technique to achieve the desired ends. That is, the likelihood of adherence is increased if clinicians take time to assess the patient's understanding of the underlying rationale, attitudes, and beliefs about cancer and early detection, perceived self-efficacy, and relevant fears and anxieties about detecting cancer. Practical constraints, such as lack of time, privacy, and the need for reminders to perform self-examination, should also be addressed. The physical and cognitive limitations of older adults should receive special attention. Once this information has been gathered, the clinician's counseling about self-examination should be tailored to the patient's concerns. This may include correcting misconceptions about cancer, reassuring the patient that his or her self-examination technique is correct, suggesting reminder systems, and altering instructions for patients with physical limitations.

Patient education materials are often useful to help patients remember when to perform self-examination and to remind them of the proper technique. Although pamphlets and websites (see "Resources—Patient Education Materials" at the end of this chapter) are often used to supplement counseling, videotapes and films are sometimes more effective in demonstrating examination techniques. With the advances in technology, personal computers and mobile devices are now equipped to offer a variety of selections in the form of apps. Self-examination can be taught in group settings, but the evidence is equivocal regarding the relative superiority of individual versus group counseling. Finally, patients need reminders and reinforcements to continue performing self-examination. Studies have shown that reassessment and retraining in BSE may achieve higher breast lump detection rates. Therefore, after teaching patients how to perform self-examination, clinicians may find it useful to reassess their performance and proficiency at a later date.

OFFICE AND CLINIC ORGANIZATION

Offices and clinics in which self-examination is taught should have private examination rooms in which the technique can be demonstrated. Some practices use models, diagrams, and illustrations as teaching aids. Patient education materials that reinforce and explain further the technique of self-examination and that define abnormal results should be easily accessible to hand to the patient, or a list of useful websites should be provided. Photographs of malignant and premalignant skin lesions, included either in office teaching aids or patient education resources, may help the patient identify important skin findings.

SUGGESTED RESOURCES AND MATERIALS

Breast Self-Examination

American Cancer Society
How to Perform a Breast Self-Examination
http://www.cancer.org/docroot/CRI/content/CRI_2_6x_How_to_perform_a_breast_self_exam_5.asp. Accessed 2007.

Skin Self-Examination

American Cancer Society
Overview: Skin Cancer—Melanoma. How is Melanoma Skin Cancer Found?
http://www.cancer.org/docroot/CRI/content/CRI_2_2_3X_How_is_melanoma_skin_cancer_found_50.asp?sitearea=. Accessed 2007.

National Cancer Institute
What You Need to Know About Skin Cancer
http://www.cancer.gov/cancertopics/wyntk/skin/page1. Accessed 2007.

National Cancer Institute
How to Do a Skin Self-Examination
http://www.cancer.gov/cancertopics/wyntk/skin/page13.

Testicular Self-Examination

American Cancer Society
Detailed Guide: Testicular Cancer. Can Testicular Cancer Be Found Early?
http://www.cancer.org/docroot/CRI/content/CRI_2_4_3X_Can_Testicular_Cancer_Be_Found_Early_41.asp?sitearea=. Accessed 2007.

REFERENCES

1. Bevers TB, Anderson BO, Bonaccio E, et al. Breast cancer screening and diagnosis. *J Natl Compr Canc Netw.* 2009;7(10):1060-1096. doi:10.6004/jnccn.2009.0070.
2. U.S. Preventive Services Task Force. *Screening for Breast Cancer: Recommendations and Rationale.* Rockville: Agency for Healthcare Research and Quality; December 2013. http://www.ahrq.gov/clinic/3rduspstf/breastcancer/brcanrr.htm.
3. U.S. Preventive Services Task Force. *Counseling to Prevent Skin Cancer: Recommendations and Rationale.* Rockville: Agency for Healthcare Research and Quality; March 2014. http://www.ahrq.gov/clinic/3rduspstf/skcacoun/skcarr.htm.
4. U.S. Preventive Services Task Force. *Screening for Testicular Cancer: Recommendation Statement.* Rockville: Agency for Healthcare Research and Quality; February 2004. http://www.ahrq.gov/clinic/3rduspstf/testicular/testiculrs.htm.
5. American Academy of Family Physicians. *Clinical Preventive Services;* 2007. http://www.aafp.org/online/en/home/clinical/exam.html.
6. Smith RA, Cokkinides V, Eyre HJ. American Cancer Society guidelines for the early detection of cancer, 2006. *CA Cancer J Clin.* 2006;56:11-25.

7. Smith RA, Andrews K, Brooks D, et al. Cancer screening in the United States, 2016: a review of current American Cancer Society guidelines and current issues in cancer screening. *CA Cancer J Clin.* 2016;66(2):95-114. doi:10.3322/caac.21336.

8. Practice Bulletin No. 179 summary: breast cancer risk assessment and screening in average-risk women. *Obstet Gynecol.* 2017;130(1):241-243. doi:10.1097/AOG.0000000000002151.

9. Foster RS, Worden JK, Costanza MC, et al. Clinical breast examination and breast self-examination. *Cancer.* 1992;69:1992-1998.

10. Miranda PY, Tarraf W, González HM. Breast cancer screening and ethnicity in the United States: implications for health disparities research. *Breast Cancer Res Treat.* 2011;128(2):535-542. doi:10.1007/s10549-011-1367-8.

11. Agency for Healthcare Research and Quality. Screening for skin cancer: summary of the evidence. *Am J Prev.* December 2013;20(3S):47-58. Rockville: Agency for Healthcare Research and Quality, Article originally in http://www.ahrq.gov/clinic/ajpmsuppl/helfand1.htm .

12. Berwick M, Begg CB, Fine JA, et al. Screening for cutaneous melanoma by skin self-examination [see comments]. *J Natl Cancer Inst.* 1996;88(1):17-23.

13. American Cancer Society. *Testicular Cancer,* 2007. http://www.cancer.org/downloads/PRO/TesticularCancer.pdf.

14. National Cancer Institute. *Testicular Cancer (PDQ®): Screening,* 2007. http://www.cancer.gov/cancertopics/pdq/screening/testicular/HealthProfessional/page2.

15. Thomas DB, Gao DL, Ray RM, et al. Randomized trial of breast self-examination in Shanghai: final results. *J Natl Cancer Inst.* 2002;94:1445-1457.

16. Semiglazov VF, Moiseenko VM, Manikhas AG, et al. Role of breast self-examination in early detection of breast cancer: Russia/WHO prospective randomized trial in St. Petersburg. *Cancer Strategy.* 1999;1:145-151.

17. UK Breast Cancer Detection Working Group. 16-year mortality from breast cancer in the UK trial of early detection of breast cancer. *Lancet.* 1999;353(9168):1909-1914.

18. Harvey BJ, Miller AB, Baines CJ, et al. Effect of breast self-examination techniques on the risk of death from breast cancer. *CMAJ.* 1997;157(9):1205-1212.

19. Kosters JP, Gotzsche PC. Regular self-examination or clinical examination for early detection of breast cancer. *Cochrane Database Syst Rev.* 2003;(2):CD003373.

20. Kearney AJ, Murray M. Evidence against breast self-examination is not conclusive: what policymakers and health professionals need to know. *J Public Health Policy.* 2006;27:282-292.

21. Humphrey LL, Chan BKS, Detlefsen S, et al. *Screening for Breast Cancer. Systematic Evidence Review No. 15, (Prepared by the Oregon Health & Science University Evidence-based Practice Center under Contract No. 290-97-0018).* Rockville: Agency for Healthcare Research and Quality; September 2002. Available on the AHRQ Web site at www.ahrq.gov/clinic/serfiles.htm: .

22. Oliveria SA, Chau D, Christos PJ, et al. Diagnostic accuracy of patients in performing skin self-examination and the impact of photography. *Arch Dermatol.* 2004;140:57-62.

23. National Cancer Institute. *AGE-adjusted SEER Incidence and U.S. Death Rates and 5-year Relative Survival Rates,* 2000–2003. http://seer.cancer.gov/csr/1975_2003/results_single/sect_01_table.04_2pgs.pdf.

24. van Dooren S, Rijnsburger AJ, Seynaeve C, et al. Psychological distress and breast self-examination frequency in women at increased risk for hereditary or familial breast cancer. *Community Genet.* 2003;6:235-241.

25. Sayger SA, Fortenberry JD, Beckman RJ. Practice patterns of teaching testicular self-examination to adolescent patients. *J Adolesc Health Care.* 1988;9:441-442.

26. Geller AC, O'Riordan DL, Oliveria SA, et al. Overcoming obstacles to skin cancer examinations and prevention counseling for high-risk patients: results of a national survey of primary care physicians. *J Am Board Fam Pract.* 2004;17:416-423.

27. Piani A, Schoenborn C. National Center for Health Statistics. Health promotion and disease prevention: United States, 1990. *Vital Health Stat.* 1993;10(185):59.
28. Frank E, Rimer BK, Brogan D, et al. U.S. women physicians' personal and clinical breast cancer screening practices. *J Womens Health Gend Based Med.* 2000;9:791-801.
29. Kaplan HG, Malmgren JA. Disease-specific survival in patient-detected breast cancer. *Clin Breast Cancer.* 2006;7(2):133-140

Please see Online Appendix: Apps and Digital Resources for additional information.

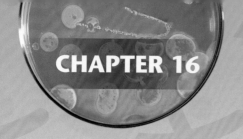
Chemoprophylaxis

MARY DIETMANN

BACKGROUND

Chemoprophylaxis (or chemoprevention) in preventive medicine is the use of drugs, nutritional and mineral supplements, or other natural substances by asymptomatic persons to prevent future disease. It does not include using such agents to treat symptomatic illnesses or in persons with a prior history of the disorder. This chapter examines the use of medications for chemoprophylaxis. (Examples of other agents used for chemoprophylaxis are iron supplements in menstruating or pregnant women or in young children to decrease the risk of iron-deficiency anemia, fluoride supplements to decrease the risk of dental caries, folic acid supplements to decrease women's risk of giving birth to children with neural tube defects, and multivitamins to reduce the risk of cancer and heart disease. Only some of these practices are fully supported by current evidence.) Chemoprophylactic agents are used in people without the condition for which they are taking the medication; therefore, great care must be taken to be certain that the benefits of the agents substantially outweigh their harms.

This chapter examines three common situations in which drugs (or classes of drugs) may (or may not) be recommended for chemoprophylaxis: selective estrogen receptor modulators to prevent breast cancer; aspirin to prevent heart disease, stroke, and possibly cancer; and postmenopausal hormone therapy to prevent chronic conditions, such as heart disease. The chapter examines the role of these drugs in primary prevention (i.e., for asymptomatic persons). It does not focus on the use of tamoxifen to treat breast cancer, the use of aspirin in patients with known cardiovascular disease, and the use of estrogen to control postmenopausal symptoms.

CHEMOPREVENTION OF BREAST CANCER

Despite improvements in the rates of screening and early detection and advances in treatment, breast cancer remains the most commonly diagnosed nonskin cancer among women in the United States. It is not possible to modify the strongest risk factors for breast cancer—increasing age and a family history. Therefore, other preventive strategies must be considered. Evidence that drugs might be able to prevent breast cancer was first recognized in trials testing tamoxifen as adjuvant chemotherapy in women with breast cancer. Tamoxifen is a member of a class of drugs called *selective estrogen receptor modulators*, compounds with both estrogen-like and antiestrogen properties. In a meta-analysis of 55 studies of adjuvant tamoxifen chemotherapy, the drug was found to reduce the risk of new cancer in the opposite breast by 47% (*P* < .001) among women who took tamoxifen for 5 years.[1]

Breast cancer prevention with tamoxifen in women at increased risk of breast cancer has been studied in four randomized clinical trials; raloxifene, another selective estrogen receptor modulator, has been studied in three trials. A meta-analysis of the tamoxifen trials showed a 38% reduction (95% confidence interval [CI], 28%–46%) in breast cancer incidence after 5 years of therapy.[2] Raloxifene was found to reduce incidence by 72% (95% CI, 54%–83%) after 4 years in a trial of postmenopausal women with osteoporosis[3] and by 44% (95% CI, 17%–62%) in a trial of postmenopausal women with coronary heart disease (CHD) or risk factors for CHD.[4] Both drugs reduce the incidence of estrogen receptor–positive tumors only. In the Study of Tamoxifen and Raloxifene (STAR) trial, a direct comparison of the two drugs in postmenopausal women at increased risk of breast cancer, the drugs were found to be equally effective and reduced expected cancers by 50%.[5] No benefit in terms of breast cancer mortality has yet been seen in any trial. Aromatase inhibitors, useful in the treatment of breast cancer, are also under consideration as chemoprophylactic agents. Tamoxifen is the only agent currently approved by the U.S. Food and Drug Administration (FDA) for primary breast cancer risk reduction (chemoprevention) in high-risk women; approval for raloxifene to be used for this indication is under review at this writing.

The use of these drugs, however, carries an increased risk of harms, a significant concern given that the women who take them do not have invasive cancer. Both tamoxifen and raloxifene are associated with a threefold higher risk for venous thromboembolic disease, especially pulmonary embolism, although the actual number of events in the studies was small.[6] Increases in stroke and deep venous thrombosis were also noted but not found to be statistically significant (except for the risk of fatal stroke in one study[4]). Tamoxifen, but not raloxifene, has been shown to increase the risk of stage I endometrial cancer and uterine sarcoma. These serious side effects occur mostly in women aged 50 years and older. In the STAR trial, however, postmenopausal women taking raloxifene not only had 36% fewer uterine cancers but also 29% fewer blood clots than the women who were assigned to take tamoxifen. Both tamoxifen and raloxifene are associated with an increased incidence of hot flashes, and tamoxifen is associated with an increased incidence of bothersome vaginal discharge. Raloxifene is also effective in reducing the risk of osteoporotic fractures in older women.

Official Recommendations

The U.S. Preventive Services Task Force (USPSTF) recommends against the routine use of tamoxifen or raloxifene for the primary prevention of breast cancer in women at low or average risk of breast cancer.[7] The USPSTF recommends that clinicians discuss chemoprevention with women at high risk of breast cancer and at low risk of adverse effects from chemoprevention. The American Society of Clinical Oncology recommends offering tamoxifen (at 20 mg/d for 5 years) to premenopausal women aged 35 years or older with a defined 5-year projected breast cancer risk of greater than or equal to 1.66%.[8] Raloxifene (60 mg/d for 5 years) or exemestane (25 mg/d for 5 years) are also recommended for discussion with postmenopausal women to reduce risk for this population.[8] The group does not recommend the use of any other selective estrogen receptive modulator or aromatase inhibitor outside of a clinical trial setting.[8]

Essentials of Counseling

Clinicians should discuss the pros and cons of breast cancer prevention with women for whom benefits would likely be greater than harms. Women with higher breast cancer risk are more likely to benefit from chemoprevention than women with lower risk, and younger women are less likely to suffer harms than older women; therefore, the group of women for whom benefits are most likely to exceed harms is younger women at higher risk of breast cancer. There is no definitive cutoff to indicate low versus high risk for breast cancer. Women are considered at high risk of breast cancer if their risk factors include a family history of breast cancer in a first-degree relative (mother, sister, or daughter), previous breast biopsy showing atypical hyperplasia, early age of menarche, or late age at first pregnancy or no pregnancy.

An estimated 5-year risk can be calculated from the Gail risk model calculator. The Gail model was developed from a large study of breast cancer screening and has been shown to be accurate in follow-up studies. Other risk assessment models, such as one developed by Claus et al., are also available; each has advantages and disadvantages. A risk level of greater than 1.66% in 5 years has been used in one of the major breast cancer chemoprevention trials as an indication of increased risk (but that level was chosen for statistical analysis reasons, not because it carried biologic significance). This approach to breast cancer chemoprevention does not apply to women with genetic abnormalities, such as *BRCA1* or *BRCA2* abnormalities, who have a much higher risk of breast cancer and require testing and preventive measures as discussed in Chapter 5.

An approximation of the balance between benefits and harms is shown in Figure 16.1. The benefits (sloped lines) increase with increasing breast cancer risk, whereas the harms (flat horizontal lines) are age dependent and not related to breast cancer risk. Keep in mind, however, that women may weigh

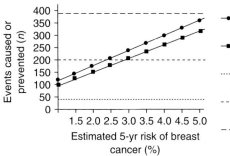

Figure 16.1   Benefits and harms of chemoprevention with tamoxifen per 10,000 women in three age groups. Harms include endometrial cancer, stroke, and pulmonary embolism combined. Adapted from Gail MH, Constantino JP, Bryant J, et al. Weighing the risks and benefits of tamoxifen treatment for prevention. *J Natl Cancer Inst*. 1999;91:1829-1846.

the importance of these outcomes differently. The possible benefit of reducing the risk of breast cancer may have more value for some women than does an increased risk of early-stage endometrial cancer (or vice versa). These estimates of benefits and harms should be applied only to white women, as the chemoprevention trials included few women of color. The trade-off between benefits and harms will likely be less favorable for African American women, who have a lower risk of breast cancer and higher background rates of adverse events. The proportion of women aged 35 to 70 years who are potentially eligible for tamoxifen chemoprevention has been estimated to be 15.5% (18.7% of white women, 5.7% of African American women, and 2.9% of Hispanic women).[9] Only a small percentage of eligible women are likely to have a positive benefit/risk index. Studies in clinical settings have found, so far, that few women are willing to take chemoprevention, citing concerns about potential adverse effects as the main limiting factor.[10]

The current recommended dose of tamoxifen is 20 mg/d for 5 years. The recommended dose for raloxifene is 60 mg/d for 5 years and for exemestane 25 mg/d for 5 years. Benefits appear to last longer than 5 years, but the total duration of effect is not known. Because the detrimental effect of tamoxifen on the endometrium is dose dependent and the drug has a long half-life, a lower dose has been suggested as a possible way to reduce side effects, but studies to determine the optimal dose have not yet been completed.

Contraindications

Women at increased risk of adverse effects from tamoxifen, raloxifene, or exemestane should carefully consider taking breast cancer chemoprevention. Women with a uterus should report any vaginal bleeding when taking tamoxifen. Women should report symptoms of chest pain, shortness of breath, or leg pain and swelling when taking either tamoxifen or raloxifene.

ASPIRIN PROPHYLAXIS

This section examines the use of low-dose aspirin (50–325 mg/d) for primary prevention of heart disease, stroke, and possibly cancer. Aspirin has been shown to reduce the risk of mortality and subsequent vascular events for patients with known cardiovascular disease (secondary prevention) and is highly recommended in that setting. The use of aspirin for primary prevention, however, is more controversial: the benefits and adverse effects in patients at lower risk are more closely balanced, and decisions about who should or should not take aspirin require careful consideration of risks and of patient preferences and values.

At this writing (2018), the effectiveness of aspirin for the primary prevention of cardiovascular events has been examined in six large randomized trials. A meta-analysis of five of these studies found that men who take aspirin daily can reduce their relative odds of coronary events by 28%.[11] The five studies included in this meta-analysis were 4 to 7 years in duration and compared doses of aspirin ranging from 75 to 500 mg/d. Three of the five trials included only men; two others included mixed populations of men and women. The results for women are discussed in the subsequent text.

In addition to its effect on total coronary events, evidence from these five trials also suggested that aspirin may reduce the risk of fatal CHD events by 13%, although the summary result did not reach statistical significance. The effect on total mortality was smaller (7% reduction) and also statistically nonsignificant, reflecting the fact that few participants died over the 4- to 7-year duration of these trials. The effect of aspirin on the development of angina is unclear—the trials that measured this outcome produced mixed results. In these five trials, aspirin did not reduce the risk of ischemic stroke, although the ascertainment of the nature of strokes in these trials (some of which predate the widespread routine use of neuroimaging for acute stroke) was suboptimal. In terms of adverse effects, aspirin increased the incidence of major gastrointestinal bleeding and hemorrhagic stroke (odds ratios of 1.7 and 1.4, respectively).[12]

Effectiveness in Women

The effectiveness of aspirin prophylaxis in women has been examined in three trials. In two, women were included in mixed populations of patients. Although the total number of women enrolled in these two studies was large, the relatively small number of cardiovascular events occurring in these women made estimates of the effects of aspirin imprecise.[9] Relevant data were published in 2005 by the large Women's Health Study, a 10-year trial of more than 39,000 women health professionals aged 45 years and older who were randomized to aspirin 100 mg every other day versus placebo.[13] The Women's Health Study found that aspirin reduced the risk of ischemic stroke by 24% but had no effect on myocardial infarction overall. The risk of adverse effects was similar to previous trials: aspirin increased the risk of major gastrointestinal bleeding and hemorrhagic stroke. In subgroup analysis, older women (65 years and older) derived greater benefit: in addition to a reduction in stroke, aspirin also reduced the risk of myocardial infarction.

The overall results of the Women's Health Study stand in contrast to previous evidence regarding aspirin prophylaxis in men (for whom myocardial infarction but not stroke was reduced) and evidence from secondary prevention (where the effects in men and women have been similar). It is currently unclear whether the observed differences are true biological differences or whether they may result from the low dosage of aspirin tested in the Women's Health Study or from the simple effects of chance.[14]

Other Effects

Beyond its effect on cardiovascular events, evidence from some observational studies suggests that aspirin may reduce the risk of colorectal cancer.[15] Aspirin also reduces headaches and can have other pain-relieving effects; on the other hand, aspirin can also cause dyspepsia and increase the risk of minor bleeding and bruising.

Official Recommendations

The USPSTF recommends that clinicians discuss aspirin with patients when the 10-year risk of CHD events is 6% or greater.[16] These discussions should include information about potential benefits and harms, and the final decision about whether to take aspirin should be informed by the relative chances of beneficial and adverse outcomes. The American Heart Association recommends aspirin prophylaxis when the 10-year risk of CHD events is greater than 10%.[17]

Essentials of Counseling

Clinicians should discuss the potential benefits and harms of routine aspirin use with men and women older than 40 years. To do so effectively, clinicians should estimate the patient's 10-year risk of cardiovascular events, using an appropriate (e.g., Framingham) risk calculator (Chapter 2).[18] Patients at low risk (men with a 10-year CHD risk less than 5% or women with a 10-year stroke risk less than 2%) should be counseled against aspirin use, as the benefits in these populations may not exceed the harms. For patients at increased CHD risk (men with a 10-year CHD risk greater than 10% or women older than 65 years with a stroke risk of 3% or greater) who are not at increased risk of adverse effects, aspirin can generally be recommended.

For patients between these risk levels, the decision about whether to take aspirin will depend on how the patient feels about the relative chances and impact of the potential benefits and harms, the extent to which taking a daily pill is onerous, and alternative means of reducing cardiovascular risk. Patients who choose to begin aspirin prophylaxis should take 75 to 325 mg daily, based on the dosages tested in most trials.

Contraindications

Routine aspirin use may not be appropriate for patients with a history of peptic ulcer disease, gastrointestinal bleeding, cerebral hemorrhage, history of uncontrolled hypertension, a bleeding diathesis, allergy to aspirin, liver or kidney disease, or diabetic retinopathy.

POSTMENOPAUSAL HORMONE THERAPY

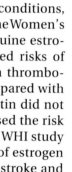

Postmenopausal use of estrogen with or without concomitant use of progestin in healthy women for the prevention of chronic conditions, such as heart disease, is no longer recommended. Results of the Women's Health Initiative (WHI) indicated that use of conjugated equine estrogen and medroxyprogesterone acetate resulted in increased risks of breast cancer, myocardial infarction, stroke, and deep vein thrombosis and reduced risks of colorectal cancer and fractures compared with placebo (see Table 16.1).[19] In addition, estrogen and progestin did not protect against mild cognitive impairment, and they increased the risk of dementia in women aged 65 years and older.[20] In a second WHI study of more than 10,000 women with prior hysterectomies, use of estrogen alone compared with placebo resulted in increased risks of stroke and deep vein thrombosis, reduced risk of fracture, and no significant effect on breast cancer, colorectal cancer, and myocardial infarction (Table 16.1).[21] Both trials were discontinued early because of lack of benefit and concern for harms. Findings from the two studies cannot be compared directly because women in the estrogen-alone study were more likely to have CHD risk factors at baseline, such as hypertension, high blood cholesterol, diabetes, and obesity.

Results of the WHI confirmed and refuted prior evidence about the effects of postmenopausal hormone therapy on multiple health outcomes.[22] Its unanticipated adverse effect on cardiovascular disease, in particular, shifted the balance of benefits and harms. As a result, recommendations changed and the FDA placed safety warnings on estrogen products and altered indications for use. Estrogen is currently approved for relief of moderate to severe hot flashes and symptoms of vulvar and vaginal atrophy, and it should be used at the lowest dose for the shortest duration needed to achieve treatment goals. Estrogen is also approved for the prevention of postmenopausal osteoporosis, but it is not considered a first-line agent. Estrogen therapy should not be taken to prevent heart disease or other chronic conditions.

TABLE 16.1 Estimates of Main Benefits and Harms From the Women's Health Initiative (WHI) trials (Number of Events per 10,000 Women per Year)

Combined Therapy Trial		Estrogen-Alone Trial	
Estrogen + Progestin	Placebo	Estrogen	Placebo
38	30	26[a]	33
37	30	49[a]	54
29	21	44	32
26	13	21	15
10	15	11	17
10	16	17[a]	16
52[a]	53	81[a]	78

Adapted from Writing Group for the Women's Health Initiative Investigators. Risks and benefits of estrogen plus progestin in healthy postmenopausal women: principal results from the Women's Health Initiative randomized controlled trial. *JAMA.* 2002;288:321-333 and Writing Group for the Women's Health Initiative Investigators. Effects of conjugated equine estrogen in postmenopausal women with hysterectomy. *JAMA.* 2004;291:1701-1712.
[a]Differences between treatment and placebo are not statistically significant using unadjusted hazard ratios.

Official Recommendations

The USPSTF recommends against the routine use of either combined estrogen and progestin or estrogen alone for the prevention of chronic conditions in postmenopausal women.[23] After review of the evidence, including results of the WHI, the USPSTF concluded that the harmful effects of either combined estrogen and progestin or estrogen alone are likely to exceed the chronic disease prevention benefits in most women. Professional societies, such as the American College of Physicians, American Academy of Obstetricians and Gynecologists,[24] American Academy of Family Physicians, and the North American Menopause Society,[25] have taken similar positions.

Essentials of Counseling

Women who use or are considering using postmenopausal hormone therapy should discuss the possible benefits and harms with their clinicians. Women should initiate postmenopausal hormone therapy only for the currently approved indications and only if potential benefits outweigh potential harms. Hormone therapy to treat hot flashes and vulvovaginal atrophy is most often initiated in women at least 10 years younger than women enrolled in the WHI trials,[26] and the generalizability of the WHI findings to guide their care is therefore unclear. Subgroup analyses of women in the WHI aged 50 to 59 years and those with menopausal symptoms are limited by small numbers of subjects and adverse events. Potential harms could be reduced by using the smallest effective dose for the shortest duration necessary.

As noted, estrogen is effective for the prevention of osteoporosis and fractures,[27,28] although other FDA-approved agents, such as bisphosphonates, are also available. Women with substantial risks for osteoporosis and fractures and who are intolerant of other medications may be appropriate candidates for estrogen. Risk estimates from the WHI may be applicable in weighing potential benefits and harms of long-term therapy depending on the candidate's age.

Women who have been taking postmenopausal hormones for a long while based on outdated information about the benefits should discontinue use. Although many women are able to discontinue estrogen easily, many others experience hot flashes and other ill effects, such as pain or stiffness, after stopping use.[29] Reducing doses in a stepwise taper may minimize symptoms. This can be done by decreasing the daily dose, reducing the numbers of days per week that estrogen is taken, or a combination of these approaches. Some women may require several weeks or months at each step. As with all patients changing or discontinuing a therapy, a woman discontinuing estrogen should follow up periodically with her clinician to assess response, monitor adverse effects, reexamine needs, and make adjustments.

Contraindications

Women considering hormone therapy for approved indications should not be prescribed estrogen if they have prior or current breast cancer, are pregnant, or have thrombophlebitis, endometrial cancer, or unevaluated abnormal vaginal bleeding.

OFFICE AND CLINIC ORGANIZATION

Offices or clinics should develop plans to routinely assess the breast cancer risk of women aged 40 years and older. Younger women (those younger than 55 years) who do not have a family history of breast cancer and who have not had a breast biopsy are not likely to be at increased risk of breast cancer, so further risk assessment is generally not necessary.[30] Women in their late 50s and older do benefit from risk assessment, however, and practices should have access to a 5-year breast cancer risk calculator, which can be used on a handheld device, smartphone, or online (http://www.cancer.gov/bcrisktool/). Patient education materials on breast cancer risk and use of chemoprevention should be available for patients.

Offices and clinics should also develop plans to routinely assess the cardiovascular risk of all men and women aged 40 years and older, as well as younger persons with other cardiovascular risk factors. Framingham risk calculators are available online at http://hp2010.nhl-bihin.net/atpiii/calculator.asp?usertype=prof, as discussed further in Chapter 2. Patients' cardiovascular risk assessments should be made available to clinicians so that appropriate counseling about chemoprophylaxis can be provided and other cardiovascular interventions considered. The office should offer relevant decision aid materials in the waiting area and in the examining room, so that the clinician can hand the brochures or website listings directly to the patient after counseling. For further reading on shared decision making, please refer to Chapter 22.

Patient education materials about postmenopausal hormone therapy should also be readily available, especially for women who have been taking these drugs and may have questions about why and how to discontinue them.

SUGGESTED RESOURCES AND MATERIALS

Breast Cancer Chemoprevention

American Cancer Society
Clifton Road
Atlanta, GA
Medicines to Reduce Breast Cancer Risk
http://www.cancer.org/docroot/CRI/content/CRI_2_6X_Tamoxifen_and_
    Raloxifene_Questions_and_Answers_5.asp.

National Cancer Institute
Bethesda, MD
1-800-4-CANCER (1-800-422-6237), 9:00 a.m. to 4:30 p.m. local time, Monday through
    Friday
Breast Cancer (PDQ): Prevention
http://www.cancer.gov/cancertopics/pdq/prevention/breast/patient.

U.S. Preventive Services Task Force
Breast Cancer Chemoprevention
http://www.ahrq.gov/clinic/uspstf/uspsbrpv.htm.

Aspirin Prophylaxis

American Heart Association
Office of Scientific Affairs
7272 Greenville Avenue
Dallas, TX 75231–4596
800-242-8721
Aspirin as a Therapeutic Agent in Cardiovascular Disease
UpToDate
Patient Information: Aspirin and Cardiovascular Disease
http://patients.uptodate.com/topic.asp?file=hrt_dis/2908.

U.S. Preventive Services Task Force
Aspirin Chemoprevention
http://www.ahrq.gov/clinic/uspstf/uspsasmi.htm.

Postmenopausal Hormone Therapy

Agency for Healthcare Research and Quality
Rockville, MD
Postmenopausal Hormone Replacement Therapy for Primary Prevention of Chronic Conditions
http://www.ahrq.gov/clinic/3rduspstf/hrt/hrtwh.htm.

Food and Drug Administration
Estrogen and Estrogen with Progestin Therapies for Postmenopausal Women
http://www.fda.gov/cder/drug/infopage/estrogens progestins/default.htm.

National Heart, Lung, and Blood Institute
Bethesda, MD
Facts About Menopausal Hormone Therapy
http://www.nhlbi.nih.gov/health/women/pht_facts.htm.

National Institute on Aging
Bethesda, MD
Hormones After Menopause
http://www.niapublications.org/agepages/hormonesafter.asp.

U.S. Preventive Services Task Force
Postmenopausal Hormone Therapy
http://www.ahrq.gov/clinic/uspstf/uspspmho.htm.

Women's Health Initiative
http://www.nhlbi.nih.gov/whi/index.html.

SUGGESTED READINGS

Cusick J, Powles T, Veronesi U, et al. Overview of the main outcomes in breast-cancer prevention trials. *Lancet.* 2003;361:296-300.
Peto R, Gray R, Collins R, et al. Randomized trial of prophylactic daily aspirin in British male doctors. *Br Med J.* 1988;296:313-316.
Steering Committee of the Physicians' Health Study Research Group. Final report on the aspirin components of the ongoing Physicians' Health Study. *N Engl J Med.* 1989;321:129-135.
Writing Group for the Women's Health Initiative Investigators. Risks and benefits of estrogen plus progestin in healthy postmenopausal women. *JAMA.* 2002;288:321-333.
Writing Group for the Women's Health Initiative Investigators. Effects of conjugated equine estrogen in postmenopausal women with hysterectomy. *JAMA.* 2004;291:1701-1712.

REFERENCES

1. Early Breast Cancer Trialists' Collaborative Group. Tamoxifen for early breast cancer: an overview of the randomized trials. *Lancet.* 1998;351:1451-1467.
2. Cusick J, Powles T, Veronesi U, et al. Overview of the main outcomes in breast-cancer prevention trials. *Lancet.* 2003;361:296-300.
3. Cauley JA, Norton L, Lippman ME, et al. Continued breast cancer risk reduction in postmenopausal women treated with raloxifene: 4-year results from the MORE trial. Multiple outcomes of raloxifene evaluation. *Breast Cancer Res Treat.* 2001;65:125-134.

4. Barrett-Conner E, Mosca L, Collins P, et al. Effects of raloxifene on cardio-vascular events and breast cancer in postmenopausal women. *N Engl J Med.* 2006;355:125-137.
5. Vogel GV, Costantino JP, Wickerham DL, et al. Effects of tamoxifen vs. raloxi-fene on the risk of developing invasive breast cancer and other disease out-comes. The NS ABP Study of Tamoxifen and Raloxifne (STAR) P-2 Trial. *JAMA.* 2006;295:2727-2741.
6. Kinsinger LS, Harris R, Woolf SW, et al. Chemoprevention of breast cancer: a summary of the evidence for the U.S. Preventive Services Task Force. *Ann Intern Med.* 2002;137:59-67.
7. Epling J. The "other" preventive services: behavioral risk factor counseling and chemoprophylaxis recommendations from the US Preventive Services Task Force. *Family Doctor.* 2014;2:17-20.
8. Visvanathan K, Hurley P, Bantug E, et al. Use of pharmacological interventions for breast cancer risk reduction: American Society of Clinical Oncology practice guidelines. *J Clin Oncol.* 2013;23:2942-2962.
9. Freedman AN, Graubard BI, Rao AR, et al. Estimates of the number of US women who could benefit from tamoxifen for breast cancer chemoprevention. *J Natl Cancer Inst.* 2003;95:526-532.
10. Melnikow J, Paternitit D, Azari R, et al. Preferences of women evaluating risks of tamoxifen (POWER) study of preferences for tamoxifen for breast cancer risk reduction. *Cancer.* 2005;103:1996-2005.
11. Hayden M, Pignone M, Phillips C, et al. Aspirin for the primary prevention of cardiovascular events: a summary of the evidence for the U.S. Preventive Services Task Force. *Ann Intern Med.* 2002;136:161-172.
12. Sudlow C. Anthithrombotic treatment. In: *Clinical Evidence.* 5th ed. London: BMJ Publishing Group; 2001.
13. Ridker PM, Cook NR, Lee IM, et al. A randomized trial of low-dose aspirin in the primary prevention of cardiovascular disease in women. *N Engl J Med.* 2005;352:1293-1304.
14. Mulrow C, Pignone M. An editorial update: should she take aspirin? *Ann Intern Med.* 2005;142:942-943.
15. Chan AT, Giovannucci EL, Meyerhardt JA, et al. Long-term use of aspirin and nonsteroidal anti-inflammatory drugs and risk of colorectal cancer. *JAMA.* 2005;294:914-923.
16. Mora S, Ames J, Manson J. Low-dose aspirin in the primary prevention of cardiovascular disease. Shared decision making in clinical practice. *JAMA.* 2016;316:709-710.
17. Pearson TA, Blair SN, Daniels SR, et al. AHA guidelines for primary preven-tion of cardiovascular disease and stroke: 2002 update: consensus panel guide to comprehensive risk reduction for adult patients without coronary or other atherosclerotic vascular diseases American Heart Association Science Advisory and Coordinating Committee. *Circulation.* 2002;106:388-391.
18. Sheridan S, Pignone M, Mulrow C. Framingham-based tools to calculate the global risk of coronary heart disease: a systematic review of tools for clinicians. *J Gen Intern Med.* 2003;18:1039-1052.
19. Writing Group for the Women's Health Initiative Investigators. Risks and ben-efits of estrogen plus progestin in healthy postmenopausal women. *JAMA.* 2002;288:321-333.
20. Shumaker S, Legault C, Thal L, et al. Estrogen plus progestin and the incidence of dementia and mild cognitive impairment in postmenopausal women: the Women's Health Initiative memory study: a randomized controlled trial. *JAMA.* 2003;289:2651-2662.

21. Writing Group for the Women's Health Initiative Investigators. Effects of conjugated equine estrogen in postmenopausal women with hysterectomy. *JAMA.* 2004;291:1701-1712.

22. Nelson HD, Humphrey LL, Nygren P, et al. Postmenopausal hormone replacement therapy: scientific review. *JAMA.* 2002;288:872-881.

23. Moyer VA. Menopausal hormone therapy for the primary prevention of chronic conditions: U.S. Preventive Services Task Force recommendation statement. *Ann of Int Med.* 2013;158:47-54.

24. ACOG Task Force on hormone therapy. Hormone therapy. *Obstet Gynecol.* 2004;104(4 suppl):1S-131S.

25. The North American Menopause Society. Recommendations for estrogen and progestogen use in peri- and postmenopausal women: October 2004 position statement of the North American Menopause Society. *Menopause.* 2004;11(6):589-600.

26. Nelson HD. Commonly used types of postmenopausal estrogen for treatment of hot flashes: scientific review. *JAMA.* 2004;291:1610-1620.

27. Torgerson DJ, Bell-Syer SE. Hormone replacement therapy and prevention of nonvertebral fractures: a meta-analysis of randomized trials. *JAMA.* 2001;285(22):2891-2897.

28. Cauley JA, Robbins J, Chen Z, et al. Effects of estrogen plus progestin on risk of fracture and bone mineral density. *JAMA.* 2003;290:1729-1738.

29. Ockene JK, Barad JH, Cochrane BB, et al. Symptom experience after discontinuing use of estrogen plus progestin. *JAMA.* 2005;294:183-193.

30. Lewis CL, Kinsinger LS, Harris RP, et al. Breast cancer risk in primary care: implications for chemoprevention. *Arch Intern Med.* 2004;164:1897-1903.

⊕ Please see Online Appendix: Apps and Digital Resources for additional information.

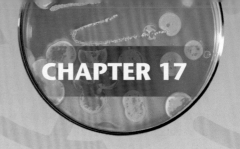

CHAPTER 17

Immunizations

NANCY C. BANASIAK

BACKGROUND

Immunization is one of the most successful examples of primary prevention. Infectious diseases that were, at the turn of the 20th century, the leading causes of childhood death and disability are now relatively rare in the United States. Vaccination programs are responsible for the global eradication of smallpox and are close to eliminating other diseases (e.g., poliomyelitis) hopefully in the near future. Decades of organized efforts to vaccinate children in the United States have very significantly reduced the incidence of diseases such as pertussis and measles. Nevertheless, incidence rates of some vaccine-preventable diseases are now rising, owing to a variety of barriers to immunization, including cost, accessibility, the increasing complexity of vaccination schedules, and a rising focus on the potential adverse effects of vaccines leading to fear in the public.[1,2]

This chapter reviews the indications and contraindications for routine childhood and adult vaccinations. It focuses on commonly used vaccines in the primary care setting and those that offer the greatest protective public health benefits among asymptomatic persons. Vaccines for selected population groups (e.g., rabies vaccine), for international travelers, and for postexposure prophylaxis are not emphasized. Patients with altered immune competence (e.g., patients with cancer, heart disease, human immunodeficiency virus [HIV] infection) require special immunization protocols[3] and are therefore beyond the scope of this chapter.

Until the 1990s, inadequate immunization coverage among preschool children had been a particular problem in the United States, which had lower early childhood immunization rates than many other industrialized and developed countries.[4] The Vaccines for Children (VFC) program was created in 1994 to ensure that uninsured children who could not pay for vaccines did not contract vaccine-preventable diseases.[5] Approximately 50% of children <19 years of age are eligible to be included in this program.[5] The vaccine rates among participants in this program is near 90% for older vaccine and improved rates with newer vaccines.[5] Healthy People

2020 target goals for immunization rates for children aged 19 to 35 months to receive recommended doses of DTaP, polio, MMR, Hib, hepatitis B, varicella, and PCV (7-vaccine series) is set at 80%.[6] In 2015, this combination of 7-vaccine series had a target rate of 72.2%, an increase from 68.4% in 2012.[7] Rates of the 7-vaccine combination series among children living below the poverty line is 5% lower or 68.7%.[7] Inadequate immunization coverage is not limited to children, however. The current burden of suffering from vaccine-preventable diseases may even be higher among adults. Approximately, 42,000 adults die each year in the United States from vaccine-preventable diseases, such as pneumococcal infection, influenza, and hepatitis B, whereas it is rare that more than 300 children die annually in the United States from the vaccine-preventable diseases of childhood.[7] Pneumococcal vaccine coverage rates are 59.7% for patients 65 years and older, which is well under the target level of 90% set forth by Healthy People 2020.[8]

The causes of inadequate immunization are multifactorial. They include systems barriers (e.g., those involving the organization/financing of the health care system), clinician barriers (e.g., inadequate clinician knowledge about vaccines and contraindications), and parent/patient barriers (e.g., fear of immunization-related adverse events).[1,2,6,7]

Problems with the supply and distribution of vaccines are among the most noticeable systems barriers. The supply of some vaccines, such as influenza vaccine, has been inadequate during recent years. Vaccine manufacturers face a variety of difficulties, including research costs, regulatory stringencies, and liability issues.[9,10] Clinician misconceptions and lack of knowledge of proper indications and contraindications to vaccine administration are surprisingly widespread. The increase in the number of vaccines now indicated for routine administration has made it difficult for clinicians to keep up with new recommendations. For example, the introduction of many new vaccines in the last four decades has quadrupled the number of immunizations that should be administered before a child's second birthday. Several studies have revealed significant knowledge deficits among clinicians regarding immunization schedules, vaccine contraindications, and vaccine side effects.[1,10,11]

"Missed opportunities," or the failure to use acute care visits for immunizations, are often cited as a common cause of a clinician failing to properly vaccinate patients. Although most clinicians will give the needed vaccinations at well child visits, the use of vaccines is much lower at visits for acute conditions. According to one study of adolescent vaccination rates for MCV, Tdap, and HVP, the researchers found that missed opportunity for vaccinations was common.[12] The most common missed opportunity was owing to visits for acute conditions.[12] Parent/patient barriers can arise from problems of logistics (lack of access to transportation), finance (inadequate insurance), or knowledge and attitude issues, such as concerns about vaccine safety issues.[1,10,11]

The recommendations in this chapter are consistent with guidelines issued by the Advisory Committee on Immunization Practices (ACIP) of the Centers for Disease Control and Prevention (CDC), a committee of 15 experts in immunization-related fields, appointed by the Secretary of the U.S. Department of Health and Human Services. Recommendations of the ACIP become CDC policy when they are accepted by the director of the CDC and are published in the CDC's *Morbidity and Mortality Weekly Report.*

Since 1994, the ACIP, American Academy of Pediatrics (AAP), and American Academy of Family Physicians (AAFP) have produced a harmonized childhood and adolescent immunization schedule (see Fig. 17.1), and the ACIP and AAFP produce a harmonized adult immunization schedule. The American College of Physicians (ACP) has not participated in the harmonized schedule, partly because ACP believes that ACIP recommendations are not sufficiently evidence based. To address this issue, the ACIP recently established an Evidence-Based Working Group, which is examining how the ACIP evaluates evidence and seeking a more consistent evidence-based approach for each ACIP recommendation. The American College of Obstetricians and Gynecologists (ACOG) has a liaison representative on the ACIP. Although its recommendations are not harmonized with the ACIP, AAFP, and AAP, ACOG has generally supported ACIP recommendations regarding adolescent and adult vaccinations for females.

Vaccine products and recommendations are frequently updated; therefore, readers are encouraged to consult up-to-date resources for current guidelines.

GENERAL PRINCIPLES

Administration of a vaccine is generally recommended for those individuals at risk of the disease at the youngest age at which the patient will develop an adequate postvaccination antibody response. Suggested ages for childhood immunizations (Fig. 17.1) have some flexibility (e.g., many immunizations recommended for infants at 2 mo of age can be given at 6 wk of age). Nonetheless, immunizations should generally be given at the earliest recommended age at which the child presents to the clinician. Partial doses or doses given too soon may dampen the antibody response and should not be counted as part of a primary series. The ACIP recommends that immunizations be given 4 days before the minimal interval or age considered as acceptable except in the case of rabies vaccine.[13] It is unnecessary to restart an interrupted series of a vaccine or toxoid or to add extra doses. Figure 17.1 provides catch-up schedules and minimum intervals between doses for children whose vaccinations have been delayed. The current schedule for adult immunization is shown in Figure 17.2.

- Consult relevant ACIP statements for detailed recommendations (www.cdc.gov/vaccines/hcp/acip-recs/index.html).
- When a vaccine is not administered at the recommended age, administer at a subsequent visit.
- Use combination vaccines instead of separate injections when appropriate.
- Report clinically significant adverse events to the Vaccine Adverse Event Reporting System (VAERS) online (www.vaers.hhs.gov) or by telephone (800-822-7967).
- Report suspected cases of reportable vaccine-preventable diseases to your state or local health department.
- For information about precautions and contraindications, see www.cdc.gov/vaccines/hcp/acip-recs/general-recs/contraindications.html.

Approved by the

Advisory Committee on Immunization Practices
(www.cdc.gov/vaccines/acip)

American Academy of Pediatrics
(www.aap.org)

American Academy of Family Physicians
(www.aafp.org)

American College of Obstetricians and Gynecologists
(www.acog.org)

This schedule includes recommendations in effect as of January 1, 2018.

CDC

U.S. Department of Health and Human Services
Centers for Disease Control and Prevention

The table below shows vaccine acronyms, and brand names for vaccines routinely recommended for children and adolescents. The use of trade names in this immunization schedule is for identification purposes only and does not imply endorsement by the ACIP or CDC.

Vaccine type	Abbreviation	Brand(s)
Diphtheria, tetanus, and acellular pertussis vaccine	DTaP	Daptacel, Infanrix
Diphtheria, tetanus vaccine	DT	No Trade Name
Haemophilus influenzae type B vaccine	Hib (PRP-T), Hib (PRP-OMP)	ActHIB, Hiberix, PedvaxHIB
Hepatitis A vaccine	HepA	Havrix, Vaqta
Hepatitis B vaccine	HepB	Engerix-B, Recombivax HB
Human papillomavirus vaccine	HPV	Gardasil 9
Influenza vaccine (inactivated)	IIV	Multiple
Measles, mumps, and rubella vaccine	MMR	M-M-R II
Meningococcal serogroups A, C, W, Y vaccine	MenACWY-D, MenACWY-CRM	Menactra, Menveo
Meningococcal serogroup B vaccine	MenB-4C, MenB-FHbp	Bexsero, Trumenba
Pneumococcal 13-valent conjugate vaccine	PCV13	Prevnar 13
Pneumococcal 23-valent polysaccharide vaccine	PPSV23	Pneumovax
Poliovirus vaccine (inactivated)	IPV	IPOL
Rotavirus vaccines	RV1, RV5	Rotarix, RotaTeq
Tetanus, diphtheria, and acellular pertussis vaccine	Tdap	Adacel, Boostrix
Tetanus and diphtheria vaccine	Td	Tenivac, No Trade Name
Varicella vaccine	VAR	Varivax
Combination Vaccines		
DTaP, hepatitis B and inactivated poliovirus vaccine	DTaP-HepB-IPV	Pediarix
DTaP, inactivated poliovirus and Haemophilus influenzae type B vaccine	DTaP-IPV/Hib	Pentacel
DTaP and inactivated poliovirus vaccine	DTaP-IPV	Kinrix, Quadracel
Measles, mumps, rubella, and varicella vaccines	MMRV	ProQuad

Figure 17.1 Recommended immunization schedule for children and adolescents aged 18 years or younger, United States, 2018.

Figure 1. Recommended Immunization Schedule for Children and Adolescents Aged 18 Years or Younger—United States, 2018.
(FOR THOSE WHO FALL BEHIND OR START LATE, SEE THE CATCH-UP SCHEDULE [FIGURE 2]).
These recommendations must be read with the footnotes that follow. For those who fall behind or start late, provide catch-up vaccination at the earliest opportunity as indicated by the green bars in Figure 1. To determine minimum intervals between doses, see the catch-up schedule (Figure 2). School entry and adolescent vaccine age groups are shaded in gray.

Vaccine	Birth	1 mo	2 mos	4 mos	6 mos	9 mos	12 mos	15 mos	18 mos	19-23 mos	2-3 yrs	4-6 yrs	7-10 yrs	11-12 yrs	13-15 yrs	16 yrs	17-18 yrs
Hepatitis B¹ (HepB)	1ˢᵗ dose	←2ⁿᵈ dose→			←———————— 3ʳᵈ dose ————————→												
Rotavirus² (RV) RV1 (2-dose series); RV5 (3-dose series)			1ˢᵗ dose	2ⁿᵈ dose	See footnote 2												
Diphtheria, tetanus, & acellular pertussis³ (DTaP: <7 yrs)			1ˢᵗ dose	2ⁿᵈ dose	3ʳᵈ dose		←———— 4ᵗʰ dose ————→					5ᵗʰ dose					
Haemophilus influenzae type b⁴ (Hib)			1ˢᵗ dose	2ⁿᵈ dose	See footnote 4		3ʳᵈ or 4ᵗʰ dose, See footnote 4										
Pneumococcal conjugate⁵ (PCV13)			1ˢᵗ dose	2ⁿᵈ dose	3ʳᵈ dose		←———— 4ᵗʰ dose ————→										
Inactivated poliovirus⁶ (IPV: <18 yrs)			1ˢᵗ dose	2ⁿᵈ dose	←———————— 3ʳᵈ dose ————————→							4ᵗʰ dose					
Influenza⁷ (IIV)								Annual vaccination (IIV) 1 or 2 doses						Annual vaccination (IIV) 1 dose only			
Measles, mumps, rubella⁸ (MMR)					See footnote 8		←———— 1ˢᵗ dose ————→					2ⁿᵈ dose					
Varicella⁹ (VAR)							←———— 1ˢᵗ dose ————→					2ⁿᵈ dose					
Hepatitis A¹⁰ (HepA)							←———— 2-dose series, See footnote 10 ————→										
Meningococcal¹¹ (MenACWY-D ≥9 mos; MenACWY-CRM ≥2 mos)							See footnote 11							1ˢᵗ dose		2ⁿᵈ dose	
Tetanus, diphtheria, & acellular pertussis¹² (Tdap: ≥7 yrs)														Tdap			
Human papillomavirus¹³ (HPV)													See footnote 14	See footnote 14			
Meningococcal B¹²															See footnote 12		
Pneumococcal polysaccharide⁵ (PPSV23)													See footnote 5				

Range of recommended ages for all children

Range of recommended ages for catch-up immunization

Range of recommended ages for certain high-risk groups

Range of recommended ages for non-high-risk groups that may receive vaccine, subject to individual clinical decision making

No recommendation

NOTE: The above recommendations must be read along with the footnotes of this schedule.

Figure 17.1 (*Continued*)

FIGURE 2. Catch-up immunization schedule for persons aged 4 months–18 years who start late or who are more than 1 month behind—United States, 2018.
The figure below provides catch-up schedules and minimum intervals between doses for children whose vaccinations have been delayed. A vaccine series does not need to be restarted, regardless of the time that has elapsed between doses. Use the section appropriate for the child's age. Always use this table in conjunction with Figure 1 and the footnotes that follow.

Vaccine	Minimum Age for Dose 1	Dose 1 to Dose 2	Dose 2 to Dose 3	Dose 3 to Dose 4	Dose 4 to Dose 5
			Children age 4 months through 6 years		
Hepatitis B[1]	Birth	4 weeks	8 weeks and at least 16 weeks after first dose. Minimum age for the final dose is 24 weeks.		
Rotavirus[2]	6 weeks Maximum age for first dose is 14 weeks, 6 days	4 weeks	4 weeks[2] Maximum age for final dose is 8 months, 0 days.		
Diphtheria, tetanus, and acellular pertussis[3]	6 weeks	4 weeks	4 weeks	6 months	6 months[3]
Haemophilus influenzae type b[4]	6 weeks	4 weeks if first dose was administered before the 1st birthday. 8 weeks (as final dose) if first dose was administered at age 12 through 14 months. No further doses needed if first dose was administered at age 15 months or older.	4 weeks[4] if current age is younger than 12 months and first dose was administered at younger than age 7 months, and at least 1 previous dose was PRP-T (ActHib, Pentacel, Hiberix) or unknown. 8 weeks and age 12 through 59 months (as final dose)[4] • if current age is younger than 12 months and first dose was administered at age 7 through 11 months; OR • if current age is 12 through 59 months and first dose was administered before the 1st birthday, and second dose administered at younger than 15 months; OR • if both doses were PRP-OMP (PedvaxHIB; Comvax) and were administered before the 1st birthday. No further doses needed if previous dose was administered at age 15 months or older.	8 weeks (as final dose) This dose only necessary for children age 12 through 59 months who received 3 doses before the 1st birthday.	
Pneumococcal conjugate[5]	6 weeks	4 weeks if first dose administered before the 1st birthday. 8 weeks (as final dose for healthy children) if first dose was administered at the 1st birthday or after. No further doses needed for healthy children if first dose was administered at age 24 months or older.	4 weeks if current age is younger than 12 months and previous dose given at <7 months old. 8 weeks (as final dose for healthy children) if previous dose given between 7–11 months (wait until at least 12 months old); OR if current age is 12 months or older and at least 1 dose was given before age 12 months. No further doses needed for healthy children if previous dose administered at age 24 months or older.	8 weeks (as final dose) This dose only necessary for children aged 12 through 59 months who received 3 doses before age 12 months or for children at high risk who received 3 doses at any age.	
Inactivated poliovirus[6]	6 weeks	4 weeks	4 weeks[6] if current age is < 4 years 6 months (as final dose) if current age is 4 years or older	6 months[6] (minimum age 4 years for final dose).	
Measles, mumps, rubella[7]	12 months	4 weeks			
Varicella[8]	12 months	3 months			
Hepatitis A[9]	12 months	6 months			
Meningococcal[11] (MenACWY-D ≥9 mos; MenACWY-CRM ≥2 mos)	6 weeks	8 weeks[11]	See footnote 11	See footnote 11	
			Children and adolescents age 7 through 18 years		
Meningococcal[11] (MenACWY-D ≥9 mos; MenACWY-CRM ≥2 mos)	Not Applicable (N/A)	8 weeks[11]			
Tetanus, diphtheria; tetanus, diphtheria, and acellular pertussis[3]	7 years[13]	4 weeks	4 weeks if first dose of DTaP/DT was administered before the 1st birthday. 6 months (as final dose) if first dose of DTaP/DT or Tdap/Td was administered at or after the 1st birthday.	6 months if first dose of DTaP/DT was administered before the 1st birthday.	
Human papillomavirus[14]	9 years		Routine dosing intervals are recommended.[14]		
Hepatitis A[9]	N/A	6 months			
Hepatitis B[1]	N/A	4 weeks	8 weeks and at least 16 weeks after first dose.		
Inactivated poliovirus[6]	N/A	4 weeks	6 months[6] A fourth dose is not necessary if the third dose was administered at age 4 years or older and at least 6 months after the previous dose.	A fourth dose of IPV is indicated if all previous doses were administered at <4 years or if the third dose was administered <6 months after the second dose.	
Measles, mumps, rubella[7]	N/A	4 weeks			
Varicella[8]	N/A	3 months if younger than age 13 years. 4 weeks if age 13 years or older.			

NOTE: The above recommendations must be read along with the footnotes of this schedule.

Figure 17.1 (Continued)

Figure 17.1 *(Continued)*

Figure 3. Vaccines that might be indicated for children and adolescents aged 18 years or younger based on medical indications

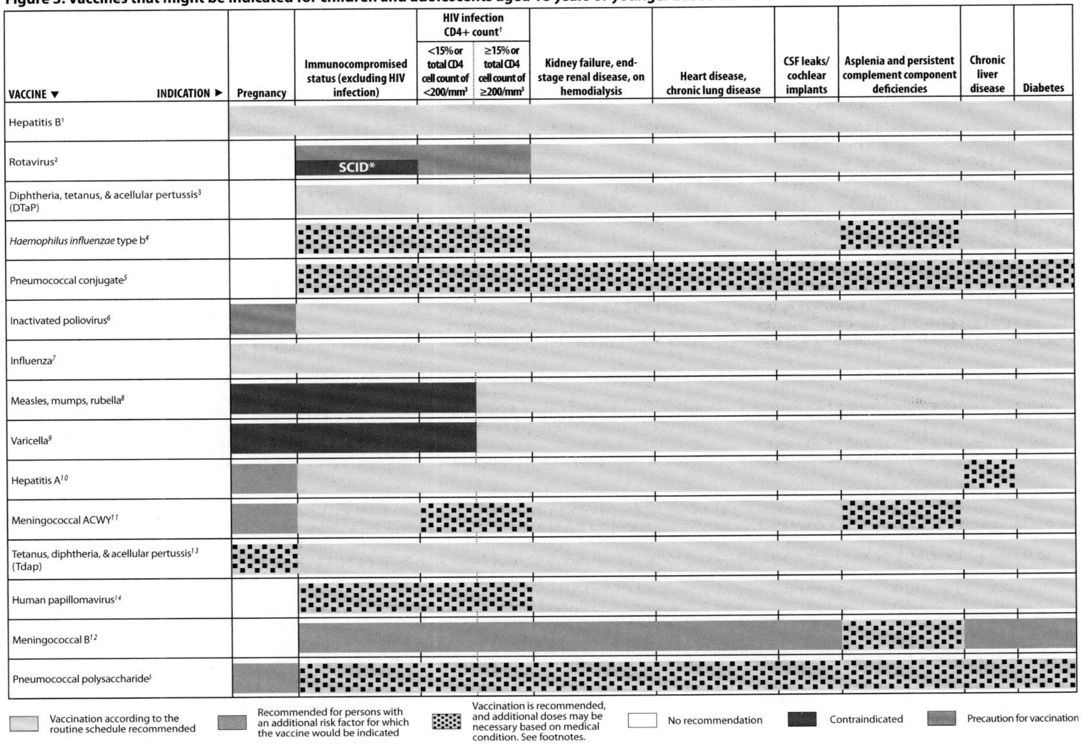

Footnotes — Recommended Immunization Schedule for Children and Adolescents Aged 18 Years or Younger, UNITED STATES, 2018

For further guidance on the use of the vaccines mentioned below, see: www.cdc.gov/vaccines/hcp/acip-recs/index.html.
For vaccine recommendations for persons 19 years of age and older, see the Adult Immunization Schedule.

Additional information

- For information on contraindications and precautions for the use of a vaccine, consult the *General Best Practice Guidelines for Immunization* and relevant ACIP statements, at www.cdc.gov/vaccines/hcp/acip-recs/index.html.
- For calculating intervals between doses, 4 weeks = 28 days. Intervals of ≥4 months are determined by calendar months.
- Within a number range (e.g., 12–18), a dash (–) should be read as "through."
- Vaccine doses administered ≤4 days before the minimum age or interval are considered valid. Doses of any vaccine administered ≥5 days earlier than the minimum interval or minimum age should not be counted as valid and should be repeated as age-appropriate. The repeat dose should be spaced after the invalid dose by the recommended minimum interval. For further details, see Table 3-1, *Recommended and minimum ages and intervals between vaccine doses, in General Best Practice Guidelines for Immunization* at www.cdc.gov/vaccines/hcp/acip-recs/general-recs/timing.html.
- Information on travel vaccine requirements and recommendations is available at www.nc.cdc.gov/travel/.
- For vaccination of persons with immunodeficiencies, see Table 8-1, *Vaccination of persons with primary and secondary immunodeficiencies, in General Best Practice Guidelines for Immunization*, at www.cdc.gov/vaccines/hcp/acip-recs/general-recs/immunocompetence.html; and Immunization in Special Clinical Circumstances, (In: Kimberlin DW, Brady MT, Jackson MA, Long SS, eds. *Red Book: 2015 report of the Committee on Infectious Diseases. 30th ed.* Elk Grove Village, IL: American Academy of Pediatrics, 2015:68-107).
- The National Vaccine Injury Compensation Program (VICP) is a no-fault alternative to the traditional legal system for resolving vaccine injury claims. All routine child and adolescent vaccines are covered by VICP except for pneumococcal polysaccharide vaccine (PPSV23). For more information; see www.hrsa.gov/vaccinecompensation/index.html.

1. **Hepatitis B (HepB) vaccine. (minimum age: birth)**

   Birth Dose (Monovalent HepB vaccine only):
   - **Mother is HBsAg-Negative:** 1 dose within 24 hours of birth for medically stable infants ≥2,000 grams. Infants <2,000 grams administer 1 dose at chronological age 1 month or hospital discharge.
   - **Mother is HBsAg-Positive:**
     o Give **HepB vaccine and 0.5 mL of HBIG** (at separate anatomic sites) within 12 hours of birth, regardless of birth weight.
     o Test for HBsAg and anti-HBs at age 9–12 months. If HepB series is delayed, test 1–2 months after final dose.
   - **Mother's HBsAg status is unknown:**
     o Give **HepB vaccine** within 12 hours of birth, regardless of birth weight.
     o For infants <2,000 grams, give **0.5 mL of HBIG** in addition to HepB vaccine within 12 hours of birth.
     o Determine mother's HBsAg status as soon as possible. If mother is HBsAg-positive, give **0.5 mL of HBIG** to infants ≥2,000 grams as soon as possible, but no later than 7 days of age.

   Routine Series:
   - A complete series is 3 doses at 0, 1–2, and 6–18 months. (Monovalent HepB vaccine should be used for doses given before age 6 weeks.)

   - Infants who did not receive a birth dose should begin the series as soon as feasible (see Figure 2).
   - Administration of **4 doses** is permitted when a combination vaccine containing HepB is used after the birth dose.
   - **Minimum age** for the final (3rd or 4th) dose: 24 weeks.
   - **Minimum Intervals:** Dose 1 to Dose 2: 4 weeks / Dose 2 to Dose 3: 8 weeks / Dose 1 to Dose 3: 16 weeks. (When 4 doses are given, substitute "Dose 4" for "Dose 3" in these calculations.)

   Catch-up vaccination:
   - Unvaccinated persons should complete a 3-dose series at 0, 1–2, and 6 months.
   - Adolescents 11–15 years of age may use an alternative 2-dose schedule, with at least 4 months between doses (adult formulation **Recombivax HB** only).
   - For other catch-up guidance, see Figure 2.

2. **Rotavirus vaccines. (minimum age: 6 weeks)**

   Routine vaccination:
   Rotarix: 2-dose series at 2 and 4 months.
   RotaTeq: 3-dose series at 2, 4, and 6 months.
   If any dose in the series is either RotaTeq or unknown, default to 3-dose series.

   Catch-up vaccination:
   - Do not start the series on or after age 15 weeks, 0 days.
   - The maximum age for the final dose is 8 months, 0 days.
   - For other catch-up guidance, see Figure 2.

3. **Diphtheria, tetanus, and acellular pertussis (DTaP) vaccine. (minimum age: 6 weeks [4 years for Kinrix or Quadracel])**

   Routine vaccination:
   - 5-dose series at 2, 4, 6, and 15–18 months, and 4–6 years.
     o **Prospectively:** A 4th dose may be given as early as age 12 months if at least 6 months have elapsed since the 3rd dose.
     o **Retrospectively:** A 4th dose that was inadvertently given as early as 12 months may be counted if at least 4 months have elapsed since the 3rd dose.

   Catch-up vaccination:
   - The 5th dose is not necessary if the 4th dose was administered at 4 years or older.
   - For other catch-up guidance, see Figure 2.

Figure 17.1 (*Continued*)

For further guidance on the use of the vaccines mentioned below, see: www.cdc.gov/vaccines/hcp/acip-recs/index.html.

4. **Haemophilus influenzae type b (Hib) vaccine.** (minimum age: 6 weeks)

Routine vaccination:
- **ActHIB, Hiberix, or Pentacel:** 4-dose series at 2, 4, 6, and 12–15 months.
- **PedvaxHIB:** 3-dose series at 2, 4, and 12–15 months.

Catch-up vaccination:
- **1st dose at 7–11 months:** Give 2nd dose at least 4 weeks later and 3rd (final) dose at 12–15 months or 8 weeks after 2nd dose (whichever is later).
- **1st dose at 12–14 months:** Give 2nd (final) dose at least 8 weeks after 1st dose.
- **1st dose before 12 months and 2nd dose before 15 months:** Give 3rd (final) dose 8 weeks after 2nd dose.
- **2 doses of PedvaxHIB before 12 months:** Give 3rd (final) dose at 12–59 months and at least 8 weeks after 2nd dose.
- **Unvaccinated at 15–59 months:** 1 dose.
- For other catch-up guidance, see Figure 2.

Special Situations:
- **Chemotherapy or radiation treatment**
  12–59 months
  o Unvaccinated or only 1 dose before 12 months: Give 2 doses, 8 weeks apart
  o 2 or more doses before 12 months: Give 1 dose, at least 8 weeks after previous dose.
  Doses given within 14 days of starting therapy or during therapy should be repeated at least 3 months after therapy completion.
- **Hematopoietic stem cell transplant (HSCT)**
  3-dose series with doses 4 weeks apart starting 6 to 12 months after successful transplant (regardless of Hib vaccination history).
- **Anatomic or functional asplenia (including sickle cell disease)**
  12–59 months
  o Unvaccinated or only 1 dose before 12 months: Give 2 doses, 8 weeks apart.
  o 2 or more doses before 12 months: Give 1 dose, at least 8 weeks after previous dose.
  Unimmunized persons 5 years or older*
  o Give 1 dose
- **Elective splenectomy**
  Unimmunized persons 15 months or older*
  o Give 1 dose (preferably at least 14 days before procedure).

- **HIV infection**
  12–59 months
  o Unvaccinated or only 1 dose before 12 months: Give 2 doses 8 weeks apart.
  o 2 or more doses before 12 months: Give 1 dose, at least 8 weeks after previous dose.
  Unimmunized persons 5–18 years*
  o Give 1 dose
- **Immunoglobulin deficiency, early component complement deficiency**
  12–59 months
  o Unvaccinated or only 1 dose before 12 months: Give 2 doses, 8 weeks apart.
  o 2 or more doses before 12 months: Give 1 dose, at least 8 weeks after previous dose.
  *Unimmunized = Less than routine series (through 14 months) OR no doses (14 months or older)

5. **Pneumococcal vaccines. (minimum age: 6 weeks [PCV13], 2 years [PPSV23])**

Routine vaccination with PCV13:
- 4-dose series at 2, 4, 6, and 12–15 months.

Catch-up vaccination with PCV13:
- 1 dose for healthy children aged 24–59 months with any incomplete* PCV13 schedule
- For other catch-up guidance, see Figure 2.

Special situations: High-risk conditions: Administer PCV13 doses before PPSV23 if possible.

Chronic heart disease (particularly cyanotic congenital heart disease and cardiac failure); chronic lung disease (including asthma treated with high-dose, oral, corticosteroids); diabetes mellitus:

Age 2–5 years:
- Any incomplete* schedules with:
  o 3 PCV13 doses: 1 dose of PCV13 (at least 8 weeks after any prior PCV13 dose).
  o <3 PCV13 doses: 2 doses of PCV13, 8 weeks after the most recent dose and given 8 weeks apart.
- No history of PPSV23: 1 dose of PPSV23 (at least 8 weeks after any prior PCV13 dose).

Age 6–18 years:
- No history of PPSV23: 1 dose of PPSV23 (at least 8 weeks after any prior PCV13 dose).

Cerebrospinal fluid leak; cochlear implant:
Age 2–5 years:
- Any incomplete* schedules with:
  o 3 PCV13 doses: 1 dose of PCV13 (at least 8 weeks after any prior PCV13 dose).
  o <3 PCV13 doses: 2 doses of PCV13, 8 weeks after the most recent dose and given 8 weeks apart.
- No history of PPSV23: 1 dose of PPSV23 (at least 8 weeks after any prior PCV13 dose).

Age 6–18 years:
- No history of either PCV13 or PPSV23: 1 dose of PCV13, 1 dose of PPSV23 at least 8 weeks later.
- Any PCV13 but no PPSV23: 1 dose of PPSV23 at least 8 weeks after the most recent dose of PCV13
- PPSV23 but no PCV13: 1 dose of PCV13 at least 8 weeks after the most recent dose of PPSV23.

Sickle cell disease and other hemoglobinopathies; anatomic or functional asplenia; congenital or acquired immunodeficiency; HIV infection; chronic renal failure; nephrotic syndrome; malignant neoplasms, leukemias, lymphomas, Hodgkin disease, and other diseases associated with treatment with immunosuppressive drugs or radiation therapy; solid organ transplantation; multiple myeloma:

Age 2–5 years:
- Any incomplete* schedules with:
  o 3 PCV13 doses: 1 dose of PCV13 (at least 8 weeks after any prior PCV13 dose).
  o <3 PCV13 doses: 2 doses of PCV13, 8 weeks after the most recent dose and given 8 weeks apart.
- No history of PPSV23: 1 dose of PPSV23 (at least 8 weeks after any prior PCV13 dose) and a 2nd dose of PPSV23 5 years later.

Age 6–18 years:
- No history of either PCV13 or PPSV23: 1 dose of PCV13, 2 doses of PPSV23 (1st dose of PPSV23 administered 8 weeks after PCV13 and 2nd dose of PPSV23 administered at least 5 years after the 1st dose of PPSV23).
- Any PCV13 but no PPSV23: 2 doses of PPSV23 (1st dose of PPSV23 to be given 8 weeks after the most recent dose of PCV13 and 2nd dose of PPSV23 administered at least 5 years after the 1st dose of PPSV23).

Figure 17.1 (*Continued*)

For further guidance on the use of the vaccines mentioned below, see: www.cdc.gov/vaccines/hcp/acip-recs/index.html.

- PPSV23 but no PCV13: 1 dose of PCV13 at least 8 weeks after the most recent PPSV23 dose and a 2nd dose of PPSV23 to be given 5 years after the 1st dose of PPSV23 and at least 8 weeks after a dose of PCV13.

Chronic liver disease, alcoholism:

Age 6–18 years:
- No history of PPSV23: 1 dose of PPSV23 (at least 8 weeks after any prior PCV13 dose).

*Incomplete schedules are any schedules where PCV13 doses have not been completed according to ACIP recommended catch-up schedules. The total number and timing of doses for complete PCV13 series are dictated by the age at first vaccination. See Tables 8 and 9 in the ACIP pneumococcal vaccine recommendations (www.cdc.gov/mmwr/pdf/rr/rr5911.pdf) for complete schedule details.

6. Inactivated poliovirus vaccine (IPV). (minimum age: 6 weeks)

Routine vaccination:
- 4-dose series at ages 2, 4, 6–18 months, and 4–6 years. Administer the final dose on or after the 4th birthday and at least 6 months after the previous dose.

Catch-up vaccination:
- In the first 6 months of life, use minimum ages and intervals only for travel to a polio-endemic region or during an outbreak.
- If 4 or more doses were given before the 4th birthday, give 1 more dose at age 4–6 years and at least 6 months after the previous dose.
- A 4th dose is not necessary if the 3rd dose was given on or after the 4th birthday and at least 6 months after the previous dose.
- IPV is not routinely recommended for U.S. residents 18 years and older.

Series Containing Oral Polio Vaccine (OPV), *either mixed OPV-IPV or OPV-only series:*
- Total number of doses needed to complete the series is the same as that recommended for the U.S. IPV schedule. See www.cdc.gov/mmwr/volumes/66/wr/mm6601a6.htm?s_cid=mm6601a6_w.
- Only trivalent OPV (tOPV) counts toward the U.S. vaccination requirements. For guidance to assess doses documented as "OPV" see www.cdc.gov/mmwr/volumes/66/wr/mm6606a7.htm?s_cid=mm6606a7_w.
- For other catch-up guidance, see Figure 2.

7. Influenza vaccines. (minimum age: 6 months)

Routine vaccination:
- Administer an age-appropriate formulation and dose of influenza vaccine annually.
  o Children 6 months–8 years who did not receive at least 2 doses of influenza vaccine before July 1, 2017 should receive 2 doses separated by at least 4 weeks.
  o Persons 9 years and older 1 dose
- Live attenuated influenza vaccine (LAIV) not recommended for the 2017–18 season.
- For additional guidance, see the 2017–18 ACIP influenza vaccine recommendations (MMWR August 25, 2017;66(2):1–20: www.cdc.gov/mmwr/volumes/66/rr/pdfs/rr6602.pdf).
(For the 2018–19 season, see the 2018–19 ACIP influenza vaccine recommendations.)

8. Measles, mumps, and rubella (MMR) vaccine. (minimum age: 12 months for routine vaccination)

Routine vaccination:
- 2-dose series at 12–15 months and 4–6 years.
- The 2nd dose may be given as early as 4 weeks after the 1st dose.

Catch-up vaccination:
- Unvaccinated children and adolescents: 2 doses at least 4 weeks apart.

International travel:
- Infants 6–11 months: 1 dose before departure. Revaccinate with 2 doses at 12–15 months (12 months for children in high-risk areas) and 2nd dose as early as 4 weeks later.
- Unvaccinated children 12 months and older: 2 doses at least 4 weeks apart before departure.

Mumps outbreak:
- Persons ≥12 months who previously received ≤2 doses of mumps-containing vaccine and are identified by public health authorities to be at increased risk during a mumps outbreak should receive a dose of mumps-virus containing vaccine.

9. Varicella (VAR) vaccine. (minimum age: 12 months)

Routine vaccination:
- 2-dose series: 12–15 months and 4–6 years.
- The 2nd dose may be given as early as 3 months after the 1st dose (a dose given after a 4-week interval may be counted).

Catch-up vaccination:
- Ensure persons 7–18 years without evidence of immunity (see MMWR 2007;56[No. RR-4], at www.cdc.gov/mmwr/pdf/rr/rr5604.pdf) have 2 doses of varicella vaccine:
  o Ages 7–12: routine interval 3 months (minimum interval: 4 weeks).
  o Ages 13 and older: minimum interval 4 weeks.

10. Hepatitis A (HepA) vaccine. (minimum age: 12 months)

Routine vaccination:
- 2 doses, separated by 6–18 months, between the 1st and 2nd birthdays. (A series begun before the 2nd birthday should be completed even if the child turns 2 before the second dose is given.)

Catch-up vaccination:
- Anyone 2 years of age or older may receive HepA vaccine if desired. Minimum interval between doses is 6 months.

Special populations:
Previously unvaccinated persons who should be vaccinated:
- Persons traveling to or working in countries with high or intermediate endemicity
- Men who have sex with men
- Users of injection and non-injection drugs
- Persons who work with hepatitis A virus in a research laboratory or with non-human primates
- Persons with clotting-factor disorders
- Persons with chronic liver disease
- Persons who anticipate close, personal contact (e.g., household or regular babysitting) with an international adoptee during the first 60 days after arrival in the United States from a country with high or intermediate endemicity (administer the 1st dose as soon as the adoption is planned—ideally at least 2 weeks before the adoptee's arrival).

11. Serogroup A, C, W, Y meningococcal vaccines. (Minimum age: 2 months [Menveo], 9 months [Menactra].

Routine:
- 2-dose series: 11-12 years and 16 years.

Catch-Up:
- Age 13-15 years: 1 dose now and booster at age 16-18 years. Minimum interval 8 weeks.
- Age 16-18 years: 1 dose.

Figure 17.1 *(Continued)*

For further guidance on the use of the vaccines mentioned below, see: www.cdc.gov/vaccines/hcp/acip-recs/index.html.

Special populations and situations:
Anatomic or functional asplenia, sickle cell disease, HIV infection, persistent complement component deficiency (including eculizumab use):
- Menveo
  ○ 1st dose at 8 weeks: 4-dose series at 2, 4, 6, and 12 months.
  ○ 1st dose at 7–23 months: 2nd dose (2nd dose at least 12 weeks after the 1st dose and after the 1st birthday).
  ○ 1st dose at 24 months or older: 2 doses at least 8 weeks apart.
- Menactra
  ○ Persistent complement component deficiency:
    — 9–23 months: 2 doses at least 12 weeks apart
    — 24 months or older: 2 doses at least 8 weeks apart
  ○ Anatomic or functional asplenia, sickle cell disease, or HIV infection:
    — 24 months or older: 2 doses at least 8 weeks apart.
    — Menactra must be administered at least 4 weeks after completion of PCV13 series.

Children who travel to or live in countries where meningococcal disease is hyperendemic or epidemic, including countries in the African meningitis belt or during the Hajj; or exposure to an outbreak attributable to a vaccine serogroup:
- Children <24 months of age:
  ○ Menveo (2-23 months):
    — 1st dose at 8 weeks: 4-dose series at 2, 4, 6, and 12 months.
    — 1st dose at 7–23 months: 2 doses (2nd dose at least 12 weeks after the 1st dose and after the 1st birthday).
  ○ Menactra (9-23 months):
    — 2 doses (2nd dose at least 12 weeks after the 1st dose. 2nd dose may be administered as early as 8 weeks after the 1st dose in travelers).
- Children 2 years or older: 1 dose of Menveo or Menactra.

Note: Menactra should be given either before or at the same time as DTaP. For MenACWY booster dose recommendations for groups listed under "Special populations and situations" and additional meningococcal vaccination information, see meningococcal *MMWR* publications at: www.cdc.gov/vaccines/hcp/acip-recs/vacc-specific/mening.html.

12. **Serogroup B meningococcal vaccines (minimum age: 10 years [Bexsero, Trumenba].**
Clinical discretion: Adolescents not at increased risk for meningococcal B infection who want MenB vaccine.
MenB vaccines may be given at clinical discretion to adolescents 16–23 years (preferred age 16–18 years) who are not at increased risk.
- **Bexsero:** 2 doses at least 1 month apart.
- **Trumenba:** 2 doses at least 6 months apart. If the 2nd dose is given earlier than 6 months, give a 3rd dose at least 4 months after the 2nd.

Special populations and situations:
Anatomic or functional asplenia, sickle cell disease, persistent complement component deficiency (including eculizumab use), serogroup B meningococcal disease outbreak
- **Bexsero:** 2-dose series at least 1 month apart.
- **Trumenba:** 3-dose series at 0, 1-2, and 6 months.

Note: Bexsero and Trumenba are not interchangeable.
For additional meningococcal vaccination information, see meningococcal *MMWR* publications at: www.cdc.gov/vaccines/hcp/acip-recs/vacc-specific/mening.html.

13. **Tetanus, diphtheria, and acellular pertussis (Tdap) vaccine. (minimum age: 11 years for routine vaccinations, 7 years for catch-up vaccination)**
Routine vaccination:
- **Adolescents 11–12 years of age:** 1 dose.
- **Pregnant adolescents:** 1 dose during each pregnancy (preferably during the early part of gestational weeks 27–36).
- Tdap may be administered regardless of the interval since the last tetanus- and diphtheria-toxoid-containing vaccine.

Catch-up vaccination:
- **Adolescents 13–18 who have not received Tdap:** 1 dose, followed by a Td booster every 10 years.
- **Persons aged 7–18 years not fully immunized with DTaP:** 1 dose of Tdap as part of the catch-up series (preferably the first dose). If additional doses are needed, use Td.

- **Children 7–10 years** who receive Tdap inadvertently or as part of the catch-up series may receive the routine Tdap dose at 11–12 years.
- **DTaP inadvertently given after the 7th birthday:**
  ○ **Child 7–10:** DTaP may count as part of catch-up series. Routine Tdap dose at 11-12 may be given.
  ○ **Adolescent 11–18:** Count dose of DTaP as the adolescent Tdap booster.
  ○ For other catch-up guidance, see Figure 2.

14. **Human papillomavirus (HPV) vaccine (minimum age: 9 years)**
Routine and catch-up vaccination:
- Routine vaccination for all adolescents at 11–12 years (can start at age 9) and through age 18 if not previously adequately vaccinated. Number of doses dependent on age at initial vaccination.
  ○ **Age 9–14 years at initiation:** 2-dose series at 0 and 6–12 months. Minimum interval: 5 months (repeat a dose given too soon at least 12 weeks after the invalid dose and at least 5 months after the 1st dose).
  ○ **Age 15 years or older at initiation:** 3-dose series at 0, 1–2 months, and 6 months. Minimum intervals: 4 weeks between 1st and 2nd dose; 12 weeks between 2nd and 3rd dose; 5 months between 1st and 3rd dose (repeat dose(s) given too soon at or after the minimum interval since the most recent dose).
- Persons who have completed a valid series with any HPV vaccine do not need any additional doses.

Special situations:
- **History of sexual abuse or assault:** Begin series at age 9 years.
- **Immunocompromised* (including HIV)** aged 9–26 years: 3-dose series at 0, 1–2 months, and 6 months.
- **Pregnancy:** Vaccination not recommended, but there is no evidence the vaccine is harmful. No intervention is needed for women who inadvertently received a dose of HPV vaccine while pregnant. Delay remaining doses until after pregnancy. Pregnancy testing not needed before vaccination.

*See *MMWR*, December 16, 2016;65(49):1405–1408, at www.cdc.gov/mmwr/volumes/65/wr/pdfs/mm6549a5.pdf.

CS270457-M

Figure 17.1 (*Continued*)

In February 2018, the *Recommended Immunization Schedule for Adults Aged 19 Years or Older, United States, 2018* became effective, as recommended by the Advisory Committee on Immunization Practices (ACIP) and approved by the Centers for Disease Control and Prevention (CDC). The adult immunization schedule was also approved by the American College of Physicians, the American Academy of Family Physicians, the American College of Obstetricians and Gynecologists, and the American College of Nurse-Midwives.

CDC announced the availability of the 2018 adult immunization schedule in the *Morbidity and Mortality Weekly Report (MMWR)*. The schedule is published in its entirety in the *Annals of Internal Medicine*.[2]

The adult immunization schedule consists of figures that summarize routinely recommended vaccines for adults by age groups and medical conditions and other indications, footnotes for the figures, and a table of vaccine contraindications and precautions. Note the following when reviewing the adult immunization schedule:

- The figures in the adult immunization schedule should be reviewed with the accompanying footnotes.
- The figures and footnotes display indications for which vaccines, if not previously administered, should be administered unless noted otherwise.
- The table of contraindications and precautions identifies populations and situations for which vaccines should not be used or should be used with caution.
- When indicated, administer recommended vaccines to adults whose vaccination history is incomplete or unknown.
- Increased interval between doses of a multidose vaccine series does not diminish vaccine effectiveness; it is not necessary to restart the vaccine series or add doses to the series because of an extended interval between doses.
- Combination vaccines may be used when any component of the combination is indicated and when the other components of the combination are not contraindicated.
- The use of trade names in the adult immunization schedule is for identification purposes only and does not imply endorsement by the ACIP or CDC.

Special populations that need additional considerations include:

- Pregnant women. Pregnant women should receive the tetanus, diphtheria, and acellular pertussis vaccine (Tdap) during pregnancy and the influenza vaccine during or before pregnancy. Live vaccines (e.g., measles, mumps, and rubella vaccine [MMR]) are contraindicated.
- Asplenia. Adults with asplenia have specific vaccination recommendations because of their increased risk for infection by encapsulated bacteria. Anatomical or functional asplenia includes congenital or acquired asplenia, splenic dysfunction, sickle cell disease and other hemoglobinopathies, and splenectomy.
- Immunocompromising conditions. Adults with immunosuppression should generally avoid live vaccines. Inactivated vaccines (e.g., pneumococcal vaccines) are generally acceptable. High-level immunosuppression includes HIV infection with a CD4 cell count <200 cells/μL, receipt of daily corticosteroid therapy with ≥20 mg of prednisone or equivalent for ≥14 days, primary immunodeficiency disorder (e.g., severe combined immunodeficiency) or complement component deficiency), and receipt of cancer chemotherapy. Other immunocompromising conditions and immunosuppressive medications to consider when vaccinating adults can be found in IDSA *Clinical Practice Guideline for Vaccination of the Immunocompromised Host*.[4] Additional information on vaccinating immunocompromised adults is in *General Best Practice Guidelines for Immunization*.[4]

Additional resources for health care providers include:

- Details on vaccines recommended for adults and complete ACIP statements at www.cdc.gov/vaccines/hcp/acip-recs/index.html
- Vaccine Information Statements that explain benefits and risks of vaccines at www.cdc.gov/vaccines/hcp/vis/index.html
- Information and resources on vaccinating pregnant women at www.cdc.gov/vaccines/adults/rec-vac/pregnant.html
- Information on travel vaccine requirements and recommendations at www.cdc.gov/travel/destinations/list
- CDC Vaccine Schedules App for immunization service providers to download at www.cdc.gov/vaccines/schedules/hcp/schedule-app.html
- Adult Vaccination Quiz for self-assessment of vaccination needs based on age, health conditions, and other indications at www2.cdc.gov/nip/adultimmsched/default.asp
- *Recommended Immunization Schedule for Children and Adolescents Aged 18 Years or Younger* at www.cdc.gov/vaccines/schedules/hcp/child-adolescent.html

Report suspected cases of reportable vaccine-preventable diseases to the local or state health department, and report all clinically significant postvaccination events to the Vaccine Adverse Event Reporting System at www.vaers.hhs.gov or by telephone, 800-822-7967. All vaccines included in the adult immunization schedule except 23-valent pneumococcal polysaccharide and zoster vaccines are covered by the Vaccine Injury Compensation Program. Information on how to file a vaccine injury claim is available at www.hrsa.gov/vaccinecompensation or by telephone, 800-338-2382. Submit questions and comments to CDC through www.cdc.gov/cdc-info or by telephone, 800-CDC-INFO (800-232-4636), in English and Spanish, 8:00am–8:00pm ET, Monday–Friday, excluding holidays.

The following abbreviations are used for vaccines in the adult immunization schedule (in the order of their appearance):

IIV	inactivated influenza vaccine
RIV	recombinant influenza vaccine
Tdap	tetanus toxoid, reduced diphtheria toxoid, and acellular pertussis vaccine
Td	tetanus and diphtheria toxoids
MMR	measles, mumps, and rubella vaccine
VAR	varicella vaccine
RZV	recombinant zoster vaccine
ZVL	zoster vaccine live
HPV vaccine	human papillomavirus vaccine
PCV13	13-valent pneumococcal conjugate vaccine
PPSV23	23-valent pneumococcal polysaccharide vaccine
HepA	hepatitis A vaccine
HepA-HepB	hepatitis A vaccine and hepatitis B vaccine
HepB	hepatitis B vaccine
MenACWY	serogroups A, C, W, and Y meningococcal vaccine
MenB	serogroup B meningococcal vaccine
Hib	*Haemophilus influenzae* type b vaccine

1. MMWR Morb Mortal Wkly Rep. 2018;66(5):xx–xx. Available at www.cdc.gov/mmwr/volumes/67/xx/xxxxxxxx.
2. Ann Intern Med. 2018;168:xxx–xxx. Available at annals.org/aim/article/doi/10.7326/M17-3439
3. Clin Infect Dis. 2014;58:e44-100. Available at www.idsociety.org/Templates/Content.aspx?id=32212256011.
4. Kroger et al. Available at www.cdc.gov/vaccines/hcp/acip-recs/general-recs/index.html

U.S. Department of Health and Human Services
Centers for Disease Control and Prevention

Figure 17.2   Recommended immunization schedule for adults aged 19 years or older, United States, 2018.

Figure 1. Recommended immunization schedule for adults aged 19 years or older by age group, United States, 2018

This figure should be reviewed with the accompanying footnotes. This figure and the footnotes describe indications for which vaccines, if not previously administered, should be administered unless noted otherwise.

Vaccine	19–21 years	22–26 years	27–49 years	50–64 years	≥65 years
Influenza[1]			1 dose annually		
Tdap[2] or Td[2]			1 dose Tdap, then Td booster every 10 yrs		
MMR[3]			1 or 2 doses depending on indication (if born in 1957 or later)		
VAR[4]			2 doses		
RZV[5] (preferred)					2 doses RZV (preferred)
or					or
ZVL[5]					1 dose ZVL
HPV–Female[6]	2 or 3 doses depending on age at series initiation				
HPV–Male[6]	2 or 3 doses depending on age at series initiation				
PCV13[7]					1 dose
PPSV23[7]		1 or 2 doses depending on indication			1 dose
HepA[8]		2 or 3 doses depending on vaccine			
HepB[9]		3 doses			
MenACWY[10]		1 or 2 doses depending on indication, then booster every 5 yrs if risk remains			
MenB[10]		2 or 3 doses depending on vaccine			
Hib[11]		1 or 3 doses depending on indication			

Recommended for adults who meet the age requirement, lack documentation of vaccination, or lack evidence of past infection

Recommended for adults with other indications

No recommendation

Figure 17.2 (*Continued*)

Figure 2. Recommended immunization schedule for adults aged 19 years or older by medical condition and other indications, United States, 2018

This figure should be reviewed with the accompanying footnotes. This figure and the footnotes describe indications for which vaccines, if not previously administered, should be administered unless noted otherwise.

Vaccine	Pregnancy[1,6]	Immuno-compromised (excluding HIV infection)[3,7,11]	HIV infection CD4+ count (cells/μL)[3,7,9,10] <200	HIV infection CD4+ count (cells/μL)[3,7,9,10] ≥200	Asplenia, complement deficiencies[7,10,11]	End-stage renal disease, on hemodialysis[7,9]	Heart or lung disease, alcoholism[7]	Chronic liver disease[7,9]	Diabetes[7,9]	Health care personnel[4,9]	Men who have sex with men[4,9]
Influenza[1]	1 dose annually										
Tdap[2] or Td[2]	1 dose Tdap each pregnancy	1 dose Tdap, then Td booster every 10 yrs									
MMR[3]	contraindicated	contraindicated	contraindicated	1 or 2 doses depending on indication							
VAR[4]	contraindicated	contraindicated	contraindicated	2 doses							
RZV[5] (preferred) or ZVL[5]	contraindicated (ZVL)				2 doses RZV at age ≥50 yrs (preferred) or 1 dose ZVL at age ≥60 yrs						
HPV–Female[6]		3 doses through age 26 yrs	3 doses through age 26 yrs		2 or 3 doses through age 26 yrs						
HPV–Male[6]		3 doses through age 26 yrs	3 doses through age 26 yrs		2 or 3 doses through age 21 yrs						2 or 3 doses through age 26 yrs
PCV13[7]					1 dose						
PPSV23[7]					1, 2, or 3 doses depending on indication						
HepA[8]					2 or 3 doses depending on vaccine						
HepB[9]					3 doses						
MenACWY[10]		1 or 2 doses depending on indication, then booster every 5 yrs if risk remains									
MenB[10]		2 or 3 doses depending on vaccine									
Hib[11]		3 doses HSCT recipients only			1 dose						

Legend:
Recommended for adults who meet the age requirement, lack documentation of vaccination, or lack evidence of past infection
Recommended for adults with other indications
Contraindicated
No recommendation

Figure 17.2 (Continued)

Footnotes. Recommended immunization schedule for adults aged 19 years or older, United States, 2018

1. Influenza vaccination
www.cdc.gov/vaccines/hcp/acip-recs/vacc-specific/flu.html

General information
- Administer 1 dose of age-appropriate inactivated influenza vaccine (IIV) or recombinant influenza vaccine (RIV) annually
- Live attenuated influenza vaccine (LAIV) is not recommended for the 2017–2018 influenza season
- A list of currently available influenza vaccines is available at www.cdc.gov/flu/protect/vaccine/vaccines.htm

Special populations
- Administer age-appropriate IIV or RIV to:
  – Pregnant women
  – Adults with hives-only egg allergy
  – Adults with egg allergy other than hives (e.g., angioedema or respiratory distress): Administer IIV or RIV in a medical setting under supervision of a health care provider who can recognize and manage severe allergic conditions

2. Tetanus, diphtheria, and pertussis vaccination
www.cdc.gov/vaccines/hcp/acip-recs/vacc-specific/tdap-td.html

General information
- Administer to adults who previously did not receive a dose of tetanus toxoid, reduced diphtheria toxoid, and acellular pertussis vaccine (Tdap) as an adult or child (routinely recommended at age 11–12 years) 1 dose of Tdap, followed by a dose of tetanus and diphtheria toxoids (Td) booster every 10 years
- Information on the use of Tdap or Td as tetanus prophylaxis in wound management is available at www.cdc.gov/mmwr/preview/mmwrhtml/rr5517a1.htm

Special populations
- Pregnant women: Administer 1 dose of Tdap during each pregnancy, preferably in the early part of gestational weeks 27–36

3. Measles, mumps, and rubella vaccination
www.cdc.gov/vaccines/hcp/acip-recs/vacc-specific/mmr.html

General information
- Administer 1 dose of measles, mumps, and rubella vaccine (MMR) to adults with no evidence of immunity to measles, mumps, or rubella
- Evidence of immunity is:
  – Born before 1957 (except for health care personnel, see below)
  – Documentation of receipt of MMR
  – Laboratory evidence of immunity or disease
- Documentation of a health care provider-diagnosed disease without laboratory confirmation is not considered evidence of immunity

Special populations
- Pregnant women and nonpregnant women of childbearing age with no evidence of immunity to rubella: Administer 1 dose of MMR if pregnant, administer MMR after pregnancy and before discharge from health care facility)

- HIV infection and CD4 cell count ≥200 cells/μL for at least 6 months and no evidence of immunity to measles, mumps, or rubella: Administer 2 doses of MMR at least 28 days apart
- Students in postsecondary educational institutions, international travelers, and household contacts of immunocompromised persons: Administer 2 doses of MMR at least 28 days apart (or 1 dose of MMR if previously administered 1 dose of MMR)
- Health care personnel born in 1957 or later with no evidence of immunity: Administer 2 doses of MMR at least 28 days apart for measles or mumps, or 1 dose of MMR for rubella (if born before 1957, consider MMR vaccination)
- Adults who previously received ≤2 doses of mumps-containing vaccine and are identified by public health authority to be at increased risk for mumps in an outbreak: Administer 1 dose of MMR
- MMR is contraindicated for pregnant women and adults with severe immunodeficiency

4. Varicella vaccination
www.cdc.gov/vaccines/hcp/acip-recs/vacc-specific/varicella.html

General information
- Administer to adults without evidence of immunity to varicella 2 doses of varicella vaccine (VAR) 4–8 weeks apart if previously received no varicella-containing vaccine (if previously received 1 dose of varicella-containing vaccine, administer 1 dose of VAR at least 4 weeks after the first dose)
- Evidence of immunity to varicella is:
  – U.S.-born before 1980 (except for pregnant women and health care personnel, see below)
  – Documentation of receipt of 2 doses of varicella or varicella-containing vaccine at least 4 weeks apart
  – Diagnosis or verification of history of varicella or herpes zoster by a health care provider
  – Laboratory evidence of immunity or disease

Special populations
- Administer 2 doses of VAR 4–8 weeks apart if previously received no varicella vaccine (if previously received 1 dose of varicella-containing vaccine, administer 1 dose of VAR at least 4 weeks after the first dose) to:
  – Pregnant women without evidence of immunity: Administer the first of the 2 doses or the second dose after pregnancy and before discharge from health care facility
  – Health care personnel without evidence of immunity
- Adults with HIV infection and CD4 cell count ≥200 cells/μL: May administer, based on individual clinical decision, 2 doses of VAR 3 months apart
- VAR is contraindicated for pregnant women and adults with severe immunodeficiency

5. Zoster vaccination
www.cdc.gov/vaccines/hcp/acip-recs/vacc-specific/shingles.html

General information
- Administer 2 doses of recombinant zoster vaccine (RZV) 2–6 months apart to adults aged 50 years or older regardless of past episode of herpes zoster or receipt of zoster vaccine live (ZVL)

- Administer 2 doses of RZV 2–6 months apart to adults who previously received ZVL at least 2 months after ZVL
- For adults aged 60 years or older, administer either RZV or ZVL (RZV is preferred)

Special populations
- ZVL is contraindicated for pregnant women and adults with severe immunodeficiency

6. Human papillomavirus vaccination
www.cdc.gov/vaccines/hcp/acip-recs/vacc-specific/hpv.html

General information
- Administer human papillomavirus (HPV) vaccine to females through age 26 years and males through age 21 years (males aged 22 through 26 years may be vaccinated based on individual clinical decision)
- The number of HPV vaccine to be administered depends on age at initial HPV vaccination
  – No previous dose of HPV vaccine: Administer 3-dose series at 0, 1–2, and 6 months (minimum intervals: 4 weeks between doses 1 and 2, 12 weeks between doses 2 and 3, and 5 months between doses 1 and 3; repeat doses if given too soon)
  – Aged 9–14 years at HPV vaccine series initiation and received 1 dose or 2 doses less than 5 months apart: Administer 1 dose
  – Aged 9–14 years at HPV vaccine series initiation and received 2 doses at least 5 months apart: No additional dose is needed

Special populations
- Adults with immunocompromising conditions (including HIV infection) through age 26 years: Administer 3-dose series at 0, 1–2, and 6 months
- Men who have sex with men through age 26 years: Administer 2- or 3-dose series depending on age at initial vaccination (see above); if no history of HPV vaccine, administer 3-dose series at 0, 1–2, and 6 months
- Pregnant women through age 26 years: HPV vaccination is not recommended during pregnancy, but there is no evidence that the vaccine is harmful and no intervention needed for women who inadvertently receive HPV vaccine while pregnant; delay remaining doses until after pregnancy; pregnancy testing is not needed before vaccination

7. Pneumococcal vaccination
www.cdc.gov/vaccines/hcp/acip-recs/vacc-specific/pneumo.html

General information
- Administer to immunocompetent adults aged 65 years or older 1 dose of 13-valent pneumococcal conjugate vaccine (PCV13), if not previously administered, followed by 1 dose of 23-valent pneumococcal polysaccharide vaccine (PPSV23) at least 1 year after PCV13; if PPSV23 was previously administered but not PCV13, administer PCV13 at least 1 year after PPSV23
- When both PCV13 and PPSV23 are indicated, administer PCV13 first (PCV13 and PPSV23 should not be administered during the same visit); additional information on vaccine timing is available at www.cdc.gov/vaccines/vpd/pneumo/downloads/pneumo-vaccine-timing.pdf

Figure 17.2 (Continued)

Special populations

• Administer to adults aged 19 through 64 years with the following chronic conditions 1 dose of PPSV23 (at age 65 years or older, administer 1 dose of PCV13, then at least 1 year after PCV13, and another dose of PPSV23 at least 1 year after PCV13 and at least 5 years after PPSV23):

- **Chronic heart disease** (excluding hypertension)
- **Chronic lung disease**
- **Chronic liver disease**
- **Alcoholism**
- **Diabetes mellitus**
- **Cigarette smoking**

• Administer to adults aged 19 years or older with the following indications 1 dose of PCV13 followed by 1 dose of PPSV23 at least 8 weeks after PCV13, and a second dose of PPSV23 at least 5 years after the first dose of PPSV23 (if the most recent dose of PPSV23 was administered before age 65 years, at age 65 years or older, administer another dose of PPSV23 at least 5 years after the last dose of PPSV23):

- **Immunodeficiency disorders** (including B- and T-lymphocyte deficiency, complement deficiencies, and phagocytic disorders)
- **HIV infection**
- **Anatomical or functional asplenia** (including sickle cell disease and other hemoglobinopathies)
- **Chronic renal failure and nephrotic syndrome**

• Administer to adults aged 19 years or older with the following indications 1 dose of PCV13 followed by 1 dose of PPSV23 at least 8 weeks after PCV13 (if the dose of PPSV23 was administered before age 65 years, at age 65 years or older, administer another dose of PPSV23 at least 5 years after the dose of PPSV23):

- **Cerebrospinal fluid leak**
- **Cochlear implant**

8. Hepatitis A vaccination

www.cdc.gov/vaccines/hcp/acip-recs/vacc-specific/hepa.html

General information

• Administer to adults who have a specific risk (see below), or lack a risk factor but want protection. 2-dose series of single antigen hepatitis A vaccine (HepA: Havrix at 0 and 6–12 months; Vaqta at 0 and 6–18 months; minimum interval: 6 months) or a 3-dose series of combined hepatitis A and hepatitis B vaccine (HepA-HepB) at 0, 1, and 6 months; minimum intervals: 4 weeks between first and second doses, 5 months between second and third doses

Special populations

• Administer HepA or HepA-HepB to adults with the following indications:

- **Travel** to or work in countries with high or intermediate hepatitis A endemicity
- **Men who have sex with men**
- **Injection or noninjection drug use**
- **Work with hepatitis A virus in a research laboratory or with nonhuman primates infected with hepatitis A virus**
- **Clotting factor disorders**
- **Chronic liver disease**

- Close, personal **contact with an international adoptee** (e.g., household or regular babysitting) during the first 60 days after arrival in the United States from a country with high or intermediate endemicity (administer the first dose as soon as the adoption is planned)
- Healthy adults **through age 40 years who have recently been exposed to hepatitis A virus**; adults older than age 40 years may receive HepA or HepA-HepB if hepatitis A immunoglobulin cannot be obtained

9. Hepatitis B vaccination

www.cdc.gov/vaccines/hcp/acip-recs/vacc-specific/hepb.html

General information

• Administer to adults who have a specific risk (see below), or lack a risk factor but want protection. 3-dose series of single antigen hepatitis B vaccine (HepB) or combined hepatitis A and hepatitis B vaccine (HepA-HepB); between doses 1 and 2 for HepB and HepA-HepB; between doses 2 and 3, 8 weeks for HepB and 5 months for HepA-HepB)

Special populations

• Administer HepB or HepA-HepB to adults with the following indications:

- **Chronic liver disease** (e.g., hepatitis C infection, cirrhosis, fatty liver disease, alcoholic liver disease, autoimmune hepatitis, alanine aminotransferase [ALT] or aspartate aminotransferase [AST] level greater than twice the upper limit of normal)
- **HIV infection**
- **Percutaneous or mucosal risk of exposure to blood** (e.g., household contacts of hepatitis B surface antigen [HBsAg]-positive persons; adults younger than age 60 years with diabetes mellitus or aged 60 years or older with diabetes mellitus based on individual clinical decision; adults in predialysis care or receiving hemodialysis or peritoneal dialysis; recent or current injection drug users; health care and public safety workers at risk for exposure to blood or blood-contaminated body fluids)
- **Sexual exposure risk** (e.g., sex partners of HBsAg-positive persons; sexually active persons not in a mutually monogamous relationship; persons seeking evaluation or treatment for a sexually transmitted infection; and **men who have sex with men** [MSM])
- **Receive care in settings where a high proportion of adults have risks for hepatitis B infection** (e.g., facilities providing sexually transmitted disease treatment, drug-abuse treatment and prevention services, hemodialysis and end-stage renal disease programs, institutions for developmentally disabled persons, health care settings targeting services to injection drug users or MSM, HIV testing and treatment facilities, and correctional facilities)
- **Travel** to countries with high or intermediate hepatitis B endemicity

10. Meningococcal vaccination

www.cdc.gov/vaccines/hcp/acip-recs/vacc-specific/mening.html

Special populations: Serogroups A, C, W, and Y meningococcal vaccine (MenACWY)

- Administer 2 doses of MenACWY at least 8 weeks apart and revaccinate with 1 dose of MenACWY every 5 years, if the risk remains, to adults with the following indications:
- **Anatomical or functional asplenia** (including sickle cell disease and other hemoglobinopathies)
- **HIV infection**
- **Persistent complement component deficiency**
- **Eculizumab use**

• Administer 1 dose of MenACWY and revaccinate with 1 dose of MenACWY every 5 years, if the risk remains, to adults with the following indications:

- **Travel to or live in countries where meningococcal disease is hyperendemic or epidemic,** including countries in the African meningitis belt or during the Hajj
- At risk from a **meningococcal disease outbreak attributed to serogroup A, C, W, or Y**
- **Microbiologists** routinely exposed to *Neisseria meningitidis*
- **Military recruits**
- **First-year college students who live in residential housing** (if they did not receive MenACWY at age 16 years or older)

General Information: Serogroup B meningococcal vaccine (MenB)

• May administer, based on individual clinical decision, to young adults and adolescents aged 16–23 years (preferred age is 16–18 years) who are not at increased risk 2-dose series of MenB-4C (Bexsero) at least 1 month apart or 2-dose series of MenB-FHbp (Trumenba) at least 6 months apart

- MenB-4C and MenB-FHbp are not interchangeable

Special populations: MenB

• Administer 2-dose series of MenB-4C at least 1 month apart or 3-dose series of MenB-FHbp at 0, 1–2, and 6 months to adults with the following indications:

- **Anatomical or functional asplenia** (including sickle cell disease)
- **Persistent complement component deficiency**
- **Eculizumab use**
- At risk from a **meningococcal disease outbreak attributed to serogroup B**
- **Microbiologists** routinely exposed to *Neisseria meningitidis*

11. *Haemophilus influenzae* type b vaccination

www.cdc.gov/vaccines/hcp/acip-recs/vacc-specific/hib.html

Special populations

• Administer *Haemophilus influenzae* type b vaccine (Hib) to adults with the following indications:

- **Anatomical or functional asplenia** (including sickle cell disease) or undergoing elective splenectomy: Administer 1 dose if not previously vaccinated (preferably at least 14 days before elective splenectomy)
- **Hematopoietic stem cell transplant** (HSCT): Administer 3-dose series with doses 4 weeks apart starting 6 to 12 months after successful transplant regardless of Hib vaccination history

Figure 17.2 *(Continued)*

Table. Contraindications and precautions for vaccines recommended for adults aged 19 years or older*

The Advisory Committee on Immunization Practices (ACIP) recommendations and package inserts for vaccines provide information on contraindications and precautions related to vaccines. Contraindications are conditions that increase the chances of a serious adverse reaction in vaccine recipients and the vaccine should not be administered when a contraindication is present. Precautions should be reviewed for potential risks and benefits for vaccine recipients.

Contraindications and precautions for vaccines routinely recommended for adults

Vaccine(s)	Contraindications	Precautions
All vaccines routinely recommended for adults	• Severe reaction, e.g., anaphylaxis, after a previous dose or to a vaccine component	• Moderate or severe acute illness with or without fever

Additional contraindications and precautions for vaccines routinely recommended for adults

Vaccine(s)	Additional Contraindications	Additional Precautions
IIV[1]		• History of Guillain-Barré syndrome within 6 weeks after previous influenza vaccination • Egg allergy other than hives, e.g., angioedema, respiratory distress, lightheadedness, or recurrent emesis; or required epinephrine or another emergency medical intervention (IIV may be administered in an inpatient or outpatient medical setting and under the supervision of a health care provider who is able to recognize and manage severe allergic conditions)
RIV[1]		• History of Guillain-Barré syndrome within 6 weeks after previous influenza vaccination
Tdap, Td	• For pertussis-containing vaccines: encephalopathy, e.g., coma, decreased level of consciousness, or prolonged seizures, not attributable to another identifiable cause within 7 days of administration of a previous dose of a vaccine containing tetanus or diphtheria toxoid or acellular pertussis	• Guillain-Barré syndrome within 6 weeks after a previous dose of tetanus toxoid-containing vaccine • History of Arthus-type hypersensitivity reactions after a previous dose of tetanus or diphtheria toxoid-containing vaccine. Defer vaccination until at least 10 years have elapsed since the last tetanus toxoid-containing vaccine • For pertussis-containing vaccine, progressive or unstable neurologic disorder, uncontrolled seizures, or progressive encephalopathy (until a treatment regimen has been established and the condition has stabilized)
MMR[2]	• Severe immunodeficiency, e.g., hematologic and solid tumors, chemotherapy, congenital immunodeficiency or long-term immunosuppressive therapy[3], human immunodeficiency virus (HIV) infection with severe immunocompromise • Pregnancy	• Recent (within 11 months) receipt of antibody-containing blood product (specific interval depends on product)[4] • History of thrombocytopenia or thrombocytopenic purpura • Need for tuberculin skin testing[5]
VAR[2]	• Severe immunodeficiency, e.g., hematologic and solid tumors, chemotherapy, congenital immunodeficiency or long-term immunosuppressive therapy[3], HIV infection with severe immunocompromise • Pregnancy	• Recent (within 11 months) receipt of antibody-containing blood product (specific interval depends on product)[4] • Receipt of specific antiviral drugs (acyclovir, famciclovir, or valacyclovir) 24 hours before vaccination (avoid use of these antiviral drugs for 14 days after vaccination)
ZVL[2]	• Severe immunodeficiency, e.g., hematologic and solid tumors, chemotherapy, congenital immunodeficiency or long-term immunosuppressive therapy[3], HIV infection with severe immunocompromise • Pregnancy	• Receipt of specific antiviral drugs (acyclovir, famciclovir, or valacyclovir) 24 hours before vaccination (avoid use of these antiviral drugs for 14 days after vaccination)
HPV vaccine		• Pregnancy
PCV13	• Severe allergic reaction to any vaccine containing diphtheria toxoid	

1. For additional information on use of influenza vaccine among persons with egg allergy, see: CDC. Prevention and control of seasonal influenza with vaccines: recommendations of the Advisory Committee on Immunization Practices—United States, 2016–17 influenza season. MMWR. 2016;65(RR-5):1–54. Available at www.cdc.gov/mmwr/volumes/65/rr/rr6505a1.htm.
2. MMR may be administered together with VAR or ZVL on the same day; separate live vaccines by at least 28 days.
3. Immunosuppressive steroid dose is considered to be daily receipt of 20 mg or more prednisone or equivalent for 2 or more weeks. Vaccination should be deferred for at least 1 month after discontinuation of immunosuppressive steroid therapy. Providers should consult ACIP recommendations for complete information on the use of specific live vaccines among persons on immune-suppressing medications or with immune suppression because of other reasons.
4. Vaccine should be deferred for the appropriate interval if replacement immune globulin products are being administered. See Best practices guidance of the Advisory Committee on Immunization Practices (ACIP). Available at www.cdc.gov/vaccines/hcp/acip-recs/general-recs/index.html.
5. Measles vaccination may temporarily suppress tuberculin reactivity. Measles-containing vaccine may be administered on the same day as tuberculin skin testing, or should be postponed for at least 4 weeks after vaccination.

* Adapted from: CDC. Table 6. Contraindications and precautions to commonly used vaccines. General recommendations on immunizations: recommendations of the Advisory Committee on Immunization Practices. MMWR. 2011;60(No. RR-2):40–1 and from: Hamborsky J, Kroger A, Wolfe S, eds. Appendix A. Epidemiology and prevention of vaccine preventable diseases. 13th ed. Washington, DC: Public Health Foundation, 2015. Available at www.cdc.gov/vaccines/pubs/pinkbook/index.html.

Abbreviations of vaccines

IIV	inactivated influenza vaccine	VAR	varicella vaccine
RIV	recombinant influenza vaccine	RZV	recombinant zoster vaccine
Tdap	tetanus toxoid, reduced diphtheria toxoid, and acellular pertussis vaccine	ZVL	zoster vaccine live
		HPV vaccine	human papillomavirus vaccine
Td	tetanus and diphtheria toxoids	PCV13	13-valent pneumococcal conjugate vaccine
MMR	measles, mumps, and rubella vaccine	PPSV23	23-valent pneumococcal polysaccharide vaccine

HepA	hepatitis A vaccine
HepA-HepB	hepatitis A and hepatitis B vaccines
HepB	hepatitis B vaccine
MenACWY	serogroups A, C, W, and Y meningococcal vaccine
MenB	serogroup B meningococcal vaccine
Hib	Haemophilus influenzae type b vaccine

Figure 17.2 *(Continued)*

C5270457-A

Intramuscular injections are generally administered in the anterolateral aspect of the thigh in infants and in the deltoid muscle in older children and adults; they should not be administered in the gluteal muscles at any age because of risk of injury to the sciatic nerve (see Figs. 17.3 and 17.4). Further details about vaccine handling and injection technique are provided in the references at the end of this chapter.

For most vaccines, simultaneous administration does not impair antibody responses or increase rates of adverse reactions.[13,14] In fact, simultaneous administration is an important public health strategy, decreasing the number of visits needed and the potential for missed doses as well as enabling earlier protection.[13,14] With the increasing number of vaccinations that are recommended for administration before the age of 18 months, combination vaccines offer many practical advantages: the avoidance of deferred immunizations due to clinician or parental concern over multiple shots with the attendant risks of missed opportunities, an increase in adherence and improved vaccination coverage rates, reduced pain, and potentially lower costs from reduced vaccine charges and reduced office visits.[14] The ACIP, AAFP, and AAP have issued a joint statement endorsing the use of combination vaccines whenever any component of the combination is indicated and its other components are not contraindicated, provided they are approved by the U.S. Food and Drug Administration (FDA) for use in children at the recommended ages.[14] Vaccines that prevent the same disease but are from different manufacturers may be interchanged when a particular antibody is known to protect against disease (called the *serologic correlate of immunity*) and when using vaccines from different manufacturers results in sufficient antibody titers.[14]

Immune globulin may interfere with viral replication and the antibody response to certain live virus vaccines. Administration of measles-mumps-rubella-varicella (MMRV) vaccine or its component vaccines should therefore be delayed for 3 to 11 months after the administration of antibody-containing blood products (such as immune globulins), depending on the type of preparation and its dose.[13] If vaccination with MMRV or its component vaccines precedes immune globulin administration, it need not be readministered if the interval between the two products is longer than 14 days. Some live virus vaccines can theoretically interfere with viral replication and the antibody response to other live virus vaccines if not administered as recommended. Measles-mumps-rubella (MMR) vaccine and varicella vaccine may be given simultaneously; otherwise their administration should be separated by at least 4 weeks. Specific guidelines for spacing administration are provided elsewhere.[13]

Appropriate indications, contraindications, and precautions for vaccination are listed in Table 17.1. According to the CDC's *Epidemiology and Prevention of Vaccine-Preventable Diseases* ("*The Pink Book*"), a *contraindication* to immunization is a condition in a recipient that increases the chance of a serious adverse reaction, such as an allergy to one of the vaccine components.[14] A vaccine should generally not be given when

Administering Vaccines:
Dose, Route, Site, and Needle Size

Vaccine	Dose	Route
Diphtheria, Tetanus, Pertussis (DTaP, DT, Tdap, Td)	0.5 mL	IM
Haemophilus influenzae type b (Hib)	0.5 mL	IM
Hepatitis A (HepA)	≤18 yrs: 0.5 mL / ≥19 yrs: 1.0 mL	IM
Hepatitis B (HepB) Persons 11–15 yrs may be given Recombivax HB (Merck) 1.0 mL adult formulation on a 2-dose schedule.	Engerix-B; Recombivax HB ≤19 yrs: 0.5 mL ≥20 yrs: 1.0 mL / Heplisav-B ≥18 yrs: 0.5 mL	IM
Human papillomavirus (HPV)	0.5 mL	IM
Influenza, live attenuated (LAIV)	0.2 mL (0.1 mL in each nostril)	Intranasal spray
Influenza, inactivated (IIV); for ages 6–35 months	Fluzone: 0.25 mL / FluLaval; Fluarix: 0.5 mL	IM
Influenza, inactivated (IIV), for ages 3 years & older; recombinant (RIV), for ages 18 years and older	0.5 mL	IM
Measles, Mumps, Rubella (MMR)	0.5 mL	Subcut
Meningococcal serogroups A, C, W, Y (MenACWY)	0.5 mL	IM
Meningococcal serogroup B (MenB)	0.5 mL	IM
Pneumococcal conjugate (PCV)	0.5 mL	IM
Pneumococcal polysaccharide (PPSV)	0.5 mL	IM or Subcut
Polio, inactivated (IPV)	0.5 mL	IM or Subcut
Rotavirus (RV)	Rotarix: 1.0 mL / Rotateq: 2.0 mL	Oral
Varicella (Var)	0.5 mL	Subcut
Zoster (Zos)	Shingrix: 0.5* mL / Zostavax: 0.65 mL	IM / Subcut
Combination Vaccines		
DTaP-HepB-IPV (Pediarix) DTaP-IPV/Hib (Pentacel) DTaP-IPV (Kinrix; Quadracel)	0.5 mL	IM
MMRV (ProQuad)	≤12 yrs: 0.5 mL	Subcut
HepA-HepB (Twinrix)	≥18 yrs: 1.0 mL	IM

* The vial might contain more than 0.5 mL. Do not administer more than 0.5 mL.

Injection Site and Needle Size

Subcutaneous (Subcut) injection
Use a 23–25 gauge needle. Choose the injection site that is appropriate to the person's age and body mass.

AGE	NEEDLE LENGTH	INJECTION SITE
Infants (1–12 mos)	5/8"	Fatty tissue over anterolateral thigh muscle
Children 12 mos or older, adolescents, and adults	5/8"	Fatty tissue over anterolateral thigh muscle or fatty tissue over triceps

Intramuscular (IM) injection
Use a 22–25 gauge needle. Choose the injection site and needle length that is appropriate to the person's age and body mass.

AGE		NEEDLE LENGTH	INJECTION SITE
Newborns (1st 28 days)		5/8"	Anterolateral thigh muscle
Infants (1–12 mos)		1"	Anterolateral thigh muscle
Toddlers (1–2 years)		1–1¼"	Anterolateral thigh muscle
		5/8–1"	Deltoid muscle of arm
Children (3–10 years)		5/8–1"*	Deltoid muscle of arm
		1–1¼"	Anterolateral thigh muscle
Adolescents and teens (11–18 years)		5/8–1"*	Deltoid muscle of arm
		1–1½"	Anterolateral thigh muscle
Adults 19 years or older			
Female or male <130 lbs		5/8–1"*	Deltoid muscle of arm
Female or male 130–152 lbs		1"	Deltoid muscle of arm
Female 153–200 lbs Male 153–260 lbs		1–1½"	Deltoid muscle of arm
Female 200+ lbs Male 260+ lbs		1½"	Deltoid muscle of arm

* A 5/8" needle may be used for patients weighing less than 130 lbs (<60 kg) for IM injection in the deltoid muscle only if the skin stretched tight, the subcutaneous tissue is not bunched, and the injection is made at a 90-degree angle.

NOTE: Always refer to the package insert included with each biologic for complete vaccine administration information. CDC's Advisory Committee on Immunization Practices (ACIP) recommendations for the particular vaccine should be reviewed as well. Access the ACIP recommendations at www.immunize.org/acip.

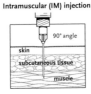
Intramuscular (IM) injection

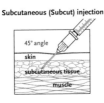
Subcutaneous (Subcut) injection

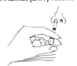
Intranasal (NAS) administration of Flumist (LAIV) vaccine

Technical content reviewed by the Centers for Disease Control and Prevention

IMMUNIZATION ACTION COALITION   Saint Paul, Minnesota · 651-647-9009 · www.immunize.org · www.vaccineinformation.org
www.immunize.org/catg.d/p3085.pdf · Item #P3085 (10/18)

Figure 17.3 Administering vaccines: dose, route, site, and needle size. Used with permission of the Immunization Action Coalition, St. Paul, MN. www.immunize.org/catg.d/p3085.pdf. Acquired from http://www.immunize.org/catg.d/p3085.pdfon 9/5/2018. We thank the Immunization Action Coalition.

a contraindication is present. A *precaution* is a condition in a recipient that *might* increase the chance or severity of a serious adverse reaction or compromise the ability of the vaccine to produce immunity (such as administering measles vaccine to a person with passive immunity to measles from a blood transfusion). The clinician may consider giving a vaccine

How to Administer Intramuscular and Subcutaneous Vaccine Injections to Adults

Intramuscular (IM) Injections

Administer these vaccines via IM route
- *Haemophilus influenzae* type b (Hib)
- Hepatitis A (HepA)
- Hepatitis B (HepB)
- Human papillomavirus (HPV)
- Influenza vaccine, injectable (IIV)
- Influenza vaccine, recombinant (RIV3; RIV4)
- Meningococcal conjugate (MenACWY)
- Meningococcal serogroup B (MenB)
- Pneumococcal conjugate (PCV13)
- Pneumococcal polysaccharide (PPSV23) – may also be given Subcut
- Polio (IPV) – may also be given Subcut
- Tetanus, diphtheria (Td), or with pertussis (Tdap)
- Zoster, recombinant (RZV; Shingrix)

Injection site
Give in the central and thickest portion of the deltoid muscle – above the level of the armpit and approximately 2–3 fingerbreadths (~2") below the acromion process. *See the diagram.* To avoid causing an injury, do not inject too high (near the acromion process) or too low.

Needle size
22–25 gauge, 1–1½" needle *(see note at right)*

Needle insertion
- Use a needle long enough to reach deep into the muscle.
- Insert the needle at a 90° angle to the skin with a quick thrust.
- Separate two injections given in the same deltoid muscle by a minimum of 1".

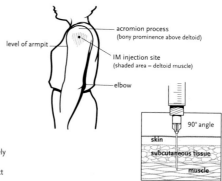

Note: A ⅝" needle is sufficient in adults weighing less than 130 lbs (<60 kg) for IM injection in the deltoid muscle **only** if the subcutaneous tissue is not bunched and the injection is made at a 90° angle; a 1" needle is sufficient in adults weighing 130–152 lbs (60–70 kg); a 1–1½" needle is recommended in women weighing 153–200 lbs (70–90 kg) and men weighing 153–260 lbs (70–118 kg); a 1½" needle is recommended in women weighing more than 200 lbs (91 kg) or men weighing more than 260 lbs (more than 118 kg).

Subcutaneous (Subcut) Injections

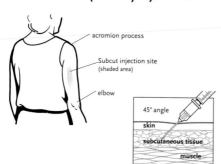

Administer these vaccines via Subcut route
- Measles, mumps, rubella (MMR)
- Pneumococcal polysaccharide (PPSV23) – may also be given IM
- Polio (IPV) – may also be given IM
- Varicella (Var; chickenpox)
- Zoster, live (ZVL; Zostavax)

Injection site
Give in fatty tissue over the triceps. *See the diagram.*

Needle size
23–25 gauge, 5/8" needle

Needle insertion
- Pinch up on the tissue to prevent injection into the muscle. Insert the needle at a 45° angle to the skin.
- Separate two injections given in the same area of fatty tissue by a minimum of 1".

immunization action coalition

IAC

immunize.org

Saint Paul, Minnesota · 651-647-9009 · www.immunize.org · www.vaccineinformation.org

Technical content reviewed by the Centers for Disease Control and Prevention

www.immunize.org/catg.d/p2020a.pdf · Item #P2020a (1/18)

Figure 17.4   Administering vaccines to adults: dose, route, site, and needle size. Used with permission of the Immunization Action Coalition, St. Paul, MN. http://www.immunize.org/catg.d/p3084.pdf Acquired from http://www.immunize.org/catg.d/p3084.pdf on 9/5/2018. We thank the Immunization Action Coaliti

TABLE 17.1 Guide to Contraindications and Precautions to Commonly Used Vaccines¹.*

Vaccine	Contraindications	Precautions
Hepatitis B (HepB)	• Severe allergic reaction (e.g., anaphylaxis) after a previous dose or to a vaccine component • Hypersensitivity to yeast	• Moderate or severe acute illness with or without fever • Infant weighing less than 2000 grams (4 lbs, 6.4 oz)²
Rotavirus (RV5 [RotaTeq], RV1 [Rotarix])	• Severe allergic reaction (e.g., anaphylaxis) after a previous dose or to a vaccine component • Severe combined immunodeficiency (SCID) • History of intussusception	• Moderate or severe acute illness with or without fever • Altered immunocompetence other than SCID • Chronic gastrointestinal disease³ • Spina bifida or bladder exstrophy³
Diphtheria, tetanus, pertussis (DTaP) Tetanus, diphtheria, pertussis (Tdap) Tetanus, diphtheria (DT, Td)	• Severe allergic reaction (e.g., anaphylaxis) after a previous dose or to a vaccine component • For pertussis-containing vaccines: Encephalopathy (e.g., coma, decreased level of consciousness; prolonged seizures) not attributable to another identifiable cause within 7 days of administration of a previous dose of DTP or DTaP (for DTaP); or of previous dose of DTP, DTaP, or Tdap (for Tdap)	• Moderate or severe acute illness with or without fever • Guillain-Barré syndrome (GBS) within 6 weeks after a previous dose of tetanus toxoid-containing vaccine • History of Arthus-type hypersensitivity reactions after a previous dose of diphtheria- or tetanus-toxoid-containing vaccine; defer vaccination until at least 10 years have elapsed since the last tetanus-toxoid containing vaccine • For DTaP and Tdap only: Progressive or unstable neurologic disorder (including infantile spasms for DTaP), uncontrolled seizures, or progressive encephalopathy; defer until a treatment regimen has been established and the condition has stabilized
Haemophilus influenzae type b (Hib)	• Severe allergic reaction (e.g., anaphylaxis) after a previous dose or to a vaccine component • Age younger than 6 weeks	• Moderate or severe acute illness with or without fever
Inactivated poliovirus vaccine (IPV)	• Severe allergic reaction (e.g., anaphylaxis) after a previous dose or to a vaccine component	• Moderate or severe acute illness with or without fever • Pregnancy
Hepatitis A (HepA)	• Severe allergic reaction (e.g., anaphylaxis) after a previous dose or to a vaccine component	• Moderate or severe acute illness with or without fever

(Continued)

TABLE 17.1 Guide to Contraindications and Precautions to Commonly Used Vaccines[1,*] (Continued)

Vaccine	Contraindications	Precautions
Measles, mumps, rubella (MMR)[4]	• Severe allergic reaction (e.g., anaphylaxis) after a previous dose or to a vaccine component • Severe immunodeficiency (e.g., hematologic and solid tumors, chemotherapy, congenital immunodeficiency or long-term immunosuppressive therapy[5]), or persons with human immunodeficiency virus [HIV] infection who are severely immunocompromised[6] • Family history of congenital or hereditary immunodeficiency in first-degree relatives (e.g., parents and siblings), unless the immune competence of the potential vaccine recipient has been substantiated clinically or verified by a laboratory test • Pregnancy	• Moderate or severe acute illness with or without fever • Recent (within 11 months) receipt of antibody-containing blood product (specific interval depends on product)[7] • For MMRV only: Family history of seizures • History of thrombocytopenia or thrombocytopenic purpura • Need for tuberculin skin testing[8]
Varicella (Var)[4]	• Severe allergic reaction (e.g., anaphylaxis) after a previous dose or to a vaccine component • Severe immunodeficiency (e.g., hematologic and solid tumors, chemotherapy, congenital immunodeficiency or long-term immunosuppressive therapy[5]), or persons with HIV infection who are severely immunocompromised[6] • Family history of congenital or hereditary immunodeficiency in first-degree relatives (e.g., parents and siblings), unless the immune competence of the potential vaccine recipient has been substantiated clinically or verified by a laboratory test • Pregnancy	• Moderate or severe acute illness with or without fever • Recent (within 11 months) receipt of antibody-containing blood product (specific interval depends on product)[7] • Receipt of specific antivirals (i.e., acyclovir, famciclovir, or valacyclovir) 24 hours before vaccination; avoid use of these antiviral drugs for 14 days after vaccination.
Pneumococcal (PCV13 or PPSV23)	• Severe allergic reaction (e.g., anaphylaxis) after a previous dose or to a vaccine component (including, for PCV13, to any diphtheria toxoid-containing vaccine)	• Moderate or severe acute illness with or without fever

Vaccine	Contraindications	Precautions
Influenza, inactivated injectable (IIV)[9]	• Severe allergic reaction (e.g., anaphylaxis) to any component of the vaccine (except egg) or to a previous dose of influenza vaccine[9]	• Moderate or severe acute illness with or without fever • History of GBS within 6 weeks of previous influenza vaccination • Egg allergy other than hives (e.g., angioedema, respiratory distress, lightheadedness, or recurrent emesis); or required epinephrine or another emergency medical intervention (IIV may be administered in an inpatient or outpatient medical setting, under the supervision of a healthcare provider who is able to recognize and manage severe allergic conditions)[9]
Influenza, recombinant (RIV)[9]	• Severe allergic reaction (e.g., anaphylaxis) to any component of the vaccine (except egg) or to a previous dose of influenza vaccine[9]	• Moderate or severe acute illness with or without fever • History of GBS within weeks of previous influenza vaccination
Influenza, live attenuated (LAIV)[2,3]	• Severe allergic reaction (e.g., anaphylaxis) to any component of the vaccine (except egg) or to a previous dose of influenza vaccine • Concomitant use of aspirin or salicylate-containing therapy in children or adolescents • Children age 2 through 4 years who have a diagnosis of asthma or had wheezing with the past 12 months, per healthcare provider statement • Children and adults who are immunocompromised due to any nbcause (including immunosuppression caused by medications or by HIV infection) • Close contacts and caregivers of severely immunosuppressed persons who required a protected environment) • Pregnancy • Receipt of influenza antivirals (amantadine, rimantadine, zanamivir, oseltamivir or peramivir) within the previous 48 hours; avoid use of these antiviral drugs for 14 days after vaccination	• Moderate or severe acute illness with or without fever • GBS within 6 weeks of previous influenza vaccination • Asthma in persons age 5 years and older • Other chronic medical conditions (e.g., other chronic lung diseases, chronic cardiovascular disease [excluding isolated hypertension], diabetes, chronic renal or hepatic disease, hematologic disease, neurologic disease, and metabolic disorders)

(Continued)

TABLE 17.1   Guide to Contraindications and Precautions to Commonly Used Vaccines[1],[·]   (Continued)

Vaccine	Contraindications	Precautions
Human papillomavirus (HPV)	• Severe allergic reaction (e.g., anaphylaxis) after a previous dose or to a vaccine component	• Moderate or severe acute illness with or without fever • Pregnancy
Meningococcal (MenACWY; MenB)	• Severe allergic reaction (e.g., anaphylaxis) after a previous dose or to a vaccine component	• Moderate or severe acute illness with or without fever

[1]The Advisory Committee on Immunization Practices (ACIP) recommendations and package inserts for vaccines provide information on contraindications and precautions related to vaccines. Contraindications are conditions that increase chances of a serious adverse reaction in vaccine recipients and the vaccine should not be administered when a contraindication is present. Precautions should be reviewed for potential risks and benefits for vaccine recipient. For a person with a severe allergy to latex (e.g., anaphylaxis), vaccines supplied in vials or syringes that contain natural rubber latex should not be administered unless the benefit of vaccination clearly outweighs the risk for a potential allergic reaction. For latex allergies other than anaphylaxis, vaccines supplied in vials or syringes that contain dry, natural rubber or natural rubber latex may be administered. Whether and when to administer DTaP to children with proven or suspected underlying neurologic disorders should be decided on a case-by-case basis.

[2]Hepatitis B vaccination should be deferred for preterm infants and infants weighing less than 2000 g if the mother is documented to be hepatitis B surface antigen (HBsAg)-negative at the time of the infant's birth. Vaccination can commence at chronological age 1 month or at hospital discharge. For infants born to women who are HBsAg-positive, hepatitis B immunoglobulin and hepatitis B vaccine should be administered within 12 hours of birth, regardless of weight.

[3]For details, see CDC. "Prevention of Rotavirus Gastroenteritis among Infants and Children: Recommendations of the Advisory Committee on Immunization Practices. (ACIP)" *MMWR* 2009; 58(No. RR–2), available at www.cdc.gov/vaccines/hcp/acip-recs/index.html.

[4]Age-appropriate parenteral vaccines (LAIV, MMR, Var, or ZVL) can be administered on the same day. If not administered on the same day, these live vaccines should be separated by at least 28 days.

[5]Immunosuppressive steroid dose is considered to be 2 or more weeks of daily receipt of 20 mg prednisone or equivalent. Vaccination should be deferred for at least 1 month after discontinuation of such therapy. Providers should consult ACIP recommendations for complete information on the use of specific live vaccines among persons on immune-suppressing medications or with immune suppression because of other reasons.

[6]HIV-infected children 5 years of age or younger should receive measles vaccine if CDT+ T-lymphocyte percentages are greater than or equal to 15% for greater than or equal to 6 months. HIV-infected children older than 5 years must have CD4+ percentages greater than or equal to 15 and CD4+ T-lymphocyte counts greater than or equal to 200 lymphocytes/cubic mm for 6 months or longer. In cases where only counts or only percentages are available for children older than 5 years, use the data that are available. In cases where percentages are not available for children 5 years of younger, use counts based on the age-specific counts at the time the counts were measured (see www.cdc.gov/vaccines/hcp/acip-recs/index.html for details). HIV-infected children younger than 8 years may receive varicella vaccine if CD4+ T-lymphocyte percentages are 15% or greater. HIV-infected children 8 years or older may receive varicella vaccine if CD4+ T-lymphocyte count is greater than 200 cells/cubic mm.

[7]Vaccine should be deferred for the appropriate interval if replacement immune globulin products are being administered (see "Table 3-5. Recommended Intervals Between Administration of Antibody-Containing Products and Measles- or Varicella-Containing Vaccine, by Product and Indication for Vaccination" found in "Best Practices Guidance of the Advisory Committee on Immunization Practices (ACIP)," available at www.cdc.gov/vaccines/hcp/acip-recs/general-recs/index.html.)

[8]Measles vaccination might suppress tuberculin reactivity temporarily. Measles-containing vaccine may be administered on the same day as tuberculin skin testing, or should be postponed for at least 4 weeks after the vaccination.

[9]For additional information on use of influenza vaccines among persons with egg allergy, see CDC. "Prevention and Control of Seasonal Influenza with Vaccines: Recommendations of the Advisory Committee on Immunization Practices (ACIP) – United States, . . ." Access links to influenza vaccine recommendations at www.cdc.gov/vaccines/hcp/acip-recs/vacc-specific/flu.html.

*Adapted from "Table 4-1. Contraindications and Precautions to Commonly Used Vaccines" found in: CDC. "Best Practices Guidance of the Advisory Committee on Immunization Practices (ACIP)" available at www.cdc.gov/vaccines/hcp/acip-recs/general-recs/index.html.

in some conditions where a precaution applies, but the benefits of giving the vaccine should outweigh the risks. It is important for the clinician to recognize that mild illnesses, low-grade fever, allergy to products not in immunizations, households where family member is pregnant or immunocompromised, breastfed infants, a history of preterm birth, family history of allergies, disease exposure or convalescence, tuberculosis skin testing, multiple immunizations, and current antibiotic therapy are generally *unfounded reasons for deferring vaccination*.[14]

Rare anaphylactic reactions to certain vaccines or vaccine components have been reported. Hypersensitivity to vaccines can occur in reaction to antigen, animal proteins, antibiotics (e.g., neomycin), preservatives, or stabilizers contained in the vaccine. The most common animal protein allergen is egg protein, which is found in the influenza and yellow fever vaccines because they are prepared using embryonated chicken eggs. Ordinarily, patients who are able to eat eggs safely may receive these vaccines. They are, however, contraindicated in persons with a history of a severe anaphylactic reactions to egg products: a history of hives, swelling of the mouth or throat, difficulty breathing, hypotension, or shock; protocols have been developed for the vaccination of such persons against influenza.[15] Although measles and mumps vaccine viruses are grown in chick embryo fibroblast tissue culture, persons with a serious egg allergy can receive measles- or mumps-containing vaccines without skin testing or desensitization to egg protein because the quantity of egg proteins found in these vaccines is not sufficient to induce immediate-type hypersensitivity reactions.[16]

Neomycin-containing antibiotics are contraindicated in persons with a history of anaphylactic reactions to neomycin. The most common allergic response to neomycin, delayed-type hypersensitivity manifested as contact dermatitis, is not a contraindication to receiving these vaccines.

Thimerosal is a preservative, containing approximately 50% ethylmercury by weight, used in some multidose vials of vaccines since the 1930s. Preservatives are not required in single-dose vials, but they were added to multidose vials because of some illness and deaths in the early 20th century caused by bacterial contamination of biologicals. Until 1999, vaccines given to infants to protect them against diphtheria, tetanus, pertussis, *Haemophilus influenzae* type b (Hib), and hepatitis B contained thimerosal as a preservative. As a result of theoretic concerns about toxicity, the U.S. Public Health Service (PHS) agencies, the AAP, and vaccine manufacturers agreed in 1999 that thimerosal levels in vaccines should be reduced or eliminated as a precautionary measure.[17] This agreement was reaffirmed in 2000 in a joint statement of the AAFP, AAP, ACIP, and PHS.[17] Currently, thimerosal has been removed from or reduced to trace levels in all vaccines routinely recommended for children 6 years and younger. Although some inactivated influenza vaccines still contain thimerosal, several brands are thimerosal-free.[17] Some groups of concerned parents and antivaccination groups have claimed that thimerosal might cause neurologic problems, particularly autism, in children. The Institute of Medicine studied this question and concluded in 2004 that there was insufficient evidence to link neurologic injury to thimerosal.[18]

PARENTAL EDUCATION AND COUNSELING

Many children do not receive vaccines because their parents or guardians do not appreciate the importance of immunizations, timely administration, or maintaining complete personal immunization records. It is therefore important for clinicians to explain the purpose of immunizations, the diseases that they prevent, and the rationale for the recommended immunization schedules. They should be counseled about the importance of obtaining immunizations at the recommended ages and should be urged to bring the child's immunization record to each visit.

In recent years, a growing minority of parents have begun to question the safety and efficacy of childhood immunizations. The extent of the problem was shown by a national survey of parental attitudes that found that, although most parents supported vaccination, 25% believed that too many vaccinations could weaken a child's immune system and 23% believed that children get too many immunizations.[19] According to a periodic survey of fellows of the AAP, 7 of 10 pediatricians reported that they had a parent refuse an immunization on behalf of a child in the 12 months preceding the survey.[20] A study of pediatricians in 2002 found that 39% reported that they would dismiss a family for refusing all vaccinations and 28% reported that they would dismiss a family for refusing certain vaccines.[21]

A number of factors may account for the increasing level of parental refusals. In part they reflect vaccine successes; the diseases that vaccines prevent are no longer present to serve as a reminder of the need for immunization.[1] Parents are also influenced by publicized controversies about vaccine safety. These concerns have been fueled by an aggressive antivaccination presence on the Internet[1] and by highly publicized controversies in the media that allege links between vaccinations and various illnesses such as autism.

All states have legal requirements that children be properly immunized before attending school. However, in addition to medical exemptions offered in every state, 47 states allow for religious exemptions and 18 states permit philosophic or personal exemptions.[22] (The vaccine requirements for school entry for each state, as well as information about state vaccine exemptions, can be found online at https://www.cdc.gov/phlp/publications/topic/vaccinations.html.) Increasing vaccine refusals for "philosophic" reasons can have a significant public health impact. A study of vaccine-preventable diseases among children who have philosophic and religious exemptions from immunization mandated by law in Colorado found that exempted children were 22.2 times more likely to acquire measles and 5.9 times more likely to acquire pertussis than were vaccinated children; furthermore, during measles outbreaks an estimated 11% of vaccinated children acquired infection through contact with an exempted child.[23]

How should a clinician approach parents who refuse vaccinations for their children? The AAP has published guidelines for counseling such parents.[24] The list of recommendations includes the following:

- Listen carefully and respectfully to the parent's concerns.
- Share honestly what is and is not known about the risks and benefits of the vaccine in question, attempt to understand the parent's concerns about immunization, and attempt to correct any misperceptions and misinformation.
- Refer parents to one of several reputable and evidence-based websites for additional information.
- Be flexible; some parents have concerns about giving multiple vaccines at a single visit and may be willing to permit a modified schedule with more visits and fewer shots at each visit.
- Explore the possibility that cost is a reason for refusing immunization.
- Revisit the immunization discussion at each subsequent appointment.
- Clinician concerns about liability should be addressed by good documentation of the discussion of the benefits of immunization and the risks associated with remaining unimmunized; clinicians may also wish to consider having the parents sign a refusal waiver.
- Explain the importance of vaccine and they save lives.
- Discuss state laws with the parents. Explain the importance of herd immunity.

As with other forms of patient education, counseling about immunizations should be culturally sensitive.

The following are websites for parents with vaccine safety concerns:

- *CDC/National Immunization Program:* https://www.cdc.gov/vaccines/index.html See sections: "Vaccine Safety" and "Why Immunize?"
- *Immunization Action Coalition:* http://www.immunize.org/
- National Network for Immunization Information: https://www.immunizationinfo.com/ See section: "Parents"

Some children with inadequate immunization coverage often come from families of low socioeconomic status; their parents may have low educational levels or may not understand the clinician's language. Clinicians should take special measures under these circumstances (e.g., obtaining assistance from translators) to ensure that parents obtain accurate information. Parental counseling is critically important to maximize immunization efforts. A CDC study found that perceived lack of information by parents was associated with negative attitudes about immunizations and toward clinicians. Basic information about the benefits and risks of vaccines presented by a trusted clinician can help maintain and/or improve confidence in the immunization process.[25]

VACCINE INFORMATION STATEMENTS

In addition to being prepared to answer patients' or parents' questions about common as well as alleged vaccine-related adverse events, clinicians must utilize "Vaccine Information Statements" (VISs) for vaccines covered under the National Vaccine Injury Compensation Program.[24,25] Federal legislation passed in 1986, the National Childhood Vaccine Injury Act, requires that adults or the parent/legal representative of child receive a copy of a specially prepared VIS developed by the CDC. VISs are required for any vaccine containing diphtheria, tetanus, pertussis, measles, mumps, rubella, polio, hepatitis A, hepatitis B, Hib, varicella, influenza, pneumococcal conjugate, meningococcal, rotavirus, human papillomavirus (HPV), or varicella vaccine. Further details are available at the CDC website at https://www.cdc.gov/vaccines/hcp/vis/current-vis.html. The mandated one-page, two-sided information sheets provide patients with information about the disease, the benefits and harms of the vaccine, the recommended immunization schedule, indications for delaying or not administering the vaccine, and potential postimmunization complications and ways to reduce them, along with addresses and telephone numbers for reporting adverse events (if the clinician fails to do so) and for obtaining federal compensation under the National Vaccine Injury Compensation Program. The pamphlets have been translated into 40 different languages. Copies are also available on the CDC website at http://www.immunize.org/vis/. VISs are also available for other vaccines, including various nonroutine vaccines such as anthrax, rabies, yellow fever, typhoid, smallpox, and Japanese encephalitis. Using the VISs for these vaccines is strongly encouraged but not required by law, although they must be used when giving vaccines purchased through a CDC contract. Physician requirements regarding VISs are provided at the CDC website.

VACCINES FOR DIPHTHERIA, TETANUS, AND ACELLULAR PERTUSSIS

Diphtheria-tetanus-pertussis (DTP) vaccine, made from a formalin-treated suspension of whole *Bordetella pertussis* cells, was introduced in the mid-1940s. Owing to concerns about possible neurologic adverse effects, a safer acellular pertussis vaccine was introduced in 1991 that used cell fragments of the pertussis bacterium. Since 1999, only formulations with acellular pertussis (diphtheria-tetanus-acellular pertussis [DTaP] and tetanus-diphtheria-acellular pertussis [Tdap]) have been used in the United States.

Tetanus and diphtheria have become rare in the United States. Between 2004 and 2015, there were two reported cases of diphtheria in the United States.[26] On average, 30 cases of tetanus are reported annually (CDC). Most cases occurred in people who had not received the tetanus vaccine or the booster every 10 years.[26,27] Both tetanus and diphtheria carry high case-fatality rates: 25% to 30% and 5% to 10%, respectively. Booster doses of the vaccines given every 10 years are recommended to maintain antibody levels.

Pertussis is also considerably less common in the United States than it was before the advent of the pertussis vaccine. Still, more than 32,971 cases were reported in the United States during 2014, one of the highest annual totals for over 50 years,[28] with many cases going undiagnosed or unreported annually in the United States. One explanation for the increase in the number of cases is that the newer, acellular form of pertussis vaccine may be less efficacious than the older whole-cell formulation. In addition, immunity to pertussis from either natural infection or vaccination wanes more rapidly than for other vaccine-preventable diseases.[28–30]

A study by Wendelhoe and colleagues found that household members accounted for 76% to 83% of the transmission of pertussis to infants who are at the highest risk of severe complications and death from pertussis infection.[30]

To attempt to reduce endemic disease in the adolescent and adult population, and thereby reduce morbidity and mortality in unimmunized infants, two new tetanus toxoids, reduced diphtheria toxoid and acellular pertussis absorbed vaccines (Tdap), were released in 2005. Boostrix (GlaxoSmithKline Biologicals, Rixensart, Belgium) was licensed for use in persons aged 10 to 18 years, and Adacel (Sanofi Pasteur, Toronto, Ontario, Canada) was licensed for use in persons aged 11 to 64 years. These agents, rather than the older tetanus-diphtheria (Td) vaccine, are recommended for use in those 11 years and older. The pertussis component of the vaccine delivers approximately one-third the antigenic dose of infant DTaP, but it produces antibody titers at least as strong, with an efficacy of 92%.[31]

Indications

DTaP vaccination is indicated in all children, except those with the contraindications listed in Table 17.1, beginning at age 6 weeks to 2 months. Pertussis immunization is currently not recommended for children aged 7 to 9 years. Tetanus toxoid is available as a single-antigen preparation, combined with diphtheria toxoid as pediatric diphtheria-tetanus (DT) or adult Td, and with both diphtheria toxoid and acellular pertussis vaccine as DTaP or Tdap. Tetanus toxoid is also available as a DTaP-inactivated poliovirus vaccine (IPV)-hepatitis B combination (Pediarix), a DTaP-Hib-IPV combination (Pentacel), and DTaP-IPV (Kinrix or Quadracel). Pediatric formulations (DT and DTaP) contain a similar amount of tetanus toxoid as do Td, but the diphtheria toxoid content is three to four times higher. Children younger than 7 years should receive either DTaP or pediatric DT (the latter if pertussis vaccine is contraindicated). Persons aged 7 to 9 years should receive the adult formulation (adult Td), even if they have not completed a DTaP or DT series. The use of single-antigen tetanus toxoid is not recommended (except in cases of a severe neurologic or hypersensitivity reaction to diphtheria toxoid). Tetanus toxoid should be combined with diphtheria toxoid, because immunologic boosting is needed for both antigens.[32]

The ACIP recommends Tdap for children aged 11 to 12 years who have completed the recommended DTP/DTaP vaccination series and have not received a Td booster dose.[32] Adolescents aged 13 to 18 years who missed the age 11- to 12-year Td/Tdap booster dose should also receive a single dose of Tdap if they have completed the recommended childhood DTP/DTaP vaccination series. It is recommended that subsequent Td or tetanus toxoid boosters be administered every 10 years.

The following ACIP recommendations for a single dose of Tdap (Adacel) apply to adults 19 to 64 years of age who have not yet received Tdap.

- **Routine.** Adults should receive a single dose of Tdap to replace a single dose of Td for booster immunization against tetanus, diphtheria, and pertussis if they received their most recent tetanus toxoid-containing vaccine (e.g., Td) 10 years before or earlier.
- **Prevention of pertussis among infants younger than 12 months by vaccinating adult contacts.** Adults who have or who anticipate having close contact with an infant younger than 12 months (e.g., parents, clinicians, childcare providers) should receive a single dose of Tdap. Also, health care personnel who work in hospitals or ambulatory care settings and have direct patient contact should receive a single dose of Tdap as soon as feasible if they have not previously received Tdap. An interval of 2 years or more since the most recent tetanus toxoid-containing vaccine is suggested; shorter intervals may be used. Ideally, Tdap should be given at least 1 month before beginning close contact with the infant. Women should receive a dose of Tdap in the immediate postpartum period if they have not previously received Tdap. Any woman who might become pregnant is encouraged to receive a single dose of Tdap. To prevent neonatal tetanus, pregnant women who have received their last tetanus-containing vaccine 10 years before or earlier should receive Td during pregnancy in preference to Tdap. Although Tdap is not contraindicated, there is some concern that antibodies acquired during pregnancy might reduce the response to DTaP vaccine in the infant at routine vaccination.

Administration

The full DTaP series consists of four doses, the first three doses given at 4-to 8-week intervals and the fourth dose given 6 to 12 months after the third dose (preferably at age 15 mo) to maintain adequate immunity during the preschool years. The booster (fifth) dose, which is normally given at age 4 to 6 years, is unnecessary if the fourth dose in the primary series is given after age 4 years. The recommended childhood immunization schedule for ages 0 to 6 years is presented in Figure 17.1.

For adolescents, routine immunization with Tdap is recommended at a preadolescent health care visit for all 11- and 12-year-olds, replacing the Td vaccine (Fig. 17.1). Children who are behind on immunizations should be vaccinated according to the schedules in Figure 17.1 depending on their age. Adults should be immunized according to the schedule in Figure 17.2.

Once the primary DTaP series is started, interruptions in the recommended schedule or delays in administering subsequent doses do not require restarting the series. Therefore, persons who received a partial series in the past need only complete the schedule. Premature infants should be vaccinated at their chronologic age from birth.

Children 6 years or younger for whom pertussis vaccination is contraindicated should complete the primary series with DT vaccine. Children aged 7 to 18 years not fully immunized with DTaP should receive one dose of Tdap, and if additional doses are needed use Td. The first two doses should be given at least 4 weeks apart, and the third dose should be given 6 months after the second dose (Fig. 17.1).

Adverse Effects

Local reactions (e.g., erythema, induration) and mild systemic reactions (e.g., fever, drowsiness, irritability, and anorexia) were common after the administration of DTP or its component antigens but are less common after the administration of DTaP. Anaphylactic reactions to DTaP vaccine are rare. Arthus-type reactions to tetanus toxoid can occur, especially in adults who have received frequent tetanus toxoid boosters. Therefore, Td boosters should be avoided in patients who have completed a primary series or have received a booster dose within the previous 5 years. They should also be avoided in patients who have experienced Arthus reactions and received a dose within the last 10 years.

Moderate or severe systemic events (such as a temperature of 105°F (40.5°C) or higher, febrile seizures, persistent crying lasting 3 hours or more, and hypotonic hyporesponsive episodes) have been reported after administration of DTaP but occur less frequently among children receiving DTaP than among children receiving whole-cell DTP (estimated occurrence is less than 1 per 10,000 doses). However, occurrence of one of these adverse reactions following DTaP vaccination in childhood is neither a contraindication nor a precaution to administration of Tdap to an adolescent or adult.

Swelling of the injection site is more common after the fourth or fifth dose of DTaP. There have been reports of swelling of the entire thigh or upper arm, sometimes accompanied by erythema, pain, and fever. Parents should be informed of the increase in reactogenicity that has been reported following the fourth and fifth doses of DTaP. The ACIP, because of the risk of pertussis in this age group, recommends that a history of extensive swelling after the fourth dose should *not* be considered a contraindication to receipt of a fifth dose at school entry.

The most common reactions reported after Tdap vaccination are local redness or swelling at the injection site. Low-grade fever and nonspecific systemic symptoms such as headache and fatigue have also been reported. Adverse reactions occur at a similar rate in recipients of Tdap and Td. A history of extensive limb swelling following DTaP is not a contraindication to Tdap vaccination.

Precautions and Contraindications

Precautions and contraindications to DTaP, DT, Tdap, and Td vaccine are listed in Table 17.1. In general, pertussis vaccine should not be given to patients with unstable neurologic conditions, such as uncontrolled seizure disorders or progressive encephalopathy. Stable neurologic conditions, such as cerebral palsy and well-controlled seizures, are not contraindications. A history of a single seizure that was not temporally related to DTaP administration does not contraindicate vaccination, especially if the seizure can be explained by other factors. A family history of seizures or other neurologic diseases or stable or resolved neurologic conditions (e.g., controlled idiopathic epilepsy, cerebral palsy, and developmental delay) are not contraindications to pertussis vaccination.

Moderate or severe acute illness is a precaution to vaccination, but children with mild illness, such as an upper respiratory infection or otitis media, should be vaccinated.

Children who have recovered from documented pertussis do not need further doses of pertussis vaccine until adolescence, when one dose of Tdap should be given (because pertussis immunity is not permanent, even from natural infection). Satisfactory documentation of pertussis infection includes recovery of *B. pertussis* on culture or typical symptoms and clinical course when these are linked epidemiologically to a culture-confirmed case. When confirmation of diagnosis is lacking, vaccination should be completed because cough may be caused by other species of *Bordetella* or by other bacteria or viruses.[28]

The only contraindications to Td/DT are a history of a severe neurologic or hypersensitivity reaction following a previous dose and moderate to severe illness.

VACCINES FOR MEASLES, MUMPS, AND RUBELLA

Measles, mumps, and rubella are all human viral diseases with no known animal reservoir. Measles can cause severe illness, often complicated by middle ear infection or bronchopneumonia. Measles is still a common and often fatal disease in developing countries. In 2016, the World Health Organization (WHO) estimates that there were 298,629 cases of measles with 89,780 deaths.[28] The incidence of measles has fallen dramatically since 1963, when the vaccine was first licensed and routine childhood vaccination instituted. In the United States in 2017, there were 118 cases of measles in mostly unvaccinated individuals.[34] It is estimated that the use of the measles vaccine from 2000 to 2016 has prevented 20.4 million deaths.[33]

Mumps is a viral disease spread by respiratory droplets. It usually begins with swelling and tenderness of one or more of the salivary glands, with >85% of persons developing unilateral or bilateral parotitis. Complications can include orchitis (12%–66% of postpubertal males infected), brain involvement including aseptic meningitis (0.2–10% of cases), and inflammation of the pancreas (2–5% of cases) and ovaries (5% of postpubertal females). Permanent deafness occurs in 1 of 20,000 cases. Mumps vaccine was introduced in 1967, following which the incidence of the disease declined from 212,000 cases in 1964 to approximately 3000 cases per year by 1985. There was a surge in the number of cases in 1986 and 1987, with almost 13,000 cases reported in 1987, which correlated with a lack of state immunization requirements and apparent incomplete immunity conferred by the original single-dose protocol. Since the two-shot MMR series was introduced, the number of reported cases has fallen steadily in the United States, with an average of 265 mumps cases reported per year between 2001 and 2005.[35] However, in 2016, a multistate outbreak of mumps occurred, with 6366 cases of mumps reported mostly on college campuses and in 2017 in a close-knit community in Arkansas.[36] The ACIP recommended a third dose of MMR for individuals who are at high risk during an outbreak of mumps.[36] Rubella (German measles) is spread by droplet infection. Although approximately half of the cases are subclinical, rubella infection may be associated with significant morbidity in adults; the greatest risk is when infection occurs in pregnant women, in whom vertical transmission to the fetus can produce congenital rubella syndrome (CRS). A rubella epidemic in the United States in 1964–65 resulted in 12.5 million cases of rubella infection and approximately 20,000 newborns with CRS. Rubella vaccination of children was introduced in 1969, after which the incidence of new cases fell from 30 per 100,000 to less than 0.5 per 100,000 by 1983. In 2003, a record low annual total of seven cases were reported. In October 2004, a CDC panel concluded that endemic rubella transmission in the United States had ceased by 2000, with all subsequent reported cases having been imported from other countries. The conquest of rubella and CRS in the United States is one of the great public health victories of the modern era. Nonetheless, it is essential that all persons, especially women of childbearing age, continue to be vaccinated or show proof of immunity to prevent a resurgence of disease.[37]

Indications

In the United States, single-antigen live virus vaccine preparations are available for measles (Attenuvax; Merck), mumps (Mumpsvax; Merck), and rubella (Meruvax II; Merck) and as combination vaccines for measles-mumps (M-M-Vax; Merck), measles-mumps-rubella (M-M-R II; Merck), and measles-mumps-rubella-varicella (ProQuad; Merck). The ACIP recommends that a combination vaccine (MMR or MMRV) be used when any of the individual components is indicated (for MMRV, the vaccine must be 12 mo through 12 yr of age). Use of single-antigen vaccines is not recommended.

All children (at least 12 mo of age) and nonpregnant adults, with the exception of those with the contraindications listed in Figure 17.1, should receive MMR vaccine if they are susceptible to measles, mumps, or rubella infection. Acceptable presumptive evidence of immunity to measles, rubella, and mumps varies by vaccine but in general such evidence requires documentation of administration, laboratory evidence of immunity, birth before 1957, or physician-diagnosed disease. The ACIP recommends the following:

- MMRV vaccine may be given to children 12 months through 12 years of age. Two doses are usually recommended:
  - First dose: 12 through 15 months of age
  - Second dose: 4 through 6 years of age
- A third dose of MMR might be recommended in certain mumps outbreak situations.[36]

Because many rashes may mimic rubella infection and many rubella infections are unrecognized, the clinical diagnosis of rubella is unreliable and should not be considered in assessing immune status. The ACIP recommends that, unless susceptible women are certain to return for vaccination, women who may be immune to rubella but lack adequate documentation of immunity should be vaccinated, rather than first performing serologic testing for rubella antibodies. Serologic testing need not be done before vaccinating for measles and rubella unless the facility considers it cost-effective.

Administration

The recommended primary immunization schedule for MMR is presented earlier. Children who are behind on immunizations should be vaccinated according to the schedule in Figure 17.1. As noted in Figure 17.1, MMR should be administered at least 14 days before, or deferred for 3 to 11 months after, administration of immune globulin because passively acquired antibodies may interfere with the response to the vaccine; guidelines for spacing the immunizations based on the type and dose of immune globulin are provided elsewhere.[13] MMR is the preferred vaccine for individuals who are susceptible to measles, mumps, or rubella and who lack contraindications.

A combination vaccine, combining MMR with varicella vaccine (MMRV), is now available (ProQuad; Merck). ProQuad is indicated for simultaneous vaccination against measles, mumps, rubella, and varicella in children aged 12 months to 12 years and may be used whenever any components of the combination vaccine are indicated and the other components are not contraindicated (Fig. 17.1). ProQuad appears to stimulate the same antibody levels as M-M-RII and varicella vaccine (Varivax; Merck) when given separately,[13] and concomitant administration of MMRV, Hib/HepB, and DTaP is well tolerated.[13] In 2010, a study was published indicating patients aged 12 to 23 months who received a dose of MMRV were at a slight increase risk of a febrile seizure.[38] The researchers recommended that the provider inform parents of the risk.[38] Because varicella vaccine is recommended to be given at the same age as MMR vaccine, MMRV is preferred over a separate injection of equivalent component vaccines.

Adverse Effects

Primary vaccination with measles vaccine may be associated with mild fever and a transient rash, beginning 7 to 12 days after vaccination and usually lasting several days. Approximately 5% to 15% of patients develop a temperature greater than 103°F (39.4°C). Neurologic complications, including encephalitis and encephalopathy, reportedly occur in less than one case per million doses administered (an incidence rate lower than the rate for encephalitis of unknown etiology). Mild, self-limited thrombocytopenia may occur in 1 of 30,000 to 40,000 doses of MMR vaccine. However, the risk of thrombocytopenia during rubella or measles infection is much greater than the risk after vaccination. On rare occasions, mumps vaccination can produce parotitis and lymphadenopathy. Allergic reactions, such as rash and pruritus, which are usually brief, are reported occasionally. Very rarely, manifestations of central nervous system involvement (e.g., febrile seizures, aseptic meningitis, unilateral nerve deafness, and encephalitis) occur; almost all of these cases resolve uneventfully, and none have been linked conclusively to vaccines used in the United States. Recipients of rubella vaccine can develop low-grade fever, a rash lasting 1 to 2 days, and lymphadenopathy that may persist 1 to 2 months after vaccination. Arthralgias and transient arthritis are more common in susceptible adults than in children, and women are more prone to this than men. Approximately 25% of women who receive the vaccine report arthralgias, and approximately 10% of recipients can develop acute arthritis-like signs and symptoms. When acute joint symptoms occur, they generally begin 1 to 3 weeks after vaccination, persist for 1 day to 3 weeks, and rarely recur. Rarely, transient peripheral neuritis is reported following rubella vaccination.

Precautions and Contraindications

Precautions and contraindications to MMR are listed in Table 17.1. MMR vaccines should not be given to women known to be pregnant or who might become pregnant within 4 weeks of vaccination. No cases of CRS have been documented among infants born to women who inadvertently received rubella vaccine during pregnancy. Therefore, although rubella vaccination should be avoided during pregnancy, there is insufficient evidence of risk to justify termination of pregnancy if a pregnant woman inadvertently receives the vaccine. Children of pregnant women can safely receive MMR vaccine without risk to the mother or fetus. Although MMR vaccination of persons with moderate or severe illness should be postponed, minor illnesses such as upper respiratory infection, with or without a low-grade fever, do not preclude vaccination.

Hypersensitivity reactions to MMR vaccine are rare. They generally consist of wheal-and-flare or urticarial reactions at the injection site. Although measles and mumps vaccines (but not rubella vaccine) are propagated in chick embryo fibroblast cells in culture, the quantity of egg proteins found in these vaccines is not sufficient to induce immediate-type hypersensitivity reactions, and these vaccines can safely be administered to children with severe egg allergies. Persons who have experienced a severe allergic reaction (i.e., hives, angioedema, difficulty breathing, and hypotension) after receiving a prior dose of MMR vaccine or a vaccine component (e.g., gelatin, neomycin) should generally not be vaccinated with MMR.

Because MMR is a live attenuated viral vaccine, it is contraindicated in persons with known severe immunodeficiency (e.g., those with hematologic and solid tumors who are receiving chemotherapy, with congenital immunodeficiency, or with HIV infection who are severely immunocompromised) (see Fig. 17.1). However, MMR can be given safely to persons with HIV infection who are asymptomatic or mildly symptomatic with age-specific CD4+ counts equal to or greater than 15%. MMR is contraindicated in persons on long-term immunosuppressive therapy (a significant immunosuppressive steroid dose is considered to be daily receipt of at least 20 mg/d [at least 2 mg/d/kg of body weight] of prednisone or its equivalent for 14 days or more).[39] Certain antibody-containing blood products can interfere with the immune response to live attenuated viral vaccines. Patients with HIV receiving immune globulin intravenously may receive MMR if given 2 weeks before the next scheduled dose of immune globulin (if it is not otherwise contraindicated).[39,40]

POLIO VACCINE

Poliomyelitis, a disease that once crippled or killed millions of persons, has become a rare disease in industrialized nations because of routine polio vaccination. In the United States, the number of cases of polio peaked in

1952, with more than 21,000 cases of paralytic polio. The last episode of the spread of wild poliovirus in this country occurred in 1979; all current U.S. cases are due to vaccine-associated paralytic poliomyelitis (VAPP). No new cases of wild-type virus have been reported in the Western Hemisphere since 1991, and global eradication of the disease may be possible.

Two forms of trivalent polio vaccines are available for use: inactivated poliovirus vaccine or IPV (introduced by Jonas Salk in 1954) and live attenuated oral poliovirus vaccine or OPV (introduced by Albert Sabin in 1961). Use of live attenuated virus vaccine can lead to mutation during viral replication in the intestine, causing VAPP. It occurs approximately once per every 6.2 million OPV doses administered to immunologically competent recipients. The risk of VAPP is 7 to 21 times higher after the first dose than after other doses in the series. To eliminate the risk for VAPP, exclusive use of IPV has been recommended for routine vaccination in the United States since 1999. OPV remains the vaccine of choice for areas where wild poliovirus is still present because it stimulates more potent intestinal immunity against wild poliovirus. Ongoing vaccination of the U.S. population against poliovirus will be required until wild poliovirus infection is eradicated worldwide.[41]

Indications

Polio vaccine should be administered to all children. Although routine immunization of adults (18 years or older) living in the United States is not recommended, some adults at higher risk of infection should be immunized.[42]

Administration

Only enhanced-potency IPV vaccine is now available for routine use in the United States. The recommended childhood immunization schedule for IPV is presented in Figure 17.1, and contraindications are listed in Table 17.1. Children who are behind on immunizations should be vaccinated according to the schedule in Figure 17.1. A polio vaccination schedule begun with OPV should be completed with IPV. If a child receives both types of vaccines, four doses of any combination of IPV or OPV by age 4 to 6 years is considered a complete poliovirus vaccination series. However, for children who receive an all-IPV or all-OPV series, a fourth dose is not necessary if the third dose was given at 4 years or older. A minimum interval of 4 weeks should separate all doses of the series.

Routine vaccination with IPV is not recommended for adults (aged 18 years or older) in the United States because most adults are already immune and have little risk of acquiring poliovirus infection. However, immunization is recommended for certain adults at higher risk, such as travelers to areas where poliomyelitis is endemic or epidemic, laboratory workers handling specimens that may contain wild-type polioviruses, and health care workers in close contact with patients who may be excreting wild poliovirus. Unimmunized adults exposed to high-risk environments should receive three doses of IPV. The first two doses should be given 1 to 2 months apart, with a third dose 6 to 12 months after the second dose. An incompletely immunized adult who started the series with OPV should receive the remaining doses using IPV; there is no need to restart the series if the schedule was interrupted. Fully immunized adults entering a high-risk situation should get one booster dose of IPV.

Adverse Effects

The administration of IPV can cause tenderness at the injection site. No serious adverse reactions to IPV have been documented. Allergic reactions may occur in persons sensitive to streptomycin, polymyxin B, and neomycin, which are present in trace amounts in IPV.

Precautions and Contraindications

Moderate or severe acute illness, or pregnancy, is a precaution in the use of IPV. However, breastfeeding is not a contraindication to the use of this vaccine. IPV is contraindicated in persons with a previous anaphylactic or neurologic reaction to the vaccine or to any of its components.

HAEMOPHILUS INFLUENZAE TYPE B VACCINE

Hib is the cause of a wide variety of serious bacterial diseases among children, such as meningitis, pneumonia, septic arthritis, epiglottitis, and sepsis. Before the development of the vaccines, Hib meningitis accounted for 50% to 65% of Hib cases. Even with the availability of antibiotic therapy, the case fatality rate was 2% to 5%, and neurologic sequelae, such as hearing impairment, occurred in 15% to 30% of survivors.

These illnesses occur primarily among children younger than 5 years. Although severe disease is most common in children aged 6 to 12 months, approximately 20% to 35% of cases of severe disease occur in children aged 18 months or older. In the United States during the 1980 to 1990 decade, the incidence of Hib disease was 40 to 100 per 100,000 among children younger than 5 years. With the routine use of Hib conjugate vaccine since 1990, the incidence of invasive Hib disease has decreased to 1.3 per 100,000 children. In 2013, 95% of the WHO states have initiated the Hib vaccine in their programs, resulting in a >90% reduction in invasive Hib disease.[43]

Indications

A complete Hib vaccination series is indicated in all infants and children, starting at age 2 months. Certain older children and adults are at higher risk of invasive Hib disease than is the general population. Such persons should receive a single dose of any pediatric Hib vaccine. This group includes persons with functional or anatomic asplenia (e.g., sickle cell disease, postsplenectomy patients), immunodeficiency (in particular, persons with immunoglobulin [IgG2] subclass deficiency), immunosuppression from cancer chemotherapy, HIV infection, and past receipt of a hematopoietic stem cell transplant.[44] Children who have had Hib disease when they were younger than 24 months should still receive Hib vaccine, because most fail to mount an immune response to clinical disease. Children aged 24 months or older who have had reliably diagnosed invasive disease do not need vaccination. Household contacts of patients with Hib disease (regardless of the contacts' age) should receive rifampin post exposure prophylaxis if one of the contacts is a child younger than 1 year who has not received the primary Hib series or a child aged 12 to 48 months who has not been fully vaccinated. Post exposure prophylaxis should also be given to all household contacts, regardless of age, if one of the child contacts (any age) is immunocompromised.[45]

Administration

Three single-antigen Hib conjugate vaccines and two combination vaccines that contain Hib conjugate are available in the United States. PRP-T (Hiberix, GlaxoSmithKline) links tetanus toxoid conjugate, PRP-T (ActHIB, Sanofi Pasteur) uses tetanus toxoid, and PRP-OMP (PedvaxHIB; Merck) uses a meningococcal protein conjugate. PRP-T requires three doses for a primary series at ages 2, 4, and 6 months followed by a single booster at age 12 to 15 months. PRP-OMP requires only two doses for the primary series, at ages 2 and 4 months, with a booster at age 12 to 15 months.

Two combination vaccines are available that contain Hib: Comvax (Merck) contains PRP-OMP (PedvaxHIB; Merck) as the Hib component plus hepatitis B vaccine (Recombivax; Merck), DtaP-IPV/Hib (Pentacel; Sanofi Pasteur), and Hib-MenCY (MenHibrix; GlaxoSmithKline). TriHIBit (Sanofi Pasteur) is no longer available in the United States. The recommended immunization schedule for Hib vaccination is presented in Figure 17.1. Children who are behind on Hib immunizations (and are younger than 5 yr) should be vaccinated according to the schedule in Figure 17.1. Adults and older children at high risk should receive a single dose of any pediatric Hib vaccine (Figs. 17.1 and 17.2).

Adverse Effects

Serious complications from Hib vaccine are unusual. Erythema, swelling, or pain at the injection site has been reported in 5% to 30% of recipients. They usually resolve within 24 hours. A temperature of 101.3°F (38.5°C) or greater occurs in approximately 1% of recipients. Severe hypersensitivity reactions are rare.

Precautions and Contraindications

Vaccination with Hib conjugate vaccine is contraindicated for persons known to have experienced an anaphylactic allergic reaction following a prior dose of that vaccine. Vaccination should be delayed for children with moderate or severe acute illnesses. Minor illnesses (e.g., mild upper respiratory infection) are not contraindications to vaccination. Hib conjugate vaccines are contraindicated for children younger than 6 weeks because of the potential for development of immunologic tolerance. Contraindications and precautions for the use of combination vaccines are the same as those for its individual component vaccines.

PNEUMOCOCCAL VACCINES

Pneumococcal disease is still a major cause of morbidity and mortality in the United States, especially in infants and the elderly. In the United States, before the introduction of pneumococcal conjugate and polysaccharide vaccines, pneumococcal disease caused an estimated 3000 cases of meningitis, 50,000 cases of bacteremia, 500,000 cases of pneumonia, and 7 million cases of otitis media each year.[46] *Streptococcus pneumoniae* is the most common cause of invasive bacterial disease in U.S. children, with the peak incidence occurring between 6 and 23 months of age. Since the disappearance of invasive Hib disease secondary to Hib vaccination, *S. pneumoniae* has now become the leading cause of bacterial meningitis in the United States. Pneumococcal disease also takes a great toll on the elderly, causing half of adult hospitalizations for pneumonia. Of those with pneumococcal pneumonia, bacteremia occurs in 25% to 30% of cases. The overall fatality rate for pneumococcal bacteremia is 20% but rises to as high as 60% in the elderly population (older than 65 yr).

There are two vaccines against pneumococcal disease: pneumococcal polysaccharide vaccine (PPSV-23) and pneumococcal conjugate vaccine (PCV-13). PPV was originally licensed in 1977 as a 13-valent vaccine against pneumococcal polysaccharide bacterial antigens. In 1983, a 23-valent polysaccharide vaccine (PPV23) was licensed. Pneumovax 23 (Merck) contains antigens against strains that account for 88% of bacteremia-causing pneumococci.

PPSV stimulates B cells to produce antibody immunity, but it does not produce T-cell immunity. This results in temporary immunity from antibody production, but immune memory is lacking, and repeated doses do not produce a boost in antibody titers. PPV is effective in older children and adults, but children younger than 2 years do not produce reliable immune responses to polysaccharide antigens. PCV, by contrast, stimulates long-term T-cell immunity, which is necessary to reduce nasal carriage and produce herd immunity. Also, in children younger than 2 years, only PCV is effective against bacteria with polysaccharide capsules, including pneumococcus, meningococcus, and Hib.

Prevnar (Wyeth) was the first pneumococcal conjugate vaccine (PCV7) licensed in the United States, in 2000. It contains purified capsular polysaccharides of seven *S. pneumoniae* serotypes (conjugated to a nontoxic diphtheria protein). Between 1978 and 1994 in the United States, among children younger than 6 years, these seven types accounted for 86% of bacteremia, 83% of meningitis, and 65% of acute otitis media.[68] A CDC study of data from 1998 to 2003 showed dramatic results from universal immunization of children with PCV7. In the United States, after the introduction of PCV7 immunization, in children younger than 5 years, invasive pneumococcal disease caused by one of the seven PCV7 pneumococcal serotypes declined by >90%.[47] Serotype 19A was not included in the PCV7 vaccine resulting in an increase after the introduction of the vaccine.[47] In 2010, a 13-valent conjugated vaccine (PCV13, Pfizer) was introduced to include the serotype 19A and five others.[47] In 2012, ACIP recommended the use of PCV13 in immunocompromised adults and patients >65 years of age to receive one dose at least 1 year after PPSV23.[48]

Indications

PPSV23 is indicated for the following:

- All patients 65 years or older
- Patients aged 2 years or older with a normal immune system who have a chronic illness, including cardiovascular disease, pulmonary disease, diabetes, alcoholism, cirrhosis, or cerebrospinal fluid leakage
- Immunocompromised patients 2 years or older at increased risk of pneumococcal disease or its complications; this includes patients with asplenia (either from disease or surgical removal), lymphoma (including Hodgkin disease), multiple myeloma, chronic renal failure, nephrotic syndrome, or conditions such as organ transplantation associated with immunosuppression. Patients who are immunosuppressed secondary to chemotherapy or high-dose corticosteroid therapy (see earlier definition) should be vaccinated
- Patients 2 years or older with asymptomatic or symptomatic HIV infection

PPV23 should also be considered for patients living in special environments or social settings with an identified increased risk of pneumococcal disease, such as certain Native American populations (i.e., Alaska Native, Navajo, and Apache).[49,50]

PCV13 is indicated for the following:

All children under 59 months of age should receive at least one dose depending on age of first vaccine (see Fig. 17.1).

All adults >65 years and patients aged 6 to 64 years with certain conditions should receive one dose of PCV13. Patients at high risk include asplenia, sickle cell disease, immunocompromising conditions such as HIV infection, cochlear implants, chronic renal failure, certain cancers, other diseases associated with immunosuppressive drugs or radiation, solid organ transplantation, or cerebrospinal fluid leaks. The PCV13 should be administered first followed by PPSV23 8 weeks later.

Administration

PPV23 can be administered either intramuscularly or subcutaneously. A one-time revaccination is recommended for patients aged 65 years or older if the first dose was given before age 65 years and if 5 years or more have elapsed since the previous dose. Revaccination is also recommended 5 years later for persons at highest risk of fatal pneumococcal infection or rapid antibody loss (e.g., renal disease).

Children aged 2 years or older who have immunocompromising conditions, HIV infection, sickle cell disease, or functional or anatomic asplenia should receive a second dose of PPV at least 3 to 5 years after the previous PPV dose if they are 10 years or younger; if they are older than 10 years, the two doses of PPV should be separated by five or more years.

The primary PCV series beginning in infancy consists of three doses routinely given at 2, 4, and 6 months of age. The vaccine is administered intramuscularly. A fourth (booster) dose is recommended at age 12 to 15 months (Fig. 17.1). Unvaccinated healthy children aged 24 to 59 months should receive one dose of PCV7. Unvaccinated children aged 24 to 59 months with sickle cell disease, asplenia, HIV infection, chronic illness, or immunocompromised conditions should receive two doses of PCV7 separated by at least 8 weeks. PCV7 is not routinely recommended for those older than 59 months.

Adverse Effects

The most common reactions after pneumococcal vaccination are local erythema and swelling, seen in 30% to 50% of PPV recipients and 10% to 20% of PCV recipients. Local reactions are seen more commonly after a second dose of PPV. Fever and myalgia have occurred in less than 1% of PPV recipients and in 15% to 24% of PCV recipients; in the latter, a temperature higher than 102.2°F (39°C) is uncommon. Severe adverse events are rare with either vaccine.

Precautions and Contraindications

Previous anaphylactic reaction to this vaccine or to any of its components is a contraindication. Moderate or severe acute illness is a precaution.

MENINGOCOCCAL VACCINE

Neisseria meningitidis spreads through exposure to aerosol droplets or contact with respiratory tract secretions. The bacterium is carried transiently in the nasopharynx of up to 10% of adolescents and adults; carriage rates in children younger than 10 years are much lower. Invasive disease occurs when the bacterium penetrates the nasal mucosa and invades the bloodstream. This occurs in less than 1% of colonized persons. The incidence of invasive disease peaks between the ages of 6 months and 2 years, with a second, lower peak occurring during adolescence. In 2016, *N. meningitidis*

caused 370 cases, with the highest rates among infants <1 year of age followed by the adolescent period. The infection in most of the patients <1 years of age (60%) was caused by serogroup B.[51,52] Meningitis occurs in up to 50% of cases of invasive disease, with a 3% to 10% fatality rate. A more serious form of invasive disease is meningococcemia, which occurs in 5% to 20% of cases and can have a fatality rate of up to 40%.[51,52] Even with antibiotic treatment, up to 20% of survivors can have permanent sequelae, such as hearing loss, neurologic damage, or loss of a limb. *N. meningitidis* has become the leading cause of bacterial meningitis in persons aged 2 to 18 years as a result of the success of Hib and pneumococcal conjugate vaccines in controlling those pathogens.

Certain groups are at higher risk of invasive disease. Host risk factors include functional or anatomic asplenia and terminal complement pathway deficiency. HIV disease is probably also a risk factor. Environmental risk factors include upper respiratory tract infection, household crowding, and both active and passive smoking. College freshmen living in dormitories have a modest increase in their risk of invasive disease.

Five serogroups (A, B, C, W-135, and Y) account for virtually all meningococcal disease. Two vaccines are available for use. Meningococcal tetravalent conjugate vaccine (MCV4 [Menactra, Sanofi Pasteur]) was licensed for use in the United States in 2005 for use in those aged 9 months to 55 years. MCV4 (Menveo, GlaxoSmithKline) also consists of four serogroups A, C, Y, and W 135 and is used for ages 2 months to 55 years of age. Each dose contains capsular polysaccharide from serogroups A, C, Y, and W-135 conjugated to diphtheria toxoid. The wide use of MCV4 is expected to reduce nasopharyngeal carriage of *N. meningitidis* and produce herd immunity.

Adolescents are at an increased risk of meningococcal disease, and in 2014, Meningococcal B vaccine was introduced. Two vaccines are available for serogroup B, including MenB (Bexero, GlaxoSmithKline) and MenB (Trumenba, Pfizer), starting at age 10 through 25 years of age.

Indications

- MCV4 should be given to all children at age 11 to 12 years and a booster at 16 years of age.
- The ACIP also recommends that MCV4 be given to the following high-risk groups starting at age 8 weeks:
- Anatomic or functional asplenia
  - Sickle cell disease
  - HIV infections
  - Persistent complement component deficiency
- Persons who travel to or reside in countries in which *N. meningitidis* is hyperendemic or epidemic, especially travelers to sub-Saharan Africa and particularly if contact with the local population will be prolonged; vaccination is required by the government of Saudi Arabia for all travelers on the annual Hajj to Mecca.

- MenB is recommended for patients who are at high risk for meningococcal disease including anatomic or functional asplenia, sickle cell disease, and persistent complement component deficiency and who are taking Soliris or during serogroup B meningococcal outbreaks. CDC does not routinely recommend serogroup B meningococcal vaccine for all adolescents.

Administration

Routine administration of MCV4 is at age 11 to 12 years and at 16 years. MCV4 is administered intramuscularly as a single 0.5-mL dose. MenB is administered starting at 10 years of age and requires two or three doses depending on the vaccine given. The vaccines are not interchangeable. See Figure 17.1.

Adverse Effects

Adverse reactions to MCV4 and MenB are similar and are generally mild. Local reactions, such as pain and erythema at the injection site, can last for 1 to 2 days. Systemic reactions, such as headache and malaise, within a week of vaccination are reported for up to 60% of recipients. Fewer than 3% of recipients characterized these systemic reactions as severe.

Precautions and Contraindications

Vaccination with MCV4 or MenB is contraindicated among persons known to have a severe allergic reaction to any component of the vaccine, including diphtheria toxoid (for MCV4).

As of 2006, 17 cases of Guillain-Barré syndrome (GBS) that had an onset within 6 weeks of MCV4 administration had been reported to the CDC and FDA.[53,54] The number of GBS cases is similar to what might have been expected to occur by chance alone (one to two cases per 100,000 population). Although the manufacturer has inserted a warning in the package insert, the CDC has not altered its recommendations for administering MCV4.

HEPATITIS B VACCINE

Hepatitis B virus (HBV) is a serious global health problem; one-third of the world's population has evidence of present or past infection, and 257 million persons are chronically infected. There are more than 887,000 deaths each year from HBV-associated acute and chronic liver disease. Approximately 1 million Americans are thought to be infectious carriers, with 21,900 acute infections or 1.1 cases per 100,000 population occurring in 2015.[55] HBV causes approximately 50% of cases of hepatocellular carcinoma, which makes it second only to tobacco among known human carcinogens.[56]

HBV infections occur through contact with infected secretions, most commonly through sexual contact, or through inoculation from infected needles. Perinatal transmission from mother to fetus is also a common route of infection. If the mother is positive for the hepatitis B surface antigen marker (HBsAg), the likelihood of transmission to the infant at birth is 10%. However, the rate increases to 70% to 90% if the mother is positive for both HBsAg and the highly infective HBeAg. Chronic HBV infection develops in 90% of infected infants, 30% to 50% of those infected between age 1 and 5 years, and 6% to 10% of those infected as adults. In Western countries, only 0.1% to 0.5% of the population are chronic HBV carriers. However, in Southeast Asia and China, most of Africa, most Pacific Islands, parts of the Middle East, and the Amazon Basin, 8% to 15% of the population carry the virus. The lifetime risk of HBV infection in these countries is greater than 60%. Most infections are acquired at birth or during early childhood, when the risk of developing chronic infection is the highest.[56,57]

In 1990, because of the failure of selective vaccination to reduce the burden of illness in persons who lack identifiable risk factors, the U.S. PHS modified its high-risk strategy and recommended universal infant vaccination and more intensive screening of adults (including universal screening of pregnant women). Following these measures, the overall incidence of reported acute HBV declined 75%, from 8.5 to 2.1 per 100,000 persons between 1990 and 2004. The most dramatic declines occurred in the cohort of children to whom recommendations for routine infant and adolescent vaccination were applied.[55-57]

Indications

The ACIP recommends vaccinating all newborns soon after birth and before hospital discharge in addition to universal HBV screening of pregnant women. Routine vaccination is also recommended for all children and adolescents through age 18 years. Children not previously vaccinated with hepatitis B vaccine should be vaccinated at age 11 to 12 years with the age-appropriate dose of vaccine.

Vaccination is also recommended for adults in high-risk groups. In general, persons at markedly increased risk of acquiring HBV include injection drug users; homosexual and heterosexual persons with multiple partners; health care workers and others with potential exposure to blood products; patients undergoing hemodialysis and those with hemophilia; recipients of certain blood products; household contacts or sexual partners of HBV carriers; inmates of long-term correctional institutions; immigrants from certain countries (e.g., China, Southeast Asian countries, African countries, the Philippines, Haiti, eastern European countries); other population groups (e.g., Alaskan Natives, Pacific Islanders) in which HBV is common; and international travelers to these regions for whom sexual contact, exposure to blood, or residence longer than 6 months is likely. The ACIP now recommends hepatitis B vaccination for all adults in settings in which a high proportion of persons are likely to be at risk of HBV infection.

Administration

The recommended immunization schedule for hepatitis B vaccine is presented in Figure 17.1 along with the pediatric catch-up schedule.

Two formulations of recombinant vaccines are available in the United States: Recombivax HB (Hep-B; Merck) and Engerix-B (Hep-B; GlaxoSmithKline). As shown in Figure 17.1, three combination vaccines containing hepatitis B vaccine are also available: Comvax (Merck), Twinrix (GlaxoSmithKline) for children >18 years of age, and Pediarix (GlaxoSmithKline). Although postvaccination testing is not routinely recommended, it should be considered for certain persons, such as health care workers in dialysis units or infants born to HBsAg-positive or HBsAg-unknown mothers. When indicated, postvaccination testing should be performed 1 to 2 months after completion of the vaccine series. All infants born to HBsAg-positive or HBsAg-unknown women should be tested 3 to 12 months after their final (third or fourth) dose of hepatitis B vaccine (i.e., at age 9–18 mo). Occasionally, vaccinated individuals will not have a detectable antibody response. Persons who do not respond to the first series of hepatitis B vaccine should complete a second three-dose series. Fewer than 5% of persons receiving six doses of hepatitis B vaccine administered in the deltoid muscle following the appropriate schedule fail to develop detectable anti-HBs antibody. An individual who remains seronegative after six doses of vaccine should be managed as a nonresponder (in such individuals HBV infection should be ruled out; details are available in the *"Pink Book,"* which can be accessed online at https://www.cdc.gov/vaccines/pubs/pinkbook/hepb.html).[56]

In certain cases, persons exposed to HBV require administration of hepatitis B immune globulin, which contains a high concentration of hepatitis B antibody. Rules for various vaccination and exposure scenarios, including the management of infants born to women who are HBsAg-positive, are complex. Detailed information can be found in the CDC's *"Pink Book"*[56] and on the CDC website.[55]

Adverse Effects

The most common side effects of hepatitis B vaccination are pain at the injection site (reported in 13%–29% of adults and 3%–9% of children) and mild fever (less than 1%). Some mild systemic symptoms, such as headache or fatigue, may also occur. The principal side effects of hepatitis B immune globulin are pain and swelling at the injection site. Urticaria, angioedema, and anaphylaxis have been reported, but their occurrence is rare.

Precautions and Contraindications

A severe allergic reaction to a vaccine component or following a prior dose of hepatitis B vaccine is a contraindication to further doses, although as noted, such reactions are rare.

Moderate or severe acute illness is a precaution against vaccination, but minor illness is not a contraindication to vaccination. Studies to date indicate that hepatitis B vaccine is probably safe for pregnant women. Since acquiring an HBV infection during pregnancy can cause severe disease for both mother and infant, hepatitis B vaccine may be administered to a pregnant woman who is otherwise eligible for it.

HEPATITIS A VACCINE

Hepatitis A viral (HAV) infection is caused by a nonenveloped RNA picornavirus. It is spread by fecal-oral transmission. After an incubation period averaging 28 days, it causes a clinical course characterized by fever, jaundice, anorexia, and malaise. In children younger than 6 years, 70% of infections are asymptomatic, but in older children and adults, more than 70% develop jaundice. In the prevaccine era, HAV epidemics occurred in 10- to 15-year cycles. Between 1980 and 1995 the attack rate in the United States was approximately 10 cases per 100,000 population, and 31% of the U.S. population had evidence of prior HAV infection. Since 1995 the total number of cases has been declining, probably due to increasing use of HAV vaccine. A record low annual total of 2800 cases was reported in 2015.[58]

HAV causes significant morbidity. Rates of hospitalization are approximately 11% to 22%. Infected adults usually miss almost a month of work. Fulminant HAV infection causes approximately 100 deaths per year in the United States.

Two inactivated whole-virus hepatitis A vaccines are available: Havrix (GlaxoSmithKline) and Vaqta (Merck). Both vaccines are manufactured in both pediatric and adult formulations, and both produce excellent immunity. In clinical trials, all vaccinees had protective levels of antibody after receiving two doses.[59]

After the vaccine was released in 1995, it was first used chiefly in individuals at high risk of acquiring disease. In 1999, the ACIP recommended routine vaccination of children aged 24 months and older in high-risk communities (attack rate more than double the national average). Success in reducing rates of HAV in these communities led the ACIP in 2005 to recommend universal vaccination at ages 12 to 23 months.

Indications

All children should be vaccinated at age 12 to 23 months. Those not vaccinated by age 2 years can be vaccinated at later visits. Vaccination is also recommended for other groups, including those older than 12 months who will be traveling to areas of increased risk, men who have sex with men, injection drug users, persons with clotting factor disorders, and persons with occupational risk of infection. Persons with chronic liver disease who are susceptible should be vaccinated. The ACIP does not recommend routine vaccination of all health care workers or food service workers.

Administration

Vaqta is quantified in antigen units (U). Children and adolescents aged 1 to 18 years should receive one dose of the pediatric formulation (25 U per dose; 0.5 mL volume), with a booster 6 to 12 months later. Adults aged 19 years or older should receive one dose of adult formulation (50 U per dose; 1 mL volume) with a booster dose 6 to 12 months later.

Havrix is quantified in ELISA units (EL.U.) per 0.5-mL dose. Children aged 1 to 18 years should receive a single dose of the pediatric formulation (720 EL.U. per 0.5-mL dose) followed by a booster dose 6 to 12 months later. Adults aged 19 years or older should receive one dose of the adult formulation (1440 EL.U. per 1.0-mL dose) followed by a booster dose 6 to 12 months later.

Since 2001, one combination vaccine, Twinrix (GlaxoSmithKline), has been available. It is approved for persons aged 18 years or older. A 1.0-mL dose of vaccine contains 720 EL.U. of inactivated HAV (equivalent to a single pediatric dose of Havrix) and 20 µg of recombinant HBsAg protein (equivalent to a single adult dose of Engerix-B). The vaccine is administered in a three-dose series at 0, 1, and 6 months. The first and second doses should be separated by at least 4 weeks, and the second and third doses should be separated by at least 5 months, with at least 6 months between the first and third doses. It is not necessary to restart the series or add doses if the interval between doses is longer than the recommended interval. In March 2007, the FDA approved an accelerated dosing schedule that consists of three doses given within 3 weeks followed by a booster dose at 12 months (at 0, 7, and 21–30 d and at 12 mo). The accelerated schedule can benefit individuals needing rapid protection, such as travelers to high-risk areas or emergency responders, especially those being deployed to disaster areas.

All hepatitis A vaccines should be administered intramuscularly into the deltoid muscle. Those vaccinated can be assumed to be immune 4 weeks after receiving the first dose of vaccine.

Prevaccination testing is not recommended for children who are expected to be susceptible. However, because HAV infection produces lifelong immunity, prevaccination testing may be indicated in certain groups at high risk of prior HAV infection, such as adults born in Africa, Asia, or South America.

Persons exposed to HAV who have not had at least one dose of hepatitis A vaccine at least 1 month before exposure may benefit from the administration of standard immune globulin therapy (IG). IG is more than 85% effective in preventing hepatitis A if given within 2 weeks of exposure. A single intramuscular dose of 0.02 mL/kg of IG confers protection for less than 3 months; 0.06 mL/kg protects for 5 months. Detailed information about this can be found in the CDC "*Pink Book*"[59] or in the AAP "*Red Book*".[13]

Adverse Effects

The most common adverse effects are pain, erythema, or swelling at the injection site, reported by 20% to 50% of recipients. These events are generally mild and self-limited. Mild systemic complaints, such as malaise, fatigue, or low-grade fever, are reported by less than 10% of recipients. No serious adverse reactions have been reported.

Precautions and Contraindications

A history of a severe allergic reaction to a vaccine component, a reaction following a prior dose of hepatitis A vaccine, hypersensitivity to alum or, in the case of Havrix, to the preservative 2-phenoxyethanol, are all contraindications to further vaccine administration. Vaccination of persons with moderate or severe acute illnesses should be deferred until recovery occurs. Because hepatitis A vaccines are inactivated, theoretically the risk of a serious adverse event in pregnant women is low. Possible risks of vaccination should be weighed against the risk of HAV infection. The vaccine is considered safe for immunocompromised persons.

INFLUENZA VACCINE

Influenza is characterized by sudden onset of fever, headache and muscle aches, fatigue, dry painful cough, and coryza. Intestinal symptoms, such as nausea and vomiting, can also occur. Influenza viruses are spread from person to person, primarily through respiratory droplet transmission, although aerosol transmission may also play a role.[60] Hand-to-mouth transmission may occur through fomites but is less important. The typical incubation period for influenza is 1 to 4 days. Adults can be infectious from 1 day before to approximately 5 days after the onset of illness; the infectious period in children may be 10 days or more, and they can shed virus before the onset of their illness. Severely immunocompromised persons can shed virus for weeks or months.[60]

In temperate climates, seasonal influenza activity peaks between late December and early March. Deaths occur not only from influenza itself but also from complications in patients with respiratory and cardiovascular diseases. In the United States, approximately 12,000 to 56,000 influenza-associated pulmonary and circulatory deaths per influenza season occurred annually after 2010, compared with approximately 36,000 deaths per season during 1990–99.[60–62] During the 2016-17 season, 101 pediatric patients died from influenza.[62] The highest rates of serious illness and death occur in persons aged 65 years or older and in children younger than 2 years, as well as in persons with certain medical conditions that are exacerbated by influenza. Pregnant women are also at increased risk of complications, especially in the second and third trimesters, when the risk of hospitalization from influenza is more than four times higher than for nonpregnant women. Two antigenic types cause epidemic human influenza: types A and B.[15] Type A influenza causes the most severe disease in all ages and also affects certain wild and domesticated birds. The three subtypes of influenza type A that are responsible for most epidemics are characterized by their different surface antigens: hemagglutinin (H1, H2, and H3) and neuraminidase (N1 and N2). Influenza type B occurs only in humans and is a milder disease that chiefly affects children. Influenza C is not a disease of humans.

Influenza vaccine is prepared each year in an attempt to anticipate antigenic variation among influenza viruses. Only three subtypes are currently circulating among humans: H1N1, H1N2, and H3N2. The choice of strains to be used by vaccine manufacturers is determined by the FDA based on recommendations from the WHO. Three strains are selected each year: a type A (H1N1), a type A (H_3N_2), and a type B. During the 2013–14 season, a fourth strain was added to the vaccine protecting against another B strain (CDC Quadrivalent influenza vaccine).[61]

Multiple types of influenza vaccines are currently available in the United States. The standard dose trivalent inactivated influenza vaccine is administered by the intramuscular route. A high-dose trivalent vaccine is approved for patients 65 years and older. The quadrivalent vaccine is approved for patients aged >6 months. The intradermal quadrivalent flu vaccine is approved for patients 18 to 64 years of age. Live attenuated influenza vaccine is not recommended for the 2017–18 season owing to concerns about efficacy.[63,64] A new FluMist quadrivalent vaccine may return for the 2018–19 season.

Indications

- Everyone aged 6 months and older should receive a yearly flu vaccine with either trivalent or quadrivalent inactivated vaccine
- Children 6 months to 8 years who did not receive at least two doses of influenza vaccines before July 1, 2017, should receive two doses 4 weeks apart
- The amount of the dose of the vaccine depends on the vaccine type and age of the patient
- All children with egg allergy can receive the influenza vaccine
- All health care workers should receive the annual flu vaccine
- Pregnant women may receive the influenza vaccine during any time during pregnancy

Administration

See CDC for details on the types and dosages of available influenza vaccines (Table 17.2A,B). Influenza vaccine should be offered beginning in September during routine patient visits.

TABLE 17.2A Influenza Vaccines—United States, 2017–18 Influenza Season[a]

Trade Name	Manufacturer	Presentation	Age Indication	Mercury (From Thimerosal, μg/0.5 mL)	Latex	Route
Inactivated Influenza Vaccines, Quadrivalent (IIV4s), Standard-Dose[b]						
Afluria Quadrivalent	Seqirus	0.5 mL prefilled syringe	≥5 yr	NR	No	IM[c]
		5.0 mL multidose vial	≥5 yr (by needle/syringe) 18 through 64 yr (by jet injector)	24.5	No	IM
Fluarix Quadrivalent	GlaxoSmithKline	0.5 mL prefilled syringe	≥6 mo	NR	No	IM
FluLaval Quadrivalent	ID Biomedical Corp. of Quebec (distributed by GlaxoSmithKline)	0.5 mL prefilled syringe	≥6 mo	NR	No	IM
		5.0 mL multidose vial	≥6 mo	<25	No	IM
Fluzone Quadrivalent	Sanofi Pasteur	0.25 mL prefilled syringe	6 through 35 mo	NR	No	IM
		0.5 mL prefilled syringe	≥3 yr	NR	No	IM
		0.5 mL single-dose vial	≥3 yr	NR	No	IM
		5.0 mL multidose vial	≥6 mo	25	No	IM
Inactivated Influenza Vaccine, Quadrivalent (ccIIV4), Standard Dose,[b] Cell Culture Based						
Flucelvax Quadrivalent	Seqirus	0.5 mL prefilled syringe	≥4 yr	NR	No	IM
		5.0 mL multidose vial	≥4 yr	25	No	IM

Inactivated Influenza Vaccine, Quadrivalent (IIV4), Standard Dose, Intradermal[d]						
Fluzone Intradermal Quadrivalent	Sanofi Pasteur	0.1 mL single-dose prefilled microinjection system	18 through 64 yr	NR	No	ID[e]
Inactivated Influenza Vaccines, Trivalent (IIV3s), Standard Dose[b]						
Afluria	Seqirus	0.5 mL prefilled syringe	≥5 yr	NR	No	IM
		5.0 mL multidose vial	≥5 yr (by needle/syringe) 18 through 64 yr (by jet injector)	24.5	No	IM
Fluvirin	Seqirus	0.5 mL prefilled syringe	≥4 yr	≤1	Yes[f]	IM
		5.0 mL multidose vial	≥4 yr	25	No	IM
Adjuvanted Inactivated Influenza Vaccine, Trivalent (aIIV3),[b] Standard Dose						
Fluad	Seqirus	0.5 mL prefilled syringe	≥65 yr	NR	Yes[f]	IM
Inactivated Influenza Vaccine, Trivalent (IIV3), High-Dose[g]						
Fluzone High-Dose	Sanofi Pasteur	0.5 mL prefilled syringe	≥65 yr	NR	No	IM
Recombinant Influenza Vaccine, Quadrivalent (RIV4)[h]						
Flublok Quadrivalent	Protein Sciences	0.5 mL prefilled syringe	≥18 yr	NR	No	IM

(Continued)

TABLE 17.2A   Influenza Vaccines—United States, 2017–18 Influenza Season[a]   (Continued)

Trade Name	Manufacturer	Presentation	Age Indication	Mercury (From Thimerosal, µg/0.5 mL)	Latex	Route
Recombinant Influenza Vaccine, Trivalent (RIV3)[h]						
Flublok	Protein Sciences	0.5 mL single-dose vial	≥18 yr	NR	No	IM
Live Attenuated Influenza Vaccine, Quadrivalent (LAIV4)[i] (Not Recommended for Use During the 2017–18 Season)						
FluMist Quadrivalent	MedImmune	0.2 mL single-dose pre-filled intranasal sprayer	2 through 49 yr	NR	No	NAS

[a]Immunization providers should check Food and Drug Administration–approved prescribing information for 2017–18 influenza vaccines for the most complete and updated information, including (but not limited to) indications, contraindications, warnings, and precautions. Package inserts for US-licensed vaccines are available at https://www.fda.gov/BiologicsBloodVaccines/Vaccines/ApprovedProducts/ucm093833.htm. Availability of specific products and presentations might change and differ from what is described in this table and in the text of this report.

[b]Standard dose intramuscular IIVs contain 15 µg of each vaccine HA antigen (45 µg total for trivalents and 60 µg total for quadrivalents) per 0.5-mL dose.

[c]For adults and older children, the recommended site for intramuscular influenza vaccination is the deltoid muscle. The preferred site for infants and young children is the anterolateral aspect of the thigh. Specific guidance regarding site and needle length for intramuscular administration is available in the ACIP General Best Practice Guidelines for Immunization, available at https://www.cdc.gov/vaccines/hcp/acip-recs/general-recs/index.html.

[d]Quadrivalent inactivated influenza vaccine, intradermal: a 0.1-mL dose contains 9 µg of each vaccine HA antigen (36 µg total).

[e]The preferred injection site is over the deltoid muscle. Fluzone Intradermal Quadrivalent is administered per manufacturer's instructions using the delivery system included with the vaccine.

[f]Syringe tip cap might contain natural rubber latex.

[g]High-dose IIV3 contains 60 µg of each vaccine antigen (180 µg total) per 0.5-mL dose.

[h]RIV contains 45 µg of each vaccine HA antigen (135 µg total for trivalent, 180 µg total for quadrivalent) per 0.5-mL dose.

[i]ACIP recommends that FluMist Quadrivalent (LAIV4) not be used during the 2017–18 season.

ACIP, Advisory Committee on Immunization Practices; *ID,* intradermal; *IM,* intramuscular; *NAS,* intranasal; *NR,* not relevant (does not contain thimerosal).

TABLE 17.2B   Contraindications and Precautions to the Use of Influenza Vaccines—United States, 2017–18 Influenza Season[a]

Vaccine Type	Contraindications	Precautions
IIV	History of severe allergic reaction to any component of the vaccine[b] or after previous dose of any influenza vaccine	Moderate to severe acute illness with or without fever History of Guillain-Barré syndrome within 6 wk of receipt of influenza vaccine
RIV	History of severe allergic reaction to any component of the vaccine	Moderate to severe acute illness with or without fever History of Guillain-Barré syndrome within 6 wk of receipt of influenza vaccine
LAIV For the 2017–18 season, ACIP recommends that LAIV not be used. Content is provided for information	History of severe allergic reaction to any component of the vaccine[b] or after a previous dose of any influenza vaccine Concomitant aspirin or salicylate-containing therapy in children and adolescents Children aged 2 through 4 yr who have received a diagnosis of asthma or whose parents or caregivers report that a health care provider has told them during the preceding 12 mo that their child had wheezing or asthma or whose medical record indicates a wheezing episode has occurred during the preceding 12 mo Children and adults who are immunocompromised owing to any cause (including immunosuppression caused by medications or by HIV infection) Close contacts and caregivers of severely immunosuppressed persons who require a protected environment Pregnancy Receipt of influenza antiviral medication within the previous 48 hr	Moderate to severe acute illness with or without fever History of Guillain-Barré syndrome within 6 wk of receipt of influenza vaccine Asthma in persons aged ≥5 yr Other underlying medical conditions that might predispose to complications after wild-type influenza infection (e.g., chronic pulmonary, cardiovascular [except isolated hypertension], renal, hepatic, neurologic, hematologic, or metabolic disorders [including diabetes mellitus])

[a]Immunization providers should check Food and Drug Administration–approved prescribing information for 2017–18 influenza vaccines for the most complete and updated information, including (but not limited to) indications, contraindications, and precautions. Package inserts for US-licensed vaccines are available at https://www.fda.gov/BiologicsBloodVaccines/Vaccines/ApprovedProducts/ucm093833.htm.

[b]History of severe allergic reaction (e.g., anaphylaxis) to egg is a labeled contraindication to the use of IIV and LAIV. However, ACIP recommends that any licensed, recommended, and appropriate IIV or RIV may be administered to persons with egg allergy of any severity (see Persons with a History of Egg Allergy).

ACIP, Advisory Committee on Immunization Practices; IIV, inactivated influenza vaccine; LAIV, live-attenuated influenza vaccine; RIV, recombinant influenza vaccine.

Certain antiviral drugs have been used for the treatment of influenza or chemoprophylaxis against influenza strains. The three drugs available in the United States are oseltamivir, zanamivir, and peramivir. Oseltamivir is approved by the FDA for infants as young as 2 weeks of age (AAP). Zanamivir is recommended for children aged ≥7 years for treatment and ≥5 years for chemoprophylaxis. Peramivir is approved for adults 18 years and older. See Table 17.3 for dosage and schedule of antiviral medication.

Clinical trials have shown a reduction in the duration of symptoms, and these antiviral drugs may reduce complications of influenza if started in the first 48 hours of symptoms.[65] Antiviral treatment is recommended for patients suspected or confirmed with influenza or at higher risk for complications.

The CDC and AAP recommend chemoprophylaxis in the following circumstances.[64,65]

- Hospitalized patient with presumed influenza or diagnosed influenza with severe, complicated, or progressive illness.
- Patients who are at high risk for influenza complications.
- Antiviral therapy should be considered in a healthy child with influenza if treatment can be initiated within 48 hours of symptoms.
- Healthy children with influenza living with a patient <6 months of age or with a medical condition that predisposes them to complications.

Control of Influenza Outbreaks in Institutions

When outbreaks occur in institutions, chemoprophylaxis should be administered to all residents, regardless of whether they received influenza vaccinations during the previous Fall, and should continue for a minimum of 2 weeks. If surveillance indicates that new cases continue to occur, chemoprophylaxis should be continued until approximately 1 week after the end of the outbreak. The dosage for each resident should be determined individually. Chemoprophylaxis can also be offered to unvaccinated staff members who provide care to persons at high risk.

Chemoprophylaxis should be considered for all employees in such institutions, regardless of their vaccination status, if the outbreak is suspected to be caused by a strain of influenza virus that is not well matched to the vaccine. If cases continue to occur despite chemoprophylaxis, it is probably ineffective and may need to be discontinued.

In addition to being used in nursing homes, chemoprophylaxis can also be considered for controlling influenza outbreaks in other closed or semiclosed settings (e.g., dormitories or other settings in which persons live in close proximity).

Details about current recommendations for influenza vaccination and antiviral drugs can be found online at http://www.cdc.gov/flu/.

TABLE 17.3 Recommended Dosage and Duration of Influenza Antiviral Medications for Treatment or Chemoprophylaxis

Antiviral Agent	Use	Children	Adults
Oral Oseltamivir	Treatment (5 d)[a]	**If younger than 1 yr old**[b]: 3 mg/kg/dose twice daily.[c,d] **If 1 yr or older, dose varies by child's weight: 15 kg or less, the dose is 30 mg twice a day** >15–23 kg, the dose is 45 mg **twice** a day >23–40 kg, the dose is 60 mg **twice** a day >40 kg, the dose is 75 mg **twice** a day	75 mg **twice** daily
	Chemopro-phylaxis (7 d)[e]	If child is younger than 3 mo, use of oseltamivir for chemoprophylaxis is not recommended unless situation is judged critical due to limited data in this age group. **If child is 3 mo or older and younger than 1 yr**[b] 3 mg/kg/dose once daily.[c] **If 1 yr or older, dose varies by child's weight: 15 kg or less, the dose is 30 mg once a day** >15–23 kg, the dose is 45 mg **once** a day >23–40 kg, the dose is 60 mg **once** a day >40 kg, the dose is 75 mg **once** a day	75 mg **once** daily
Inhaled Zanamivir[f]	Treatment (5 d)	10 mg (two 5-mg inhalations) **twice** daily **(FDA approved and recommended for use in children 7 yr or older)**	10 mg (two 5-mg inhalations) **twice** daily
	Chemopro-phylaxis (7 d)[e]	10 mg (two 5-mg inhalations) **once** daily **(FDA approved for and recommended for use in children 5 yr or older)**	10 mg (two 5-mg inhalations) **once** daily

(Continued)

TABLE 17.3 Recommended Dosage and Duration
of Influenza Antiviral Medications for Treatment or
Chemoprophylaxis   (Continued)

Antiviral Agent	Use	Children	Adults
Intravenous Peramivir[g]	Treatment (1 d)[a]	(2–12 yr of age) One 12 mg/kg dose, up to 600 mg maximum, via intravenous infusion for a minimum of 15 min **(FDA approved and recommended for use in children 2 yr or older)**	(13 yr and older) One 600 mg dose, via intravenous infusion for a minimum of 15 min
	Chemoprophylaxis	N/A	N/A

[a]Longer treatment duration may be needed for severely ill patients.

[b]Oral oseltamivir is approved by the FDA for treatment of acute uncomplicated influenza within 2 d of illness onset with twice-daily dosing in persons 14 d and older, and for chemoprophylaxis with once-daily dosing in persons 1 yr and older. Although not part of the FDA-approved indications, use of oral oseltamivir for treatment of influenza in infants less than 14 day old, and for chemoprophylaxis in infants 3 mo to 1 yr of age, is recommended by the CDC and the American Academy of Pediatrics (Committee on Infectious Diseases, 2017).

[c]This is the FDA-approved oral oseltamivir treatment dose for infants 14 d and older and less than 1 year old, and provides oseltamivir exposure in children similar to that achieved by the approved dose of 75 mg orally twice daily for adults, as shown in two studies of oseltamivir pharmacokinetics in children (Kimberlin, 2013 [CASG 114], EU study WP22849, FDA Clinical Pharmacology Review). The American Academy of Pediatrics has recommended an oseltamivir treatment dose of 3.5 mg/kg orally twice daily for infants aged 9–11 mo, on the basis of data that indicated that a higher dose of 3.5 mg/kg was needed to achieve the protocol-defined targeted exposure for this cohort as defined in the CASG 114 study (Kimberlin, 2013). It is unknown whether this higher dose will improve efficacy or prevent the development of antiviral resistance. However, there is no evidence that the 3.5-mg/kg dose is harmful or causes more adverse events to infants in this age group.

[d]Current weight-based dosing recommendations are not appropriate for premature infants. Premature infants might have slower clearance of oral oseltamivir because of immature renal function, and doses recommended for full-term infants might lead to very high drug concentrations in this age group. CDC recommends dosing as also recommended by the American Academy of Pediatrics (Committee on Infectious Diseases, 2017): limited data from the National Institute of Allergy and Infectious Diseases Collaborative Antiviral Study Group provide the basis for dosing preterm infants using their postmenstrual age (gestational age + chronological age): 1.0 mg/kg/dose, orally, twice daily, for those <38 wk postmenstrual age; 1.5 mg/kg/dose, orally, twice daily, for those 38 through 40 wk postmenstrual age; 3.0 mg/kg/dose, orally, twice daily, for those >40 wk postmenstrual age.

[e]See Special Considerations for Institutional Settings section below for details regarding duration of chemoprophylaxis for outbreaks in institutional settings.

[f]Inhaled zanamivir is approved for treatment of acute uncomplicated influenza within 2 d of illness onset with twice-daily dosing in persons aged 7 yr and older, and for chemoprophylaxis with once-daily dosing in persons aged 5 yr and older.

[g]Intravenous peramivir is approved for treatment of acute uncomplicated influenza within 2 d of illness onset with a single dose in persons aged 2 yr and older. Daily dosing for a minimum of 5 d was used in clinical trials of hospitalized patients with influenza (de Jong, 2014; Ison, 2014).

N/A, not applicable.

Adverse Effects

Adverse reactions to flu vaccine are generally mild, consisting of discomfort at the injection site for up to 2 days. Immediate allergic reactions (e.g., urticaria, angioedema) are rare and are usually related to allergies to egg proteins. Fever, malaise, and myalgia, usually lasting 6 to 48 hours, have been infrequently reported. Although GBS was associated with the use of the "swine flu" vaccine in 1976, annual surveillance in subsequent years has not demonstrated a clear association between influenza vaccination and neurologic complications. The estimated risk of GBS is approximately one additional case per 1 million persons vaccinated (if GBS was found to be associated with influenza vaccine). This risk is, in any case, much less than the health risk of severe influenza, which is vaccine preventable.

Precautions and Contraindications

Contraindications and precautions to vaccination with influenza vaccines are listed in Table 17.1.

VARICELLA VACCINE

Varicella is a highly contagious disease caused by the varicella zoster virus (VZV). It usually lasts 4 to 5 days and is characterized by fever, malaise, and a generalized vesicular rash typically consisting of 250 to 500 lesions. Secondary attack rates among close contacts may be as high as 90%.

Complications of varicella infection include secondary bacterial infections of the skin, pneumonia, and complications involving the central nervous system, especially meningitis and encephalitis. The complication rate increases with age: adults account for only 5% of cases of varicella but 35% of deaths.[66] Immunocompromised persons have a particularly high rate of varicella complications and disseminated disease. A late complication of VZV infection, herpes zoster (HZ) (shingles), carries a lifetime risk of 10% to 20% and can cause serious illness in elderly persons. Maternal varicella infection in the first 20 weeks of pregnancy can also cause congenital varicella syndrome in up to 2% of exposed fetuses, characterized by segmental areas of skin loss or scarring, limb hypoplasia, and reduced birth weight.[66] No cases of congenital varicella syndrome have been reported from the use of varicella vaccine.

Because of the high rate of infectivity, and because communicability through aerosol droplets begins 1 to 2 days before the appearance of the rash, a universal vaccination program is necessary to prevent the spread of VZV. Varicella vaccine was first licensed for use in the United States in 1995. The current vaccine (Varivax; Merck) is a live attenuated vaccine derived from the Oka strain of VZV and is approved for vaccination of children aged 12 months or older. A combined MMR and varicella vaccine (MMRV [ProQuad; Merck]) was approved for use in 2005 for children aged 12 months to 12 years in cases when both MMR and varicella vaccine are due.

After one dose of Varivax, detectable antibody titers develop in 97% of children aged 1 to 12 years. More than 90% of responders maintain antibody for at least 6 years. In Japanese studies, 97% of children maintained antibody 7 to 10 years after vaccination. Postlicensure studies have shown that vaccine efficacy is usually 80% to 85% against infection (range of 44%–100%) and more than 95% against moderate or severe disease.[66] An average of 78% of adolescents and adults develop antibody after one dose, and 99% develop antibody after a second dose given 4 to 8 weeks later. Antibody has persisted for at least 1 year in 97% of vaccinated patients who received the second dose (4–8 weeks after the first dose).[66] ProQuad (MMRV) appears to stimulate the same antibody levels as M-M-RII and Varivax when given separately,[13,66] and concomitant administration of MMRV, Hib/HepB, and DTaP is well tolerated.[13,66]

Before the widespread use of varicella vaccine, there were approximately 4 million cases of VZV infection in the United States every year, causing approximately 11,000 hospitalizations (rate of 5 cases per 1,000), and 100 deaths each year (approximately 1 in 60,000 cases). Since the varicella vaccine was introduced in the United States, varicella cases, hospital admissions, and deaths have been reduced by more than 80% in children, with lesser reductions in infants and adults from indirect effects (herd immunity).[66] A mild form of varicella can occur in 1% to 4% of vaccinees per year following exposure to wild-type VZV. Such illness is usually shorter and less severe than naturally occurring varicella (less than 50 lesions with minimal or no fever).

Initially, the ACIP recommended one dose for children younger than 13 years and two doses for those aged 13 years and older. However, subsequent studies have found that 15% to 20% of children who have received one dose of the vaccine were not fully protected and were susceptible to develop chickenpox after exposure to VZV. Also, there was concern that one dose of the vaccine might not provide protection into adulthood when chickenpox is more severe. As noted, in 2006 the ACIP recommended a two-dose schedule for all children in the United States.

Indications

Routine immunization with varicella vaccine is recommended for all susceptible children and adolescents without a contraindication. As noted, in 2006 the ACIP recommended that the vaccine be administered to all children and to all other people aged 13 years or older without evidence of immunity. See Figure 17.2 for revised criteria of evidence of immunity to varicella in adults.

Administration

Two doses of varicella virus vaccine are administered at an interval of at least 3 months for patients aged 12 months to 12 years and at an interval of 4 to 8 weeks for people aged 13 years or older. In children, the first dose should be administered at age 12 to 15 months and the second dose at age

4 to 6 years (i.e., before entering kindergarten or first grade). The second dose can be administered at an earlier age provided the interval between the first and second dose is at least 3 months. However, if the second dose is administered at least 28 days following the first dose, the second dose need not be repeated. Because it is recommended that varicella vaccine be given at the same age as MMR vaccine, MMRV is preferred over a separate injection of equivalent component vaccines, unless contraindicated.

A second-dose, catch-up varicella vaccination is recommended for children, adolescents, and adults who previously had received one dose, to improve individual protection against varicella and for more rapid impact on school outbreaks. Catch-up vaccination can be implemented during routine visits to the clinician and through school and college entry requirements. The catch-up second dose can be administered at any interval longer than 3 months after the first dose.

Children with chronic illness or who are immunocompromised should see schedule 1 for the recommended vaccine schedule.

The ACIP recommends assessing pregnant women for evidence of varicella immunity. Clinicians should not vaccinate women who are pregnant or might become pregnant within 4 weeks of receiving the vaccine. Women who do not have evidence of immunity should receive the first dose of varicella vaccine upon completion or termination of pregnancy and before discharge from the health care facility. The second dose should be given 4 to 8 weeks after the first dose.

A dose of varicella vaccine used as postexposure prophylaxis is 70% to 100% effective at preventing or reducing the severity of varicella if given within 3 days of exposure. It may also be effective up to 5 days after exposure. The ACIP also recommends a second dose of varicella vaccine during outbreaks: persons who have received one dose of varicella vaccine should receive a second dose (resources permitting), provided the appropriate vaccination interval has elapsed since the first dose.

Oral acyclovir is recommended by some experts for postexposure prophylaxis and should be started between day 7 and 10 after exposure for a total of 7 days of therapy. Other antiviral agents, such as valacyclovir and famciclovir, can be used for prophylaxis in susceptible adults who have been exposed.

Varicella immune globulin contains high titers of VZV antibody and is recommended for postexposure prophylaxis in certain high-risk individuals, such as immunocompromised patients, susceptible pregnant women without evidence of immunity, infants of mothers who develop chickenpox from 5 days before to 2 days after delivery, and certain premature infants exposed during the neonatal period.[66] It is most effective when administered within 96 hours of exposure. The only available varicella immune globulin (as of early 2007) is VariZIG (Aptevo), which is a purified lyophilized human immune globulin preparation made from plasma containing high levels of anti-varicella antibodies (immunoglobulin class G). For the management of uncomplicated cases of varicella in healthy children the AAP does not recommend routine use of oral acyclovir therapy. However, certain groups at increased risk of complicated disease should be considered for oral acyclovir therapy, including healthy, nonpregnant persons aged 13 years and older; children older than 12 months with chronic cutaneous or respiratory disorders and those receiving long-term salicylate therapy; and children receiving short, intermittent, or aerosolized courses of corticosteroids. Some experts advise using oral acyclovir for secondary cases within a household. For maximum benefit, oral acyclovir therapy should be started within 24 hours of the appearance of the rash. Intravenous acyclovir therapy is recommended for the treatment of immunocompromised children with primary varicella or recurrent HZ and for otherwise healthy individuals suffering from viral-mediated complications of varicella (e.g., pneumonia).

Adverse Effects

The most common adverse reactions following varicella vaccine are usually mild and self-limited: injection site irritation, such as pain, erythema, and swelling. Such local reactions are reported by approximately 20% of vaccinated persons. A varicella-like rash (usually several maculopapular lesions) at the injection site is reported by 3% of children, and by 1% of adolescents and adults, following the second dose. A generalized varicella-like rash, which is usually maculopapular rather than vesicular, is reported by 4% to 6% of recipients of varicella vaccine (1% after the second dose in adolescents and adults). Fever within 6 weeks of vaccination is reported by 15% of children and 10% of adolescents and adults; however, fever occurs in a similar percentage of persons receiving placebo and may be due to other infections rather than the vaccine.

Varicella vaccine, containing a live virus, can theoretically cause a mild latent infection. The rate of HZ after vaccination appears to be less than the rate after wild-virus infection. Unpublished CDC data indicate a rate of 2.6 cases of HZ per 100,000 varicella vaccine doses administered versus a rate of 68 cases per 100,000 person-years in healthy persons aged 20 years or older. Not all these cases have been confirmed as having been caused by the vaccine virus, and many may in fact be due to wild virus. Cases of zoster after vaccination appear to be milder than after natural infection, with fewer sequelae such as postherpetic neuralgia.[67]

Transmission of vaccine-borne virus appears to be a rare event. Cases of suspected secondary transmission of vaccine virus have been reported, and in studies of household contacts, several instances of asymptomatic seroconversion have been observed. It appears that transmission occurs mainly, and perhaps only, when the vaccinated patient develops a rash. If a vaccinated child develops a rash, close contact should be avoided with persons who do not have evidence of varicella immunity and who are at high risk of complications of varicella, such as immunocompromised persons, until the rash in the vaccinated patient has resolved.[66]

Serious adverse events, such as encephalitis, ataxia, erythema mul-tiforme, Stevens-Johnson syndrome, pneumonia, thrombocytopenia, seizures, neuropathy, and death, have been reported rarely in temporal association with varicella vaccine. In some cases, wild-type VZV or another causal agent has been identified. In most cases, data are insufficient to determine a causal association.

Precautions and Contraindications

Contraindications and precautions to varicella vaccine can be found in Table 17.1.

HERPES ZOSTER VACCINE

HZ, or shingles, is caused by reactivation of VZV, which remains latent in the dorsal root (sensory) ganglia after a primary chickenpox infection. HZ is characterized by a vesicular rash and radicular pain, usually along a sin-gle dermatome. Pain usually occurs 2 to 3 days before the rash appears. Vesicles from HZ typically crust over in 7 to 10 days but may take up to a month to heal. VZV infection can be spread by contact with lesions.

Persons at higher risk of HZ include the elderly and immunosuppressed persons, apparently because they experience a decline in cell-mediated immunity. The overall incidence of disease is 3 to 4 per 1,000 in developed countries, but the incidence increases markedly after age 50 years and rises to 10 per 1000 after age 75 years. Some studies suggest that lifetime incidence is 32% and may be as high as 50% among individuals older than 85 years.[66] Estimates of the number of new HZ cases in the United States vary from 500,000 to 1,000,000 annually.[66] Up to 10% of patients older than 65 years who develop HZ require hospitalization.

A common, debilitating complication of HZ is postherpetic neural-gia, which is pain along the affected cutaneous nerves that persists more than 90 days after the lesions have healed. Postherpetic neuralgia is more common with increasing age, occurring in 25% to 50% of patients with HZ older than 50 years, and it may persist for months or years. Other severe complications include keratitis, uveitis, retinitis, and blindness from HZ in the ophthalmic nerve; motor paresis or paralysis; GBS; and skin complica-tions, including bacterial skin infections, gangrene, and sepsis.

A live attenuated HZ vaccine, Zostavax (Merck), was developed to boost cell-mediated immunity against VZV in older individuals and was licensed by the FDA in 2006. Zostavax has 14 times the antigenicity of pediatric varicella vaccine. In a study involving 38,546 participants aged 60 years or older, the vaccine, compared with placebo, reduced the burden of illness caused by HZ by 61.1%, the incidence of postherpetic neuralgia by 66.5%, and the incidence of HZ by 51.3%. Adverse events were similar in the vaccine and the placebo groups; injection-site reactions (erythema, pain, and tenderness) were more common among vaccine recipients but were generally mild.[66] The cost-effectiveness of the vaccine is uncertain, with estimates ranging from 2000 to more than 100,000 per quality-adjusted life-year gained, depending on the method of calculation.[66,68]

Indications

In 2006, the ACIP recommended the administration of Zostavax (Merck) to all people aged 50 years and older, whether or not they report a previous episode of shingles. Zostavax is not indicated for the treatment of HZ or postherpetic neuralgia. In 2017, Shingrix (GlaxoSmithKline) was approved for patients 50 years and older as a two-dose series.

Administration

The CDC prefers the use of Shingrix vaccine. The vaccine is a two-dose series administered intramuscularly 2 to 6 months a part is the preferred vaccine by CDC. The Zostavax is a single-dose (0.65-mL) vaccine and intended for subcutaneous administration (preferably in the upper arm). It should be given immediately after reconstitution to minimize loss of potency. Unused reconstituted vaccine should be discarded after 30 minutes.

Adverse Effects

Side effects reported more often include redness, pain, tenderness, and swelling at the injection site and headache.

Because zoster vaccine, like varicella vaccine, is an attenuated live virus, transmission to other individuals is theoretically possible. Although further data will be needed to confirm this risk, it seems reasonable to follow the guidelines for varicella vaccine, in which viral transmission seems to occur only if the recipient develops a rash. If this occurs, it would be prudent for the patient to avoid contact with persons who do not have evidence of varicella immunity and who are at high risk of complications of varicella, such as immunocompromised persons, until the rash has resolved.

Precautions and Contraindications

Zoster vaccine should not be administered to the following individuals: patients with a history of anaphylactic/anaphylactoid reaction to gelatin, neomycin, or any other component of the vaccine; those with a history of primary or acquired immunodeficiency states, including leukemia, lymphomas of any type, or other malignant neoplasms affecting the bone marrow or lymphatic system; patients with AIDS or other clinical manifestations of HIV infection; patients on immunosuppressive therapy, including high-dose corticosteroids; patients with active untreated tuberculosis; and women who are or may be pregnant.[66]

ROTAVIRUS VACCINE

Rotavirus affects virtually all children by age 5 years. Prevaccine in the United States, rotavirus causes an estimated million episodes of diarrhea, with 400,000 clinic visits, 55,000 to 70,000 hospitalizations, and 20 to 60 deaths in children younger than 5 years.[69] The financial burden of rotavirus infections in the United States is estimated at more than 1 billion dollars annually. It is responsible for 500,000 diarrheal deaths worldwide.[69]

In 1998, the first rotavirus vaccine was licensed in the United States, and it appeared to offer excellent protection against this disease. However, the vaccine was withdrawn from the market in 1999 because it caused intussusception, at an estimated rate of one case per 10,000 vaccinated infants. In early 2006, placebo-controlled clinical trials for two new rotavirus vaccines showed excellent vaccine efficacy without an increased risk of intussusception and the ACIP approved a new pentavalent live attenuated oral rotavirus vaccine, RotaTeq (Merck), containing human serotypes G1, G2, G3, G4, and P[8]. In a study of 68,038 infants, the vaccine reduced hospitalizations and emergency department visits related to G1 to G4 rotavirus gastroenteritis by 95%. Efficacy against any G1 to G4 rotavirus gastroenteritis through the first full rotavirus season after vaccination was 74%, and efficacy against severe gastroenteritis was 98%; the vaccine reduced clinic visits for G1 to G4 rotavirus gastroenteritis by 86% and produced no increase in intussusception.[70]

Also, in 2008, a second rotavirus vaccine, Rotarix (GlaxoSmithKline), was approved and licensed in the United States. Rotarix is an attenuated monovalent vaccine derived from the most common human rotavirus strain, G1P[8]. It is administered in two oral doses 1 to 2 months apart. In a study of 63,225 infants in Finland and Latin America, two oral doses given at age 2 and 4 months reduced severe rotavirus gastroenteritis and rotavirus-associated hospitalization by 85%, with no increase in the incidence of intussusception.[71]

Indications

RotaTeq and Rotarix vaccine are indicated for all infants.

Administration

RotaTeq and Rotarix vaccines are both given orally. The ACIP recommends that infants receive three doses of the RotaTeq at age 2, 4, and 6 months and two doses of Rotarix at 2 and 4 months. Infants should receive the first dose between age 6 and 12 weeks, with the subsequent doses administered at 4- to 10-week intervals. The third dose should be administered by age 32 weeks, and no doses of rotavirus vaccine should be given after this time. Although the ACIP recommends not initiating vaccination in infants older than 14 weeks 6 days, Rotarix may be given off label to maximum age of 32 weeks (ACIP).

Adverse Effects

Mild adverse effects have been reported with both vaccines, including diarrhea, vomiting, cough, rhinorrhea, irritability, and flatulence.

Precautions and Contraindications

Rotavirus vaccine is contraindicated in infants with a history of hypersensitivity to any component of the vaccine or have a history of intussusception or severe combined immunodeficiency. Rotarix applicator contains latex so infants with latex allergy should not receive Rotarix. ACIP recommends that patients who are immunocompromised consult with an infectious disease specialist before administration of the rotavirus.

HUMAN PAPILLOMAVIRUS VACCINE

HPV is the most common sexually transmitted infection in the United States. An estimated 79 million Americans are currently infected with HPV, with an incidence of more than 14 million new cases per year. On the basis of present estimates, 75% to 80% of all sexually active people will become infected with HPV at some point during their lifetime.

Although the immune system eliminates the vast majority of HPV infections, in a minority of women persistent HPV infection may lead to the development of cervical cancer. HPV is thought to cause all cervical cancer, particularly types 16 and 18 are associated with 70% of cervical cancer.[72] Worldwide, cervical cancer causes a significant disease burden, with approximately 270,000 deaths each year. An estimated 12,820 women in the United States develop cervical cancer each year, with approximately 4200 deaths. Screening and treatment of cervical cancer are estimated to cost 6 billion annually in the United States. Prevention of HPV infection is difficult without changes in sexual behavior. Use of condoms has not been shown to be effective in eliminating transmission of the HPV virus.[72] A vaccine against high-risk HPV types could significantly reduce not only cervical cancer but also HPV-related cancers of the vulva, penis, and anus.

Three HPV vaccines have been developed. Gardasil (Merck) was approved by the FDA in 2006 for use in females aged 9 to 26 years and is designed to prevent HPV types 16 and 18—the leading vectors of cervical cancers—as well as HPV types 6 and 11, which are linked to roughly 90% of genital warts. One study showed the vaccine to be 89% effective in preventing infection with these viral strains and 100% effective in preventing cervical cancer, precancerous lesions, or genital warts.[73] However, the vaccine does not protect women against HPV strains with which they have already been infected before vaccination, nor is it designed to protect against less common HPV types. The second vaccine, Cervarix (GlaxoSmithKline), also protects against the two HPV strains that cause most cervical cancers. Cervarix has been shown to be 100% effective in preventing HPV strains 16 and 18; it is 100% effective for more than 4 years, according to data presented to the ACIP in 2006. The manufacturer applied for FDA approval in March 2007.

In the United States, the Gardasil-9 (Merck) is the only vaccine available. It targets HPV types 6, 11, 16, 18, 31, 33, 45, 52, and 58.

Indications

In March 2007, the ACIP published its recommendation for routine HPV vaccination for children aged 11 to 12 years. The ACIP recommendation also allows for vaccination beginning at age 9 years as well as catch-up vaccination of girls and women aged through 26 years and males through 21 years of age. Men aged 22 to 26 years may be vaccinated in special population. The vaccine should be administered before onset of sexual activity.

Routine and catch-up age groups. ACIP recommends routine HPV vaccination at age 11 or 12 years. Vaccination can be given starting at age 9 years. ACIP also recommends vaccination for females through age 26 years and for males through age 21 years who were not adequately vaccinated previously. Men aged 22 through 26 years may be vaccinated. (See Fig. 17.1: Special populations, Medical conditions.)

Dosing schedules. For persons initiating vaccination before their 15th birthday, the recommended immunization schedule is two doses of HPV vaccine. The second dose should be administered 6 to 12 months after the first dose (0, 6–12 mo schedule) (Fig. 17.1).

For persons initiating vaccination on or after their 15th birthday, the recommended immunization schedule is three doses of HPV vaccine. The second dose should be administered 1 to 2 months after the first dose, and the third dose should be administered 6 months after the first dose (0, 1–2, 6 mo schedule) (Fig. 17.1).

Administration

HPV vaccine (Gardasil-9 [Merck]) is available in single-dose vials (0.5 mL). It is administered intramuscularly in a two- or three-dose schedule. Persons vaccinated before their 15th birthday receive two doses 6 to 12 months apart. For persons 15 years and older, a three-dose schedule is recommended. The second and third doses should be administered 2 and 6 months after the first dose.

Adverse Effects

The most commonly reported side effects include pain, swelling, itching, and redness at the injection site. Fever, nausea, and dizziness have also been reported. Difficulty in breathing (bronchospasm) has been reported very rarely.

Precautions and Contraindications

See Table 17.1 for precautions and contraindications. Administration of HPV vaccine is not recommended during pregnancy but may be safely given to lactating mothers.

COMBINATION VACCINES

The Standards for Child and Adolescent Immunization Practices call for clinicians to administer simultaneously all vaccine doses for which a child is eligible at the time of each visit.[13,14] However, most parents and clinicians are concerned about the administration of multiple injections at a single visit and hesitate to administer more than two or three simultaneous injections. These factors have created a demand for new combination vaccines that include multiple unrelated antigens. Combination vaccines have certain practical benefits: they reduce the psychological burden of the parents and office staff brought about by the concern that the infant experiences greater pain when receiving multiple injections; they lead to more efficiency in the office setting by decreasing shipping, handling, and vial storage needs; less time is needed to prepare vaccines and document their administration; handling fewer syringes reduces the potential for accidental needle sticks; administration costs are reduced; and the immunization schedule is simplified, which may lead to increased adherence and fewer missed opportunities for vaccination.[13,14] For these reasons, the use of licensed combination vaccines is preferred over separate injection of their equivalent component vaccines.[13,14]

Some parents, in part influenced by antivaccination activism in the media and on the Internet, express concerns about the use of multiple antigens in a single injection. There is no scientific evidence to support such concerns.[13,14] Nonetheless, clinicians should be aware of these sentiments and should offer parents clear and concise information about the benefits of combination vaccines. Resources for counseling parents on vaccination can be accessed at https://www.cdc.gov/vaccines/parents/tools/parents-guide/parents-guide-part4.html.

Table 17.4 lists the currently available combination vaccines in the United States. This can significantly reduce the number of shots given by age 2 years.

IMMUNIZATIONS FOR TRAVELERS

Patients traveling to other countries may require special immunizations against endemic diseases and/or chemoprophylaxis against malaria and other diseases. Some countries require an International Certificate of Vaccination against yellow fever. Vaccination against hepatitis A and hepatitis B, meningococcal disease, Japanese encephalitis, polio, plague, rabies, or typhoid fever may be indicated for travelers to certain countries. Depending on their destination, patients may also require counseling about measures to protect themselves against exposure to mosquitoes and arthropod vectors, risks from water and food, swimming and animal-related hazards, traveler's diarrhea, and motion sickness.

TABLE 17.4 Currently Available Combination Vaccines in the United States

Vaccine	Trade Name	Abbreviation	Manufacturer	Type/Route	Approved	Comments
Adenovirus	Adenovirus type 4 & type 7		Barr Labs Inc.	Live viral/oral (tablets)	2011	Approved for military populations 17 through 50 yr
Anthrax	BioThrax	AVA	Emergent BioSolutions	Inactivated bacterial/IM	1970	Age range 18 through 65 yr
Cholera	Vaxchora		PaxVax	Live bacterial/oral	2016	Age range 18 through 64 yr
DTaP	Daptacel	DTaP	Sanofi	Inactivated toxoids and bacterial/IM	2002	Age range 6 wk through 6 yr
	Infanrix	DTaP	GlaxoSmithKline	Inactivated toxoids and bacterial/IM	1997	Age range 6 wk through 6 yr
DT	Generic	DT	Sanofi	Inactivated bacterial toxoids/IM	1978	Age range 6 mo through 6 yr
Haemophilus influenzae type b (Hib)	ActHIB	Hib (PRP-T)	Sanofi	Inactivated bacterial/IM	1993	3-dose primary series
	Hiberix	Hib (PRP-T)	GlaxoSmithKline	Inactivated bacterial/IM	2009	3-dose primary series
	PedvaxHIB	Hib (PRP-OMP)	Merck	Inactivated bacterial/IM	1989	2-dose primary series

(Continued)

TABLE 17.4 Currently Available Combination Vaccines in the United States (Continued)

Vaccine	Trade Name	Abbreviation	Manufacturer	Type/Route	Approved	Comments
Hepatitis A	Havrix	HepA	GlaxoSmithKline	Inactivated viral/IM	1995	Pediatric & adult formulations. Minimum age = 1 yr
	Vaqta	HepA	Merck	Inactivated viral/IM	1996	Pediatric & adult formulations. Minimum age = 1 yr
Hepatitis B	Engerix-B	HepB	GlaxoSmithKline	Recombinant viral/IM	1989	Pediatric & adult formulations. Minimum age = birth
	Recombivax HB	HepB	Merck	Recombinant viral/IM	1986	Pediatric & adult formulations. Minimum age = birth
Herpes Zoster (Shingles)	Zostavax	LZV	Merck	Live attenuated viral/SC	2006	One dose: Minimum age = 50 yr
	Shingrix	RZV	GlaxoSmithKline	Recombinant viral/IM	2017	Two doses: Minimum age = 50 yr
Human pap-illomavirus (HPV)	Gardasil 9	9vHPV	Merck	Inactivated viral/IM	2014	Approved for males and females 9 through 26 yr

Disease	Brand	Abbreviation	Manufacturer	Type/Route	Year	Notes
Influenza	Afluria	IIV3 IIV4	Seqirus	Inactivated viral/IM	2007 2016	Minimum age = 5 yr
	Fluad	IIV3	Seqirus	Inactivated viral/IM	2015	Adjuvented minimum age = 65 yr
	Fluarix	IIV4	GlaxoSmithKline	Inactivated viral/IM	2012	Minimum age = 3 yr
	Flublok	RIV3 RIV4	Protein Sciences Corp.	Recombinant viral/IM	2013	Egg free minimum age = 18 yr
	Flucelvax	ccIIV4	Seqirus	Cell-culture viral/IM	2016	Minimum age = 4 yr
	FluLaval	IIV4	GlaxoSmithKline	Inactivated viral/IM	2013	Minimum age = 6 mo
	FluMist	LAIV4	Medimmune	Live attenuated viral/intranasal (spray)	2003	Age range 2 through 49 yr
	Fluvirin	IIV3	Seqirus	Inactivated viral/IM	1988	Minimum age = 4 yr
	Fluzone	IIV3 IIV4	Sanofi	Inactivated viral/IM	1980 2013	Minimum age = 6 mo
	Fluzone High-Dose	IIV3	Sanofi	Inactivated viral/IM	2009	Minimum age = 65 yr
	Fluzone Intradermal	IIV4	Sanofi	Inactivated viral/Intradermal	2011	Age range 18 through 64 yr
Japanese encephalitis	Ixiaro	JE	Valneva	Inactivated viral/IM	2009	Minimum age = 2 mo

(Continued)

TABLE 17.4   Currently Available Combination Vaccines in the United States   (Continued)

Vaccine	Trade Name	Abbreviation	Manufacturer	Type/Route	Approved	Comments
Measles, mumps, rubella	M-M-R II	MMR	Merck	Live attenuated viral/ SC	1978 (First MMR, 1971)	Minimum age = 12 mo
Meningococcal	Menactra	MCV4 MenACWY	Sanofi	Inactivated bacterial/ IM	2005	Age range 9 mo through 55 yr
	Menveo	MCV4 MenACWY	GlaxoSmithKline	Inactivated bacterial/ IM	2010	Age range 2 mo through 55 yr
	Trumenba	MenB	Pfizer	Recombinant bacterial/ IM	2014	Age range 10 through 25 yr
	Bexsero	MenB	GlaxoSmithKline	Recombinant bacterial/ IM	2015	Age range 10 through 25 yr
Pneumococcal	Pneumovax 23	PPSV23	Merck	Inactivated bacterial/ SC or IM	1983	Minimum age = 2 yr
	Prevnar 13	PCV13	Pfizer	Inactivated bacterial/ IM	2010 (PCV7 – 2000)	Minimum age = 6 wk
Polio	Ipol	IPV	Sanofi	Inactivated viral/SC or IM	1990 (IPV-1955)	Minimum age = 6 wk
Rabies	Imovax Rabies		Sanofi	Inactivated viral/IM	1980	All ages
	RabAvert		GlaxoSmithKline	Inactivated viral/IM	1997	All ages

Rotavirus	RotaTeq	RV5	Merck	Live viral/oral (liquid)	2006	3-dose series 1st dose 6 through 14 wk 3rd dose max age 8 mo 0 d
	Rotarix	RV1	GlaxoSmithKline	Live viral/oral (liquid)	2008	2-dose series 1st dose 6 through 14 wk 2nd dose max age 8 mo 0 d
Tetanus, (reduced) diphtheria	Tenivac	Td	Sanofi	Inactivated bacterial toxoids/IM	2003	Minimum age 7 yr
	(Generic)	Td	Massachusetts Biological Labs	Inactivated bacterial toxoids/IM	1967	Minimum age 7 yr
Tetanus, (reduced) diphtheria, (reduced) pertussis	Boostrix	Tdap	GlaxoSmithKline	Inactivated bacterial/IM	2005	Age range 10 through 64 yr
	Adacel	Tdap	Sanofi	Inactivated bacterial/IM	2005	Age range 10 through 64 yr
Typhoid	Typhim Vi		Sanofi	Inactivated bacterial/IM	1994	Minimum age = 2 yr
	Vivotif		PaxVax	Live attenuated bacterial/oral (4 capsules)	1989	Minimum age = 6 yr
Varicella	Varivax	VAR	Merck	Live attenuated viral/SC	1995	Minimum age = 12 mo

(Continued)

TABLE 17.4   Currently Available Combination Vaccines in the United States   (Continued)

Vaccine	Trade Name	Abbreviation	Manufacturer	Type/Route	Approved	Comments
Vaccinia (smallpox)	ACAM2000		Sanofi	Live attenuated viral/percutaneous	2007	All ages
Yellow fever	YF-Vax	YF	Sanofi	Live attenuated viral/SC	1978	Minimum age = 9 mo
DTaP, polio	Kinrix	DTaP-IPV	GlaxoSmithKline	Inactivated bacterial & viral/IM	2008	Approved for 5th (DTaP) and 4th (IPV) booster at 4–6 yr
	Quadracel™	DTaP-IPV	Sanofi	Inactivated bacterial & viral/IM	2015	Approved for 5th (DTaP) and 4th (IPV) booster at 4–6 yr
DTaP, hepatitis B, polio	Pediarix	DTaP-HepB-IPV	GlaxoSmithKline	Inactivated bacterial & viral/IM	2002	Age range 6 mo through 6 yr

DTaP, polio, *Haemophilus influenzae* type b	Pentacel	DTaP-IPV/Hib	Sanofi	Inactivated bacterial & viral/IM	2008	Age range 6 mo through 4 yr
Hepatitis A, hepatitis B	Twinrix	HepA-HepB	GlaxoSmithKline	Inactivated/recombinant Viral/IM	2001	Pediatric HepA + adult HepB minimum age = 18 yr
Measles, mumps, rubella, varicella	ProQuad	MMRV	Merck	Live attenuated viral/SC	2005	Age range 1 through 12 yr

The abbreviations in this table (Column 3) were standardized jointly by staff of the Centers for Disease Control and Prevention, ACIP Work Groups, the editor of the *Morbidity and Mortality Weekly Report* (*MMWR*), the editor of *Epidemiology and Prevention of Vaccine-Preventable Diseases* (the *Pink Book*), ACIP members, and liaison organizations to the ACIP.

These abbreviations are intended to provide a uniform approach to vaccine references used in ACIP Recommendations and Policy Notes published in the *MMWR*, the *Pink Book*, and the American Academy of Pediatrics *Red Book*, and in the U.S. immunization schedules for children, adolescents, and adults.

In descriptions of combination vaccines, dash (-) indicates products in which the active components are supplied in their final (combined) form by the manufacturer; slash (/) indicates: products in which active components must be mixed by the user.

Clinicians who are unfamiliar with current recommendations for travel to specific countries can consult the CDC's *Traveler's Health* website at https://wwwnc.cdc.gov/travel/, which is updated continuously. Not all clinicians have access to all travel vaccines. Clinicians can refer patients to community referral resources, such as local public health departments, many of which operate travel medicine clinics, other health care facilities in the community offering immunization services for international travelers, and local infectious disease specialists with expertise in travel medicine.

OTHER IMMUNIZATIONS

Rabies infection is spread by contact with the saliva of infected animals. Worldwide, an estimated 35,000 to 50,000 human deaths from rabies occur every year. Before 1960, most of the U.S. cases occurred in domestic animals; at present, more than 90% of all animal cases reported annually occur in wildlife. Raccoons continue to be the most frequently reported rabid wildlife species (37.2% of all animal cases during 2001), followed by skunks (30.7%), bats (17.2%), foxes (5.9%), and other wild animals, including rodents and lagomorphs (0.7%). The number of rabies-related human deaths in the United States has declined from more than 100 annually at the turn of the century to one to two per year in the 1990s. Modern day prophylaxis has proved approximately 100% successful. Rabies vaccination is indicated as preexposure prophylaxis for persons whose occupations, travel, or recreational activities expose them to potentially rabid animals, and (along with human rabies immune globulin) as postexposure prophylaxis following certain bite wounds.

Tetanus prophylaxis with tetanus immune globulin and/or toxoid is indicated in certain patients with wounds that are potentially contaminated with tetanus spores (see Table 17.5). Travelers to areas where postexposure tetanus immunization might be unavailable should consider receiving a booster dose of Td or Tdap before departure if five or more years have elapsed since their last vaccination. Measles, mumps, and rubella are still common throughout the world; travelers without evidence of adequate immunity should receive boosters (see "Suggested Readings" for guidance on MMR requirements for international travelers). The Bacille Calmette-Guérin vaccine is a live antituberculosis vaccine used in more than 100 countries throughout the world, primarily to prevent serious disease from *Mycobacterium tuberculosis*. It is more than 80% effective in protecting against meningeal and miliary tuberculosis in children. It is recommended in the United States only for certain children and health care workers in certain high-risk settings.[74] It is not recommended for HIV patients.

TABLE 17.5 Tetanus Wound Management

Vaccination history	Clean, Minor Wounds		All Other Wounds[a]	
	Tdap or Td[b]	TIG	Tdap or Td[b]	TIG
Unknown or fewer than 3 doses	Yes	No	Yes	Yes
3 or more doses	No[c]	No	No[d]	No

[a]Such as, but not limited to, wounds contaminated with dirt, feces, soil, and saliva; puncture wounds; avulsions; and wounds resulting from missiles, crushing, burns, and frostbite.
[b]Tdap is preferred to Td for adults who have never received Tdap. Single antigen tetanus toxoid (TT) is no longer available in the United States.
[c]Yes, if more than 10 years since the last tetanus toxoid-containing vaccine dose.
[d]Yes, if more than 5 years since the last tetanus toxoid-containing vaccine dose.
Centers for Disease Control and Prevention. Tetanus. In: Hamborsky J, Kroger A, Wolfe S, eds. *Epidemiology and Prevention of Vaccine-Preventable Diseases*. 13th ed. Washington DC: Public Health Foundation; 2015.

OFFICE AND CLINIC ORGANIZATION

In spite of many advances in vaccine delivery, many national goals for universal immunization have not been reached. For clinicians, a number of organizational and logistical issues can interfere with adequate delivery of vaccination services. In response to this problem, Standards for Child and Adolescent Immunization Practices (SCAIP)[75] and objectives for adult immunization[76] have been issued by the National Vaccine Advisory Committee (see "Suggested Readings"). These standards suggest organizational practices to help clinicians ensure timely and comprehensive immunization of all appropriate patients. The SCAIP has been endorsed by the AAP, AAFP, American Medical Association, and 40 other health-related organizations. Although these recommendations were developed to improve the delivery of childhood and adolescent immunizations, the same office procedures can also enhance the delivery of adult immunizations. Many SCAIP recommendations are cited in the following discussion:

- **Vaccine product management.** Office or clinic procedures for handling and storage of vaccines should be designed to comply with the recommendations in the manufacturer's package inserts. The SCAIP recommends daily monitoring of the temperature at which vaccines are stored and the expiration date of each vaccine. CDC-recommended storage and handling procedures are available at http://www.cdc.gov/vaccines/recs/storage/default.htm.

- **Use of appropriate contraindications.** Systems should be in place to ensure that parents are asked routinely about adverse events following prior immunizations and proper precautions or contraindications are considered before administering any vaccine (Table 17.1). The SCAIP recommends posting up-to-date immunization protocols at all locations where vaccines are administered. Vaccines should be administered only by individuals with proper training and/or supervision.
- **Maintenance of vaccination records.** SCAIP recommends that vaccination records be "accurate, complete, and easily accessible." Vaccination records should be recorded on a standard form or flow sheet in the medical record to help the clinician quickly determine whether the patient's immunizations are up to date. Unfortunately, clinicians may be faced with incomplete or confusing immunization records because many patients change clinicians often as their health insurance coverage changes. Patient-held records, or immunization cards, can be helpful, but these may be unavailable or incomplete.

A key plan to ensure the availability and completeness of the immunization record is the use of immunization registries. Immunization registries are confidential, computerized information systems that collect vaccination data from multiple clinicians, generate reminder and recall notifications, and assess vaccination coverage within a defined geographic area.[75,76] A registry with added capabilities, such as vaccine management, adverse event reporting, lifespan vaccination histories, and linkages with electronic data sources, is called an immunization information system. State registries receive funding under section 317b of the Public Health Service Act. Among the many benefits of such systems are consolidation of immunization records from many clinicians into one central location that can be accessed on demand by parents or clinicians; identification of due or overdue immunizations and generation of reminder notices; and the use of advanced centralized computer support to help clinicians determine needed immunizations at routine and catch-up visits, as well as to facilitate the integration of new vaccines into the recommended schedules.[75,76]

The widespread use of electronic billing systems and electronic health records (EHRs) will not necessarily improve completeness of the vaccination record. A study of clinicians who submitted immunization data electronically from computerized billing records to an immunization registry in Philadelphia found that almost a fourth of the immunizations given were not submitted. At their present stage, EHRs do not use a standard format that allows communication with other EHR systems and do not uniformly offer immunization decision support. Furthermore, frequent updates in ACIP recommendations are unlikely to be distributed throughout the many proprietary EHR systems in a timely manner. An AAP task force recommended that "the ability [of EHRs] to flexibly format immunization data and support electronic data interchange with registries is vital." Enhanced data exchange between EHRs and state registries would greatly increase the likelihood that immunization records would be accurate and available when needed.

SCAIP recommends that all administered vaccinations should be reported to state or local immunization registries, where available, to ensure that each patient's vaccination history remains accurate and complete. More information about vaccine registries can be found at the National Immunization Program website at http://www.cdc.gov/vaccines/programs/iis/default.htm.

- **Reminder systems.** Reminder systems can be helpful in ensuring that children return on time for their next immunization. Manual or automated systems can be used to trigger postcard, letter, or telephone reminders for parents to schedule their next vaccination appointment. Reminders, incorporated into EHRs, could also notify clinicians about overdue immunizations during acute care visits.
- **Medical record documentation.** Physicians are required by statute to record the following information about childhood immunizations: name of vaccine, date of administration, manufacturer, lot number, signature and title of person administering the vaccine, and address where the vaccine was given. Adverse reactions to immunizations should be described in detail in the medical record. Vaccine refusal should also be documented.

For vaccines requiring a VIS, the clinician should document which VIS was given, its date of publication, and the date the VIS was given. There is no federal requirement for written informed consent for vaccinations, and VISs are not informed consent documents, but some states do have such requirements. In such cases the clinician should have the recipients or their parents (or legal representatives) sign a separate "informed consent" form.

According to SCAIP, clinicians should be aware of and report selected adverse events occurring after vaccination through the Vaccine Adverse Event Reporting System, a national vaccine safety surveillance program operated by the CDC and FDA. The National Childhood Vaccine Injury Act requires clinicians to report any event listed by the vaccine manufacturer as a contraindication to subsequent doses of the vaccine and any event listed in the Reportable Events Table that occurs within a certain period after vaccination. Reportable events, which are specified, are generally those that require the patient to seek medical attention. Vaccines listed in the Reportable Events Table are tetanus in any combination; pertussis in any combination; measles, mumps, and rubella in any combination; rubella in any combination; measles in any combination; OPV; IPV; hepatitis A;

hepatitis B; Hib conjugate; varicella; rotavirus; pneumococcal conjugate; and influenza vaccines. Report forms and assistance can be obtained by calling 1-800-822-7967. Report forms can be downloaded from http://vaers.hhs.gov/pubs.htm. The Reportable Events Table can be viewed or downloaded from http://vaers.hhs.gov/reportable.htm.

SCAIP also recommends that clinicians should be familiar with the National Vaccine Injury Compensation Program. This is a no-fault, federally funded system designed to compensate persons who may have been injured by childhood vaccines. Any new vaccine recommended by the CDC for routine administration to children is covered. Vaccines currently covered under this program are DTP, DTaP, DT, tetanus toxoid, Tdap, Td, MMR or its components, OPV, IPV, hepatitis A, hepatitis B, Hib, varicella, rotavirus, trivalent inactivated influenza vaccine, and live attenuated influenza vaccine, whether administered individually or in combination. Information about the Vaccine Injury Compensation Program can be obtained online at http://www.hrsa.gov/vaccinecompensation/or by calling 1-800-338-2382. It should be noted that this program is separate from the Vaccine Adverse Event Reporting System; a claim initiated in the former does not automatically generate an adverse event report, or vice versa.

Minimization of vaccine costs for children. Charges for vaccinations have become a major barrier to immunizations, especially among poor parents. The SCAIP recommends that patient costs should be kept as low as possible, and that "no child or adolescent should be denied vaccination because of inability to pay." One of the main publicly funded sources of low-cost vaccinations is the VFC Program. This is an entitlement program for children up to age 18 years, started in 1994 and paid for by federal funding, which supplies vaccines free of charge to participating clinicians. VFC is administered by the CDC, which contracts with vaccine manufacturers to buy vaccines at reduced rates and then distributes them to VFC providers. Children are eligible for VFC vaccines if they

- are 18 years or younger
- are eligible for Medicaid
- have no health insurance
- are Native American or Alaskan Native
- have health insurance that does not cover immunizations. In these cases, children must go to a federally qualified health center or rural health clinic for immunizations.

Further information about the VFC program can be obtained at http://www.cdc.gov/vaccines/programs/vfc/default.htm or by calling the CDC at 1-800-CDC-INFO (1-800-232-4636) (TTY [hearing impaired]: 1-888-232-6348).

Some companies also offer patient assistance programs for certain individuals who cannot afford the vaccine and lack medical coverage (Merck for all adult vaccines, e.g., HPV vaccine, Zostavax, Pneumovax 23;

Sanofi Pasteur for rabies vaccine/immune globulin and meningococcal polysaccharide vaccine).

The SCAIP includes other recommendations that may help improve immunization practices but that, although often difficult, can be important for clinicians to implement. These include regular chart reviews to assess the effectiveness of vaccination coverage; working with other community organizations such as public health departments, health plans, and other clinicians to determine local needs and develop community vaccination programs; and allowing sufficient time during each visit to discuss with parents (or guardians) and adolescent patients the benefits and risks of vaccines in a culturally appropriate and easy-to-understand manner.

SUGGESTED RESOURCES AND MATERIALS

Vaccine Information Statements are available online at:
https://www.cdc.gov/vaccines/hcp/vis/index.html and

Immunization Action Coalition web site at:
http://www.immunize.org/vis/

National Immunization Program Publications: Immunization Educational and Training Materials.
https://www.cdc.gov/vaccines/ed/courses.htmlImmunization Action Coalition has a collection of free print materials.

REFERENCES

1. Esposito S, Principi N, Cornaglia G. Barriers to the vaccination of children and adolescents and possible solutions. *Clin Microbiol Infect.* 2014;20(suppl. 5):25-31.
2. Gingold JA, Briccetti C, Zook K, et al. Context matters: practitioner perspective on immunization delivery quality improvement efforts. *Clin Pediatr.* 2016;55(9):825-837.
3. Advisory Committee on Immunization Practices. Altered immunocompetence. https://www.cdc.gov/vaccines/hcp/acip-recs/general-recs/immunocompetence.html. Updated 21 February 2018. Accessed 21 March 2018.
4. Zimmerman RK, Giebink GS. Childhood immunizations: a practical approach for clinicians. *Am Fam Physician.* 1992;45(4):1759-1772.
5. Centers for Disease Control and Prevention. Benefits from immunization during the vaccines for children program era – United States, 1994–2013. *MMWR Morb Mortal Wkly Rep.* 2014;63(16):352-355.
6. Healthy People 2020. Washington, DC: U.S. Department of Health and Human Services, Office of Disease Prevention and Health Promotion. https://www.healthypeople.gov/node/4722/data_details#revision_history_header. Accessed 2 April 2018.
7. Hill HA, Elam-Evans LD, Yankey D, et al. Vaccination coverage among children aged 19-35 months – United States, 2015. *MMWR.* 2016;65(39):1065-1071.
8. Kim DK, Bridges CB, Harriman KH. Advisory committee on immunization practices recommended immunization schedule for adults aged 19 years or older—United States, 2015. *MMWR.* 2015;64(4):91-92.
9. Régnier SA, Huels J. Drug versus vaccine investment: a modelled comparison of economic incentives. *Cost Eff Resour Alloc.* 2013;11:23. doi:10.1186/1478-7547-11-23.

10. Philipson TJ, Thornton SJ, Chit A, et al. The social value of childhood vaccination in the United States. *Am J Manag Care.* 2017;23(1):41-47.
11. Zweigoron RT, Roberts JR, Levin M, et al. Influence of office systems on pediatrics vaccination rates. *Clin Pediatr.* 2017;56(3):231-237.
12. Wong CA, Taylor JA, Wright JA, et al. Missed opportunities for adolescent vaccination, 2006–2011. *J Adolesc Health.* 2013;53(4):492-497.
13. American Academy of Pediatrics. *Redbook 2015 Report of the Committee of Infectious Diseases.* 30th ed. Elk Grove Village, IL: American Academy of Pediatrics; 2015.
14. Centers for Disease Control and Prevention. General recommendations on immunizations. In: Hamborsky J, Kroger A, Wolfe S, eds. *Epidemiology and Prevention of Vaccine-preventable Diseases.* 13th ed. Washington, DC: Public Health Foundation; 2015:9-31.
15. Grohskopf LA, Sokolow LZ, Broder KR, et al. Prevention and control of seasonal influenza with vaccines: recommendations of the advisory committee on immunization practices – United States, 2017–18 influenza season. *MMWR.* 2017;66(RR-2):1-20. doi:10.15585/mmwr.rr6602a1.
16. Centers for Disease Control and Prevention. Measles. In: Hamborsky J, Kroger A, Wolfe S, eds. *Epidemiology and Prevention of Vaccine-preventable Diseases.* 13th ed. Washington, DC: Public Health Foundation; 2015.
17. Hurley AM, Tadrous M, Miller ES. Thimerosal-containing vaccines and autism: a review of recent epidemiologic studies. *J Pediatr Pharmacol Ther.* 2010;15(3):173-181.
18. Stratton K, Gable A, McCormick MC, et al. *Immunization Safety Review: Thimerosal-Containing Vaccines and Neuro-Developmental Disorders.* Washington, DC: National Academy Press; 2001.
19. Gellin BG, Maibach EW, Marcuse EK. Do parents understand immunizations? A national telephone survey. *Pediatrics.* 2000;106(5):1097-1102.
20. Diekema DS, Committee of Bioethics. Reaffirmation: responding to parental refusals of immunization of children. *Pediatrics.* 2013;131(5):e1696.
21. Flanagan-Klygis EA, Sharp L, Frader JE. Dismissing the family who refuses vaccines: a study of pediatrician attitudes. *Arch Pediatr Adolesc Med.* 2005;159(10):929-934.
22. Barraza L, Schmit C, Hoss A. The latest in vaccine policies: selected issue in school vaccinations, healthcare workers vaccinations, and pharmacist vaccination authority laws. *J Law Med Ethics.* 2017;16-19.
23. Feikin DR, Lezotte DC, Hamman RF, et al. Individual and community risks of measles and pertussis associated with personal exemptions to immunization. *JAMA.* 2000;284(24):3145-3150.
24. Kimmel SR, Wolfe RM. Communicating the benefits and risks of vaccines. *J Fam Practice.* 2005;54:S51-S57.
25. Edwards KM, Hackell JM, Committee of Infectious Diseases, et al. Countering vaccine hesitancy. *Pediatrics.* 2016;138(3):e20162146.
26. Centers for Disease Control and Prevention. Diphtheria 2016. https://www.cdc.gov/diphtheria/. Updated 15 January 2016. Accessed 12 April 2018.
27. Centers for Disease Control and Prevention. Tetanus 2017. https://www.cdc.gov/tetanus/clinicians.html. Updated 1 September 2017. Accessed 21 March 2018.
28. Centers for Disease Control and Prevention. Pertussis 2016. https://www.cdc.gov/pertussis/about/index.html. Updated 7 April 2017. Accessed 21 March 2018.
29. Parker JL, Conner RS. Advocating for childcare employee single-dose Tdap vaccination to combat infant pertussis. *J Pediatr Health Care.* 2017;31(2):241-245.
30. Wendelhoe AM, Njamkepo E, Bourillon A, et al, Transmission of *Bordetella pertussis* to young infants. *Pediatr Infect Dis J.* 2007;26(4):293-299.
31. Ward JI, Cherry JD, Chang S-J, et al. Efficacy of an acellular pertussis vaccine among adolescents and adults. *N Engl J Med.* 2005;353(15):1555-1563.

32. Centers for Disease Control and Prevention. Tetanus. In: Hamborsky J, Kroger A, Wolfe S, eds. *Epidemiology and Prevention of Vaccine-preventable Diseases.* 13th ed. Washington, DC: Public Health Foundation; 2015.
33. World Health Organization. Measles Fact Sheet. http://www.who.int/mediacentre/factsheets/fs286/en/. Updated January 2018. Accessed 28 March 2018.
34. Centers for Disease Control and Prevention. Measles. https://www.cdc.gov/measles/stats-surv.html. Updated 5 February 2018. Accessed 28 March 2018.
35. Centers for Disease Control and Prevention. Mumps epidemic-Iowa, 2006. *MMWR Morb Mortal Wkly Rep.* 2006;55(13):366-368.
36. Marin M, Marlow M, Moore KL, et al. Recommendation of the advisory committee on immunization practices for use of a third dose of mumps virus–Containing vaccine in persons at increased risk for mumps during an outbreak. *MMWR Morb Mortal Wkly Rep.* 2018;67:33-38. doi:10.15585/mmwr.mm6701a7.
37. Centers for Disease Control and Prevention. Prevention of measles, rubella, congenital rubella syndrome, and mumps, 2013, Summary recommendations of the advisory committee on immunization practices. *MMWR.* 2013;62(RR-4):1-34.
38. Klein NP, Fireman BW, Yih WK, et al. Measles-mumps-rubella-varicella combination vaccine and the risk of febrile seizures *Pediatrics.* 2010;126(1):e1-e8.
39. Rubin L, Levin M, Ljungman P, et al. 2013 IDSA clinical practice guideline for vaccination of the immunocompromised host. *Clin Infect Dis.* 2014;58(3):e44-e100.
40. Centers for Disease Control and Prevention. Altered immunocompetence general best practice guidelines for immunization: Best practices guidance of the advisory committee on immunization practices. https://www.cdc.gov/vaccines/hcp/acip-recs/general-recs/immunocompetence.pdf. Updated 21 February 2018. Accessed 30 March 2018.
41. World Health Organization. Polio. http://www.who.int/mediacentre/factsheets/fs114/en/. Updated March 2018. Accessed 30 March 2018.
42. Centers for Disease Control and Prevention. Polio. In: Hamborsky J, Kroger A, Wolfe S, eds. *Epidemiology and Prevention of Vaccine-preventable Diseases.* 13th ed. Washington, DC: Public Health Foundation; 2015.
43. World Health Organization. Haemophilus influenzae type b (Hib) 2009. http://www.who.int/immunization/topics/hib/en/. Updated 19 August 2009. Accessed 30 March 2018.
44. Centers for Disease Control and Prevention. *Haemophilus influenzae type* b In: Hamborsky J, Kroger A, Wolfe S, eds. *Epidemiology and Prevention of Vaccine-preventable Diseases.* 13th ed. Washington, DC: Public Health Foundation; 2015.
45. World Health Organization. Haemophilus influenzae type b (Hib) vaccination position paper – July 2013. *Wkly Epidemiol Rec.* 2013;88(39):413-426.
46. Centers for Disease Control and Prevention. Prevention of pneumococcal disease: recommendations of the advisory committee on immunization practices (ACIP). *MMWR Recomm Rep.* 1997;46(RR-8):1-24.
47. Moore MR, Link-Gelles R, Schaffner W, et al. Effectiveness of 13-valent pneumococcal conjugate vaccine for prevention of invasive pneumococcal disease in children in the USA: a matched case-control study. *Lancet Resp Med.* 2016;4(5):399-406.
48. Pilishvile T, Bennett NM. Pneumococcal disease prevention among adults: strategies for the use of pneumococcal vaccines. *Vaccine.* 2015;33(suppl 4);d60-65.
49. Advisory Committee on Immunization Practices. Use of PCV-13 and PPSV-23 vaccine among children aged 6-18 years with immunocompromising conditions. *MMWR.* 2013;62(25);521-524.
50. Centers for Disease Control and Prevention. Pneumococcal. In: Hamborsky J, Kroger A, Wolfe S, eds. *Epidemiology and Prevention of Vaccine-preventable Diseases.* 13th ed. Washington, DC: Public Health Foundation; 2015.

51. Centers for Disease Control and Prevention. Meningococcal. In: Hamborsky J, Kroger A, Wolfe S, eds. *Epidemiology and Prevention of Vaccine-preventable Diseases.* 13th ed. Washington, DC: Public Health Foundation; 2015.

52. Centers for Disease Control and Prevention. Meningococcal Disease Surveillance. https://www.cdc.gov/meningococcal/surveillance/index.html. Updated 2 February 2018. Accessed 3 April 2018.

53. Centers for Disease Control and Prevention. Update: Guillain-Barre syndrome among recipients of Menactra meningococcal conjugate vaccine-United States, June 2005–September 2006. *MMWR Morb Mortal Wkly Rep.* 2006;55(41):1120-1124.

54. Gardner P. Clinical practice. Prevention of meningococcal disease. *N Engl J Med.* 2006;355(14):1466-1473.

55. Centers for Disease Control and Prevention. Hepatitis B. https://www.cdc.gov/hepatitis/hbv/hbvfaq.htm#overview. Updated 11 January 2018. Accessed 10 April 2018.

56. Centers for Disease Control and Prevention. Hepatitis B. In: Hamborsky J, Kroger A, Wolfe S, eds. *Epidemiology and Prevention of Vaccine-preventable Diseases.* 13th ed. Washington, DC: Public Health Foundation; 2015.

57. Abara WE, Qaseem A, Schillie S, High Value Care Task Force of the American College of P, et al. Hepatitis B vaccination, screening, and linkage to care: Best practice advice from the American College of Physicians and the Centers for Disease Control and Prevention. *Ann Intern Med.* 2017;167(11):794-804.

58. Centers for Disease Control and Prevention. Viral Hepatitis Surveillance in US-2015. https://www.cdc.gov/hepatitis/statistics/2015surveillance/pdfs/2015HepSurveillanceRpt.pdf. Accessed 30 March 2018.

59. Centers for Disease Control and Prevention. Hepatitis A. In: Hamborsky J, Kroger A, Wolfe S, eds. *Epidemiology and Prevention of Vaccine-preventable Diseases.* 13th ed. Washington, DC: Public Health Foundation; 2015.

60. Centers for Disease Control and Prevention. Key Facts about Influenza 2017. https://www.cdc.gov/flu/keyfacts.htm. Updated 3 October 2017. Assessed 1 March 2018.

61. Shang M, Blanton L, Brammer L, et al. Influenza-associated pediatric deaths in the United States, 2010–2016. *Pediatrics.* 2018;141(4);1-9.

62. Centers for Disease Control and Prevention. Weekly US Influenza Surveillance Report. https://www.cdc.gov/flu/weekly/. Updated 6 April 2018. Assessed 7 April 2018.

63. Centers for Disease Control and Prevention. About Flu. https://www.cdc.gov/flu/about/index.html. Updated 3 October 2017. Assessed 1 March 2018.

64. American Academy of Pediatrics, Committee of Infectious Diseases. Recommendation for prevention and control of influenza in children, 2017–2018. *Pediatrics.* 2017;140(40);1-20.

65. Centers for Disease Control and Prevention. Influenza Antiviral Medications: Summary for Clinicians. https://www.cdc.gov/flu/professionals/antivirals/summary-clinicians.htm. Updated 23 February 2018. Assessed 10 March 2018.

66. Centers for Disease Control and Prevention. Varicella. In: Hamborsky J, Kroger A, Wolfe S, eds. *Epidemiology and Prevention of Vaccine-preventable Diseases.* 13th ed. Washington, DC: Public Health Foundation; 2015.

67. Gershon AA. Is chickenpox so bad, what do we know about immunity to varicella zoster virus, and what does it tell us about the future? *J Infection.* 2017;74(suppl 1);s27–s33.

68. Centers for Disease Control and Prevention. Herpes zoster. https://www.cdc.gov/shingles/hcp/index.html. Updated 17 October 2017. Assessed 12 March 2018.

69. Centers for Disease Control and Prevention. Rotavirus. In: Hamborsky J, Kroger A, Wolfe S, eds. *Epidemiology and Prevention of Vaccine-preventable Diseases.* 13th ed. Washington, DC: Public Health Foundation; 2015.

70. Vesikari T, Matson DO, Dennehy P, et al. Safety and efficacy of a pentavalent human-bovine (WC3) reassortant rotavirus vaccine. *N Engl J Med.* 2006;354(1):23-33.

71. Ruiz-Palacios GM, Perez-Schael I, Velazquez FR, et al. Safety and efficacy of an attenuated vaccine against severe rotavirus gastroenteritis. *N Engl J Med.* 2006;354(1):11-22.

72. Centers for Disease Control and Prevention. Human papillomavirus. In: Hamborsky J, Kroger A, Wolfe S, eds. *Epidemiology and Prevention of Vaccine-Preventable Diseases.* 13th ed. Washington, DC: Public Health Foundation; 2015.

73. Villa LL, Costa RL, Petta CA, et al. Prophylactic quadrivalent human papillomavirus (types 6, 11, 16, and 18) L1 virus-like particle vaccine in young women: a randomised double-blind placebo-controlled multicentre phase II efficacy trial. *Lancet Oncol.* 2005;6(5):271-278.

74. Centers for Disease Control and Prevention. BCG Vaccine. https://www.cdc.gov/tb/publications/factsheets/prevention/bcg.htm. Updated 12 September 2016. Assessed 12 March 2018.

75. National Vaccine Advisory Committee. Standards for child and adolescent immunization practices. *Pediatrics.* 2003;112(4):958-963.

76. National Vaccine Advisory Committee. A pathway to leadership for adult immunization: recommendations of the national vaccine advisory committee. *Public Health Rep.* 2012;127(suppl 1); 1-42.

Please see Online Appendix: Apps and Digital Resources for additional information.

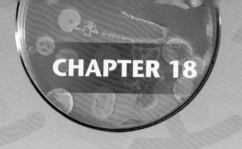

CHAPTER 18

Health Promotion and Disease Prevention for Children and Adolescents

NANCY C. BANASIAK | ALISON MORIARTY DALEY

BACKGROUND

Primary care providers deliver the foundation of care to pediatric patients with the goal of promotion of health and disease prevention. Social determinants of health as defined by the World Health Organization is "The conditions in which people are born, grow, live, work and age. These circumstances are shaped by the distribution of money, power and resources at global, national and local levels."[1] Given the limited time and other resources, how can a clinician best promote optimal growth and development of a child and support the family and community that surround the child? This chapter briefly reviews health promotion and disease prevention in children, focusing on the ways it may differ from that in adults and on the specific interventions that are reasonably well supported by research evidence. In addition, the chapter offers a special focus on two special populations of children: newborns and adolescents.

Early in the 20th century well child care made its appearance in the form of public child health fairs (sometimes called milk fairs) and free-standing, publicly supported well baby clinics run mostly by women pediatricians and public health nurses. Starting in the 1920s, political action on the part of the American Medical Association to prevent what it viewed as a socialist scheme, as well as the recognition by academic pediatricians of the importance of care of the well child, resulted in the movement of well child care to private physicians.[2] By the 1950s, well child care was firmly established as a part of primary care in the United States.

The content of well child visits has changed significantly since the days of clean milk and immunization fairs. Infectious diseases and premature birth are no longer the primary causes of morbidity and mortality in children; ill health related to environmental and social problems has become the "new morbidities"[3] of childhood and adolescence. Childhood obesity, diabetes, asthma, injuries, mental illness, and behavioral disorders may be devastating to children and have lifelong implications for children and their families, as affected children become adults whose potential contributions to society are impaired by chronic disease.

Current views about the important outcomes of child health have evolved from the prevention of specific conditions to a broader view based on the concept of healthy development across the life span.[4] The Children's Health, the Nation's Wealth report defines health as follows:

> "Children's health should be defined as the extent to which individual children or groups of children are able or enabled to (a) develop and realize their potential, (b) satisfy their needs, and (c) develop the capacities that allow them to interact successfully with their biological, physical, and social environments."[4]

Each child has an optimal developmental trajectory that is subject to both upward and downward pressure, so that small changes in the trajectory at an early age may result in very large differences in outcomes at a later age (see Fig. 18.1). What have traditionally been called risk factors *threaten* the child's health and development. Other factors can be identified that *promote* optimal health and development. The former should be identified and mitigated, and the latter should be identified and supported. Unfortunately, one of the most important stressors children experience is associated with living in poverty.[5]

Helping Families With Limited Resources

For disadvantaged families, paying for preventive health care may take a back seat to meeting other expenses. After early infancy, parents may dispense with preventive visits except to obtain required interventions such as the immunizations required for school attendance and mandatory sports or camp physicals. The negative effects of this situation can be mitigated if prevention is incorporated into every health care visit, no matter what the presenting complaint. These "opportunistic" discussions should focus on expressed parental concerns, issues noted on the physical examination, and the most common threats to the child's health at that age.

This chapter reviews the approach to the well child visit in children and adolescents in the order suggested by the "real-time" sequence of that visit: from taking the history through the physical examination and appropriate laboratory or other screening tests, to the provision of immunizations and the delivery of anticipatory guidance to the child and family. The end of the chapter gives special consideration to newborns and adolescent populations.

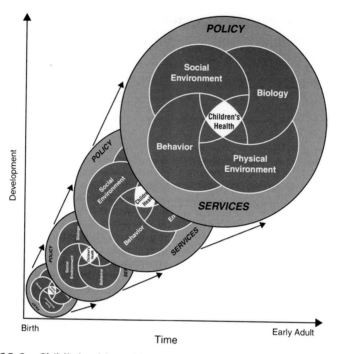

Figure 18.1   Child's health and its influences. From the National Research Council and Institute of Medicine. *Committee on Evaluation of Children's Health. Children's Health, the Nation's Wealth: Assessing and Improving Child Health.* Washington, DC: National Academies Press; 2004.

GENERAL CONSIDERATIONS

The Maternal and Child Health Bureau granted the American Academy of Pediatrics (AAP) to lead the third edition of the Bright Futures initiative. The initiative was to address the needs of all children, promoting health, preventing disease, providing anticipatory guidance for patients and families, and recommending appropriate screening. Figure 18.2 lists the recommendations for preventive health care developed by the AAP and Bright Future.[6] The optimal number and frequency of scheduled child health maintenance visits has not yet been fully determined. Many agencies, including state Medicaid programs and private insurance companies, mandate both the visit schedule and specific health interventions and screenings by age and often link provider reimbursement to documentation of these services. More frequent visits are appropriate during periods of rapid growth and development, such as infancy and adolescence, than during the relative stability of middle childhood. However, it is important

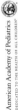

Figure 18.2 Recommendations for Preventive Pediatric Health Care. From the American Academy of Pediatrics.

to carefully tailor both the schedule and the visit to the individual child and family and to avoid a one-size-fits-all approach. The evidence base is somewhat slim for much of what is routine in well child care. Discussion with families and patients regarding what we know and what we do not know about preventive health care in children, in the context of shared decision making, will be best when the balance of benefits and harms is either unknown or close (see discussion of "Shared Decision Making" in Chapter 22).

CONTENT OF THE WELL CHILD VISIT

The well child visit is aimed at disease detection and prevention, along with health promotion and anticipatory guidance. The history and physical examination and selected screening tests are intended to detect existing conditions and risk factors for disease. Health promotion and anticipatory guidance are intended to prevent future illness and injury and to optimize development.

Pediatric History Taking

Every family arrives at the well child visit with an agenda—sometimes quite a long one. Determining what is on this agenda is essential to successfully engage both the patient and the family in the health supervision process. The concerns of the family can then be integrated with the clinician's agenda for health supervision so that a shared agenda guides the visit and so that both patient/family and clinician will be satisfied that the goals of the visit have been met.

Much like the taking of the history discussed in Chapter 3, the history taken during a well child visit is geared to discovering current problems and potential threats to the child's health, including inherited conditions, environmental risks, and psychosocial risks. As noted in Chapter 3, printed or online questionnaires, which can be completed before arriving for the visit or in the waiting room, are useful to obtain the new patient's medical history, family history, and social history as well as information about nutrition, diet, school performance, psychosocial adjustment, and health concerns. Examples of questionnaires designed for use with children are listed in the "Suggested Readings" at the end of this chapter.

A targeted pediatric history requires special attention to birth and perinatal history, childhood immunizations, developmental and school history, and a family history tailored to childhood-onset illnesses, such as asthma, seizure disorders, learning disabilities, cardiovascular disease, hypertension, and diabetes. Clinicians using a "waiting room questionnaire" should be mindful of the literacy rates and relevant language or cultural barriers of their patient populations and should be prepared to review the questionnaire during the visit.

Some questionnaires (e.g., Vanderbilt scale for attention deficit hyperactivity disorder; see "Suggested Readings") have been developed to aid in screening for specific health risk behaviors, developmental status, and behavioral issues when they are identified as concerns during the course of the patient encounter. Others are considered a part of the standard assessment of a child and include lists of developmental "milestones" (such as the Modified Checklist for Autism in Toddlers for autism screening) and risk factors for tuberculosis (TB) exposure, environmental lead exposure, and the like. Alternatively, the interview with the family may be used by the clinician to evaluate these risks. The clinician should be alert for high-risk situations, such as the child's exposure to incarcerated persons (for which TB testing may be indicated), or substandard living conditions or diet, in which screening for lead toxicity or anemia, respectively, may be indicated.

The Physical Examination

The physical examination at each well child visit is an important part of each well child visit. It is an opportunity for clinicians to reassure and teach the parents as they examine the child, generally assessing the overall state of the child's health and pace of development, and noting the interaction between the parent(s) and the child. For children beyond infancy, the physical examination can trigger a conversation about health issues with the child. Specific, formalized screening maneuvers as a part of the physical examination should be differentiated from surveillance. *Surveillance* is an ongoing process in which the clinician's conscientious, skilled observation permits detection of *obvious* abnormalities or concerns, whereas screening is a formal process applied to a patient in whom surveillance has not revealed a concern. Readers should consult a pediatric reference for detailed instructions on the nuances of physical examination in the infant and child; the discussion here focuses only on a few prevention-oriented aspects of the standard physical examination.

The focus of the routine physical examination in children varies with age, and it differs in important respects from the focus of the physical examination in adults. If the child presents with complaints, the examination should focus on these, but most infants and children have few or no physical complaints. Fair- to good-quality evidence is available for some aspects of the pediatric physical examination, which are discussed next. A comprehensive review of the evidence supporting these maneuvers, and the rationale for advising against other forms of screening, is beyond the scope of this chapter. The reader may consult the "Suggested Readings" for further discussion of the science supporting the physical examination.

Growth Measurements

Growth is usually monitored at health maintenance visits. Weight, length, and head circumference (for children younger than 2 years and older children with developmental concerns) should be plotted on standardized gender-specific growth charts (http://www.cdc.gov/growthcharts). Growth since the last visit should be noted, and any deviations from expected growth investigated.[7] If a clinician intends to monitor these parameters, they should be measured consistently in the following manner.

Before the second birthday, weight should be obtained with the child completely undressed, length should be measured with a reclining stadiometer, and head circumference should be measured with a nonelastic tape measure at the largest point. Taking three measurements and using the largest of the three is often advised. The toddler and older child should be weighed unclothed or in underwear only. Beginning at age 2 years, standing height rather than reclining length should be recorded, and it should be measured with the child standing firmly against a wall-mounted device that has a fixed right angle at the head. Special growth curves have been developed for children with common syndromes that affect growth, such as Down syndrome, achondroplasia and Turner syndrome, which are available from the AAP website (www.aap.org).

Body mass index (BMI) is calculated as (weight [in kilograms]) divided by (height [in meters]^2); measured in pounds and inches the formula is (weight [in pounds]) divided by (height [in inches]^2) multiplied by 703. An online calculator can be found at: https://www.cdc.gov/healthyweight/assessing/bmi/childrens_bmi/about_childrens_bmi.html.   Reference ranges for BMI change significantly as children grow; therefore, obesity in children is defined by BMI percentile rather than by a single cutoff as it is in adults. Gender-specific BMI percentile growth charts are available for children starting at age 2 years, but the usefulness of this measure has not been confirmed in young children. BMI percentiles in young children are poor predictors of adult obesity, and data are lacking to demonstrate a benefit of monitoring BMI in young children. In children with obvious obesity, BMI percentile is a reasonable measure to follow the child's weight status. BMI percentile in adolescents is a better predictor of adult obesity, and BMI above the 85th percentile is also associated with insulin intolerance and other adverse health effects, making calculation and plotting of BMI in adolescents a more useful tool. A link from the calculator page provides the reference ranges for children: https://www.cdc.gov/healthyweight/assessing/bmi/childrens_bmi/about_childrens_bmi.html.

Vital Signs

If vital signs are routinely obtained, age-based normal values such as those found in *The Harriet Lane Handbook* (see "Suggested Readings") should be used. Although evidence from trials is lacking, blood pressure screening has been recommended starting at age 3 years, as noted in Chapter 3. The clinician should measure blood pressure using a cuff of the appropriate size (see Chapter 4, Table 4.2), recalling that use of too small a cuff may result in a falsely elevated measurement. The clinician should also be careful to interpret blood pressure according to gender-, age-, and height-based norms (see Chapter 4, Table 4.3).[8]

Ophthalmic Examination

Funduscopy in children is difficult at best and rarely yields useful information in a child who has no visual complaints and normal visual acuity. In early infancy, the detection of symmetric red retinal reflexes may be useful in excluding retinoblastoma or congenital cataracts. To perform this test, the examiner should stand 2 to 3 feet from the patient and look through the direct ophthalmoscope with the largest white-light circle aimed at the face, then use the dial to focus on the face, illuminating both eyes simultaneously. With the infant looking at the light, the color of the red reflex (which may vary normally from yellow to orange or red) should be the same in both eyes. If the color is significantly different, or the reflex is absent in one eye, the infant should be referred to an ophthalmologist for further evaluation.

Young children should also be screened for amblyopia, strabismus, and defects in visual acuity. In infants and toddlers, the cover test and the Hirschberg light reflex test can be used to detect strabismus. To perform the cover test, the clinician should have the child look at an object 10 feet away (such as a colorful toy) and cover one of the child's eyes. Children may not cooperate with keeping one eye covered, in which case an eye patch can be taped over the eye. As the examiner covers the eye, he or she notes whether the uncovered eye moves to remain focused on the toy; this is repeated with the other eye. Movement of either eye suggests that the eyes are not aligned and requires referral. In the Hirschberg test, the examiner points a light source at the eyes and checks for an asymmetric light reflex. Convergent strabismus ("crossed eyes") may be seen in healthy infants until 6 months of age, but divergent strabismus is usually pathologic at any age.

Visual acuity screening in very young children typically requires specialized training and equipment. Visual acuity testing is often performed qualitatively during infancy by observing the patient's ability to fixate on a target and, by 3 months of age, to follow a moving object. By 6 months of age, the child should be able to grasp objects and recognize faces.

By age 3 years, most children can cooperate with office-based tests. Children who do not understand the instructions can sometimes participate if they are given a card with a large E and told to turn the card in the direction of the letter on the chart ("tumbling E" test). The "tumbling E" and similar tests, which are ideal for children aged 3 to 5 years, are performed with the child standing 10 feet from the chart and covering one eye. The child "reads" each line until reaching the line at which fewer than four of the symbols are identified correctly; the test is then repeated for the other eye. If the acuity is less than 20/40 in either eye *or* if there is a two-line difference between the eyes, the child should be referred for further evaluation.

Cardiovascular Examination

Auscultation of the chest is often difficult in the child who is distressed by the examination and is crying. Therefore, it is useful to examine the chest when the child is quiet and to perform the chest examination before relatively more invasive examinations of the eyes, ears, and oropharynx. Familiarity with functional or innocent murmurs is important to avoid alarming the parents and to avoid an unnecessary workup for the child. Most children with significant congenital heart disease present with cyanosis or symptoms related to heart failure early in life. Identification of children with structural heart disease who are hemodynamically stable is still important from the standpoint of prophylaxis for endocarditis. Therefore, the clinician should be skilled in detecting valvular heart disease, including mitral valve prolapse, as well as septal defects.

Genitourinary Examination

Examination of the external genitalia is often omitted from well child visits owing to concerns about invasion of privacy. This is a good example of an instance in which inclusion of the examination serves not only to detect abnormalities such as undescended testis or inguinal hernia but also to offer an opportunity to discuss issues such as modesty, prevention of sexual molestation, and information about normal development. This discussion may be as important as the examination itself. It should be noted that most children who allege child sexual abuse have normal physical examinations without evidence of penetration.

Scoliosis Examination

Screening for scoliosis (using a scoliometer or inclinometer, or using the forward bending test) by the clinician or in school-based screening is not recommended, as it results in overdetection of minor curvature or postural abnormalities. Most adolescents with mild scoliosis are not candidates for intervention as they approach the end of linear growth. An unclothed examination to rule out asymmetry (specifically of the scapulae or the iliac crests) is sufficient and is more important for the diagnosis of scoliosis in early to middle childhood. Plain spine films are not useful for the diagnosis of scoliosis.

Developmental and Behavioral Assessment

Developmental and behavioral assessment can begin in the waiting room with parent questionnaires, as discussed previously. Although developmental and language delay are important problems, and studies suggest that earlier intervention is likely to result in improved outcomes, formal screening has not been shown to result in improved outcomes. Validated tools include the Parents Evaluation of Developmental Status and Ages and Stages Questionnaire instruments (see "Suggested Readings"). Even under optimal circumstances, false-positive and false-negative results may occur. Parental concern is a sensitive indicator of developmental delay, so clinicians should be alert to issues raised by the parents, and their concerns should not be ignored or "brushed off."[9] Any concern about delay on the part of the parent or clinician should result in immediate referral for evaluation.

Speech delay is the single most common form of delay in children with otherwise normal development. In the past, some clinicians have falsely reassured parents who are concerned about delayed speech, calling such children "late bloomers." It is now clear that many children benefit from early referral for delayed speech milestones. Children with delayed language development may have either hearing loss or language delay, and both of these possible explanations should be investigated.

The apparent increase in the prevalence of autism concerns many parents and physicians. The two hallmarks of autism are impaired communication, for which speech delay may be the heralding sign, and impaired relationships, marked by a lack of "shared attention" with the parent or caretaker. If a child has deficiencies in speech acquisition or personal social skills, the primary care clinician may wish to use a screening instrument, such as the Modified Checklist for Autism in Toddlers (see "Suggested Readings"), or may wish to immediately refer the child for further evaluation. Some experts recommend routine screening for autism, although the efficacy of this practice is not known.

Laboratory Screening

Laboratory screening tests that have been recommended during childhood include newborn metabolic screening and screening for anemia, lead poisoning, TB, lipid disorders, and urinary tract abnormalities if indicated. See Newborn metabolic screening.

Anemia Screening

Screening during infancy for lead poisoning and anemia is mandated by many state Medicaid programs and is often recommended by other authorities. Although screening using venous blood samples is simple and straightforward for both conditions, what to do with the results is much less clear. The theoretic basis for screening for anemia or lead poisoning is the known adverse effects of elevated lead levels and of iron deficiency (even without anemia) on the developing brain. However, treatment of elevated lead levels (by abatement or chelation) has not been shown to improve developmental outcomes. Treatment of iron deficiency (the most common cause of anemia in childhood) improves hemoglobin levels but has not been shown to improve clinical outcomes. In both cases, it may be that treatment comes too late, and resources would be better spent on community-based efforts to prevent these conditions. All infants should receive an iron-rich diet, including iron-fortified formula (if formula fed) and infant cereals. If screening for either lead poisoning or anemia is mandated, sampling by venipuncture is more accurate and less painful than sampling by fingerstick.

Tuberculosis Screening

As noted in Chapter 5, TB skin testing is recommended only for children at high risk of exposure. Risk factors include recent immigration of the patient or household contacts from a country with a high prevalence of TB infection and exposure to a person with known infectious TB, to an adult with chronic cough and no other underlying diagnosis, to a person who has been incarcerated, to an injection drug user, or to a person with known immunosuppressive disease, especially human immunodeficiency virus (HIV) infection. Children with HIV infection must also be screened for TB. Testing should be performed using the Mantoux test, with interpretation of the skin test determined by the Centers for Disease Control and Prevention at https://www.cdc.gov/tb/publications/factsheets/testing/skintesting.htm.

Lipid Screening

Cholesterol screening of the general pediatric population has been a subject of controversy, and recommendations vary widely. Currently the AAP, American Heart Association, and National Heart, Lung and Blood Institute do not recommend routine screening of well children without personal or family risk factors. Cholesterol screening (especially isolated cholesterol screening with no further lipid profile analysis) is sometimes done at health fairs. The discovery of elevated serum lipid levels is likely to result in anxiety for the parents, which is unnecessary unless there are comorbid disorders such as hypertension, obesity, or diabetes risk. In the context of the child's primary care setting, judicious evaluation may be warranted when children have a strong family history of cardiovascular disease, including cardiac death before age 55 years in first-degree relatives or relevant risk factors such as hypertension, obesity, or diabetes. There is little evidence that dietary change or the use of cholesterol-lowering drugs in childhood affect health outcomes during adulthood or that these drugs are safe for long-term use in children. However, families with familial hyperlipidemia may represent a special case, hence the importance of an accurate family history. Normal lipid values for children differ from those for adults (see Table 18.1).[10]

Screening Urinalysis

In 2010, the AAP recommended against routine urinalysis for asymptomatic children and adolescents.[11] They also do not recommend a urinalysis for sport preparticipation physical examinations.

TABLE 18.1   Classification of Serum Cholesterol Levels in High-Risk[a] Children and Adolescents

	Total Cholesterol (mg/dL)	LDL Cholesterol (mg/dL)
Acceptable	<170	<110
Borderline	170–199	110–129
High	≥200	≥130

[a]Children and adolescents from families with hypercholesterolemia or premature cardiovascular disease.
LDL, low-density lipoprotein.
Reproduced from the National Cholesterol Education Program. https://www.nhlbi.nih.gov/files/docs/peds_guidelines_sum.pdf.

Anticipatory Guidance in Pediatrics

Providing "anticipatory guidance" is a time-honored tradition in pediatric care. Many pediatric clinicians believe that their greatest contribution is in educating and guiding parents, especially first-time parents, with regard to their child's health. Rapid changes in a child's developmental status mean rapid changes in the most important threats to the child's health and safety. Therefore, specific counseling interventions change with the patient's age and individual circumstances. As the child gradually advances toward physical, cognitive, and emotional independence, the target of the counseling intervention will gradually shift from the parent(s) to the child and parent(s) together, and eventually to the patient alone in late adolescence.

For many specific counseling interventions, there is clear evidence that the recommended behavior change will lead to the desired outcome (e.g., wearing bicycle helmets decreases head injuries) but it is less clear that the clinician's advice has a causal role in changing the behavior. The clinician's advice is probably most effective when it is part of a multifaceted, community-based effort to change behavior.

Car Safety Seats

One of the most effective interventions in child safety has been the introduction and use of automobile safety seats. Until the infant is at least 2 years old and weighs the maximum amount allowed by the care seat manufacture, the car seat should face the back of the vehicle and preferably be placed in the middle of the back seat. It should never be placed on a seat within range of an airbag. Older children should wear seat belts in a booster seat, sized as appropriate, until they are approximately 8 to 12 years and 57 in tall. Discussing child safety seats is a good opportunity to emphasize to parents the importance of wearing seat belts themselves, for their own benefit and to model good car safety behavior, to say nothing

TABLE 18.2	Types of Car Seats	
Age Group	**Type of Seat**	**General Guidelines**
Infants and toddlers	• Rear facing only • Rear-facing convertible	All infants and toddlers should ride in a **rear-facing seat** until they are at least **2 yr of age** or reach the highest weight or height allowed by their car seat manufacturer
Toddlers and pre-schoolers	• Convertible • Forward facing with harness	Children who have outgrown the rear-facing weight or height limit for their convertible seat should use a **forward-facing seat** with a harness for as long as possible, up to the highest weight or height allowed by their car safety seat manufacturer
School-aged children	• Booster seats	All children whose weight or height exceeds the forward-facing limit for their car safety seat should use a **belt-positioning booster** seat until the vehicle seat belt fits properly, typically when they have reached 4 ft 9 in in height and are 8 through 12 yr of age. All children younger than 13 yr should ride in the back seat
Older children	• Seat belts	When children are old enough and large enough for the vehicle seat belt to fit them correctly, they should always use **lap and shoulder seat belts** for the best protection. All children younger than 13 yr should ride in the back seat

AAP Healthy Children. Accessed 2018 from: https://www.healthychildren.org/English/safety-prevention/on-the-go/Pages/Car-Safety-Seats-Information-for-Families.as.

of complying with traffic safety laws. Table 18.2 provides child car seat guidelines, but clinicians should familiarize themselves with applicable regulations in their state.

Injury Prevention

The leading fatal events in the home are poisonings, falls, fires and burns, and suffocation by an ingested object. Discussion by the clinician about the use of baby walkers, smoke alarms, safe water heater temperature, and the importance of keeping small objects away from young children who may choke on them may help reinforce what parents hear on such matters from public health campaigns. Parents who ride bicycles should be encouraged to use helmets for themselves (especially as it may be mandated by local law) and to insist that their children always wear helmets for activities such as bicycling, skateboarding, skating, and skiing. Use of helmets during these activities has been shown to reduce significant head injury by 88%.[12]

Encouraging Literacy

Emerging evidence suggests that at the child health visit in late infancy through early childhood, physician-supported attention to early literacy through provision of books and encouragement of reading may be beneficial in achieving a measurable increase in vocabulary in early school years.[13]

Dental Care

Every child should begin to receive oral health risk assessments by 6 months of age from a pediatrician or a qualified pediatric health care professional. Risk factors for caries include family history of caries (which may represent both genetic factors and the vertical transmission of cariogenic bacteria from caregivers), bottle-feeding, drinking juice, lack of an adequate fluoride source in the diet, and recent immigrant or low socioeconomic status. The AAP recommends establishing a dental home early when their first tooth erupts or on the first birthday.[7]

Parents may clean the teeth of older infants and toddlers with a clean washcloth in plain water at the beginning of bath time. The American Academy of Pediatric Dentistry recommends age-appropriate toothbrush and for children at high risk for caries using a smear of fluoridated toothpaste for children less than 2 years of age and a pea size for children aged 2 to 5 years. Fluoride administration can help prevent caries, but its risks include fluorosis or staining of the teeth from overzealous use of topical or dietary fluoride.

Exogenous fluoride supplementation should not be prescribed for infants younger than 6 months. Fluoride supplementation should be prescribed for older infants if the community water supply has inadequate fluoride content.[7]

Immunizations

The eradication or near eradication of vaccine-preventable disease means that many 21st century clinicians will not see any cases of illnesses that were commonplace in the 20th century. Continued dedication to the provision of recommended immunizations is one of the hallmarks of primary care, not only for young children but also increasingly for adolescents and young adults. The recommended immunization schedule changes frequently as new immunizations and combination vaccines are developed. The reader is directed to Chapter 16 for a complete discussion of immunizations. "Best practice" for ensuring high vaccination rates entails review of the immunization record and a policy of "no missed vaccine opportunities" with regard to office visits for minor illness or injury.

Some parents, not having seen firsthand the burden of illnesses such as polio, chickenpox, pertussis, and measles, may question the need or advisability of providing immunizations for their children. Of course, it is those very vaccines that have prevented the outbreaks that older clinicians can vividly remember. Helpful resources for patient and parent education about vaccines can be found at https://www.cdc.gov/vaccines/hcp/conversations/resources-parents.html. See also the resources and guidelines provided in Chapter 17.

SPECIAL POPULATIONS

Early infancy and adolescence are the times of greatest risk during childhood; perhaps this is why more evidence on evaluation and intervention has been developed for these age groups than for the relatively quiet years in between.

THE NEWBORN

History and Risk Assessment

Evaluation of the newborn begins with a review of the child's prenatal course, including the mother's prenatal care, ultrasonography and laboratory screening results (if available), and perinatal events. Infants of adolescent mothers, mothers with a history of depression or substance abuse, and mothers with no prenatal care are at increased risk of neonatal problems and require closer follow-up.

Physical Examination

About 2% to 3% of children are born with congenital defects, some of which are not immediately obvious; furthermore, a newborn with one congenital abnormality is at increased risk of a second abnormality. The initial physical examination should be thorough, with particular attention to the most common and significant congenital abnormalities. A careful oral examination is required to detect submucous cleft palate, which may be associated with future respiratory and speech problems. A normal cardiac examination in the immediate newborn period does not rule out the presence of congenital heart disease, as the adaptation to extrauterine circulation continues for the first several weeks of life. An undescended testis increases the risk of both infertility and later testicular cancer. If the testis does not descend spontaneously in the first year of life, the infant should be referred for evaluation; bilateral undescended testes should be evaluated immediately.

Identification of developmental dysplasia of the hip (now known to not always be "congenital" but in some instances to first manifest itself in early infancy) remains important because this condition may result in lifelong difficulties with ambulation and in arthritis. However, the natural history of this disorder is poorly understood and evidence for the efficacy of screening examinations with the Ortolani or Barlow maneuver or with ultrasonography is lacking. Spontaneous resolution occurs in the newborn period in most (60%–80%) cases identified as abnormal or suspicious on physical examination and in greater than 90% of those cases so identified on ultrasonography. The common surgical and nonsurgical interventions are associated with a risk of avascular necrosis of the hip. Given the lack of evidence for routine screening, the best path may be attention to known risk factors for developmental dysplasia of the hip (such as female gender and breech positioning at birth) and careful follow-up of infants at risk.[14]

Although extreme hyperbilirubinemia is very rare, and jaundice in the first 24 hours of life is always of concern, moderate jaundice is a common finding after the first 24 hours of life. Risk factors for extreme hyperbilirubinemia include gestational age below 37 weeks, blood group incompatibility, cephalohematoma, East Asian origins, a previous infant with severe hyperbilirubinemia, and exclusive breastfeeding, especially if breastfeeding has not gone well. Newborns should be assessed for jaundice and risk factors for developing jaundice before hospital discharge. If a serum bilirubin is obtained, a nomogram for interpreting the result based on age is available at www.bilitool.org.

Laboratory and Other Screenings

Newborn screening using dried blood spots on filter paper is mandated in all 50 states and includes (at a minimum) screening for phenylketonuria and congenital hypothyroidism. Most states also require screening for sickle cell anemia and galactosemia. The evidence that screening for these conditions leads to improved outcomes is quite strong. The evidence in support of screening for cystic fibrosis or congenital adrenal hyperplasia is less strong, whereas the usefulness of dramatically expanded newborn screening panels made possible by tandem mass spectrometry has not yet been studied. Clinicians should have a thorough understanding of their state's screening policies and of systems for follow up of abnormal screens, and they should ensure that a normal screen has been reported within the first month.

Screening for congenital hearing loss is also mandated in most states and is provided in most hospitals before the newborn's discharge. The screening typically involves otoacoustic emission testing and/or auditory brainstem response. Such screening has led to earlier identification and intervention in children with congenital hearing loss, which is associated with improved language skills during childhood. The results of this test should be reviewed during the first month of life so that infants who are identified can be evaluated and intervention undertaken as early as possible.

Screening for congenital heart disease in the newborn is also recommended. The screening is recommended after 24 hours of life and before discharge. Pulse oximeters should be taken from the right hand and either foot.[15]

Anticipatory Guidance

The initial in-hospital visit by the pediatric caregiver is a uniquely "teachable" moment for new parents. The clinician should be sure to admire the baby and help the parents understand the emotional roller coaster of new parenthood. The health benefits of breastfeeding, such as decreased rates of infant diarrhea and otitis media, are discussed in Chapter 8. As noted in that chapter, the clinician's support for breastfeeding, especially in concert with hospital programs, improves the rate and duration of breastfeeding.

The clinician should also emphasize the importance of supine sleep to decrease the risk of sudden infant death syndrome. Infants should be placed on their back for sleep in the first year of life. Parents should be warned that the side position is unstable and is therefore not recommended. Skull deformities resulting from prolonged supine positioning (positional plagiocephaly) are reported. However, this complication can be avoided by allowing the child plenty of "tummy time" when awake and by alternating to which side the child's head is positioned for sleep.

The clinician should discuss the importance of avoiding the child's exposure to cigarette smoke, which is associated with sudden infant death syndrome, otitis media, asthma, and other disorders. See Chapter 10 for a further discussion of smoking by parents and passive exposure to "sidestream" environmental tobacco smoke. The clinician should also take the opportunity to begin counseling about the importance of using car safety seats for the first ride home from the hospital and every ride thereafter.

Newborn Follow-up

With the shortening of postpartum hospital stays, "early follow-up" visits are now routinely recommended to assess weight gain and breastfeeding and to detect neonatal jaundice and assess for physical signs suggestive of congenital cardiac or metabolic defects. It is recommended that these visits take place within 72 hours of discharge. The examination should include the following elements: infant weight, assessment of maternal/infant bonding, assessment of maternal lactation and infant feeding, and a targeted physical examination looking for ductal dependent congenital cardiac abnormalities, neonatal jaundice, evidence of normal hydration, and intact neuromuscular function. Newborns should be seen again at age 2 weeks to 1 month to assess weight gain, feeding, residual jaundice (which requires evaluation for cholestasis if it persists to the third week of age), the cardiac examination, and the general well-being of the infant and caretaker.

THE ADOLESCENT

Adolescent well visits focus on the prevention and early detection of risky behaviors and accidents.[16] Teenagers enter into adolescence and make the transition to adulthood at different rates and assume a primary role in their health care. Adolescent-focused health services foster increased independence and decision making, with parents remaining involved to varying degrees.[17] As teens mature, the encounter with the clinician (regardless of whether it was originally precipitated by an illness/injury or for health maintenance) must be structured to meet the needs of the patient primarily and the parent secondarily. This is a paradigm shift for many clinicians, and it can also be difficult for parents to accept.

Consent and Confidentiality

Confidentiality is a critical aspect of care for adolescents. It allows teens to seek care for sensitive or private issues in a timelier manner. Unfortunately, there are many potential threats to an adolescent's confidentiality, including health-related bills, explanations of benefits, medical records, even reminder calls from the health care agency for upcoming appointments, and computer-generated calls from pharmacies reminding teens of their prescriptions.[18] Confidentiality and agreements about confidentiality should be discussed with the adolescent and the parent or guardian. In general, information shared between the clinician and the adolescent is confidential unless the teen intends to harm himself or herself (e.g., suicide), harm someone else (e.g., homicide), or is being harmed by someone else (abuse).[19]

For most health conditions, permission for health care of an adolescent is provided by the parent or legal guardian. The legal rights of adolescents vary from state to state.[20] All states have specific laws related to certain aspects of care that the teen may consent to without a parent or guardian's permission. Every state allows teens to have testing and treatment of sexually transmitted infections without parental consent.[21] Adolescents in some states can receive reproductive care, pregnancy-related care, mental health services and counseling, and treatment for substance or alcohol abuse.[20] Some states require parental notification before an abortion.[22] The Mature Minor Doctrine allows unemancipated teens in a few states (Pennsylvania, Tennessee, Illinois, Maine, and Massachusetts) to consent for their own care if the clinician feels the teen exhibits the maturity to consent for his or her own care.[23] Legally emancipated minors are able to consent for their own medical care. Teens may also be emancipated under certain circumstances. For example, when adolescents marry or join the armed forces before age 18 years (with parental consent and permission from the court), they become emancipated from their parents. In general, if adolescents can consent to treatment for a condition, they have a legal right to confidentiality about that treatment. Chapter 13 also discusses the potential for parents to learn inadvertently about visits through insurance billing.[24]

Although parents must (legally) give permission for most treatments, adolescents who are capable of understanding can (and should) assent to any planned treatment. Certainly, coercing the adolescent to undergo testing (such as a drug screen or pregnancy test) or to accept treatment they object to is very likely to damage the relationship between the clinician and the patient. Clinicians should determine the limits of confidentiality based on the specific laws of their state and their own comfort level. State laws concerning confidentiality and consent may be found at http://www.law.cornell.edu/topics/Table_Emancipation.htm.[25]

The Adolescent Health Maintenance Visit

For young adolescents or new patient visits it is often helpful for the clinician to meet with the teen and parent/guardian initially to review the reason for the appointment, social history, family medical history, and the teen's medical history (hospitalizations, surgery, allergies, medications, etc.). An overview of what will occur during the wellness visit is often helpful to both the teen and parent. Once these elements of history have been obtained and the parents' concerns are heard, the remainder of the adolescent examination should be conducted without the parents in the examination room. Teens should not be placed in the position of making the decision for the parent to stay or leave, rather the clinician should explain the importance of the teen having time to discuss their concerns with the clinician privately and ask the parent to step out of the room. In some situations, the teen may want the parent to remain present or to return to the examination room later in the visit.

The adolescent patient should be reassured at the beginning of each visit that the conversation is confidential. The HEEADSSS assessment is helpful in taking the adolescent psychosocial history (Table 18.3) and allows the clinician to rapidly assess a teen's psychosocial development and behavior, moving from less sensitive areas, such as their home environment, to more sensitive topics, such as suicidal feelings.[26] Although this chapter discusses anticipatory guidance after the physical examination and laboratory screening, counseling can be woven into the visit by allowing the history and physical examination to provide an opening for discussion of particular issues. For example, questions about activities provide an opportunity to promote physical activity, and questions about sexual activity provide an opportunity to discuss the prevention of sexually transmitted infections and contraceptive options.

The comprehensive review of systems follows the HEEADSSS assessment. Medical jargon should be avoided. Targeted screening for depression, cardiovascular risk, and sexually transmitted infections will be guided by the information gathered in the family medical history, past medical history, HEEADSSS assessment, and review of systems. Multiple mental health screening tools are available for use in primary care settings. See Chapters 11 and 14 for further details about screening for substance abuse and depression, respectively.

TABLE 18.3 HEEADSSS Psychosocial Assessment and Focus Areas	
Home	Who lives at the home, where the teen lives, recent changes, moves, relationships
Education/ employment	School (grade, grades), connectedness to school, peer relationships, supportive school faculty/staff, future education and employment goals, current employment and number of hours
Eating	Feelings related to body shape or weight, weight changes, dieting, how many meals, exercise patterns
Activities	Activities enjoys or does for fun, who the teen spends time with, screen time, Internet use
Drugs	Use of tobacco, electronic cigarettes, drugs, or alcohol by family, friends, or teen, CRAFFT
Sexuality	Like boys, girls, or both? Relationship status, sexual activity, birth control use, condom use
Suicide/ depression	Feelings of stress, anxiety, sadness, boredom? Past or present suicidal thoughts/feelings PHQ-2
Safety	History of injuries, seatbelt use (front and back), helmet use, texting while driving, feeling safe at home/school/neighborhood

Adapted from Klein DA, Goldenring JM, Adelman WP. HEEADSSS 3.0: The psychosocial interview updated for a new century fueled by media. *Contemp Pediatr.* 2014. Retrieved from: www.contemporarypediatrics.com/contemporary-pediatrics/content/tags/adolescent-medicine/heeadsss-30-psychosocial-interview-adolesce?page=full.

Physical Examination

Annual wellness examinations are recommended for all adolescents.[6] The Advisory Committee on Immunization Practices provides guidance on recommended immunizations for adolescents.[27] These guidelines are updated annually. Physical examination and immunization requirements for adolescents to attend school, camp, or college; participate in sports or other activities; and volunteer vary by state, institution, and agency. Adolescents may also have specific religious or cultural factors that may need to be carefully considered before the examination. Teens may be more comfortable with a provider of the same gender.

Adolescents who are new to an agency or provider may also be nervous about meeting a new clinician. Younger adolescents may be anxious about whether their bodies are normal and about the pace of their pubertal development. The assessment of Tanner staging for sexual maturity is part of the wellness examination and provides the patient and the clinician an opportunity to discuss their concerns and provide anticipatory guidance about pubertal changes. All adolescents should have growth parameters (height, weight, and BMI) and blood pressure measured and

TABLE 18.4   Key Elements of the Adolescent Physical Examination

General appearance	Consistency with previous visits, anxiety, interaction with clinician
Head/neck	Vision, hearing, thyroid, lymphadenopathy, teeth (caries, erosion of enamel, wisdom teeth eruption), mouth/gums (evidence of smokeless tobacco use, gingivitis)
Chest	Wheezing, murmur, clicks Tanner stage (female), symmetry, gynecomastia (male), masses, discharge, or galactorrhea
Abdomen	Tenderness, masses, hepatosplenomegaly
Musculoskeletal	Range of motion, symmetry, evidence of injury or overuse, scoliosis
Neurological	Deep tendon reflexes, strength, coordination
Genitalia Male Female	Tanner staging (pubic hair, penis, and testes), evidence of STIs (discharge, lesions, or sores), hernia, foreskin Tanner staging of pubic hair Pelvic examination if abnormal vaginal discharge or pelvic pain Pap smear annually beginning at age 21 yr (adolescents with HIV or other immune deficiency before age 21 yr per guidelines)[28,29]
Skin	Acne, rashes, scars, warts, moles, birthmarks, changes in pigmentation, piercings, tattoos

HIV, human immunodeficiency virus; STI, sexually transmitted infection.
Adapted from Jasik CB, Ozer EM. Chapter 5: Preventive care for adolescents and young adults. In Neinstein LS, Katzman DK, eds. *Neinstein's Adolescent and Young Adult Health Care: A Practical Guide*, 6th ed. New York, NY: Wolters Kluwer, 2016:50–68.

compared with age-based norms at each annual wellness visit (see Table 4.3). Heart rate and temperature are also typically measured. Table 18.4 provides a list of specific areas of focus for the physical examination of the adolescent.

The "Sports Physical" and Other Preparticipation Evaluations

Healthy People 2020 has identified physical activity in adolescents as an important factor in improving bone health and cardiorespiratory fitness and decreasing body fat and depression.[30] Participation in team sports has been shown to have additional benefits, including the lower incidence of teen pregnancy and greater self-esteem among female adolescents and lower rates of overweight/obesity in males.[31,32] The preparticipation sports evaluation is performed annually to identify conditions that would make participation unsafe, screening for underlying illness and identifying and ameliorating existing patterns of injury in the young athlete. The Council on Sports Medicine and Fitness and the AAP provide clinicians with resources specific to the preparticipation sports history and physical examination.[33] The family history should include evaluation for premature cardiac death and inherited cardiac conditions, such as prolonged QT or Marfan syndrome. The patient should be asked about symptoms associated with exertion, including excessive breathlessness, fatigue, chest pain, lightheadedness, or syncope, and should be asked about prior injuries, particularly musculoskeletal injuries and concussion (whether from sports or other causes) that may place the adolescent at risk for additional injuries.[33] A comprehensive list of medical conditions affecting sports participation and guidelines for what types of activity are recommended depending on various medical conditions can be found at https://www.healthychildren.org/English/health-issues/injuries-emergencies/sports-injuries/Pages/Medical-Conditions-That-May-Rule-Out-Sports-Participation.aspx. Disqualification from participation in athletic activities most commonly result from cardiovascular conditions.[33–35] Consultation with a pediatric cardiologist is recommended for any adolescent with cardiovascular disease.[34] Any condition that is not well controlled, places the teen at risk for injury or death, or places team mates or competitors at risk needs further evaluation and/or disqualification.[3,33]

The preparticipation sports physical examination focuses on the cardiovascular and musculoskeletal systems and includes documentation of blood pressure, cardiac examination (both supine and upright), inspection for stigmata of Marfan syndrome, and examination of bones and joints for prior injury.[34,35] The clinician should be alert for nutritional issues, including the use of supplements and the appearance of eating disorders, which are associated with weight-class sports (e.g., wrestling) and aesthetic sports (e.g., gymnastics). Highly conditioned female athletes may develop amenorrhea, especially if they have markedly decreased body fat. Although the young athlete may not be seeing the clinician for general health maintenance, the sports physical is a good opportunity to ask about and discuss smoking and drug use, because they relate directly to sports performance. As with adults (see Chapter 20), screening electrocardiograms or echocardiograms have not been shown to be useful in adolescent preparticipation evaluations.[35]

Laboratory Screening
Tuberculosis

Screening for TB is based on individual risk factors and/or requirements of employment, volunteering, or school. Typically testing for TB is indicated for adolescents with a known exposure, immune deficiency, HIV, or drug use; those living in or visiting a high-risk area of the world; or in persons with symptoms of active infection.[36]

Diabetes Screening

As with adults, universal screening of children and adolescents for diabetes is not recommended (see Chapter 20). However, children with *both* a family history of insulin resistance *and* physical evidence of obesity, acanthosis nigricans, or other risk factors may benefit from early screening by glucose tolerance testing. Screening guidelines are updated annually.[37]

Screening for Sexually Transmitted Infections and Human Immunodeficiency Virus

As discussed in Chapters 5 and 13, screening for chlamydia and gonorrhea is recommended for sexually active adolescent females and adolescent males receiving care in high-incidence communities and settings.[6,38] HIV testing should be offered to all adolescents with a history of sexual activity or sexually transmitted infection. The first Pap smear should take place at age 21 years unless the teen has HIV or other immunodeficiency.[28,29]

Counseling and Anticipatory Guidance

Sexual Behavior

Abstinence, condom use, and increased access to highly effective contraceptive methods have contributed to the significant decrease in teen pregnancy in the United States since 1991.[39,40] Urine-based screening for gonorrhea and chlamydia make it easier for teens to be tested and treated.[38] The Centers for Disease Control and Prevention and Bright Futures advocate for sexual risk assessments and appropriate screening for adolescents.[6,38] See Chapter 12 for details on how to counsel patients about contraceptive choices and use of emergency contraception. Chapter 13 provides guidance on condom use and the prevention of sexually transmitted infections.

Alcohol and Tobacco Screening

As discussed in Chapters 10 and 11, avoiding tobacco use and ethanol abuse early in life will reduce the risk of a wide host of diseases in later years. The majority of adult smokers began smoking during adolescence. Physician counseling of young people appears to have a modest effect on tobacco cessation.[41] Direct evidence of its effect on substance use is lacking. See Chapters 10 and 11, respectively, for detailed guidance on how to counsel patients about smoking and about alcohol and drug abuse.

Injury Prevention

Wearing safety belts has been clearly shown to reduce injury and death in motor vehicle accidents, but it is not clear whether guidance from clinicians regarding this intervention helps promote this practice.[42]

However, motor vehicle accidents remain a significant source of morbidity and mortality for adolescents.[43] Law enforcement and school and community efforts may be chiefly responsible for compliance when it occurs. Similarly, use of safety gear (e.g., helmets) when riding bicycles or motorcycles, skateboarding, and skiing reduces injury during accidents involving rapid deceleration.[12] Clinician counseling for injury prevention is probably most effective when offered in combination with reinforcing messages from community and school-based health promotion programs.

Lastly, the absence (or locked storage) of firearms in the home prevents access to both guns and ammunition and is associated with lower risk of youth suicide, homicide, and unintentional shootings. It is not known whether brief counseling by clinicians is likely to influence handgun safety practices.[42] Unless evidence emerges that doing so is counterproductive, it seems prudent for clinicians to continue to address gun safety in discussions with young people and their parents.

OFFICE AND CLINIC ORGANIZATION

The organization of the office in which children are seen should be somewhat different from that of the office where adults are seen exclusively. Separate waiting areas for sick children or even areas or procedures for caring for patients with known infections (e.g., chickenpox) may be useful in some practices. Age-appropriate reading material is important and conducive to literacy development in young children.[9] Toys provided for a waiting area or examination room should be child safe and diminish hazardous play. Adolescents are most comfortable when either a section of the waiting room relates to their interests or they are promptly moved to an area not decorated and equipped for young children.

Some practices use the waiting room time and experience to foster anticipatory guidance, to deliver other useful health information with proprietary video or television programming for patients and parents, and to display health information and periodicals relevant to the patient population. For example, the pediatric waiting room might have brochure racks with information about newborn care, adolescent health concerns, immunizations, safety, and the like. As previously discussed, much information can be elicited before the initial child health maintenance visit through questionnaires that address both the general patient history and information targeted to the purpose of the visit if indicated.

Examination room furnishings should be equally safe and comfortable for children and should minimize potential for falls (e.g., rolling stools may be a hazard). Private areas to discuss issues such as adolescent sexuality, perinatal infections, and child abuse allegations are frequently needed.

A separate supervised area for children to play while parents discuss issues with the clinician may be useful. The use of an office without an examination table or other medical equipment may be useful for the follow-up of children with behavioral or other concerns and may be less threatening once the medical examination has finished.

CONCLUSION

The philosophy of caring for the pediatric population has always been that "the child is not a little adult." As well child health care continues to progress toward evidence-based interventions, the pediatric health care provider will remain pivotal as an advocate and participant, along with schools and community organizations, in improving the health of children. The clinician also plays a role in working with the community to develop those resources, advocating for change when evidence suggests it will better children's environment, and encouraging early childhood education for young children and support for their parents. Policy initiatives to promote health and prevent disease, combined with efforts by clinicians in their individual relationships with patients and their parents, offer the best opportunity for advancing the health of today's children and enhancing their well-being as tomorrow's adults.

SUGGESTED RESOURCES AND MATERIALS

American Academy of Family Physicians
Health information for the whole family
https://familydoctor.org/family-health/infants-and-toddlers/.

American Academy of Pediatrics
Parenting corner
https://www.healthychildren.org/English/Pages/default.aspx.

Bright Futures.
https://brightfutures.aap.org/families/Pages/Resources-for-Children-and-Teens.aspx.

Pediatric screening tests
http://www.pedstest.com/default.aspx.

National Association of Pediatric Nurse Practitioners
Teen Proofing Your Home https://www.napnap.org/teen-proofing-your-home

Adolescent Health: Think, Act, Grow® (TAG) https://www.hhs.gov/ash/oah/tag/index.html.

SUGGESTED READINGS

Ages and Stages Questionnaire. One of several evidence-based developmental assessment questionnaires available in English and Spanish in hard copy or on CD-ROM. https://agesandstages.com/.
Bright Futures Guidelines for Health Supervision for Infants, Children and Adolescents, American Academy of Pediatrics in conjunction with the Maternal and Child Health Bureau, 2017. A collection of materials (manuals and pocket guides) including guidelines for health supervision visits for children of all ages

and materials regarding nutrition, physical activity, and other patient and family instructional material in English and Spanish. https://shop.aap.org/bright-futures-guidelines-for-health-supervision-of-infants-children-and-adolescents-4th-edition-1/. Kahl L, Hughes H, eds. *The Harriet Lane Handbook*, 21st ed. The Johns Hopkins Hospital: Elsevier Science; 2017.

Modified Checklist for Autism in Toddlers (MCHAT). Available at several websites, including https://m-chat.org/. Neinstein LS. *Adolescent Health Curriculum. Includes Discussion of the HEEADSSS Exam.* http://learn.pediatrics.ubc.ca/body-systems/general-pediatrics/approach-to-a-routine-adolescent-interview/ Parents Evaluation of Developmental Status. A computer-based or hard copy questionnaire to evaluate parental concern about children's development. Pediatric Symptom Checklist (PSC). This waiting room questionnaire may be used as an initial instrument for detecting problems outside the realm of normal childhood behavioral and emotional disturbances, although care must be taken with any "broad" screening tool to use it only as a screen before using other instruments such as depression inventories or before treatment or referral for depression. Available in the public domain at https://www.brightfutures.org/mentalhealth/pdf/professionals/ped_sympton_chklst.pdf. See Chapter 13 for further details about screening for depression.

Screening tools. Accessed 2018. https://screeningtime.org/star-center/#/screening-tools.

U.S. Preventive Services Task Force. *Counseling About Proper Use of Motor Vehicle Occupant Restraints* and *Avoidance of Alcohol Use While Driving: U.S. Preventive Services Task Force Recommendation Statement;* August 2007. First published in *Ann Intern Med.* 2007;147:187–193. Agency for Healthcare Research and Quality, Rockville, MD. https://www.ahrq.gov/professionals/clinicians-providers/guidelines-recommendations/guide/section2c.html#Motor.

Vanderbilt scale for ADHD. This questionnaire also includes subtests for screening for anxiety and oppositional behavior comorbid with ADHD. Available at the National Institute for Child Health Quality website: https://www.nichq.org/resource/nichq-vanderbilt-assessment-scales.

REFERENCES

1. World Health Organization. Social Determinants of Health. http://www.who.int/gender-equity-rights/understanding/sdh-definition/en/. Accessed 4/10/2018.
2. Baker J. Women and the invention of well child care. *Pediatrics.* 1994;94(4):527-531.
3. American Academy of Pediatrics Committee on Psychosocial Aspects of Child and Family Health. The pediatrician and the "new morbidity". *Pediatrics.* 1993;92(5):731-733.
4. National Research Council and Institute of Medicine. *Committee on Evaluation of Children's Health. Children's Health, the Nation's Wealth: Assessing and Improving Child Health.* Washington, DC: National Academies Press; 2004.
5. Halfon N, Verhoef PA, Kuo AA. Childhood antecedents to adult cardiovascular disease. *Peds in Review.* 2012;33(2);1-19.
6. America Academy of Pediatrics. *Bright Futures;* 2017. https://brightfutures.aap.org/materials-and-tools/Pages/default.aspx. Accessed 3/20/2018.
7. Tanski S, Garfunkel LC, Duncan PM, Weitzman M. *Performing Preventive Services: A Bright Futures Handbook.* Elk Grove Village, IL: American Academy of Pediatrics; 2010.
8. Flynn JT, Kaelber DC, Baker-Smith CM, et al. Subcommittee on screening and management of high blood pressure in children. Clinical practice guideline for screening and management of high blood pressure in children and adolescents. *Pediatrics.* 2017;140(3):e20171904.

9. Centers for Disease Control and Prevention. *Developmental Monitoring and Screening*, 2018. https://www.cdc.gov/ncbddd/childdevelopment/screening. html. Accessed 3/28/2018.

10. *Expert Panel on Integrated Guidelines for Cardiovascular Health and Risk Reduction in Children and Adolescents: Full Report*, 2011. Available at:www.nhlbi. nih.gov/guidelines/cvd_ped/index.htm . Accessed 5 January 2012.

11. Primack W. AAP does not recommend routine urinalysis for asymptomatic youths. *AAP News*. 2010. http://www.aappublications.org/content/31/12/16.1. Accessed 4/10/2018

12. American Academy of Pediatrics. Bicycle Helmets. Committee on injury and poison prevention. *Pediatrics*. 2001;108(4):1030-1032.

13. Counsel of Early Childhood. Literacy promotion: an essential component of primary care practice. *Pediatrics*. 2014;134:404-409.

14. Shipman SA, Helfand M, Moyer VA, et al. Screening for developmental dysplasia of the hip: a systematic literature review for the U.S. Preventive Services Task Force. *Pediatrics*. 2006;117:e557-e576.

15. Harold JD. Screening for critical congenital heart disease in newborns. *Circulation*. 2014;130:e79-e81.

16. Miniño AM. *Mortality Among Teenagers Aged 12-19 Years: United States, 1999–2006*. NCHS Data Brief, No. 37http://www.cdc.gov/nchs/data/databrief/db37. pdf. Hyattsville, MD: National Center for Health Statistics; 2010. Retrieved from:http://www.cdc.gov/nchs/data/databrief/db37.pdf

17. Hofmann A. Managing adolescents and their parents: avoiding pitfalls and traps. *Adolesc Med*. 1992;3(1);1-11.

18. Guttmacher Institute. https://www.guttmacher.org/news-release/2017/confidentiality-concerns-may-deter-us-adolescents-and-young-adults-obtaining.

19. Ford CA, Thomsen SL, Compton B. Adolescents' interpretations of conditional confidentiality assurances. *J Adolesc Health*. 2001;29(3);156-159.

20. Guttmacher Institute. *An Overview of Minors' Consent Law*, 2018. Retrieved from:https://www.guttmacher.org/print/state-policy/explore/overview-minors-consent-law .

21. Guttmacher Institute. *Minors' Access to STI Services*, 2018. Retrieved from:https://www.guttmacher.org/state-policy/explore/minors-access-sti-services .

22. Guttmacher Institute. Parental Involvement in Minors' Abortions. 2018. Retrieved from:https://www.guttmacher.org/print/state-policy/explore/parental-involvement-minors-abortion .

23. Coleman DL, Rosoff PM. The legal authority of mature minors to consent to general medical treatment. *Pediatrics*. 2013:131;786-793.

24. Ford C, English A, Sigman G. Confidential health care for adolescents: position paper of the Society for Adolescent Medicine. *J Adolesc Health*. 2004;35(2):160-167.

25. English A, Bass L, Boyle AD, Eshragh F. *State Minor Consent Laws: A Summary*, 3rd ed. Chapel Hill, SC: Center for Adolescent Health & Law; 2010.

26. Klein DA, Goldenring JM, Adelman WP. HEEADSSS 3.0: the psychosocial interview updated for a new century fueled by media. *Contemp Pediatr*. 2014. Retrieved from:www.contemporarypediatrics.com/contemporary-pediatrics/content/tags/adolescent-medicine/heeadsss-30-psychosocial-interview-adolesce?page=full .

27. Centers for Disease Control and Prevention. Advisory Committee on Immunization Practices recommended immunization schedules for persons aged 18 years and younger — United States. *MMWR*. 2018;67(5):156-157. Retrieved from:https://www.cdc.gov/vaccines/schedules/hcp/child-adolescent.html .

28. Saslow D, Solomon D, Lawson HW, et al. American Cancer Society, American Society for Colposcopy and Cervical Pathology, and American Society for Clinical Pathology Screening guidelines for the prevention and early detection of cervical cancer. *CA Cancer J Clin*. 2012;62(3):147-172.

29. Panel on Opportunistic Infections in HIV-Infected Adults and Adolescents. Guidelines for Prevention and Treatment of Opportunistic Infections in HIV-infected Adults and Adolescents: Recommendations from the Centers for Disease Control and Prevention, the National Institutes of Health, and the HIV Medicine Association of the Infectious Diseases Society of America. 2018. Available at http://aidsinfo.nih.gov/contentfiles/lvguidelines/adult_oi.pdf .

30. U.S. Department of health and Human Services. *Healthy People 2020: Physical Activity*; 2014. Retrieved from https://www.healthypeople.gov/2020/topics-objectives/topic/physical-activity.

31. Drake KM, Beach ML, Longacre MR, et al. Influence of sports, physical education, and active commuting to school on adolescents' weight status. *Pediatrics.* 2012;130(2):e296-e304.

32. Sabo DF, Miller KE, Farell M, et al. High school athletic participation, sexual behavior, and adolescent pregnancy: a regional study. *J Adolesc Health.* 1999;25(3):207-216.

33. Peterson AR, Bernhardt DT. The preparticipation sports evaluation. *Pediatr Rev.* 2011;32:e53-e64.

34. Rice SG; The Council on Sports Medicine and Fitness. Medical conditions affecting sports participation. *Pediatrics.* 2008;121:841-848.

35. Maron BJ, Levine BD, Washington RL et al. Eligibility and disqualification recommendations for competitive athletes with cardiovascular abnormalities: task force 2: preparticipation screening for cardiovascular disease in competitive athletes. A scientific statement from the American Heart Association and American College of Cardiology. *Circulation.* 2015;132:e267-e272.

36. Lewinsohn DM, Leonard MK, LoBue PA et al. Official American Thoracic Society/Infectious Diseases Society of America/Centers for Disease Control and Prevention clinical practice guidelines: diagnosis of tuberculosis in adults and children. *Clin Infect Dis.* 2017;64(2):111-115. Retrieved from:https://www.cdc.gov/tb/publications/guidelines/pdf/ciw778.pdf .

37. American Diabetes Association. Standards of medical care in diabetes. *Diabetes Care.* 2018;41(Supp 1):1-159. Retrieved from:http://care.diabetesjournals.org/content/41/Supplement_1 .

38. Centers for Disease Control and Prevention. Sexually transmitted diseases treatment guidelines 2015. *MMWR.* 2015;64(3):1-137.

39. Santelli JS, Lindberg LD, Finer LB, Singh S. Explaining recent declines in adolescent pregnancy in the United States: the contribution of abstinence and improved contraceptive use. *Am J Public Health.* 2007;97(1):150-156.

40. Boostra H. What is behind the declines in teen pregnancy rates. *Guttmacher Policy Rev.* 2014;17(3):1-21. Retrieved from:https://www.guttmacher.org/gpr/2014/09/what-behind-declines-teen-pregnancy-rates .

41. Grimshaw GM, Stanton A. Tobacco cessation interventions for young people. *Cochrane Database Syst Rev.* 2006;(4):CD003289.

42. Stevens MM, Olson AL, Gaffney CA, et al. A pediatric, practice-based randomized trial of drinking and smoking prevention and bicycle helmet, gun and seatbelt safety promotion. *Pediatrics.* 2002;109(3):490-497.

43. Heron M. Deaths: leading causes for 2015. *National Vital Statistics Rep.* 2017;66(5):1-76. Retrieved from:http://www.cdc.gov/nchs/data/nvsr/nvsr66_05.pdf .

Please see Online Appendix: Apps and Digital Resources for additional information.

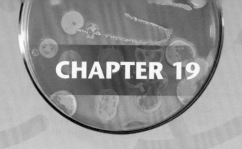

CHAPTER 19

What to Do With Abnormal Screening Test Results?

LESLIE ANN KOLE

INTRODUCTION

This chapter examines what clinicians should do when they find abnormal results arising from screening tests, as recorded in the history, physical examination, and laboratory procedures (see Chapters 3–5). The tests specifically considered in this chapter are those that identify lipid disorders, hypertension, abdominal aortic aneurysm, asymptomatic coronary artery disease, certain cancers (breast, colorectal, cervical, prostate, lung), diabetes, osteoporosis, hepatitis C infection, and tuberculosis (TB). Approaches to abnormal results for screening for sexually transmitted infections and for neonatal screening are discussed in Chapters 13 and 18, respectively. Topics not addressed in this book are the evaluation of abnormalities found through prenatal screening, nonrecommended screening interventions, tests used to evaluate specific patient complaints (e.g., thyroid function studies to evaluate fatigue), and chronic disease monitoring.

This chapter presents the recommended steps for initiating appropriate management. The reader should consult the references and "Suggested Readings" at the end of this chapter for more detailed information. For the most part, the "Suggested Readings" contain or reflect formal guidelines produced by relevant national medical organizations. With medical advances over time, recommended workups will change and guidelines will be updated. By performing literature and Internet searches using the "Suggested Readings" as a starting point, the reader should be able to easily update outdated references.

A general limitation of recommendations concerning the evaluation and management of abnormalities detected by screening tests is that the supporting evidence for intervention may be less rigorous than the evidence justifying screening itself. Management recommendations often rely on expert opinion or only apply to select patient populations rather than being totally evidence based. This chapter compiles and combines recommendations from many sources.

Screening tests do not necessarily lead directly to the alleviation of symptoms but instead are focused on the immediate goal of identifying patients at increased risk of disease, either for further testing to clarify the diagnosis or for identifying a modifiable risk factor that affects the probability of developing disease. For example, blood pressure (BP) screening is meant to identify hypertension, a risk factor for cardiovascular disease. Patients may not necessarily derive an immediate benefit from treating hypertension; they may not feel better with a lower BP. For benefits to occur (i.e., a reduction in cardiovascular risks), treatments must be maintained and monitored for long periods. Most often, patient education and a long-term relationship centered on patient-clinician collaboration are essential to ensure that management of the condition identified by the screening test results in an improved health outcome.

In addition, risk factors are interdependent. Interpretation of one test result and appropriate next steps may be influenced by the awareness of other coexisting risk factors (e.g., the appropriate goal for lipid-lowering therapy depends on the patient's overall cardiovascular risk profile). Often, management must extend beyond dealing with the identified condition (e.g., in a hypertensive patient the priority is not only BP control but also the control of other cardiovascular disease risk factors, such as smoking, diet, physical inactivity, and serum lipid levels).

Although the results of some screening tests are binary—"positive" or "negative"—they do not necessarily determine whether the patient has or does not have the target condition. False positives often occur more frequently than true positives, for two reasons: First, screening tests are designed to "cast a wide net" to ensure that patients with the target condition are not missed (i.e., some tests have relatively high sensitivity, but low specificity). Second, the disease prevalence in asymptomatic populations is often low. For example, the positive predictive value of a positive fecal occult blood test (FOBT)—the chance that a patient with a positive test has colorectal cancer or a polyp—is only 10%[1] (90% of positive results are falsely positive). The intent of the FOBT is not to diagnose disease but rather to identify patients most likely to benefit from the more definitive but invasive test, colonoscopy. Likewise, a negative bimodal screening test rarely rules out the target condition; the FOBT test detects only about one-third of colorectal cancers or abnormal polyps.

Other types of screening tests measure continuous variables (e.g., BP or prostate-specific antigen [PSA] concentration). For these conditions, the risk increases as the abnormal value changes, but not necessarily in a linear manner. A threshold or "cutoff" value is used to define "normal" and "abnormal." The cutoff value at which intervention is recommended is often selected arbitrarily, depending on epidemiologic information, the morbidity of the disease, the risks of further intervention, and the efficacy of the interventions contemplated. For example, a common definition of an abnormal PSA test is a value greater than 4 ng/mL. Patients with lower PSA values can also have prostate cancer, but the risk that they do is lower. The likelihood that a patient will have a positive biopsy for prostate cancer is 15% with a PSA value less than 4 ng/mL, whereas the likelihood is 25% for values equal to or greater than 4 ng/mL.[2] A slight change in a result that carries little biological significance may cross the threshold and make the difference in labeling the patient as having the target condition. For example, a BP of 120/70 is normal but a slightly higher reading (e.g., 130//80) now classifies the patient as being hypertensive.

Steps in Responding to an Abnormal Screening Result

Responses to an abnormal screening test result should include the following:

1. Verifying the accuracy of the result
2. Interpreting the result's significance in the context of the individual patient
3. Applying the result to the diagnostic criteria for the target condition
4. Developing a plan for assessment of other risk factors for the target condition
5. Setting treatment goals
6. Recommending a treatment plan
7. Implementing longitudinal follow-up and monitoring

Steps 1 and 2 may include repeating the test or looking for clinical factors that may influence the significance of the result. It may include verifying that the patient was fasting when the blood was drawn, had been following proper dietary restrictions, or had not been taking medications that might interfere with the test result. Step 3 emphasizes that an abnormality on screening is not tantamount to a diagnosis. Step 4 places the findings in the broader context of the patient's overall risks and other priorities. Steps 5 and 6 apply only if the results represent true disease or indicate that the patient is at greater risk of developing disease and if there is evidence that treatment is beneficial. They also present an opportunity for patient education about risk reduction. Step 7 is often necessary regardless of whether the results are abnormal, although the frequency and method of follow-up depend on prior test findings. There are many barriers to reaching appropriate closure on normal and abnormal test results (see Table 19.1). The ability of screening to achieve its proven health benefits may ultimately be lost if these barriers are inadequately addressed and managed.

TABLE 19.1 Barriers to Closure in Appropriately Responding to Screening Test Results

Results of Test Not Reviewed by Clinician

- Test recommended by clinician but not obtained by patient because of disinterest, resistance, or lack of barriers
- Test obtained in another setting but results not forwarded to clinician
- Results filed in patient's chart without review by clinician

Knowledge Deficit

- Clinician unaware of guidelines, recommendations, or the current literature
- Clinician unaware of other patient factors that influence patient's risk profile

Resistance to Diagnosis by Patient or Clinician (Clinical Inertia)

GENERAL PATIENT EDUCATION

Because an abnormal result on a screening test may for the first time label a previously well individual as ill, the clinician should address the patient's readiness to accept the label or recommended interventions. Ideally, much of the groundwork required to help patients understand abnormal screening test results should be accomplished before the performance of the test. Patients should not be asked to undergo a test without understanding the implications of an abnormal result. In practice, however, it is quite common for patients to be subjected to testing without a full understanding of the downstream consequences. It is therefore necessary to educate the patient about the chances that an abnormal result is falsely positive, the diagnostic steps that will follow, initial treatments if the diagnosis is confirmed, and any prognostic implications. Even when clinicians attempt to provide this information before performing tests, patients may only partially grasp or retain the details. To assist patients and clinicians in managing these considerations, high-quality, accessible patient education and motivation tools are essential. Recommended resources are listed at the end of this chapter (see "Resources—Patient Education Materials").

SCREENING TESTS FOR CARDIOVASCULAR RISK FACTORS

The modifiable risk factors for coronary artery disease—hypertension, hyperlipidemia, smoking, diabetes, and obesity—are both continuous and additive. Identification of any risk factor for cardiovascular disease should prompt a search for the presence of other risk factors. This will allow for a more accurate estimation of the patient's total cardiovascular risk, the adoption of appropriate therapeutic targets, and a determination of the proper intensity of therapy for risk factor modification. The principal cardiovascular abnormalities considered here involve BP, serum lipids, and metabolic syndrome. Screening for diabetes is covered on Chapter 5. Chapters that discuss counseling about other cardiovascular risk factors include those on exercise, nutrition, obesity, and smoking (see Chapters 7–10).

An increased risk of cardiovascular disease is associated with other biochemical markers, including elevated high-sensitivity C-reactive protein, homocysteine, and uric acid levels. The use of high-sensitivity C-reactive protein to screen the general population for atherosclerotic cardiovascular disease (ASCVD) is controversial. However, these tests may have a role in determining therapeutic options for patients with borderline lipid values or for those with early cardiovascular disease but no identifiable risk factors.[3]

Hypertension

Abnormal Screening Results

In 2017, the American College of Cardiology (ACC) and the American Heart Association (AHA) released a new comprehensive practice guideline on the prevention, detection, evaluation, and management of hypertension in adults.[4] Using evidence from randomized controlled clinical trials, the guideline updated the 2003 Seventh Report of the Joint National Committee and the 2013 Expert Panel Report (Fig. 19.1).

The guideline gives uniform definitions for elevated BP and hypertension for all patients, without regard to age or comorbid condition status. Normal BP is now categorized as systolic BP (SBP) under 120 mm Hg and diastolic BP (DBP) under 80 mm Hg, elevated is SBP 120 to 129 mm Hg *or* DBP 80 to 89 mm Hg, state 1 hypertension is SBP 130 to 139 mm Hg *or* DBP 80 to 89 mm Hg, and state 2 hypertension is SBP over or equal to 140 mm Hg *or* DBP over or equal to 90 mm Hg. Stage 1 hypertension was formerly classified as "prehypertension." Reclassifying patients who were previously deemed healthy as having hypertension increases the percentage of U.S. adults diagnosed with hypertension from 32% to 46% of the population.[5]

Initial Diagnostic Strategy

Clinicians should encourage home or ambulatory BP monitoring to both establish the diagnosis of hypertension and adjust antihypertensive medications. The new guidelines emphasize the importance of out-of-office BP measurements and educating patients how to accurately accomplish and record this.

Risk factors for ASCVD, such as smoking, diabetes, hyperlipidemia, obesity, low fitness, poor diet, low fitness, and sleep apnea, should be

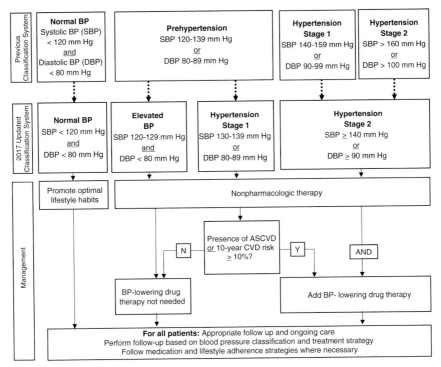

Figure 19.1 Updated classification and management of high blood pressure (BP) in adults. *ASCVD*, atherosclerotic cardiovascular disease; *CVD*, cardiovascular disease. Reprinted with permission Whelton PK, Carey RM, Aronow WS, et al. 2017. ACC/AHA/AAPA/ABC/ACPM/AGS/APhA/ASH/ASPC/NMA/PCNA guideline for the prevention, detection, evaluation, and management of high blood pressure in adults: a report of the American College of Cardiology/American Heart Association Task Force on Clinical Practice Guidelines. *Hypertension*. 2017. *J Am Coll Cardiol*. doi:10.1016/k.jacc.2017.11.006.

screened for. Basic laboratory testing in patients with elevated BP or stage 1 hypertension includes fasting blood glucose, complete blood count, fasting lipid panel, basic metabolic panel, thyroid stimulating hormone, urinalysis, and electrocardiogram.

Screening for secondary causes of hypertension (Table 19.2) should be considered in patients with new-onset or uncontrolled hypertension, patients who have a spike of BPs with no apparent cause after being well controlled, failure to achieve target BPs despite appropriate medication management, failure to control high BP when on three or more medications. A secondary cause may also be suspected based on the patient's age, pertinent findings on the history or physical examination, the severity of hypertension, or initial laboratory findings.

TABLE 19.2 Evaluation for Secondary Causes of Hypertension

Cause	Suggestive Findings	Evaluation
Renovascular disease	Onset before age 30 yr or after age 55 yr, abdominal bruit	Doppler flow study; magnetic resonance angiography
Chronic kidney disease	Risk factors for renal disease	Estimated glomerular filtration rate
Pheochromocytoma	Abrupt factors for renal disease	Estimated glomerular filtration rate
Coarctation of aorta	Early onset, characteristic murmur	Computerized tomographic angiography
Sleep apnea	Obesity, history from sleep partner	Sleep study with monitoring of oxygen saturation
Cushing syndrome	Obesity, striae, glucose intolerance	History, dexamethasone suppression
Primary aldosteronism	Hypokalemia	24-hr aldosterone level
Drug or substance induced[a]	History of use	History, observation when not using substance
Thyroid or parathyroid disease	Tachycardia; skin, hair, or nail changes; anxiety; tremor	Thyroid-stimulating hormone and serum parathyroid hormone levels

[a]Examples of suspect drugs include sympathomimetics (e.g., cocaine, amphetamines, ephedra), steroids, overuse of alcohol, licorice, tobacco, oral contraceptives, nonsteroidal anti-inflammatory drugs, erythropoietin, tacrolimus, cyclosporine.

Adapted from National Heart, Lung, Blood Institute. *Complete Report: The Seventh Report of the Joint National Committee of Prevention, Detection, Evaluation, and Treatment of High Blood Pressure.* National Heart, Lung, and Blood Institute. Available at: http://nhlbi.nih.gov/guide-lines/hypertension/. Accessed February 2007.

Treatment Options

All patients should be counseled about hypertension-ameliorating lifestyle modifications, which include smoking cessation, normalizing weight to a body mass index less than $25 \text{ kg}/\text{m}^2$, increasing physical activity to 30 minutes a day or moderate exercise most days of the week, limiting alcohol consumption to maximum of two drinks a day in most men and one drink a day in women, and adopting the Dietary Approach to Stop Hypertension (DASH) diet (Table 19.3).

TABLE 19.3   Best Proven Nonpharmacologic Interventions for Prevention and Treatment of Hypertension

Nonpharmacologic Intervention	Dose	Approximate Impact on SBP	
		Hypertension (mm Hg)	Normotension (mm Hg)
Weight loss	Weight/body fat	Ideal weight is best goal but at least 1 kg reduction in body weight for most adults who are overweight. Expect about 1 mm Hg for every 1 kg reduction in body weight	−5	−2/3
Healthy diet	DASH dietary pattern	Diet rich in fruits, vegetables, whole grains, and low-fat dairy products with reduced content of saturated and trans fat	−11	−3
Reduced intake of dietary sodium	Dietary sodium	<1500 mg/d is optimal goal but at least 1000 mg/d reduction in most adults	−5/6	−2/3
Enhanced intake of dietary potassium	Dietary potassium	3500–5000 mg/d, preferably by consumption of a diet rich in potassium	−4/5	−2

(Continued)

TABLE 19.3   Best Proven Nonpharmacologic Interventions for Prevention and Treatment of Hypertension   (Continued)

	Nonpharmacologic Intervention	Dose	Approximate Impact on SBP	
			Hypertension (mm Hg)	Normotension (mm Hg)
Physical activity	Aerobic	• 120–150 min/wk • 65%–75% heart rate reserve	–5/8	–2/4
	Dynamic resistance	• 90–150 min/wk • 50%–80% 1 rep maximum • 6 exercises, 3 sets/exercises, 10 repetitions/set	–4	–2
	Isometric resistance	• 4 × 2 min (hand grip), 1 min rest between exercises, 30%–40% maximum voluntary contraction, 3 sessions/wk • 8–10 wk	–5	–4
Moderation in alcohol consumption	Alcohol consumption	• In individuals who drink alcohol, reduce alcohol[a] to: • Men: <2 drinks daily • Women <1 drink daily	–4	–3

Type dosage and expected impact on BP in adults with a normal BP with hypertension.
[a]In the Unites states, one "standard" drink contains roughly 14 g of pure alcohol, which is typically found in 12 oz of regular beer (usually 5% alcohol), 5 oz of wine (usually 12% alcohol), and 1.5 oz of distilled spirits (usually 40% alcohol).
SBP, systolic blood pressure.
Reprinted with Permission J. Am Coll Cardiol. 2017:23976. doi:10.1016/j.jacc.2017.07.745.

The current ACC/AHA guideline calls for more aggressive thresholds and goals for treatment compared with previous guidelines. Treatment decisions are based on an individual's underlying ASCVD risk, comorbid conditions, and hypertension classification. By focusing on underlying 10-year estimated ASCVD risk and BP elevation, clinicians and patients will have coherent goals to achieve. Focusing on cardiovascular risk reduction using ASCVD risk calculators combined with the new definition of stage 1 hypertension will hopefully translate into earlier interventions and lower cardiovascular event rates. Patients with stage 1 hypertension, who have an estimated 10-year ASCVD of 10% or higher, should be given pharmacotherapy, along with lifestyle modifications. For patients with stage 1 hypertension with lower ASCVD risk, lifestyle modifications should be advised and medication started if the patient reaches stage 2 hypertension (140/90 mm Hg).

Patients with stage 1 hypertension who have known ASCVD or diabetes should be given antihypertensive medication, regardless of 10-year ASCVD risk calculation. Initial first-line treatment options are thiazide diuretics (guideline recommends chlorthalidone (12.5–25 mg because of the long half-life and proven reduction of cardiovascular disease [CVD] risk), angiotensin-converting enzyme inhibitors, angiotensin-receptor blockers, and calcium channel blockers. Beta-blockers are no longer considered first-line therapy for hypertensive patients with any coexisting conditions requiring beta-blocker therapy.

For stage 2 hypertensive patients, two first-line medications are recommended. The new guideline advocates for initial combination medications to improve adherence. Initial agents for black hypertensive patients include calcium channel blockers and thiazide diuretics over renin-angiotensin system blockers (Table 19.4).

A useful table detailing all the available oral antihypertensive agents can be accessed at Guidelines Made Simple, a Selection of Tables and Figures at http://www.acc.org/education-and-meetings/image-and-slide-gallery/media-detail?id=BDA0F36F3160426FAB2E784B82E2629A.

Specific treatment recommendations for hypertensive patients with other comorbidities such as chronic kidney disease, previous stroke, and cerebral vascular disease are beyond the scope of this chapter, but guidance can be found in the ACC/AHA complete report.

Follow-up

For stage 1 high BP with less than 10% ASCVD risk, recommendations include lifestyle changes, out-of-office BP monitoring, and repeat BP evaluation within 3 to 6 months. For stage 1 hypertension with 10% or greater ASCVD risk, recommendations include combination lifestyle changes and antihypertensive medications, out-of-office BP monitoring and logging, and repeat BP monitoring in 1 month. Annual validation of patients' home BP monitoring machines is also recommended by the new guideline.

TABLE 19.4   Strategies to Dose Antihypertensive Drugs

Strategy	Description	Detail
A	Start one drug, titrate to maximum dose, and then add a second drug	If goal blood pressure (BP) is not achieved with the initial drug, titrate the dose of the initial drug up to the maximum recommended dose to achieve goal BP. If goal BP is not achieved with the use of one drug despite titration to the maximum recommended dose, add a second drug from the list (thiazide-type diuretic, CCB, ACEI, or ARB) and titrate up to the maximum recommended dose of the second drug to achieve goal BP. If goal BP is not achieved with 2 drugs, select a third drug from the list (thiazide-type diuretic, CCB, ACEI, or ARB), avoiding the combined use of ACEI and ARB. Titrate the third drug up to the maximum recommended dose to achieve goal BP
B	Start one drug and then add a second drug before achieving maximum drug dose of the initial drug	Start with one drug, then add a second drug before achieving the maximum recommended dose of the initial drug, then titrate both drugs up to the maximum recommended doses of both to achieve goal BP. If goal BP is not achieved with 2 drugs, select a third drug from the list (thiazide-type diuretic, CCB, ACEI, or ARB), avoiding the combined use of ACEI and ARB. Titrate the third drug up to the maximum recommended dose to achieve goal BP
C	Begin with 2 drugs at the same time, either as 2 separate pills or as a single pill combination	Initiate therapy with 2 drugs simultaneously, either as 2 separate drugs or as a single pill combination. Some committee members recommend starting therapy with ≥2 drugs when SBP is >160 mm Hg and/or DBP is >100 mm Hg, or if SBP is >20 mm Hg above goal and/or DBP is >10 mm Hg above goal. If goal BP is not achieved with 2 drugs, select a third drug from the list (thiazide-type diuretic, CCB, ACEI, or ARB), avoiding the combined use of ACEI and ARB. Titrate the third drug up to the maximum recommended dose

This table is not meant to exclude other agents within the classes of antihypertensive medications that have been recommended but reflects those agents and dosing used in randomized controlled trials that demonstrated improved outcomes.

ACEI, angiotensin-converting enzyme inhibitor; ARB, angiotensin receptor blocker; BP, blood pressure; CCB, calcium channel blocker; DBP, diastolic blood pressure; SBP, systolic blood pressure.

Reprinted with permission. James PA, Oparil S, Carter BL, et al. 2014 Evidence-based guideline for the management of high blood pressure in adults. Report from the panel members appointed to the eighth Joint National Committee (JNC 8). *JAMA*. 2014;311(5):507-520. doi:10.1001/jama.2013.284427.

Treatment target BP goals for high-risk hypertensive patients with known ASCVD or patients with a 10-year ASCVD risk estimate greater than 10% are less than 130/80 mm Hg.

Before the release of the adjusted classification for hypertension, only 50% of treated hypertensive patients could be considered "under control."[6] By lowering the threshold for what is considered normal BP, clinicians will be further challenged to keep an acceptable proportion of their patients' BPs within acceptable levels.

Lipid Disorders

Initial Diagnostic Strategy

Risk of ASCVD in the population appears to rise steadily with increasing cholesterol levels. Because the benefits of lipid management depend on a patient's overall risk for cardiovascular disease, no single "abnormal" lipid level applies to all patients.

There are numerous guidelines for cholesterol screening with differing recommendation about what age to start screening, how frequently to screen, and when to stop. Unlike previous recommendations, the most recent ACC/AHA guidelines no longer recommend for or against specific target levels for low-density lipoprotein-cholesterol (LDL-C) or non-high-density lipoprotein-cholesterol (HDL-C) in the primary or secondary prevention of ASCVD. Instead they suggest statins for all adults at risk for ASCVD, regardless of LDL-C levels. Secondary causes of hyperlipidemia should be routinely ruled out.

Initial Management Strategy

Lifestyle modifications are essential to reducing cardiovascular event risks, including eating a heart healthy diet, exercising regularly, abstaining from tobacco and avoiding excess weight. The ACC/AHA and the U.S. Preventive Services Task Force (USPSTF) guidelines recommend that clinicians and patients discuss adverse effects, drug interactions, potential benefits, and patient preferences when deciding about statin therapy.[7,8]

With the release of the latest USPSTF's Final Recommendation Statement on Statin Use for the Primary Prevention of Cardiovascular Disease in Adults, the question has shifted from asking which patients should be screened for hyperlipidemia to which patients should be prescribed statin therapy? USPSTF recommends prescribing patients a low to moderate intensity statin if they are between ages 40 and 75 years, without a history of ASCVD, but with at least one CVD risk factor (diabetes, hypertension, smoking, hyperlipidemia) and a calculated 10-year CVD event risk of 10% or greater. Furthermore, they recommended selectively offering a low-intensity to moderate-intensity statin to patients in this same age group, who have no history of ASCVD, at least one CVD risk factor, and a calculated 10-year CVD 10-year event risk of 7.5% to 10%.

The ACC/AHA guidelines support the concept of matching therapy for patient's absolute risk. Four population groups were designated for statin therapy: (1) patients who already have ASCVD, (2) patients with primary LDL-C levels of 190 mg/dL or greater; (3) patients with diabetes mellitus aged 40 to 75 years who have LDL-C levels of 70 to 189 mg/dL but who do not have clinical ASCVD, and (4) patients with an estimated 10-year ASCVD risk of 7.5 mg or greater who do not have clinical ASCVD or diabetes who have LDL-C levels of 70 to 189 mg/dL.

In the first group, patients below the age of 75 years without safety concerns should be maintained on a high-intensity statin; those above 75 years should be on a moderate-intensity statin. In the second group, the goal is to reduce the current LDL-C level by 50%, so a high-intensity statin is recommended. The third group comprising patients with diabetes should be given a moderate-intensity statin except if they have a 10-year ASCVD event risk of over 7.5%; then, they should be offered a high-intensity statin. In the fourth group, estimate the 10-year ASCVD risk every 4 to 6 years and let that result guide treatment choice. Shared decision making should be embraced.

High-intensity statin regimens include atorvastatin at 40- to 80-mg doses or rosuvastatin at 20- to 40-mg doses. The low-intensive and moderate-intensity agents can be found in Table 19.5. The ACC/AHA cholesterol

TABLE 19.5   Statin Regimens Used in Available Trials

Statin	Dose, mg[a]		
	Low	Moderate	High
Atorvastatin		10–20	40–80
Fluvastatin	20–40	40 twice daily	
Fluvastatin extended release		80	
Lovastatin	20	40	
Pitavastatin	1	2–4	
Pravastatin	10–20	40–80	
Rosuvastatin		5–10	20–40
Simvastatin	10	20–40	

[a]Dose categories are from the American College of Cardiology/American Heart Association 2013 guidelines on the treatment of blood cholesterol to reduce atherosclerotic cardiovascular risk in adults.

Reprinted with permission Statin use for the primary prevention of cardiovascular disease in adults US preventive services task force recommendation statement. *JAMA*. 2016;316(19):1997-2007. doi:10.1001/jama.2016.15450.

treatment guidelines found no evidence for any benefit from adding a second lipid-lowering medication to try to reduce LDL-C target levels.

For patients attempting lifestyle modification for hyperlipidemia, serum lipid levels should be rechecked in 3 to 6 months. Once a patient starts taking a lipid-lowering medication, serum cholesterol should be rechecked in 4 to 6 weeks, allowing the regimen time to achieve its full effect. Once the serum cholesterol target has been reached, it is reasonable to monitor lipid levels and liver function every 6 months.

Metabolic Syndrome

Diagnostic Strategy

Metabolic syndrome is a constellation of abnormalities caused by insulin resistance accompanying excessive adipose deposition and function. Think of this diagnosis if a patient has at least three of the following conditions:

- Fasting glucose >100 mg/dL (or receiving drug therapy for hyperglycemia)
- Waist measurement >35 in in women and >40 in in men
- Elevated BP or receiving treatment for hypertension
- Elevated triglycerides or receiving treatment for hypertriglyceridemia
- Low HDL-C: <40 mg/dL in men; <50 mg/dL in women

Management Strategy

Therapy for metabolic syndrome is focused on individual risk factors and begins with therapeutic lifestyle changes.

Abdominal Aortic Aneurysm

Abnormal Screening Results

The USPSTF recommends one-time ultrasound screening for abdominal aortic aneurysm (AAA) in men 65 to 74 years of age who have ever smoked.[9] They recommend against screening in women of any age who have never smoked. The ultrasound measurement of the abdominal aorta diameter over 3 cm or greater is abnormal.

Diagnostic Strategy and Management Recommendations

Most AAAs are asymptomatic until they rupture. Mortality associated with AAA rupture can be as high as 75% to 90%.[10] Depending on a patient's overall health status, an aneurysm equal to or greater than 4.5 cm warrants referral to a vascular specialist for consideration of surgical options. Decisions regarding further imaging and endovascular versus open repair depend on clinical circumstances and local resources and expertise. Patients with symptomatic aneurysms and those whose aneurysms increase in diameter by 0.5 cm or greater within 6 months, regardless of aneurysm diameter should be referred to vascular surgery.[11] Patients with AAA of 3 to 4 cm should undergo ultrasonography either annually or every several years to monitor for size. Smoking cessation should be advised for all patients. The proper management (intervention or surveillance) of small aneurysms (4–5.5 cm) is controversial. Treatment with lipid-lowering medications appears to slow AAA growth rates. However, the efficacy and role of beta-blockers remains unclear; further research is needed.

Tests for Asymptomatic Coronary Artery Disease

Tests to detect asymptomatic coronary artery disease, for example, resting electrocardiography, exercise stress testing, and electron beam coronary artery calcium scoring, are available but are not recommended for asymptomatic average-risk populations. Nonetheless, the clinician will frequently encounter patients who present with abnormalities found on one or more of these tests, and further follow-up with more invasive testing may be necessary. Exercise stress testing, stress echocardiography, myocardial perfusion scintigraphy, or cardiac catheterization can clarify the presence of significant disease. Treatment and follow-up should be dictated by the presence of significant clinical findings. Consultation with a cardiologist is frequently necessary.

SCREENING RESULTS SUGGESTIVE OF CANCER

Clinicians can encounter a range of findings from cancer screening tests that include negative results, the presence of an abnormal finding that *suggests* the possibility of malignancy (e.g., positive FOBT), or a result that is diagnostic of cancer (e.g., a biopsy report indicating invasive carcinoma). In a patient diagnosed with cancer, coordination among numerous health professionals may be necessary in both the evaluation of abnormal cancer screening test results and the delivery of the indicated medical care. The potential team includes medical specialists (e.g., surgeons, pulmonologists, gynecologists, gastroenterologists, urologists, medical oncologists, and radiation oncologists), pain specialists, dieticians, home care staff, social service workers, and counseling and support groups. The patient struggling with cancer evaluation or treatment may be overwhelmed by and tends to focus solely on that problem. The primary care clinician should also address the other aspects of primary care, including other preventive services, and is responsible for the long-term care of cancer survivors.

Breast Cancer

Abnormal Screening Tests

Abnormal findings on a clinical breast examination that might indicate malignancy include a palpable mass; dimpling; nipple retraction or discharge; rashes and change in skin texture, such as peau d'orange; and axillary lymphadenopathy. Potential abnormal findings on a mammogram include calcification, cystic masses, and solid masses.

TABLE 19.6 Indications for Breast Ultrasound as Diagnostic Adjunct to Mammography

- To better characterize mass seen on mammogram
- To identify cystic mass and guide fine needle biopsy or core biopsy
- In patients with dense breasts, to elucidate a lesion when mass is palpable on physical examination but not seen on mammogram
- To measure and clip a lesion before neoadjuvant chemotherapy in patients with large or locally advanced tumors

Diagnostic Strategy

Most breast cancers are detected with abnormal mammograms but not all abnormal findings end up being cancer. A new type of mammogram, referred to as "3D mammography" or breast tomosynthesis gives the radiologist a three-dimensional view of the breast. When the results of a screening mammogram are abnormal, additional testing is necessary, usually comprising additional mammographic views or targeted ultrasonography (Table 19.6) or breast MRI to establish the necessity for biopsy. Interpreting the radiographic criteria that define abnormalities on a mammogram is beyond the purview of primary care clinicians and is not discussed here. Because mammograms have a poor positive predictive value, patients should be counseled that an abnormal mammogram usually does not mean that breast cancer is present. In community settings, only 8% to 21% of abnormal mammograms are indicative of breast cancer.[12]

The evaluation of a palpable breast mass depends on the patient's age, the history of the lesion, and characteristics of the lesion on examination. Further diagnostic tests that can be undertaken include imaging (ultrasonography or mammography) and obtaining a tissue sample (fine needle aspiration, core needle biopsy, or incisional or excisional surgical biopsy). Because mammography fails to detect 10% of breast cancers, tissue diagnosis of a palpable mass should be pursued even if a mammogram is normal.

Women who are identified as having breast cancer on the basis of tissue diagnosis will need a staging evaluation to determine the next appropriate treatment steps. This evaluation includes a comprehensive history and physical examination, chest radiography, liver function tests, the measurement of serum tumor markers, and breast MRI in select patients.

Treatment Options

Noncancerous breast lesions may not require further treatment. Treatment for localized lobular and ductal breast carcinomas entails some combination of surgical excision, lymph node dissection, radiation, and hormonal therapy (e.g., tamoxifen). Radiation therapy and chemotherapy may also be beneficial for women with more extensive breast cancers. For many women, either breast conserving therapy (lumpectomy and radiation therapy) or a modified radical mastectomy may be equally appropriate. Less aggressive therapy may be warranted for in situ breast disease, but this is an area of ongoing controversy.

Colorectal Cancer

Abnormal Screening Tests

Detection of a polyp (hyperplastic, adenomatous, or villous) by colonoscopy, a positive FOBT or fecal immunochemical test (FIT), or a positive stool DNA requires further investigation to rule out cancer.[13]

Diagnostic Strategy

All patients who have positive FOBT, FIT, or stool DNA should have a colonoscopy. Patients who refuse screening colonoscopy should be educated that they need to be screened every year with FIT. All colonic polyps encountered on colonoscopy should be completely removed and sent for pathologic evaluation.

Although 80% of colorectal cancers arise from adenomatous polyps, an adenomatous polyp of less than 1 cm in diameter has less than 1% chance of progressing to cancer in 10 years. An adenomatous polyp greater than 1 cm has a 10% chance of becoming malignant in the same period. Hyperplastic polyps, which are normal variants, are not precancerous, nor do they portend an increased risk for precancerous polyps or cancer elsewhere in the colon. The American Cancer Society and a consortium of gastroenterological organizations have issued recommendations on when to repeat a colonoscopy following abnormal endoscopy findings[14] (Table 19.7).

The number, size, and histological features of adenomas must be weighed when considering postpolypectomy surveillance. Colonoscopy follow-up in 3 years is recommended in patients with three or more adenomas. Polyp size classification includes diminutive (<5 mm), small (between 6 and 9 mm), and large (>10 mm). Patients with adenomas larger than 10 mm, any serrated polyp larger than 10 mm, any tubulovillous or villous adenoma, or any adenoma with high-grade dysplasia should have follow-up colonoscopy in 3 years.

Individuals with normal screening tests or hyperplastic polyps can be retested using any of the recommended colorectal cancer screening tests at the same intervals recommended for low-risk individuals.

Patients with colorectal masses should have a partial or complete surgical biopsy to rule out malignancy. Patients diagnosed with malignancy will need a further evaluation for staging, which may include surgical resection for the determination of the depth and extent of lesion penetration, blood work (complete blood count, liver function tests, and carcinoembryonic antigen), and imaging studies to determine metastasis.

TABLE 19.7   Postpolypectomy Surveillance

Colonoscopy findings and recommended scheduling of follow-up colonoscopy are as follows:

No polyps	10 yr
Small (<10 mm) hyperplastic polyps in rectum or sigmoid	10 yr
3–10 small (<10 mm) tubular adenomas	5–10 yr
3–10 tubular adenomas	3 yr
10 adenomas	<3 yr
One or more tubular adenomas >10 mm	3 yr
One or more villous adenomas	3 yr
Adenoma with high-grade dysplasia	3 yr

For serrated lesions, recommended surveillance intervals are as follows:

Sessile serrate polyp(s) <10 mm with no dysplasia	5 yr
Sessile serrated polyp(s) >10 mm with no dysplasia	3 yr
Sessile serrated polyp with dysplasia	1 yr
Traditional serrated adenoma	1 yr
Serrated polyposis syndrome	1 yr

Adapted with permission from Lieberman DA et al. Guidelines for colonoscopy surveillance after screening and polypectomy: a consensus update by the US multi-society task force on colorectal cancer. *Gastroenterology*. 2012;143(3):844-857.

Treatment Options

Patients who have localized resectable colon cancer should have colectomy with en bloc removal of regional lymph nodes. Whether adjuvant chemotherapy and/or chemoradiation therapy is advised depends on the stage of colon cancer. The surveillance for patients with resected colon cancer (stage II and III) entails review of medical history, physical examination, carcinoembryonic antigen assays, colonoscopy, and abdominal and chest computed tomography (CT).

Follow-up

It is common to find polyps during a colonoscopy; they are present in 25% of persons by age 50 years and in 50% by age 75 years. Accordingly, an essential role of the primary care clinician is to ensure that patients receive the appropriate follow-up after abnormal findings. Repeating colonoscopy too infrequently may create an opportunity for invasive cancer to progress, but repeating the colonoscopy too frequently may subject patients to unnecessary risks.

Cervical Cancer

Abnormal Screening Results

Red or white lesions found on cervical inspection raise concerns about the presence of either cervical atypia or cancer. PAP smear abnormalities include reactive and inflammatory changes (variants of normal); squamous cell abnormalities, such as atypical cells of unknown significance (ASCUS); low-grade squamous intraepithelial lesions (LGSIL); high-grade squamous intraepithelial lesions; and glandular abnormalities, such as atypical glandular cells of unknown significance. The connection of cervical intraepithelial neoplasia, grades 2 and 3 (CIN 2,3), to cervical cancer and to human papillomavirus (HPV) infection is well established. Since 2014, when the U.S. Food and Drug Administration approved HPV DNA testing for primary cervical cancer screening, some authorities recommend cotesting with PAP cytology and HPV testing every 5 years for women between the ages of 30 and 65 years.[15]

Diagnostic Strategy

As surveillance strategies for cervical cancer screening are based on a patient's age, screening history, risk factors, and individual choice, the determination of further workup is also influenced by these considerations.

For women with an ASCUS PAP test who are 25 years or older, HPV DNA test should be performed if cotesting was not done. In patients with ASCUS or LGSIL, HPV status helps determine whether a patient should undergo colposcopy or early repeat PAP testing. If high-risk HPV is positive, the patient should undergo colposcopy. If colposcopy is inconclusive, endocervical sampling may be necessary. Patients who test negative for HPV with an LGSIL PAP test can wait 1 year for another PAP test and high-risk HPV test.

Conservative follow-up (cotesting in 12 mo) is acceptable with women with a positive HPV test and negative cytology. If the HPV testing remains positive and/or if cytology shows ASCUS or greater cytologic abnormality, colposcopy is advisable (Fig. 19.2). Atypical glandular cells of unknown significance found on PAP smear heightens concern for malignancy and requires endometrial and endocervical sampling and colposcopy.

Treatment Options

Observation versus treatment are the two strategies for treating CIN, based on the risk of the patient developing cancer. Surveillance using cervical cytology, HPV testing, and colposcopy are acceptable for patients with lesions that are likely to regress (CIN 1).

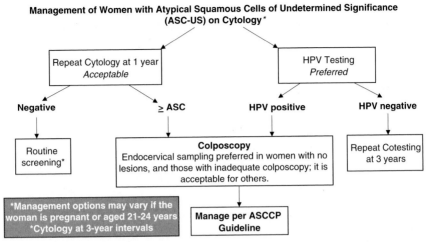

Figure 19.2 Management of women with atypical squamous cells of undetermined significance (ASC-US) on cytology. *HPV,* human papillomavirus. From *J Lower Genital Tract Dis.* 17(5), with the permission of ASCCP © American Society for Colposcopy and Cervical Pathology; 2013.

Treatment decisions are usually based on the pathology results from colposcopic biopsy. CIN 2,3 are more likely to be treated with cervical excision or ablation, although observation is an option in patients of childbearing age wishing future children.

Patients with high-grade squamous intraepithelial lesions have a high likelihood of having CIN 2,3 and may warrant an immediate excisional procedure or colposcopy with endocervical sampling. With the exception of young women and pregnant women, patients with CIN 2,3 should have excision or ablation of the cervical transformation zone, assuming that the colposcopy is adequate. Hysterectomy is infrequently indicated. An excisional procedure should be performed for patients who have had inadequate colposcopies or recurrent CIN 2,3 or endocervical sampling with CIN 2,3. Clinicians are advised to refer to the guidelines from the American Society for Colposcopy and Cervical Pathology for information about management of young women and pregnant women.[16]

Follow-up

Patients aged 25 years or older with CIN 1 should have repeat PAP and HPV cotesting in 12 months. If both are normal, they can go back to routine cytology and HPV screening every 3 years. If either of the cotests is abnormal, the patient should be referred for colposcopy.

Following excision or ablation, patients with CIN 2,3 should have PAP and HPV cotesting every 12 to 24 months. If both tests are negative, the interval for next testing is 3 years. At that time, if both tests are negative, the patient can resume routine screening, which should continue for at least 20 years, even if the patient is older than 65 years. If there is a positive high-risk HPV or abnormal cytology in patients who have been treated for CIN 2,3, they should have another colposcopy with endocervical sampling.[17]

Prostate Cancer

Abnormal Screening Tests

A prostate nodule palpable on digital rectal examination and a PSA value of 4 ng/mL or greater are considered abnormal. A PSA velocity, or rate of increase, greater than 0.7 to 1.0 ng/mL/yr is also considered abnormal.

Diagnostic Strategy

The evaluation of a prostate mass includes measuring the PSA level and considering a prostate biopsy. The evaluation of an abnormal PSA value can include (1) observation (doing nothing immediately), (2) measuring the free to total PSA ratio, (3) rechecking the PSA in 3 to 6 months, or (4) performing a prostate biopsy. The most appropriate diagnostic step should be determined jointly between a patient and clinician. The clinician should use a shared or informed decision-making process to review the false-positive rate of PSA screening and the downstream implications of the workup and to gauge how aggressively the patient wishes to evaluate the abnormal results.

Considerations influencing next steps include, but are not limited to, patient preferences and beliefs (e.g., beliefs about the benefits of early treatment, beliefs about the harms of treatment, and comfort with uncertainty), the likelihood that the elevated value could represent another condition (e.g., benign prostatic hypertrophy), and the patient's overall health and life expectancy. More aggressive diagnostic steps (such as prostate biopsy) may be warranted for patients who are at increased risk of prostate cancer (e.g., marked elevation in PSA concentration, suspicious symptoms, a family history of prostate cancer, or African American race), men with a relatively long life expectancy (and therefore at greater risk of developing complications from prostate cancer), and patients who are particularly concerned that they might have prostate cancer (and are willing to tolerate the risks associated with diagnosis and treatment of prostate cancer).

For patients at lower risk of experiencing complications from prostate cancer, or for those with greater apprehensions about unnecessary diagnostic or therapeutic procedures, a more cautious approach is indicated. For example, the clinician might initially measure the free to total PSA ratio and, if it is normal, recheck the PSA level in 3 to 6 months. This less aggressive approach is supported by evidence that men with prostate cancer who defer treatment demonstrate no increase in mortality from prostate cancer for 8 to 15 years.[18] A 6- to 12-month observation period to assess the persistence of a PSA elevation over time appears reasonable.

Treatment Options

Treatments for prostate cancer are dictated by the Gleason score assigned to the biopsy specimen (the score is a rating of cell pathology based on histologic characteristics, ranging from 2 to 10, with higher scores assigned to more aggressive cancers), whether the cancer has expanded beyond the prostatic capsule, the age of the patient, and the patient's personal preferences. For cancers confined to the prostate, treatment options include watchful waiting, implantation of radioactive seeds, external beam radiation, or prostatectomy. More aggressive treatments have greater risks of side effects, such as incontinence or impotence. Radiation, chemotherapy, and/or antitestosterone therapy may be indicated for cancers that have extended beyond the prostatic capsule. Side effects of various forms of treatment should be considered in selecting the appropriate management.

Follow-up

Men with PSA abnormalities should have their PSA rechecked every 3 to 6 months until the value has normalized, an alternative diagnosis is established (e.g., benign prostate hypertrophy), or a determination is made to proceed further with diagnostic evaluation(s). Similarly, men treated for prostate cancer should have their PSA rechecked every 3 to 6 months for 1 to 2 years. Beyond that time, it is sufficient to recheck the PSA annually. Further research is needed to establish evidence-based models of follow-up care for men with prostate cancer.

Lung Cancer

Lung cancer is the leading cause of death from cancer in both men and women. Annual low-dose computed tomography (LDCT) of the lungs is currently recommended to screen for lung cancer in adults aged 55 to 80 years who have a 30-pack-year smoking history and currently smoke or have quit within the past 15 years. LDCT is useful in detecting early-stage non–small cell lung cancer (NSCLC). Patients have a better prognosis if NSCLC is caught early and treated with surgical resection.[19]

Diagnostic Strategy

If a small lesion is visualized on LDCT and the patient is considered low risk for lung cancer, repeat testing is determined by the size of the nodule. If the nodule is between 6 and 8 mm, repeat CT scan to reassess the nodule is usually ordered in 6 to 12 months. If there is no increase in size, CT scan can be delayed for 18 to 24 months. For low-risk patients with a nodule over 8 mm in diameter, there are three diagnostic options: (1) repeat CT scan in 3 months, (2) consider positron-emission tomography/CT scan, (3) consider biopsy instead of CT scan.

For patients at high risk for lung cancer (smokers; exposure to asbestos, radon, uranium), the size of the lesion also determines the next diagnostic tests. If a nodule is smaller than 6 mm, repeat CT scan in 12 months. If there is no increase in size, no further routine follow-up is recommended.

Treatment Options

The most important intervention to prevent NSCLC is smoking cessation. Screening for lung cancer is viewed as an adjunct to quitting smoking.[20] The Centers for Disease Control and Prevention and the National Institutes of Health have useful websites that contain numerous resources, including smoking "quit lines," that provide behavioral counseling and support at https://www.cdc.gov/tobacco/quit_smoking/index.htm and https://smokefree.gov/. Combining medications with counseling has shown to increase cessation rates. If the results of screening LDCT are suspicious for cancer, referral to oncology and thoracic surgery is necessary.

Follow-up

Diligent follow-up is important in this high-risk population; they should be screened annually by LDCT. False-positive LDCT occurs in a significant proportion of screened patients, necessitating further imaging and periodically invasive procedures.

SCREENING RESULTS SUGGESTIVE OF ENDOCRINE AND METABOLIC DISORDERS

Diabetes

Abnormal Screening Results

A fasting blood glucose level of 126 mg/dL or greater or a random plasma glucose level of 200 mg/dL or greater are considered abnormally high. A1C of equal or greater than 6.5% is diagnostic of diabetes. In patients who are symptomatic, a random plasma glucose level of 200 mg/dL or higher is diagnostic. Prediabetes describes patients who have elevated glucose levels that do not meet the criteria for diabetes. A fasting glucose level of 100 to 125 mg/dL or A1C of 5.7% to 6.4% indicates prediabetes (Table 19.8).

Diagnostic Strategy

Typically type 1 diabetes mellitus can be differentiated from type 2 diabetes based on age and history alone. Some studies suggest that testing islet autoantibodies in relatives of patients with type 1 diabetes can identify people who are at risk for developing the disease. Ascertaining the presence of other comorbid conditions, such as hyperlipidemia, hypertension, and coronary artery disease, is essential at the beginning stages of assessing and treating patients with diabetes.

TABLE 19.8   Criteria for Testing for Diabetes or Prediabetes in Asymptomatic Adults

1. Testing should be considered in overweight or obese (BMI >25 kg or >23 kg/m² in Asian American) adults who have one or more of the following risk factors:
   - First-degree relative with diabetes
   - High-risk race/ethnicity (e.g., African American, Latino, Native American, Asian American, Pacific Islander)
   - History of CVD
   - Hypertension (>140/90 mm Hg or on therapy for hypertension)
   - HDL-C level <35 mg/dL and/or a triglyceride level >250 mg/dL
   - Women with polycystic ovary syndrome
   - Physical inactivity
   - Other clinical conditions associated with insulin resistance (e.g., severe obesity, acanthosis nigricans)

2. Patients with prediabetes (A1C > 5.7%)

3. Women who were diagnosed with GDM should have lifelong testing at least every 3 yr

4. For all others, testing should begin at age 45 yr

5. If results are normal, testing should be repeated at a minimum of 3-yr intervals with consideration of more frequent testing depending on initial results and risk status

BMI, body mass index; CVD, cardiovascular disease; GDM, gestational diabetes mellitus; HDL, high-density lipoprotein.
Reprinted with permission American Diabetes Association. 2. Classification and diagnosis of diabetes standards of medical care in diabetes—2018. *Diabetes Care.* 2018;41(suppl 1):S16.

The American Diabetes Association recommends confirmation of a diagnosis of diabetes with a repeated fasting plasma glucose test on a separate day, especially for patients with borderline results and for patients with normal fasting plasma glucose for whom suspicion of diabetes is high. If patients have test results near the margins of the diagnostic threshold, the clinician should follow the patient closely and repeat the test in 3 to 6 months. In asymptomatic adults of any age who are overweight or obese (body mass index >25 kg/m²) and who have one or more risk factors for diabetes, screening for diabetes should be pursued. Consider testing for prediabetes in children and adolescents who are overweight or obese.

A complete medical evaluation should be performed at the initial visit to:

- Confirm the diagnosis and classify diabetes.
- Evaluate for diabetes complications and potential comorbid conditions.
- Begin patient engagement in the formulation of a care management plan.
- Develop a plan for continuing care.

Treatment Options

Aggressive interventions to establish and maintain regular exercise, healthy diet, and normal weight should be emphasized for patients at increased risk for developing diabetes, especially those who are overweight or obese, have a family history of diabetes, or have a racial or ethnic background associated with an increase risk (e.g., Native Americans). Intensive dietary and physical activity programs should be considered for patients who have impaired fasting glucose or impaired glucose tolerance. Good quality evidence from large trials has demonstrated that these programs can reduce the incidence of diabetes in these at-risk patients.[21]

Patients with type 1 diabetes require insulin therapy. Refer to the latest American Diabetes Association guidelines for specific updated recommendations pertaining to insulin administration.[22]

Metformin is the drug of choice for patients with type 2 diabetes. In newly diagnosed, symptomatic patients with A1C >10% and/or blood glucose >300 mg/dL, insulin therapy should be initiated, with or without metformin. Numerous new medications (in a variety of novel drug classes) are now available to add to the regimen for a patient who does not have acceptable glucose levels after taking metformin. If the A1C target is not achieved after 3 months of metformin administration and the patient does not have ASCVD, consider a combination of metformin and any one of the preferred six treatment options: sulfonylureas, thiazolidinedione, DPP-4 inhibitor, GLP-1 receptor agonist, or basal insulin.

If A1C is not reached after 3 months of dual therapy, proceed to a three-drug combination. If A1C is not achieved after another 3 months of triple therapy, move to combination injectable therapy. Avoid clinical inertia when patients are not reaching their A1C goals.

It is important to reduce the risk for cardiovascular events in diabetics, especially those who also have ASCVD, who should be initiated on statin medications.[23] Two agents in the SGLT2 inhibitor class (empagliflozin and canagliflozin) and one drug in the GLP-1 receptor agonist class (liraglutide) have shown statistically significant reductions in major adverse cardiovascular events.

Along with medications, a cornerstone of management is lifestyle modification. Patients need to adhere to a diabetic diet and engage in a program of regular exercise. Clinicians should be vigilant about keeping their diabetic patients up to date with immunizations.

Follow-up

Type 1 and type 2 diabetes is a lifelong condition hampered by a myriad of challenging complications. Utilizing a multidisciplinary team has been shown to yield the best outcomes, minimize macrovascular and microvascular complications, and reduce costs, the frequency of hospitalization, and the development of ASCVD. A follow-up visit

TABLE 19.9 Components of the Comprehensive Diabetes Medical Evaluation Initial and Follow-up Visits

		Initial Visit	Every Follow-up Visit	Annual Visit
Past medical and family history	**Diabetes history**			
	• Characteristics at onset (e.g., age, symptoms)	✓		
	• Review of previous treatment regimens and response	✓		
	• Assess frequency/ cause/severity of past hospitalizations	✓		
	Family history			
	• Family history of diabetes in a first-de-gree relative	✓		
	• Family history of autoimmune disorder	✓		
	Personal history of complications and common comorbidities			
	• Macrovascular and microvascular	✓		
	• Common comorbidities	✓		
	• Presence of hemo-globinopathies or anemias	✓		✓
	• High blood pressure or abnormal lipids	✓		
	• Last dental visit	✓		✓
	• Last dilated eye examination	✓	✓	✓
	• Visits to specialists	✓		

(Continued)

TABLE 19.9   Components of the Comprehensive Diabetes Medical Evaluation Initial and Follow-up Visits   (Continued)

		Initial Visit	Every Follow-up Visit	Annual Visit
Social history	**Assess lifestyle and behavior patterns**			
	• Eating patterns and weight history	✓		
	• Sleep behaviors and physical activity	✓		
	• Familiarity with carbohydrate counting in type 1 diabetes	✓	✓	✓
	• Tobacco, alcohol, and substance use	✓	✓	✓
	• Identify existing social supports	✓		
	Interval history			
	• Changes in social history since last visit		✓	✓
Medications and vaccinations	• Medication-taking behavior	✓	✓	✓
	• Medication intolerance or side effects	✓	✓	✓
	• Complementary and alternative medicine use	✓	✓	✓
	• Vaccination history and needs	✓	✓	✓
Technology use	• Assess use of health apps, online education, patient portals, etc.	✓		✓
	• Glucose monitoring (meter/CGM): results and data use	✓	✓	✓
	• Review insulin pump settings	✓	✓	✓

TABLE 19.9 Components of the Comprehensive Diabetes Medical Evaluation Initial and Follow-up Visits (Continued)

		Initial Visit	Every Follow-up Visit	Annual Visit
Screening	**Diabetes self-manage-ment education and support**			
	• History of dietitian/ diabetes educator visits	✓	✓	✓
	• Screen for barriers to diabetes self-management	✓		✓
	• Refer or offer local resources and support as needed	✓	✓	✓
	Hypoglycemia			
	• Timing of episodes, awareness, frequency, and causes	✓	✓	✓
Physical examination	• Height, weight, and BMI; growth/pubertal development in children and adolescents	✓	✓	✓
	• Blood pressure determination	✓	✓	✓
	• Orthostatic blood pressure measures (when indicated)	✓		✓
	• Funduscopic examination (refer to eye specialist)	✓		✓
	• Thyroid palpation	✓		✓
	• Skin examination (e.g., acanthosis nigricans, insulin injection or insertion sites, lipodystrophy)	✓	✓	✓
	• Comprehensive foot examination	✓	✓	✓

(Continued)

TABLE 19.9 Components of the Comprehensive Diabetes Medical Evaluation Initial and Follow-up Visits (Continued)

		Initial Visit	Every Follow-up Visit	Annual Visit
Laboratory evaluation	• AIC, if the results are not available within the past 3 mo	✓	✓	✓
	If not performed/available within the past year:	✓		✓[d]
	• Lipid profile, including total, LDL, and HDL cholesterol and triglycerides[c]	✓		✓
	• Liver function tests[c]	✓		✓
	• Spot urinary albumin-to-creatinine ratio	✓		✓
	• Serum creatinine and estimated glomerular filtration rate[b]	✓		✓
	• Thyroid-stimulating hormone in patients with type 1 diabetes[c]	✓		✓
	• Vitamin B$_{12}$ if on metformin (when indicated)	✓		✓
	• Serum potassium levels in patients on ACE inhibitors, ARBs, or diuretics[b]	✓		✓

TABLE 19.9   Components of the Comprehensive Diabetes Medical Evaluation Initial and Follow-up Visits   (Continued)

		Initial Visit	Every Follow-up Visit	Annual Visit
Assessment and plan	**Goal setting**			
	• Set AIC/blood glucose target and monitoring frequency	✓	✓	✓
	• If hypertension diagnosed, establish blood pressure goal	✓		✓
	• Incorporate new members to the care team as needed	✓	✓	✓
	• Diabetes education and self-management support needs	✓	✓	✓
	Cardiovascular risk assessment and staging of CKD			
	• History of ASCVD	✓	✓	✓
	• Presence of ASCVD risk factors	✓	✓	✓
	• Staging of CKD[b]	✓	✓	✓
	Therapeutic treatment plan			
	• Lifestyle management	✓	✓	✓
	• Pharmacologic therapy	✓	✓	✓
	• Referrals to specialists (including dietitian and diabetes educator) as needed	✓	✓	✓
	• Use of glucose monitoring and insulin delivery devices	✓	✓	✓

[a]>65 yr.
[b]May be needed more frequently in patients with known chronic kidney disease or with changes in medications that affect kidney function and serum potassium.
[c]May also need to be checked after initiation or dose changes of medications that affect these laboratory values (i.e., diabetes medications, blood pressure medications, cholesterol medications, or thyroid medications).
[d]In people without dyslipidemia and not on cholesterol lowering therapy, testing may be less frequent.
ACE, angiotensin-converting enzyme; ARB, angiotensin receptor blockers; ASCVD, atherosclerotic cardiovascular disease; BMI, body mass index; CGM, continuous glucose monitoring; CKD, chronic kidney disease; HDL, high-density lipoprotein; LDL, low-density lipoprotein.
Adapted with permission from American Diabetes Association. 3. Comprehensive medical and assessment of comorbidities: standards of medical care and diabetes. *Diabetes Care.* 2018;41(suppl 1):S31-S32.

should include most components of the initial comprehensive medical evaluation, including interval medical history; assessment of medication-taking behavior and intolerance/side effects; physical examination; laboratory evaluation as appropriate to assess attainment of A1C and metabolic targets; and assessment of risk for complications, diabetes self-management behaviors, nutrition, psychosocial health, and the need for referrals, immunizations, or other routine health maintenance screening (Table 19.9). Long-term management extends beyond glycemic control and includes treating cardiovascular comorbid disorders, lifestyle counseling, and close monitoring for diabetic complications. Ophthalmologists, neurologists, nephrologists, cardiologists, podiatrists, and endocrinologists join the primary care providers in augmenting care and managing the potential complications of the disease.

Osteoporosis

Abnormal Screening Results and Diagnostic Strategy

Decreased bone density as measured by dual-energy x-ray absorptiometry (DEXA) scans or ultrasonography can be diagnostic for osteopenia and osteoporosis. Patients who sustain a "fragility fracture," defined as a fracture occurring with less intense trauma than the equivalent of falling from a standing position (e.g., a spontaneous vertebral fracture), also deserve evaluation for osteoporosis. The occurrence of a fragility fracture can be diagnostic for osteoporosis.

The DEXA's T score, which is a measure of the standard deviation of a patient's bone mineral density compared with the peak bone density of a gender- and ethnically matched young adult ascertains whether a patient has osteopenia or osteoporosis. A T score between −2.5 and −1.0 is diagnostic for osteopenia; a T-score less than −2.5 standard deviations is diagnostic for osteoporosis.

Risk scores that consider clinical risk factors such as low weight, smoking, previous fracture, excessive alcohol use, or the use of steroids combined with DEXA results, such as those generated from the World Health Organization's Fracture Risk Assessment Tool (FRAX), can help estimate 10-year fracture risk among untreated patients with low bone density. This tool can be accessed at https://www.sheffield.ac.uk/FRAX/tool.aspx?country=9.

Treatment Options

The most recent guidelines for the treatment of low bone density or osteoporosis to prevent fractures in men and women come from the American College of Physicians (ACP).[24] The first recommendation was that clinicians offer pharmacotherapy to all osteoporotic women for 5 years, to reduce the risk of hip or vertebral fracture. Medications options include the bisphosphonates, alendronate, risedronate, or zoledronic acid, or a biologic agent, denosumab. The ACP also recommended against bone density monitoring during the 5-year treatment period in women. Men who have clinically recognized osteoporosis should be offered bisphosphonates to decrease the risk of vertebral fracture. The use of menopausal estrogen plus progesterone or raloxifene is no longer advocated in the treatment of osteoporosis in women.

Traditionally weight-bearing physical activity and supplementation with vitamin D (400–800 IU daily) and calcium (1500 mg/daily) have been recommended to reduce the risk of fracture in osteopenic and osteoporotic individuals. The ACP did not find evidence to conclusively show the effect of physical activity on fracture risk.

Clinicians should engage patients in a shared decision-making process to select the most appropriate treatment regimen. Potential risks from the medication, along with the patient's overall risk for osteoporotic fracture, should be considered. For osteopenic women over 65 years, the ACP advises that clinicians discuss with their patients about their personal preferences and the benefits, harms, and costs of medications, along with the fracture risk profile before deciding whether to start medication.

Screening for Hepatitis C Virus
Abnormal Screening Results
An anti–hepatitis C virus (HCV) antibody test reactivity suggests HCV infection. A qualitative measurement of HCV RNA should be ordered to verify current infection.

Diagnostic Strategies
If the anti-HCV antibody test is nonreactive in a patient who might have been exposed to HCV in the last 6 months, monitor HCV RNA levels every 4 to 8 weeks for at least 6 months. Patients who have a positive HCV test and negative HCV RNA test do not carry the diagnosis of HCV infection[25] (Table 19.10).

Patients who have been diagnosed with HCV infection should have a quantitative HCV RNA test to ascertain the baseline viral load and a test for the HCV genotype before treatment decisions are made. Evaluation of the liver, usually by liver biopsy, is necessary to determine the degree of liver fibrosis and cirrhosis, which estimates clinical outcomes and disease progression. Patients who have chronic HCV infection should be tested for HIV and hepatitis B because these infections are additional threats to the liver. Liver imaging is recommended to rule out hepatocellular carcinoma. If cirrhosis is found, endoscopic evaluation may be advisable to rule out portal hypertension.

TABLE 19.10   Interpretation of Results of Tests for Hepatitis C Virus (HCV) Infection and Further Actions

Test Outcome	Interpretation	Further Action
HCV antibody nonreactive	No HCV antibody detected	Sample can be reported as nonreactive for HCV antibody. No further action required. If recent HCV exposure in person tested is suspected, test for HCV RNA[a]
HCV antibody reactive	Presumptive HCV infection	A repeatedly reactive result is consistent with current HCV infection, or past HCV infection that has resolved, or biologic false positivity for HCV antibody. Test for HCV RNA to identify current infection
HCV antibody reactive, HCV RNA detected	Current HCV infection	Provide person tested with appropriate counseling and link person tested to medical care and treatment[b]
HCV antibody reactive, HCV RNA not detected	No current HCV infection	No further action required in most cases. If distinction between true positivity and biologic false positivity for HCV antibody is desired, and if sample is repeatedly reactive in the initial test, test with another HCV antibody assay. In certain situations,[c] follow up with HCV RNA testing and appropriate counseling

[a]If HCV RNA testing is not feasible and person tested is not immunocompromised, do follow-up testing for HCV antibody to demonstrate seroconversion. If the person tested is immunocompromised, consider testing for HCV RNA.
[b]It is recommended before initiating antiviral therapy to retest for HCV RNA in a subsequent blood sample to confirm HCV RNA positivity.
[c]If the person tested is suspected of having HCV exposure within the past 6 mo, or has clinical evidence of HCV disease, or if there is concern regarding the handling or storage of the test specimen.

Treatment Options

Chronic infection develops in 50% to 80% of patients.[26] Of those patients, 20% will progress to cirrhosis, end-stage liver disease, and/or hepatocellular carcinoma. Antiviral therapy is the mainstay of therapy and aims at preventing long-term complications, such as cirrhosis, liver failure, and hepatocellular carcinoma.[27] New treatment regimens and recommendations are constantly emerging; patients with HCV infections may consider enrolling in clinical trials. Clinicians experienced in treating HCV infections should be involved in therapeutic decisions considering genotype, extent of fibrosis or cirrhosis, possible side effects, previous treatments, and comorbidities.

Abstinence from alcohol and illicit drugs is mandatory. Referrals for counseling and substance abuse/addiction treatment should occur before initiating pharmacologic therapy. Behavioral risks factors for transmission and reinfection should be identified and patients' mental health assessed.

Combination direct-acting antivirals have optimized treatment, allowing for better tolerability and efficacy in a shorter duration of time. PEGylated interferon and ribavirin, previously central to multidrug pharmacologic regimens, are not as frequently used. These newer direct-acting antivirals target specific proteins of the viral genome to inhibit viral replication. For patients who have never been treated before, the duration is 8 to 12 weeks. For patients with advanced liver disease, a 24-week treatment duration is necessary.

Follow-up

Patients undergoing treatment for HCV infection should be evaluated, at every visit, for adherence to therapy, adverse effects to medication, mental health issues, and alcohol and substance abuse. Measurement of HCV RNA viral load assesses treatment effectiveness and is typically done at the end of week 4 and at the end of therapy. A sustained viral response is defined by the absence of HCV RNA on polymerase chain reaction testing 24 weeks after cessation of treatment. Sustained viral response 12 weeks after treatment is a new primary end point in many recent drug trials.

Some treatment-emergent resistance is occurring as more patients are being treated. The complete blood count and comprehensive metabolic panel should be periodically checked to ascertain safety and tolerability.

Patients should be educated that they will always be anti-HCV antibody positive; this finding does not mean that they have been reinfected. Viral load testing is the approach for retesting for HCV in treated patients.

Tuberculosis

Abnormal Screening Results

New clinical practice guidelines recommend using interferon-γ release assay (IGRA), e.g., Quantiferon TB Gold or T-SPOT, instead of a tuberculin skin test to diagnose active or latent TB in patients 5 years or older. IRGAs measure a patient's immune reactivity to *Mycobacterium tuberculosis*.[28] Patients who have been infected with *M. tuberculosis* have white blood cells that will release interferon-gamma (IFN-g) when mixed with antigens derived from *M. tuberculosis*. IGRA interpretations are based on the amount of IFN-g that is released or on the number of cells that release IFN-g. The standard qualitative test reports positive, negative, or indeterminate results.

A positive tuberculin skin test (TST) is an acceptable alternative. The TST is assessed by determining the number of millimeters of induration (not erythema) in the transverse diameter perpendicular to the long axis of the arm at the site of application. An induration of five or more millimeters is considered positive in HIV-infected patients, those with a recent contact with a person with known TB, persons with fibrotic changes on chest radiograph consistent with prior TB, patients with organ transplants, or patients who are immunosuppressed for other reasons. Induration of 10 or more millimeters is considered positive in recent immigrants from high-prevalence countries; injection drug users; residents and employees of high-risk, congregate settings; mycobacteriology laboratory personnel; persons with clinical conditions that place them at high risk; and children less than 4 years of age. Induration of 15 or more millimeters is considered positive in any person, including persons with no known risk factors for TB.

Although prior immunization with Bacillus Calmette-Guérin can cause a false-positive TST result, this effect wanes over a few years. For practical purposes, Bacillus Calmette-Guérin administration more than 1 year before the TST has no bearing on the interpretation of the TST result.

For patients at low risk for TB, a second confirmatory test (either IGRA or TST) is often recommended if the initial test is positive in patients 5 years or older. The patient is considered infected if both tests are positive.

Diagnostic Strategies

Neither IGRA nor TST can differentiate between active TB and latent TB. Clinicians must investigate whether active TB is likely by elucidating whether signs and symptoms of disease are present, by reviewing chest x-rays for signs of active TB (pleural effusions, cavities, air-space opacities, and if necessary obtaining sputum specimens for acid-fast bacilli smear microscopy and both liquid and solid mycobacterial cultures. A diagnostic nucleic acid amplification test should also be performed on initial respiratory specimens in patients suspected of having pulmonary TB. Consultation with a pulmonary specialist and infectious disease specialist, particularly if bronchoscopy is considered, is prudent.

Treatment Options

There are two phases of antituberculosis therapy: the 2-month intensive phase and the 4-month continuous phase.[29] During the intensive phase, four medications are given daily: isoniazid, rifampin, pyrazinamide, and ethambutol. The continuous phase consists of two daily medications, usually isoniazid and rifampin. If possible, directly observed therapy is recommended to prevent emergency of drug resistance and to promote adherence.

Sputum for acid-fast bacilli smear and culture should be obtained at monthly intervals until two consecutive cultures are negative.

Follow-up

Patients should be advised to avoid regular alcohol consumption. They should be assessed monthly for symptoms and signs of hepatotoxicity and for medication adherence. Routine laboratory monitoring is not recommended, except in patients at increased risk of hepatitis. Once the continuation phase of the therapy is finished, a chest x-ray should be ordered for a baseline comparison for future imaging studies.

OFFICE AND CLINIC ORGANIZATION

Practices should establish reminder and referral systems to identify patients overdue for follow-up tests and to ensure that the clinician receives test results, that patients return for repeat visits and testing at recommended intervals, and that patients with positive results receive appropriate follow-up and treatment. For patients screened for infectious diseases, reminder systems should also ensure that infected patients receive appropriate antibiotic therapy; that potential contacts of infected patients are notified, tested, and treated according to guidelines; and that the public health department is notified of reportable cases. Patient education materials, such as those listed in the subsequent text, should be available to help patients learn more about these disorders and related diagnostic tests and treatments and to facilitate shared decision making.

CONCLUSION

The clinician's ability to respond appropriately to the results of abnormal screening tests ultimately determines the value of a screening program. Clinicians who deliver preventive care must understand not only the evaluation of abnormal results but also the range of therapeutic options. By definition, the process of screening involves an asymptomatic patient. Any potential future health benefit must be weighed against the assured expense, inconvenience, anxiety, and risk of the workup prompted by an abnormal screening test. Particularly when the potential benefits are small or unproven, it is essential to elicit and include the patient's values in making both screening and evaluation recommendations.

Clinicians should expect that the guidelines for appropriate evaluation of an abnormal screening test will continually evolve as diagnostic tests improve and treatment options expand. Clinicians delivering preventive care must remain vigilant for changes in screening, evaluation, and treatment recommendations for a broad range of clinical topics.

SUGGESTED RESOURCES AND MATERIALS

Hypertension

https://familydoctor.org/condition/high-blood-pressure/.
https://medlineplus.gov/highbloodpressure.html.

Metabolic Syndrome

https://familydoctor.org/condition/metabolic-syndrome/.
https://medlineplus.gov/metabolicsyndrome.html.

Lipids

https://familydoctor.org/condition/cholesterol/.
https://medlineplus.gov/ency/article/000403.htm.

Coronary Artery Disease

https://familydoctor.org/condition/coronary-artery-disease-cad/.
https://medlineplus.gov/coronaryarterydisease.html.

Abdominal Aortic Aneurysm

https://familydoctor.org/condition/abdominal-aortic-aneurysm/.
https://medlineplus.gov/aorticaneurysm.html.

Breast Cancer

https://familydoctor.org/condition/breast-cancer/.
https://medlineplus.gov/breastcancer.html.
NIH National Cancer Institute Breast Cancer Treatment (PDQ)-Patient Version.
    Accessed at: https://www.cancer.gov/types/breast/patient/breast-treatment-pdq.
Susan G. *Komen Follow-up After an Abnormal Mammogram.*
https://ww5.komen.org/BreastCancer/FollowingUpanAbnormalMammogram.html.

Colorectal Cancer

https://familydoctor.org/condition/colorectal-cancer/.
https://medlineplus.gov/colorectalcancer.html.

Cervical Cancer

https://familydoctor.org/how-to-interpret-abnormal-pap-smear-results/.
https://familydoctor.org/condition/cervical-cancer/.
https://medlineplus.gov/cervicalcancer.html.

Prostate Cancer

https://familydoctor.org/condition/prostate-cancer/.
https://familydoctor.org/risks-benefits-common-prostate-cancer-treatments/.
https://medlineplus.gov/prostatecancer.html.

Lung Cancer

https://familydoctor.org/condition/lung-cancer/.
https://medlineplus.gov/lungcancer.html.

NCCN Guidelines for Patients: Lung Cancer-Non-small Cell 2018

https://www.nccn.org/patients/guidelines/lung-nsclc/116/.
https://www.cdc.gov/cancer/lung/basic_info/screening.htm.
https://www.cdc.gov/tobacco/quit_smoking/index.htm.

Diabetes

https://familydoctor.org/diabetes-and-heart-disease/.
https://familydoctor.org/condition/diabetes/.
https://familydoctor.org/diabetes-and-nutrition/.
https://medlineplus.gov/diabetestype2.html.

Osteoporosis

https://familydoctor.org/condition/osteoporosis/.
https://medlineplus.gov/osteoporosis.html.

Hepatitis C

https://familydoctor.org/condition/hepatitis-c/.
https://medlineplus.gov/hepatitisc.html.

Tuberculosis

https://familydoctor.org/condition/tuberculosis/.
https://medlineplus.gov/tuberculosis.html.
https://medlineplus.gov/tuberculosis.html.

Hypertension

James PA, Oparil S, Carter BL, et al. 2014 Evidence-based guideline for the management of high blood pressure in adults. Report from the panel members appointed to the eighth joint national committee (JNC 8). *JAMA*. 2014;311(5):507-520.

Whelton PK, Carey RM, Aronow WS, et al. 2017 ACC/AHA/AAPA/ABC/ACPM/AGS/APhA/ASH/ASPC/NMA/PCNA Guideline for the prevention, detection, evaluation, and management of high blood pressure in adults: executive summary. *J Am Coll Cardiol*. 2017. doi:10.1016/jack.2017.11.005.

Cifu AS, Davis AM. JAMA clinical guidelines synopsis: prevention, detection, evaluation, and management of high blood pressure in adults. *JAMA*. 2017;318(21):2132-2134.

Greenland P, Peterson E. The new 2017 ACC/AHA guidelines "up the pressure" on diagnosis and treatment of hypertension. *JAMA*. 2017;318(21):2083-2084.

CardioSmart: What to Tell your Patients: New High Blood Pressure Guidelines. Accessed at: https://www.cardiosmart.org/For-Clinicians/Content/High-Blood-Pressure.

Lipids

Final Recommendation Statement: Statin Use for the Primary Prevention of Cardiovascular Disease in Adults: Preventive Medication. U.S.Preventive Services Task Force; November 2016. https://www.uspreventiveservicestaskforce.org/Page/Document/RecommendationStatementFinal/statin-use-in-adults-preventive-medication1.

Stone NJ, Robinson JG, Lichtenstein AH, et al; American College of Cardiology/American Heart Association Task Force on practice guidelines. 2013 ACC/AHA guideline of the treatment of blood cholesterol to reduce atherosclerotic cardiovascular risk in adults: a report of the American College of Cardiology/American Heart Association Task Force on practice guidelines. *Circulation*. 2014;129(25 suppl 2):S1-S45.

Jellinger PS, Handelsman Y, Rosenblit PD, et al. American Association of clinical endocrinologists and American College of Endocrinology guidelines for management of dyslipidemia and prevention of cardiovascular disease. *Endocr Prac*. 2017;23(suppl 2):1-87.

Ngo-Metzger Q, Gottfredson R. Stain use for the primary prevention of cardiovascular disease in adults. *Am Fam Physician*. 2017;96(12):895-806.

Coronary Artery Disease

Chou R; High Value Care Task Force of the American College of Physicians. Cardiac screening with electrocardiography, stress echocardiography, or myocardial perfusion imaging: advice for high-value care from the American College of Physicians. *Ann Intern Med.* 2015;162(6):438-447.

Metabolic Syndrome

U.S. Preventive Services Task Force. Final Recommendation Statement, Obesity in Adults: Screening and Management; June 2012. http://www.uspreventiveservicestaskforce.org/Page/Document/RecommendationStatementFinal/obesity-in-adults-screening-and-management.

Jensen MD, Ryan DH, Apovian CM, et al. 2013 AHA/ACC/TOS guideline for the management of overweight and obesity in adults: a report of the American College of Cardiology/American Heart Association Task Force on practice guidelines and the obesity society. *Circulation.* 2014;129(25 suppl 2):S102-S138. http://circ.ahajournals.org/content/129/25_suppl_2/S102.

Abdominal Aortic Aneurysm

Final Recommendation Statement: Abdominal Aortic Aneurysm: Screening. U.S. Preventive Services Task Force; June 2014. https://www.uspreventiveservicestaskforce.org/Page/Document/RecommendationStatementFinal/abdominal-aortic-aneurysm-screening.

Cancer

Smith FA, Andrews KA, Brooks D, et al. Cancer screening in the United States, 2017: a review of current American Cancer Society guidelines and current issues in cancer screening. *CA Cancer J Clin.* 2017;67:100-121.

Breast Cancer

Siu AL on behalf of the US Preventive Services Task Force. Screening of breast cancer: USPSTF recommendation statement. *Annals Int Med.* 2016;164(4):279-296.

Shieh Y, Eklund M, Madlensky L, et al. Breast cancer screening in the precision medicine era: risk-based screening in a population-based trial. *J Natl Cancer Inst.* 2017;109.

Colorectal Cancer

Rex DK, Boland RB, Dominitz JA, et al. Colorectal cancer screening: recommendations for physicians and patients from the U.S. Multi-society Task Force on colorectal cancer. *Am J Gastroenterol.* 2017;112(7):116-1030.

Final Recommendation Statement: Colorectal Cancer Screening. U.S. Preventive Services Task Force; June 2017. https://www.uspreventiveservicestaskforce.org/Page/Document/RecommendationStatementFinal/colorectal-cancer-screening2.

Cervical Cancer

Algorithms from consensus guidelines American Society for Colposcopy and Cervical Pathology in collaboration with American College of Obstetricians and Gynecologists, the Society of Obstetricians and Gynaecologists of Canada, the Society of Gynecologic Oncology, the American Cancer Society, Centers for Disease Control and Prevention and US Food and Drug Administration can be found. http://www.asccp.org/asccp-guidelines.

Apgar BS, Kittendorf AL, Bettcher CM, Wong J, et al. Update on ASCCP consensus guidelines for abnormal cervical screening tests and cervical histology. *Am Fam Physician.* 2009;80(2):147-155.

Prostate Cancer

National Comprehensive Cancer Network: Prostate Cancer Version 1.2018. National Comprehensive Cancer Network; 2018. https://www.nccn.org/professionals/physician_gls/pdf/prostate.pdf.

Parker C, Gillessen S, Heidenreich A, et al. Cancer of the prostate: ESMO clinical practice guidelines. *Ann Oncol.* 2015:26(suppl 5):69-77.

Lung Cancer

Moyer VA on behalf of the U.S. Preventive Services Task Force. Screening for lung cancer: U.S. Preventive Task Force recommendation statement. *Ann Intern Med.* 2014;160:330-338.

Mulshine JL. Status of lung cancer screening. *J Thoracic Dis.* 2017;9(11):4311-4314.

Diabetes Mellitus

American Diabetes Association. Standards of medical care in Diabetes—2018. Abridged for primary care providers. *Clin Diabetes.* 2018;36(1):14-37.

Osteoporosis

Quaseem AQ, Forcia MA, McLean RM, et al; for the Clinical Guidelines Committee of the American College of Physicians. Treatment of low bone density or osteoporosis to prevent fractures in men and women: a clinical practice guideline update from the American College of Physicians. *Ann Int Med.* 2017;166:818-839.

Hepatitis C

American Association for the Study of Liver Diseases and the Infectious Diseases Society of America. *HCV Guidance: Recommendations for Testing, Managing, and Treating Hepatitis C;* 2016. www.hcvguidelines.org/full-report/monitoring-patients-who-are-starting-hepatitis-c-treatment-or-havehttps://www.hcvguidelines.org/evaluate/monitoring.

Moyer VA; on behlf of the U.S. Preventive Services Task Force. Screening for hepatitis C virus infection in adults: U.S. Preventive services Task Force recommendation statement. *Ann Intern Med.* 2013;159:349-357.

Tuberculosis

Nahid P, Dorman SE, Alipanah N, et al. Official American Thoracic Society/Centers for Disease Control and Prevention/Infectious Diseases Society of America clinical practice guidelines: treatment of drug-susceptible tuberculosis. *Clin Infect Dis.* 2016;63:e147.

Lewinsohn DM, Leonard MK, LeBue PA, et al. Official American Thoracic Society/Infectious Disease Society of America/Centers for Disease Control and Prevention clinical practice guidelines: diagnosis of tuberculosis in adults and children. *Clin Infect Dis.* 2017;64:111-115.

REFERENCES

1. Lin JS, Piper M, Perdue LA, et al. *Screening for Colorectal Cancer: A Systematic Review for the U.S. Preventive Services Task Force. Evidence Synthesis No. 135. AHRQ Publication No. 14-05203-EF-1.* Rockville, MD: Agency for Healthcare Research and Quality; 2016.
2. Thompson IM, Pauler DK, Goodman PJ, et al. Prevalence of prostate cancer among men with a prostate-specific antigen level < or =4.0 ng per milliliter. *N Engl J Med.* 2004;350:2239-2246.

3. Yeboah J, McClelland RL, Polonsky TS, et al. Comparison of novel risk markers for improvement in cardiovascular risk assessment in intermediate-risk individuals. *JAMA.* 2012;308:788.
4. Whelton PK, Carey RM, Aronow WS, et al. 2017. ACC/AHA/AAPA/ABC/ACPM/AGS/APhA/ASH/ASPC/NMA/PCNA guideline for the prevention, detection, evaluation, and management of blood pressure in adults: a report of the American College of Cardiology/American Heart Association Task Force on clinical practice guidelines. *J Am Coll Cardiol.* 2017. doi:10.1016/j.jacc.2017.11.006.
5. Bakris G, Sorrentino M. Redefining hypertension-assessing the new blood pressure guidelines. *N Engl J Med.* 2018;378:497-499.
6. Merai R, Siegel C, Rakotz M, et al. CDC Grand Rounds: a public health approach to detect and control hypertension. *MMWR Morb Mortal Wkly Rep.* 2016;65(45):1261-1264.
7. Stone NJ, Robinson JG, Lichtenstein AH, et al; American College of Cardiology/American Heart Association Task Force on Practice Guidelines. 2013 ACC/AHA guideline of the treatment of blood cholesterol to reduce atherosclerotic cardiovascular risk in adults: a report of the American College of Cardiology/American Heart Association Task Force on practice guidelines. *Cirulation.* 2014;129(25 suppl 2):S1-S45.
8. U.S. Preventive Services Task Force. Statin use for the primary prevention of cardiovascular disease in adults. U.S. Preventive services Task Force recommendation statement. *JAMA.* 2016;316(19):1997-2007.
9. Guirguis-Blake JM, Beil TL, Senger CA, Whitlock EP. Ultrasonography screening for abdominal aortic aneurysms: a systematic evidence review for the U.S. Preventive Services Task Force. *Ann Intern Med.* 2014;160:321-329.
10. *Final Recommendation Statement: Abdominal Aortic Aneurysm: Screening. U.S. Preventive Services Task Force;* June 2011. https://www.uspreventive-servicestaskforce.org/Page/Document/RecommendationStatementFinal/abdominal-aortic-aneurysm-sceening.
11. Galyfos G, Voulalas G, Stamatatos I, et al. Small abdominal aortic aneurysms. *Vasc Disease Management.* 2015;12(8):E152-E159.
12. Hofvind S. Patnick PA, Ascence N, et al. False positive results in mammographic screening for breast cancer in Europe: a literature review and survey of service screening programmes. *J Med Screen.* 2012;19(suppl 1):57-66.
13. US Preventive Services Task Force. Bibbins-Domingo K, Grossman DC, Curry SJ et al Screening for colorectal cancer: US preventive services task force recommendation statement. *JAMA.* 2016;315(23):2564-2575.
14. Lieberman DA, Rex DK, Winawer SJ, Giardiello FM, Johnson DA, Levin TR. Guidelines for colonoscopy surveillance after screening and polypectomy: a consensus update by the US multi-society task force on colorectal cancer. *Gastroenterology.* 2012;143:844-857.
15. Committee on Practice Bulletins—Gynecology. Practice Bulletin No. 168: cervical cancer screening and prevention. *Obstet Gynecol.* 2016;128(4):111-130.
16. Saslow D, Solomon D. Lawson HW, et al. American Cancer Society, American Society for Colposcopy and Cervical Pathology and American Society for Clinical Pathology screening guides for the prevention and early detection of cervical cancer. *CA Cancer J Clin.* 2012;62:147-172.
17. Massad LS, Einstein MH, Huh WK, at al. 2012 Updated consensus guidelines for the management of abnormal cervical cancer screening tests and cancer precursors. *J Low Genit Tact Dis.* 2013;17:S1.

18. Johansson JE, Andren O, Andersson SO, et al. Natural history of early, localized prostate cancer. *JAMA*. 2004;291:2713-2719.
19. Moyer VA, on behalf of the U.S. Preventive Services Task Force. Screening for lung cancer: U.S. preventive task force recommendation statement. *Ann Intern Med*. 2014;160:330-338.
20. Pastorino U, Boffi R, Marchiaino A, et al. Stopping smoking reduced mortality in low-dose computed tomography screening participants. *J Thorac Oncol*. 2016;11(5):693-699.
21. American Diabetes Association. 2. Classification and diagnosis of diabetes: standards of medical care in diabetes. *Diabetes Care*. 2018;41(suppl 1):S13-S27.
22. American Diabetes Association. 8. Pharmacologic approaches to glycemic treatment: Standards in Diabetes—2018. *Diabetes Care*. 2018;41(suppl 1):S73-S85.
23. American Diabetes Association. 9. Cardiovascular disease and risk management: standards of medical care in Diabetes—2018. *Diabetes Care*. 2018;41(suppl. 1P):S86-S104.
24. Quaseem AQ, Forcia MA, McLean RM, Denberg TD; for the Clinical Guidelines Committee of the American College of Physicians. Treatment of low bone density or osteoporosis to prevent fractures in men and women: a clinical practice guideline update from the American College of Physicians. *Ann Intern Med*. 2017;166(11):818-839.
25. Wilkins T, Akhtar M, Gititu E. Diagnosis and management of hepatitis C. *Am Fam Physician*. 2015;91(12):835-842.
26. Pawlotsky JM. Pathophysiology of hepatitis C virus infection and related liver disease. *Trends Microbiol*. 2004;12(2):96-102.
27. Moyer VA, on behalf of the U.S. Preventive Services Task Force. Screening for hepatitis C virus infection in adults: U.S. preventive services task force recommendation statement. *Ann Intern Med*. 2013;159:349-357.
28. Lewinsohn DM, Leonard MK, LeBue PA, et al. Official American Thoracic Society/Infectious Disease Society of America/Centers for disease control and prevention clinical practice guidelines: diagnosis of tuberculosis in adults and children. *Clin Infect Dis*. 2017;64:111-115.
29. Nahid P, Dorman SE, Alipanah N, et al. Official American Thoracic Society/Centers for disease control and prevention/infectious diseases society of America clinical practice guidelines: treatment of drug-susceptible tuberculosis. *Clin Infect Dis*. 2016;63:e147.

Please see Online Appendix: Apps and Digital Resources for additional information.

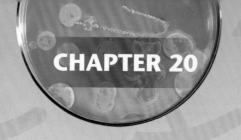

CHAPTER 20

What Not to Do and Why: The Arguments Against Some Forms of Screening and Chemoprevention

JANELLE GUIRGUIS-BLAKE AND RUSSELL HARRIS

INTRODUCTION

As the patient-clinician relationship has changed over time, new complexity has emerged regarding which preventive services are offered and how advice is delivered to patients. No longer is this solely a clinician-determined decision; patients want and deserve information and a share in decision making about preventive services, just as other medical services. Such transparency with shared decision making, however, must be balanced with the clinician's responsibility to prioritize and offer only those services that have a reasonable probability of providing more benefit than harm, at reasonable cost.

HIGH-VALUE SERVICES

The clinician should prioritize the limited time of an office encounter to make sure that "high-value" services are brought to each patient's attention. High-value services are those that clearly have a reasonable probability of providing substantially more benefit than harm for the individual patient at reasonable cost, based on our best available evidence. Beyond high value, however, are other types of preventive services: low value, uncertain value, and close calls. In this context, value refers to the benefit accrued against the expenditure (harms, time, resources); it is important to recognize that value and cost are not necessarily inversely proportional, as high-cost services may have high value if they bring a substantial benefit to many individuals and low-cost services of no or minimal benefit are low value.[1,2] Table 20.1

TABLE 20.1 Value Categories for Clinical Services	
Value Category	**Definition**
High value, including reasonable cost	Evidence is clear that there is a high probability that benefits substantially outweigh harms; the great majority of informed people would want the service
Low value	Evidence is clear that there is a reasonable probability that benefits do not outweigh harms; most informed people would not want the service
Close call, including reasonable cost	Evidence is clear that there is a reasonable probability that benefits and harms are aligned closely enough so that many informed people would disagree about value; many reasonably informed people would want the service, whereas many others would not
Uncertain value	Either benefits and/or harms are uncertain; value cannot be determined

gives a brief summary of the definitions of these value categories. These value categories roughly translate to the U.S. Preventive Services Task Force recommendation grades: A and many B recommendations are more likely to be high-value services; D recommendations are almost always low-value services; C recommendations are most likely close calls, and I recommendations are of uncertain value.[3] Different from the U.S. Preventive Services Task Force, however, we do specify that high-value and close call services must have "reasonable cost." A more careful examination of cost is needed to determine value for borderline services.[4]

High-value preventive services are the subject of other chapters in this book. This chapter focuses on those preventive services that fall within the other 3 categories of value. In general, we recommend against spending time discussing low-value and uncertain-value services unless the services are high visibility or the patient specifically raises the issue. If there is time with the patient after considering high-value services, then close-call services could be discussed. Most important is not to allow lower- or uncertain-value services to take time away from discussing those that are high value.

LOW-VALUE SERVICES

Low-value services signify those services for which there is at least a moderate probability that harm equals or outweighs benefit, given current evidence. Uncertain-value services are those services for which the evidence is unclear about the balance between benefit and harm. The following circumstances predispose to low or uncertain value:

1. Unacceptably high harms: The service is associated with an unacceptably high probability that harms are either too frequent or too severe (or both). These harms may be physical, psychological, or other. In some cases, the harms are serious, even though infrequent; in others, the harms are less serious but more frequent. The important consideration is whether the combination of severity and frequency adds up to overall harms that outweigh overall benefits. This may involve services that do have benefits, although either the importance or frequency of the benefit does not match the accompanying magnitude of harms.
2. Modest or no benefit for the target population
   a. Minimal or no clinical benefit: The service is associated with few or no benefits but at least some clear harms. There are some preventive services for which science has shown no benefit in the general population. Others may have shown some improvement in an intermediate outcome (e.g., a blood test) that likely leads to a smaller, modest benefit in actual health.
   b. Small number of individuals could benefit owing to low disease prevalence: Although the population undergoing the service is large, the actual number of people who could potentially benefit is small. Thus, many are exposed to the potential harms, whereas few actually gain improved quality or quantity of life.
3. Uncertain net benefits
   a. Insufficient evidence base: There is either little relevant evidence, or the available evidence is conflicting, biased, or not applicable such that it is not possible with any certainty to determine the benefits and harms. For example, early evidence for services often overstates the actual benefit to society (small-study effect, early-extremes effect; regression to the mean; selectively citing the literature; healthy screenee effect; indication creep). This evidence may be from less certain research designs, may involve less generalizable populations or medical care systems, or may overstate benefit by random chance. Services should only be offered when the magnitude of benefits for a population are clearly established and clearly outweigh the magnitude of harms. The proper response is more research rather than widespread implementation.

b. Unfocused target condition: The service has no clear target disease; it is actually a hunting expedition with no specified benefit. It may intuitively seem to offer benefit, but exactly what type or degree of benefit is unclear.

We will offer further discussion and examples of these situations in the sections that follow.

The Harms of Preventive Services

Not all preventive services result in improved health. In fact, as is noted in several chapters in this book, almost all preventive services (like almost all medical services in general) have a downside. For example, screening can cause physical harm in several ways, including by the screening test itself (e.g., colonoscopy), by the downstream diagnostic workup of a positive screening test (e.g., lung biopsy), or by the overtreatment of people with overdiagnosed disease (e.g., low-risk prostate cancer). Screening can also cause psychological distress in ways such as anxiety from a false-positive screening test, labeling from a premature or unnecessary diagnosis, extended concern from postscreening surveillance, financial consequences of future care, or worry about an incidental finding. Time spent on ineffective screening can also displace other preventive or chronic care management activities that could contribute more to a person's health. Likewise, chemoprevention carries potential physical harms (medication side effects) and psychological harms, including the daily reminder of risk and the nonbeneficial effects of the medication.

THE MAGNITUDE OF HARMS IS UNACCEPTABLY HIGH

Screening is often thought of as a single test; it is actually a cascade of events that result from the screening test. Harms can occur at every level of the cascade: the screening test itself, workup of positive screening results, uncertainty from indeterminate results, incidental findings, physical and psychological harm from workup of positive results, and labeling and overtreatment from unnecessary early diagnosis. Throughout the process, patients and families go through psychosocial turmoil and financial worry and are distracted from normal lives. Importantly, these harms occur sooner, during the screening process, whereas any benefit is delayed until after the patient would have suffered from the target condition.

Hormone Replacement Therapy

Certain previously popular preventive services have proved harmful for patients. For example, for many years asymptomatic postmenopausal women were advised to take hormone replacement therapy. Such therapy was thought to prevent a number of chronic diseases as well as to improve the quality of life. As detailed in Chapter 16 evidence from the Women's Health Initiative,[5] a large randomized controlled trial, has since shown that for most women combined hormone replacement therapy actually *increases* the risk of the very diseases that were once thought to be prevented by hormone therapy, such as cardiovascular disease (CVD) and dementia.[6]

Prostate Cancer Screening

Another example of excessive harms is prostate cancer screening. In this case, although some men may benefit from screening, many more men would suffer impotence and incontinence from various treatments. Similarly, screening for carotid artery stenosis to prevent stroke can lead to carotid endarterectomy surgery that actually causes stroke. Primary prevention of CVD with aspirin prophylaxis for older individuals increases the risk of intracerebral hemorrhage and major bleeding events. Screening for genital herpes virus causes psychosocial problems for many people. Screening women or lower-risk men for abdominal aortic aneurysm (AAA) exposes them to the concern about a "ticking time bomb" for those small-sized aneurysms as well as risky invasive surgical treatment when those aneurysms expand to a surgical threshold. Screening for ovarian cancer often leads to invasive workups and treatment but has not been shown to decrease ovarian cancer–specific mortality. Likewise, tamoxifen chemoprevention to prevent breast cancer carries serious potential harms when our ability to discriminate those women who could benefit from those unlikely to benefit is poor.

OVERDIAGNOSIS AND OVERTREATMENT

Two important harms of screening that are frequently overlooked are overdiagnosis and overtreatment. Overdiagnosis refers to detection of conditions through screening that would never have led to important clinical problems within a reasonable period of time. For example, screening for prostate cancer detects many actual prostate cancers that would never have caused problems for the patients. Similarly, screening women older than 70 years for breast cancer would detect cancers that, because of the woman's competing risks from other conditions, would never have caused clinical problems within the woman's lifetime. Overdiagnosis causes two types of harms: labeling with its psychosocial consequences and overtreatment with its physical and psychological effects.[7] Overdiagnosis is a problem with many types of screening services, including diabetes, cervical cancer, skin cancer, and bladder cancer.

Screening can also cause harm by precipitating overtreatment. *Overtreatment* refers to the treatment of conditions that would never have become clinically important (e.g., radical prostatectomy or radiation therapy for prostate cancers that would never have progressed). The risk of overtreatment is greatest in situations in which there are "borderline" conditions that are neither completely normal nor completely pathologic (e.g., small colonic polyps, ductal carcinoma in situ of the breast, and cervical intraepithelial neoplasia I and II) or in which there is great heterogeneity in the natural history of conditions that appear to be pathologic (e.g., breast cancer, prostate cancer, and bladder cancer). As it is often not possible to know which persons with these conditions will experience clinically meaningful progression, all are usually treated.

BENEFITS OF SCREENING AND PREVENTION

For some preventive services, harm can be reduced by offering the service selectively to subgroups of patients. The trade-off between benefits and harms is usually most favorable among people who are at increased risk for the target condition but at low risk for harms. For example, aspirin prophylaxis net benefits would be maximized if its use is targeted to a group at higher risk for CVD events but lower risk for bleeding complications.[8]

When screening is offered to a population with a higher prevalence of the condition, more patients have the potential to benefit and harm may be reduced. For example, screening women aged 65 to 69 years for osteoporosis would prevent more hip fractures than screening younger women aged 50 to 54 years. Yet whether younger women would still face the harm of labeling and the effect of earlier treatment when risk is lower, or benefit from later treatment when risk is higher, is uncertain. Small potential benefit from treatment at a younger age may reduce larger potential benefit from treatment at an older age, producing a net harm.

Modest or No Benefit

There are at least two reasons why a screening or chemoprevention program might benefit few or no people:

- The service carries minimal or no benefit for the target population.
- The target condition has low prevalence in the target population, and thus few people can benefit.

Minimal or No Net Benefit

We refer here to services for which there is *evidence of minimal or no net benefit*, which is distinguished from *insufficient evidence of benefit*. The latter refers to a gap in the research, whereas the former refers to good-quality evidence that a service does not work. There are some preventive services for which science has shown no benefit in the general population. For example, studies find no benefit from routine screening for asymptomatic bacteriuria or pyuria in average- or high-risk adults by urinalysis, urine microscopy, or urine culture.[9] Vitamin supplements are used by many people, yet the evidence is clear that there are few or no benefits from their use.[10]

Another factor in considering benefit is screening or chemoprevention in patients with short life expectancy, such as the "frail" elderly or patients with severe comorbid disease. Since the benefit from screening or chemoprevention often occurs some years after starting the preventive service, many of these patients will not live long enough to benefit from the service. For example, screening for colorectal cancer in those older than 80 years, mammography in women older than 75 years, and cervical cancer screening of women older than 65 years are examples of services that are unlikely to be beneficial. As noted in Chapter 5, guidelines for many of these screening tests recommend discontinuation when the average life expectancy is less than 10 to 15 years.

So-called baseline screening is yet another form of screening without benefit. For example, baseline electrocardiograms are commonly ordered as a part of the periodic health examination with the rationale that they may be useful if the patient has chest pain in the future. The value of any test as a comparison for the future, however, rapidly decreases as the time from the provision of the "baseline" test increases. To maintain their usefulness, such "baseline" tests need to be repeated regularly. If there are benefits to such periodic screening, then the salient question is at what age such screening has been shown to yield benefits.

As benefit is measured in improved quality or quantity of life, screening sometimes detects conditions when there is little or no evidence that the detection improves health. For example, screening for obstructive sleep apnea may lead to a diagnosis, but the evidence of benefit from early treatment is poor.[11] Similarly, screening for carotid artery stenosis may find narrowed carotid arteries and even a higher risk of stroke, but evidence indicates that any benefit from early endarterectomy is small at best.[12] Screening for testicular cancer or pancreatic cancer sometimes detects these conditions, but there is no evidence that earlier treatment improves either the quality or quantity of people's lives.[13] Screening for hypothyroidism may find people with higher thyroid stimulating hormone levels, but the benefit from treatment of this in asymptomatic people is scant.[14] Although annual screening pelvic examinations in asymptomatic women could potentially detect a host of gynecologic conditions, it is either inaccurate or has minimal to no clinical benefit.[15,16]

In some cases, there may be small benefits and apparently small harms. Yet another type of harm, opportunity costs, puts these situations in the minimal or no-net-benefit category. Opportunity costs are the services that will be crowded out and not performed because of the time and effort required to deliver the service in question.

Clinicians, patients, and society can experience opportunity costs. For clinicians, an unnecessary preventive service to discuss and monitor consumes time and effort that the clinician and the clinician's staff could use for more effective services. As discussed in Chapters 1, 3, and 6, lack of time is a barrier to the delivery of preventive care. In today's world of limited time availability, in the course of a day it can prove impossible to provide even those services known to be effective.[17] For every minute spent on ineffective prevention, 1 minute is lost from implementing effective prevention. Therefore, during a 15-minute office visit, the clinician has a choice: whether to offer a preventive service for which there is limited evidence of benefit (e.g., screening for thyroid disorders) or to discuss a service for which there is good evidence of a substantial benefit (e.g., colorectal cancer screening). It is important for clinicians to realize that prioritization of services based on available evidence is not a way to ration but rather a way to maximize the benefit to patients. Prioritization of preventive services is discussed further in Chapters 1, 3, and 6. Chapter 21 examines how practices can set their own priorities in identifying the preventive services to emphasize.

For patients, the opportunity costs of services with limited effectiveness include time, effort, and often financial cost. Given other demands, patients are able to attend to a limited number of health issues at any one time and often choose to focus on urgent symptomatic issues rather than prevention. Offering patients relatively ineffective services may result in an unfavorable trade-off, such as foregoing other, more effective, services.

For society, using scarce resources such as medical personnel and dollars to deliver services that provide minimal return is a poor investment. Routinely providing ineffective services drives up the cost of health care without improving the health of the public. Providing services that offer few benefits reduces the time and effort devoted to services that are higher value, resulting in a negative impact on the health of the population.

Small Number of Individuals Could Benefit due to Low Disease Prevalence

This category includes preventive services applied to low-prevalence populations and would include examples such as screening women <50 years for breast cancer, screening low-risk nonsmokers for lung cancer or AAA, screening the general population for hepatitis B and C, and screening low-risk populations for gonorrhea or chlamydia. Although some of these services may carry more benefit when targeted to a narrower, higher-prevalence population, expansion of the populations offered such services results in minimal additional benefit. For example, most women in their 40s have a lower risk of being diagnosed with or dying from breast cancer within the coming 10 years than women in their 50s or 60s. Screening these women, at best, reduces breast cancer mortality by about 1 in 1000 women screened for 10 years and followed for 15 to 20 years.[18] Most informed people would consider this a small benefit.

Screening and Prevention for Target Groups

When screening or chemoprevention is applied to target groups in which the type of condition that is likely to cause serious health problems has low prevalence, many people must undergo the service and be exposed to risk to benefit a very few. Even services that carry benefits may have a high "number needed to treat" (NNT) or "number needed to screen" (NNS) if used in a population in which few have the potential to benefit (see Box 20.1).

Box 20.1   Measures of Treatment and Screening Effectiveness

Number needed to treat (NNT)	Average number of patients that need to be treated over a given period to have an impact on one person	Calculated as the inverse of the absolute risk reduction: 1 ÷ (control group event rate minus the experimental group event rate)
Number needed to screen (NNS)	Average number of patients that need to be screened over a given period to have an impact on one person	

For example, if a chemoprevention service has a number needed to treat of 250 over 10 years, this means that 249 of the people taking the medication for 10 years would not benefit but be exposed to the harms regardless. Similarly, a screening strategy with a number needed to screen of 250 over 10 years would subject 249 people to screening harms with no benefit over 10 years. Thus, the vast majority of patients may unnecessarily suffer harms with no benefit (e.g., as noted earlier, tamoxifen for those women at low risk for breast cancer). Also, as noted earlier, the harms from false-positive results are more likely to outweigh the benefits when screening is conducted in populations with a low prevalence of the target condition. Screening average-risk women in their 50s for osteoporosis benefits few women and is not recommended.[19] For similar reasons, screening for gonorrhea is not recommended in low-risk groups[20] (e.g., monogamous women older than 25 years in low-prevalence settings) and screening for cancer is rarely advocated in young adults (see Chapter 5).

Likewise, only a small fraction of breast cancer cases is attributable to the *BRCA* genetic mutation. Screening of the general population would benefit very few women and create anxiety for many more. Moreover, because the *BRCA* gene is large, general screening would detect multiple mutations, most of which are not clinically important.[21]

Uncertain Benefit

There are at least two reasons why a screening or chemoprevention program might have uncertain benefit:

- The current evidence base is insufficient to determine the benefits and/or harms with any reasonable degree of certainty.
- The preventive service is not focused to screen or prevent any single specific target condition.

Insufficient Evidence Base

Some preventive services should be avoided because there is uncertainty about the balance between their benefits and harms. This occurs because there is an insufficient evidence base (no studies, few small studies, poor-quality studies with high risk of bias, or conflicting studies) about the benefits and/or harms of the interventions. The potential upper and lower limits of benefit therefore cannot be estimated with reasonable certainty. Further research may be necessary to obtain the data to quantify the actual benefits and harms of routinely offering the preventive services that fall into this category.

Some examples of such services with uncertain benefits include screening for AAA in women aged 65 to 75 years with a smoking history,[22] screening for celiac disease[23] or hypothyroidism,[24] use of electrocardiogram to detect heart disease or atrial fibrillation,[25] and ankle-brachial index or coronary calcium scores for cardiac risk assessment.[26] Statin use in those >75 years has an unclear benefit because none of the primary prevention trials included adults in this age group and there is some observational evidence that very low cholesterol levels are associated with increased mortality in advanced age.[27] The net benefit associated with the use of aspirin to prevent CVD events in older adults >70 years is likewise uncertain.[8] Although there is evidence that older adults can have a substantial decrease in their CVD events with aspirin use, risk of bleeding (gastrointestinal bleeding and hemorrhagic stroke) increases with age. Thus, although there is reasonable certainty that older patients will derive at least a moderate benefit from aspirin, it is not clear whether or not this benefit will be mitigated by the higher bleeding risk; thus, the balance between benefits and harms is uncertain.

Unfocused Target

This is a subcategory of uncertain benefits and includes either screening or chemoprevention services without a specific disease detection or prevention aim and includes examples such as whole-body computerized tomography scan, routine urinalysis, and serum panels such as liver function tests, chemistry, or complete blood counts. Unfocused prevention, particularly with serum-based screening tests, is easy to do. During annual prevention visits, young healthy patients often inquire what routine screening laboratory tests are needed, erroneously assuming that annual complete blood counts and chemistries are beneficial. Certainly, "casting a wide net" will detect many abnormalities. The problem with unfocused prevention is that the laboratory abnormalities or preclinical conditions detected through the screening are often not clinically important, nor is their detection beneficial to patients. When ordering a multicomponent blood chemistry panel, for example, it is important to be aware that an abnormal result is much more likely to be a false positive than a true positive. An unfocused blood chemistry panel with 20 independent variables has a 64% probability of producing an abnormal result, even when no abnormality exists. The risk of false-positive results is especially high in a population of healthy individuals for which the suspicion and probability of disease are low.

Direct-to-consumer advertisements for whole-body positron emission testing, spiral computed tomography, and multiple vascular ultrasound scans have become increasingly common. As a result, patients have come to believe that this new technology can detect any occult cancer or CVD and thereby allay any underlying fears of undetected disease. Such screening is often applied to inappropriate populations (i.e., those with low disease prevalence) and finds many conditions of uncertain significance; such detection is likely to be of little overall benefit. If there are benefits from such broad-based, unfocused screening, they are likely to be outweighed by the harms of downstream testing and overtreatment of insignificant conditions, as discussed earlier. False-positive and incidental findings from whole-body scans often precipitate anxiety. False negatives are also common, perhaps giving patients a false sense of security that everything is normal, with the risk of discouraging patients from undergoing specific screening tests that have been shown to be effective and help save lives (e.g., colonoscopy, mammography) or engaging in healthy lifestyle behaviors (e.g., smoking cessation, healthy eating, exercise).

Likewise, patients inquire what their clinician thinks about their use of multiple vitamins and herbal supplements to maintain their health. As opposed to targeted chemoprevention using supplements with known benefit (e.g., folic acid supplementation in pregnant women) or therapeutic use of supplements in those with known specific vitamin or mineral deficiencies (e.g., iron supplementation for iron-deficiency anemia), such unfocused use of multivitamins likely has little or no benefit to individuals. Toxicity from overuse of these supplements ("more is better") is a potential harm (see Chapter 15 on chemoprevention).[28]

Intensity of Screening

Although some screening and chemoprevention issues involve whether to recommend the service or not, in many other cases the issue is rather how intensive the recommended strategy should be. Higher-intensity screening strategies are those that screen a wider population (e.g., younger age to start, older age to stop, lower risk to meet screening criteria), use more sensitive screening methods (e.g., prostate-specific antigen cutoff at 2.6 ng/mL rather than 4.0 ng/mL), and screen more frequently (e.g., Pap smears annually versus every 3 or 5 yr). More intensive chemoprevention strategies are those that use a higher dose in a wider population for a longer duration.

It is important to understand that higher intensity does not mean higher value; indeed, increasing intensity beyond an optimal level actually decreases value. This is because, at high intensity levels, harms and costs rise more quickly than benefits. Thus, we should seek to find that intensity that best balances benefits against harms and costs, not that intensity that provides the highest level of benefit. Throughout this book, there are examples of reducing the intensity of the recommended screening strategy. In considering what not to do, it is important to avoid overly intensive screening and chemoprevention strategies.

IMPLEMENTING EVIDENCE-BASED PREVENTION PROGRAMS IN CLINICAL PRACTICE

Clinicians face two opposing errors in deciding which preventive strategies to recommend in clinical practice: adopting a service too early, before the balance of benefits and harms is established by properly conducted research, or adopting a service too late, after many missed opportunities for improving health. Clinicians are more vulnerable to the first risk if they immediately adopt new technologies before evidence of benefits and harms is confirmed. Clinicians are more vulnerable to the second risk if they require direct evidence from randomized controlled trials for every intervention they implement.

Finding the middle ground between these two extremes is crucial. Clinicians must determine when the evidence is sufficient to justify action—whether positive (e.g., offering the intervention) or negative (e.g., not offering the intervention). The answer depends partly on the service and the condition. Services with little potential for harm and a large potential for benefit may be offered with less definitive evidence than services with a greater potential for harm and a lower potential for benefit. The opportunity costs discussed in the preceding text lead us to discourage the investment of time on services with uncertain benefits and harms.

As mentioned throughout this chapter, focusing limited time and resources on preventive services with a known and substantial net benefit is more likely to improve health outcomes for a clinician's panel of patients. Further suggestions are provided in Table 20.2. These strategies may not be immediately satisfactory to patients. It is always appropriate to discuss these issues with patients and families who request services of limited effectiveness. Clinicians should communicate to patients the uncertainty

TABLE 20.2	How to Appropriately Provide Preventive Services
1.	Routinely offer patients high-value services: those for which the magnitude of benefits clearly justifies the associated harms and costs
2.	Target prevention to those with a high chance of benefiting from intervention (e.g., high-risk groups)
3.	Discourage patients from getting "parking lot van" or shopping mall testing (e.g., whole-body scans)
4.	Do not routinely offer preventive services for which there is insufficient evidence of effectiveness. If patients request such services, engage in shared decision making (see Chapter 22)
5.	Do not offer preventive services for which there is evidence of unacceptable harms; if patients request such services, discourage their use; be ready to negotiate
6.	Even high-value prevention requires up-front discussion with patients, helping them to understand potential benefits and harms. See related chapters in this book

of the likely outcomes and help them to appreciate how they will benefit by focusing on a limited number of preventive services that carry substantially greater benefits than harms. If feasible, it is best to deliver this important message in small doses, using multiple examples over a number of patient encounters. A clinician's willingness to discuss issues over time and negotiate mutually agreeable solutions to prevention is an attribute that most patients appreciate.

It is important that clinicians prioritize their time in the interaction to focus on high-value services. Discussion of low- and uncertain-value services should not take time away from high-value services. When patients request low- or uncertain-value services, clinicians should be ready to discuss the limited or uncertain benefits and the concern about potential harms. In many situations, the patient will accept the clinician's recommendation against using the service. In some cases, there may be a need for further negotiation. Clinicians should pursue continued efforts to provide accurate information to the patient, including information about how screening and chemoprevention services can cause harm. As discussed in Chapter 22, there are an increasing number of decision aids appropriate for primary care practices that facilitate this process, save time, and provide accurate information in an understandable format.[29]

CONCLUSION

This chapter specifically focuses on those services that should not be routinely offered to the general population. Some of the services discussed in this chapter may have benefit in high-risk populations only (e.g., chlamydia/gonorrhea screening in high-risk populations, screening for AAAs in male smokers older than 65 years, and screening for the *BRCA* mutation in women with high-risk family histories). Differentiating those services that provide benefit to the general population, those that provide benefit in high-risk populations, and those that provide no benefit (or harm) in any population is critical to providing quality preventive care in clinical practice. Table 20.3 provides a selected list of preventive services and target groups that should not be routinely offered or prioritized. The list is hardly exhaustive, for example, it does not include routine magnetic resonance imaging of the breasts, which is recommended only for high-risk women (see Chapters 5 and 15). New preventive services that emerge after publication of this book and that also lack supporting evidence of net benefit should also join the list, whereas some services in Table 20.3 may become more important as supporting evidence accumulates.

TABLE 20.3   Discouraged Preventive Services and the Target Groups to Which They Apply

Service	Population in Which Service Is Discouraged	Rationale for Discouraging Service[a]	Primary Exclusion Category[b]
Endocrine			
Bone mineral density testing (e.g., DEXA scans)	Young women	Young women (<60 yr of age) have relatively low prevalence of osteoporosis. See https://www.uspreventiveservicestaskforce.org/Page/Document/UpdateSummaryDraft/osteoporosis-screening1	2
Hormone therapy to prevent chronic disease	General population	Increased incidence of cardiovascular events, dementia, and breast cancer outweighs benefit of prevention of osteoporotic fractures. See Chapter 16 and https://www.uspreventiveservicestaskforce.org/Page/Document/UpdateSummaryFinal/menopausal-hormone-therapy-preventive-medication1	1

(Continued)

TABLE 20.3 Discouraged Preventive Services and the Target Groups to Which They Apply   (Continued)

Service	Population in Which Service Is Discouraged	Rationale for Discouraging Service[a]	Primary Exclusion Category[b]
Routine measurement of thyroid-stimulating hormone	General population	Clinical harm caused by overtreatment of subclinical disease and clinical improvement after treatment of sub-clinical disease are not known. See https://www.uspreventive-servicestaskforce.org/Page/Document/UpdateSummaryFinal/thyroid-dysfunc-tion-screening	2
Diabetes screening	General population (without risk factors)	Unknown magnitude of incremental benefit from earlier detection and treatment in terms of patient-oriented outcomes due to microvascular disease. See Chapter 5 and https://www.uspreventiveser-vicestaskforce.org/Page/Document/UpdateSummaryFinal/screening-for-abnor-mal-blood-glucose-and-type-2-diabetes	3
Celiac disease screening	General population	Insufficient evidence to determine the accu-racy of screening in the general population as well as to assess the overall health benefits and harms of screening. https://www.uspreventive-servicestaskforce.org/Page/Document/UpdateSummaryFinal/celiac-disease-screen-ing	3

TABLE 20.3   Discouraged Preventive Services and the Target Groups to Which They Apply   (Continued)

Service	Population in Which Service Is Discouraged	Rationale for Discouraging Service[a]	Primary Exclusion Category[b]
Hematology			
Screening for hemochromatosis	General population	Prevalence of clinical disease owing to hemochromatosis in the general population is likely low; the natural history of people with increased iron stores is unknown; overtreatment is likely	2
Cardiovascular and Pulmonary			
Beta-carotene supplements and vitamin E to prevent heart disease	General population	No health benefit; smokers harmed by beta-carotene. See https://www.uspreventiveservicestaskforce.org/Page/Document/UpdateSummaryFinal/vitamin-supplementation-to-prevent-cancer-and-cvd-counseling	2
Routine chest radiography or computed tomography scans for lung cancer screening	General population	High false-positive rate; diagnostic workup (bronchoscopy, mediastinoscopy with biopsy) is invasive and potentially harmful. Screening may be of higher yield in specific high-risk populations. See https://www.uspreventiveservicestaskforce.org/Page/Document/UpdateSummaryFinal/lung-cancer-screening	1,2

(Continued)

TABLE 20.3 Discouraged Preventive Services and the Target Groups to Which They Apply   (Continued)

Service	Population in Which Service Is Discouraged	Rationale for Discouraging Service[a]	Primary Exclusion Category[b]
Routine electrocardiograms	General population	In average-risk population, no known benefit and minimal potential yield based on many false positives (nonspecific electrocardiographic findings have little clinical significance) and false negatives. See https://www.uspreventiveservicestaskforce.org/Page/Document/UpdateSummaryDraft/cardiovascular-disease-risk-screening-with-electrocardiography	2
Routine pulmonary function testing	General population or high-risk asymptomatic individuals	Little or no potential benefit in asymptomatic individuals as treatment benefit in asymptomatic stage of COPD/asthma would be minimal. https://www.uspreventiveservicestaskforce.org/Page/Document/UpdateSummaryFinal/chronic-obstructive-pulmonary-disease-screening	2
Screening for abdominal aortic aneurysms	Women and non-smoking men	Surgical repair has high morbidity/mortality; women have lower prevalence. See Chapter 5 and https://www.uspreventiveservicestaskforce.org/Page/Document/UpdateSummaryFinal/abdominal-aortic-aneurysm-screening	1, 2

TABLE 20.3 Discouraged Preventive Services and the Target Groups to Which They Apply   (Continued)

Service	Population in Which Service Is Discouraged	Rationale for Discouraging Service[a]	Primary Exclusion Category[b]
Routine aspirin chemoprophylaxis	Populations at low risk for CVD	Net harms from increased gastro-intestinal bleeding and hemorrhagic stroke. See Chapter 16 and https://www.uspreventiveser-vicestaskforce.org/Page/Document/UpdateSummaryFinal/aspirin-to-prevent-car-diovascular-dis-ease-and-cancer	1
Tamoxifen in women	Women at low risk of breast cancer	Few women benefit; net harms from increased venous thromboembolic disease. See Chapter 16 and https://www.uspreventiveser-vicestaskforce.org/Page/Document/UpdateSummaryFinal/breast-cancer-medica-tions-for-risk-reduction	1, 2
Infectious Disease			
Screening for asymp-tomatic bacteriuria	Nonpregnant women	No health benefit as few health consequences of asymptomatic condition (in non-pregnant individuals). See https://www.uspreventiveser-vicestaskforce.org/Page/Document/UpdateSummaryFinal/asymptomatic-bacte-riuria-in-adults-screen-ing	2

(Continued)

TABLE 20.3   Discouraged Preventive Services and the Target Groups to Which They Apply   (Continued)

Service	Population in Which Service Is Discouraged	Rationale for Discouraging Service[a]	Primary Exclusion Category[b]
Screening for syphilis	Low-risk populations	Patients without risk factors have minimal potential benefit owing to low prevalence and resulting false-positive results, which lead to unnecessary treatment. Screening in high-risk populations can lead to important health benefits. See Chapter 13, and https://www.uspreventive-servicestaskforce.org/Page/Document/UpdateSummaryFinal/syphilis-infec-tion-in-nonpreg-nant-adults-and-ado-lescents	2
Screening for gonor-rhea or chlamydia	Low-risk populations	Low-risk patients (>25 yr of age without risk factors) have mini-mal potential benefit owing to low prevalence; false-positive results lead to unnecessary treat-ment. See Chapter 13, and https://www.uspreventive-servicestaskforce.org/Page/Document/UpdateSummaryFinal/chlamydia-and-gonor-rhea-screening	2

TABLE 20.3 Discouraged Preventive Services and the Target Groups to Which They Apply (Continued)

Service	Population in Which Service Is Discouraged	Rationale for Discouraging Service[a]	Primary Exclusion Category[b]
Screening for hepatitis C	General population	Yield of screening low in the general population that has low prevalence, whereas treatment carries important harms. See https://www.uspreventiveservicestaskforce.org/Page/Document/UpdateSummaryFinal/hepatitis-c-screening	1, 2
Screening for genital herpes	General population	Detection does not alter care and confers little health benefit. See Chapter 13 and https://www.uspreventiveservicestaskforce.org/Page/Document/UpdateSummaryFinal/genital-herpes-screening1	2
Screening for hepatitis B infection	General population	Yield of screening low in the general population. Screening in high-risk populations may have benefits. See https://www.uspreventiveservicestaskforce.org/Page/Document/UpdateSummaryFinal/hepatitis-b-virus-infection-screening-2014	2
Cancer			
Screening for pancreatic cancer	General population	No treatment has been shown to improve outcomes. See https://www.uspreventiveservicestaskforce.org/Page/Document/UpdateSummaryFinal/pancreatic-cancer-screening	1, 2

(Continued)

TABLE 20.3 Discouraged Preventive Services and the Target Groups to Which They Apply   (Continued)

Service	Population in Which Service Is Discouraged	Rationale for Discouraging Service[a]	Primary Exclusion Category[b]
Screening for testicular cancer	General population	Treatment is effective even when the condition is detected clinically, so there is little incremental benefit from earlier detection through screening. See Chapter 15 and https://www.uspreventiveservicestaskforce.org/Page/Document/UpdateSummaryFinal/testicular-cancer-screening	2
Screening for *BRCA* mutations	General population	Minimal potential benefit in the general population, as a minority of breast cancer cases is linked to this specific genetic mutation. See Chapter 5 and https://www.uspreventiveservicestaskforce.org/Page/Document/UpdateSummaryFinal/brca-related-cancer-risk-assessment-genetic-counseling-and-genetic-testing	2
Screening for bladder cancer	General population	Minimal potential benefit, uncertain effectiveness of early detection, and harms due to overtreatment. See https://www.uspreventiveservicestaskforce.org/Page/Document/UpdateSummaryFinal/bladder-cancer-in-adults-screening	1, 2

TABLE 20.3   Discouraged Preventive Services and the Target Groups to Which They Apply   (Continued)

Service	Population in Which Service Is Discouraged	Rationale for Discouraging Service[a]	Primary Exclusion Category[b]
Screening for thyroid cancer	General population	Thyroid cancer is relatively rare; there are some studies showing lack of difference in health outcomes between treatment and surveillance of common thyroid cancer subtypes and observational study of a mass screening program showing no mortality improvements; thus the maximum potential benefit would be no greater than small. See https://www.uspreventiveservicestaskforce.org/Page/Document/UpdateSummaryFinal/thyroid-cancer-screening1	
Routine screening for prostate cancer (prostate-specific antigen, digital rectal examination)	General population	Important harms from overtreatment; uncertainty about benefits of earlier detection and treatment. See Chapter 5 and https://screeningforprostatecancer.org/	1, 2
Colonoscopy	Low-risk populations younger than 50 yr	Net harms. See Chapter 5 and https://www.uspreventiveservicestaskforce.org/Page/Document/UpdateSummaryFinal/colorectal-cancer-screening2	1, 2

(Continued)

TABLE 20.3   Discouraged Preventive Services and the Target Groups to Which They Apply   (Continued)

Service	Population in Which Service Is Discouraged	Rationale for Discouraging Service[a]	Primary Exclusion Category[b]
Mammography	Women younger than 50 yr	Minimal potential benefit as prevalence of invasive disease is relatively low and false-positive rate from mammography is high, leading to overdiagnosis and invasive workup; discuss appropriateness and balance of benefits and harms with women aged 40–50 yr. See Chapter 5 and https://www.uspreventiveservicestaskforce.org/Page/Document/UpdateSummaryFinal/breast-cancer-screening1	1, 2
Screening for ovarian cancer with ultrasonography or CA-125	General population	Screening inaccurate, with high false-positive rate leading to invasive workup with laparoscopy. See https://www.uspreventiveservicestaskforce.org/Page/Document/UpdateSummaryFinal/ovarian-cancer-screening1	1, 2
Screening for skin cancer	General population	Uncertain benefits; requires much time and effort. See Chapter 15, and https://www.uspreventiveservicestaskforce.org/Page/Document/UpdateSummaryFinal/skin-cancer-screening2	3

Service	Population in Which Service Is Discouraged	Rationale for Discouraging Service[a]	Primary Exclusion Category[b]
TABLE 20.3 Discouraged Preventive Services and the Target Groups to Which They Apply (Continued)			
Teaching breast self-examination	General population	Lack of evidence that teaching improves health outcomes; increases risk of diagnostic procedures. See Chapter 15.	1, 2
Vision			
Glaucoma screening	General population	Unknown balance of benefits and harms: earlier detection and treatment does improve vision-related function and quality of life but treatment involves some risks. See https://www.uspreventiveservicestaskforce.org/Page/Document/UpdateSummaryFinal/glaucoma-screening	3
Mental Health			
Dementia screening	General population	Unknown balance of benefit and harms: current treatments have limited effectiveness in modifying instrumental activities of daily living. See Chapter 14 and https://www.uspreventiveservicestaskforce.org/Page/Document/UpdateSummaryFinal/cognitive-impairment-in-older-adults-screening	2, 3

(Continued)

TABLE 20.3 Discouraged Preventive Services and the Target Groups to Which They Apply   (Continued)

Service	Population in Which Service Is Discouraged	Rationale for Discouraging Service[a]	Primary Exclusion Category[b]
Unfocused Screening			
Screening pelvic examinations	General population	Population-based RCTs show that screening for ovarian cancer using bimanual pelvic examinations does not improve health outcomes. Although there are a host of other gynecologic diseases that could be detected, given the epidemiology of these diseases, yield would be low and not more than a low-value service overall. https://www.uspreventive-servicestaskforce.org/Page/Document/UpdateSummaryFinal/gynecological-conditions-screening-with-the-pelvic-examination	2
Routine complete blood counts	General population	Identifies multiple hematologic abnormalities; detection of the most common disorders not associated with improved health outcomes in asymptomatic adults; false-positive results common	2
Routine chemistry panels	General population	Screens for dozens of abnormalities, many of which are rare; evidence of benefit scant, and false-positive results common. See Chapter 5	2

TABLE 20.3   Discouraged Preventive Services and the Target Groups to Which They Apply   (Continued)

Service	Population in Which Service Is Discouraged	Rationale for Discouraging Service[a]	Primary Exclusion Category[b]
Routine liver function panel	General population	Screens for liver dysfunction, but there is no effective treatment for isolated abnormalities in liver function tests in asymptomatic population; false-positive results common	2
Whole-body scans	General population	Whole-body ultrasonography, computed tomography, positron emission testing offered by mobile vans, senior centers, or shopping mall outlets do not provide targeted screening for those selected populations for which early detection improves outcomes (e.g., screening for abdominal aortic aneurysms in male smokers older than 65 yr); high rate of false-positive and false-negative results	1, 2
Routine urinalysis	General population	Urinalysis detects asymptomatic bacteriuria, hematuria, and pyuria, but these findings are nonspecific; bacteriuria not known to cause harms in asymptomatic adults; false-positive results common	2

[a]Space limitation precludes detailed explanations. In most cases the table provides the current website address for more detailed rationale statements from the U.S. Preventive Services Task Force.
[b]**1, Unacceptably high harms; 2, modest or no benefit; 3, uncertain benefits or harms.**
COPD, chronic obstructive pulmonary disease; CVD, cardiovascular disease; DEXA, dual x-ray absorptiometry; RCT, randomized control trial.

On-Line Resources

https://www.uspreventiveservicestaskforce.org/.
https://epss.ahrq.gov/PDA/index.jsp.
https://www.acponline.org/clinical-information/high-value-care.

REFERENCES

1. Qaseem A, Alguire P, Dallas P, et al. Appropriate use of screening and diagnostic tests to foster high-value, cost-conscious care. *Ann Intern Med.* 2012;156(2):147-149.
2. Owens DK, Qaseem A, Chou R, Shekelle P. Clinical guidelines committee of the American College of Physicians. High-value, cost-conscious health care: concepts for clinicians to evaluate the benefits, harms, and costs of medical interventions. *Ann Intern Med.* 2011;154(3):174-180.
3. US Preventive Services Task Force. *USPSTF Procedure Manual*; 2015. https://www.uspreventiveservicestaskforce.org/Page/Name/procedure-manual. Accessed 1 March 2018.
4. Maciosek MV, LaFrance AB, Dehmer SP, et al. Updated priorities among effective clinical preventive services. *Ann Fam Med.* 2017;15(1):14-22.
5. Manson JE, Aragaki AK, Rossouw JE, et al; WHI Investigators. Menopausal hormone therapy and long-term all-cause and cause-specific mortality: the women's health initiative randomized trials. *JAMA.* 2017;318(10):927-938.
6. Gartlehner G, Patel SV, Feltner C, et al. Hormone therapy for the primary prevention of chronic conditions in postmenopausal women evidence report and systematic review for the US preventive services task force. *JAMA.* 2017;318(22):2234-2249.
7. Cotter A, Viong K, Mustelin L, et al. Labeling: a systematic review of an under-appreciated and understudied harm of screening. *BMJ.* 2017. http://bmjopen.bmj.com/content/bmjopen/7/12/e017565.draft-revisions.pdf. Accessed 1 March 2018.
8. Bibbins-Domingo K; U.S. Preventive Services Task Force. Aspirin use for the primary prevention of cardiovascular disease and colorectal cancer: U.S. preventive services task force recommendation statement. *Ann Intern Med.* 2016;164(12):836-845.
9. Harding GKM, Zhanel GG, Nicolle LE, et al. Antimicrobial treatment in diabetic women with asymptomatic bacteriuria. *N Engl J Med.* 2002;347(20):1576-1583.
10. Moyer VA; U.S. Preventive Services Task Force. Vitamin, mineral, and multivitamin supplements for the primary prevention of cardiovascular disease and cancer: U.S. preventive services task force recommendation statement. *Ann Intern Med.* 2014;160(8):558-564.
11. Bibbins-Domingo K, Grossman DC, et al; U.S. Preventive Services Task Force. Screening for obstructive sleep apnea in adults: US preventive services task force recommendation statement. *JAMA.* 2017;317(4):407-414.
12. LeFevre ML; U.S. Preventive Services Task Force. Screening for asymptomatic carotid artery stenosis: U.S. preventive services task force recommendation statement. *Ann Intern Med.* 2014;161(5):356-362.
13. U.S. Preventive Services Task Force. Screening for testicular cancer: U.S. preventive services task force reaffirmation recommendation statement. *Ann Intern Med.* 2011;154(7):483-486.
14. LeFevre ML; U.S. Preventive Services Task Force. Screening for thyroid dysfunction: U.S. preventive services task force recommendation statement. *Ann Intern Med.* 2015;162(9):641-650.
15. Bloomfield HE, Olson A, Wilt TJ. Screening pelvic examinations in asymptomatic, average-risk adult women. *Ann Intern Med.* 2014;161(12):924-925.

16. Guirguis-Blake JM, Henderson JT, Perdue LA. Periodic screening pelvic examination: evidence report and systematic review for the US preventive services task force. *JAMA.* 2017;317(9):954-966.

17. Yarnall KS, Pollak KI, Ostbye T, et al. Primary care: is there enough time for prevention? *Am J Public Health.* 2003;93(4):635-641.

18. U.S. Preventive Services Task Force. Screening for breast cancer: U.S. preventive services task force recommendation statement. *Ann Intern Med.* 2016;164:279-296.

19. U.S. Preventive Services Task Force. Screening for osteoporosis: U.S. preventive services task force recommendation statement. *JAMA.* 2018;319(24):2521-2531.

20. LeFevre ML; U.S. Preventive Services Task Force. Screening for chlamydia and gonorrhea: U.S. Preventive services task force recommendation statement. *Ann Intern Med.* 2014;161(12):902-910.

21. Moyer VA; U.S. Preventive Services Task Force. Risk assessment, genetic counseling, and genetic testing for BRCA-related cancer in women: U.S. preventive services task force recommendation statement. *Ann Intern Med.* 2014;160(4):271-281.

22. LeFevre ML; U.S. Preventive Services Task Force. Screening for abdominal aortic aneurysm: U.S. preventive services task force recommendation statement. *Ann Intern Med.* 2014;161(4):281-290.

23. Bibbins-Domingo K, Grossman DC, Curry SJ, et al; US Preventive Services Task Force. Screening for celiac disease: U.S. preventive services task force recommendation statement. *JAMA.* 2017;317(12):1252-1257.

24. Bibbins-Domingo K, Grossman DC, Curry SJ, et al; US Preventive Services Task Force. Screening for thyroid cancer: U.S. preventive services task force recommendation statement. *JAMA.* 2017;317(18):1882-1887.

25. Curry SJ, Krist AH, Owens DK, et al. Screening for cardiovascular disease risk with electrocardiography: US preventive services task force recommendation statement. *JAMA.* 2018;319(22):2308-2314.

26. Curry SJ, Krist AH, Owens DK, et al. Risk Assessment for cardiovascular disease with nontraditional risk factors: US preventive services task force recommendation statement. *JAMA.* 2018;320(3):272-280.

27. Bibbins-Domingo K, Grossman DC, Curry SJ, et al; US Preventive Services Task Force. Statin use for the primary prevention of cardiovascular disease in adults: U.S. preventive services task force recommendation statement. *JAMA.* 2016;316(19):1997-2007.

28. Moyer VA; U.S. Preventive Services Task Force. Vitamin D and calcium supplementation to prevent fractures in adults: U.S. preventive services task force recommendation statement. *Ann Intern Med.* 2013;158(9):691-696.

29. Mayo Clinic Shared Decision Making National Resource Center. https://shared-decisions.mayoclinic.org/. Accessed 1 March 2018.

Please see Online Appendix: Apps and Digital Resources for additional information.

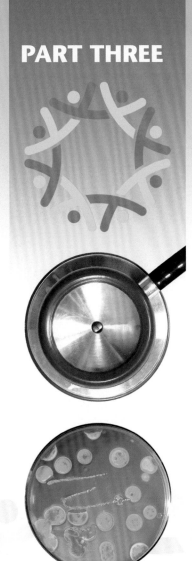

PART THREE

Putting Prevention Recommendations into Practice

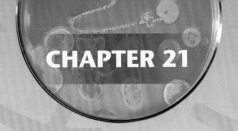

CHAPTER 21

Developing a Health Maintenance Schedule

KELLY F. HOLTZ AND GERALDINE F. MARROCCO

BACKGROUND

Primary care clinicians are responsible for providing medical care to both sick and well patients. Their most challenging task may be the delivery of preventive services as recommended in current guidelines. Such guidelines are useless unless the services they advocate are routinely offered to eligible patients and are accepted by these patients. Clinicians encounter many barriers to implementation of preventive guidelines and often lack the motivation to incorporate preventive services into their practices owing to the lack of direct incentives. The consequences of not treating an illness are more immediately apparent to the clinician than are the consequences of not offering recommended preventive services. For example, the failure to prescribe antibiotics for bacterial pneumonia creates immediate consequences, such as clinical deterioration or the need for referral to the emergency department. Forgetting to recommend health maintenance interventions, however, has deferred consequences, months or years in the future, and produces little effect in the near term to motivate clinicians to behave differently.

The proven benefits of preventive services cannot be fully realized unless practices develop systems to ensure their delivery. As shown in Figure 21.1, the organized delivery of preventive services in primary care settings requires a written health maintenance schedule—a protocol that describes the preventive services a practice intends to offer—and a system to ensure that the schedule is implemented. A health maintenance schedule defines the primary or secondary preventive services that should be offered to patients and their recommended periodicity. Interventions can include screening for disease, counseling patients about lifestyle changes, immunizations, and chemoprophylaxis. These services are indicated based on the patient's age, gender, and risk factors. The health maintenance schedule is a general guide for clinicians that can be modified based on the circumstances, characteristics, and needs of individual patients.

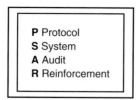

P Protocol
S System
A Audit
R Reinforcement

Figure 21.1   Process for implementing prevention.

An explicit written health maintenance schedule is the foundation for developing an effective system of implementing prevention in patient care. It defines the goals of the practice for delivery of preventive services. The health maintenance schedule should be a written document so that there are no uncertainties about what the group is trying to achieve. Having a clearly stated standard for the practice does not mean, however, that individual clinicians cannot deviate from the basic protocol to accommodate their own preferences or the circumstances of individual patients. It does mean that the group's minimum standards are clearly stated. The health maintenance schedule is not a static document. It needs to be revised periodically based on changing evidence or group preference.

Carefully constructing a health maintenance schedule can be an intimidating task. For one thing, it takes time. It is an important task, however, because incorporating health promotion and disease prevention into the provision of acute medical care is a large part of what distinguishes primary care from specialty medicine. Designing the health maintenance schedule is also challenging because of conflicting expert recommendations, clinician preferences, expectations, time constraints, and costs that the clinician or group incurs in designing the schedule.

The system and tools for implementing the health maintenance schedule include the following components: a plan for offering preventive services, a process for delivering the preventive services, a person responsible for making sure the goals of the practice are met, a clinician and patient reminder plan, and a plan for engaging patients in their own preventive care. Audits are necessary to monitor the progress of the practice in achieving its goals. Artificial reinforcements such as peer review and cajoling or more formal reinforcements such as monetary incentives may also be needed, because the natural reinforcements that are found in acute care may not pertain to implementing a prevention program. Many tools can be helpful in implementing the preventive system, for example, flow charts, computer-based reminders, patient handouts, and Web-based information resources, but tools alone do not ensure effective implementation of preventive medicine in practice. Tools should not be confused with a system.

This chapter focuses on the first step in adopting a system: reaching agreement on a health maintenance schedule. The discussion begins with an examination of barriers to the implementation of preventive

TABLE 21.1 Pearls for Developing a Health Maintenance Schedule
Get maximum clinician input in the developmental process
Develop a minimum, not a maximum, schedule
Allow individual clinician variation above the minimum
Make the schedule relevant to the local patient population and feasible to implement in the practice
Remember that the development of the schedule is an ongoing dynamic process
Remember that screening frequency is determined by the rate of progression of the disease and the sensitivity of the screening test
Remember that a person's risk status influences the cost-effectiveness of screening for a given disease, not screening frequency

services in practice. This is important primarily because the design of the health maintenance schedule must be sensitive to these barriers and deal with them constructively to be acceptable to clinicians and applicable to patient care. The chapter then discusses the three steps necessary to develop a health maintenance schedule: establishing a group process, determining which interventions to include in the schedule, and deciding on the recommended frequency for each of the interventions. Table 21.1 summarizes the important take-home points regarding this process.

BARRIERS TO PREVENTION

Barriers to implementing preventive services that affect the development of a health maintenance schedule include lack of time, uncertainty about the value of preventive services, conflict among expert groups that issue recommendations, lack of good systems to facilitate delivery of preventive services, and social barriers.[1]

Lack of time is of paramount concern in primary care. A busy clinician sees 25 to 35 patients per day, and at each patient visit the question must be asked, "Is preventive care up to date?" Time does not permit clinicians to offer unlimited preventive services to all patients. Yarnall et al. estimated that a clinician would have to spend 7.4 hours of each work day to optimally implement all of the preventive services recommended by the U.S. Preventive Services Task Force (USPSTF) in 1996. Two hours each day would be required of an average primary care clinician to implement only the strongest ("A" grade) USPSTF recommendations.[2] The health maintenance schedule must be sensitive to these time constraints by including only proven interventions that are feasible in the practice setting. In developing the schedule, the practice should prioritize interventions as essential or optional; it should include all the essential interventions and be selective about including the optional ones. In addition, the health maintenance schedule should be organized to enable clinicians to quickly determine which preventive services are indicated at any given patient visit.

Uncertainty about the value of preventive services is another barrier to effective implementation. For example, clinicians are unlikely to order a screening test if they do not believe it to be worthwhile. The practice should adopt and adhere to criteria of effectiveness that preventive interventions must meet to be considered worthwhile and appropriate for the health maintenance schedule. Clinicians and the practice must be comfortable with the criteria they adopt. An example of such criteria is provided in Table 21.2. Evidence-based guidelines explicitly state the evidence on which recommendations are based, allowing the group to discuss and debate the appropriateness of specific interventions. It is important for preventive service recommendations to assess the balance of evidence and harms based on evidence in an efficient manner.[4]

Conflict among expert groups provides a further obstacle to preventive medicine. Although there is usually a core of agreement between the recommendations of different expert groups, there are often significant disagreements. For example, specialists often recommend intensive preventive efforts for conditions in their particular specialty, even

TABLE 21.2   Criteria for Appropriate Screening Programs
The condition must have a significant effect on the quality or quantity of life
Acceptable methods of treatment must be available
Facilities for diagnosis and treatment should be available[3]
The condition must have an asymptomatic period in which detection and treatment significantly reduce morbidity and/or mortality
Treatment in the asymptomatic phase must yield a superior result to that obtained by delaying treatment until symptoms appear
Tests that are acceptable to patients must be available at a reasonable cost to detect the condition in the asymptomatic period
The natural history of the condition should be understood[3]
The incidence of the condition must be sufficient to justify the cost of screening
There should be an agreed policy on whom to treat as patients
The cost of case finding should be economically balanced; a continuing process therefore limiting "single-occasion screening"[3]

Adapted from Frame PS, Carlson SJ. A critical review of periodic health screening using specific screening criteria: part 1. Selected diseases of respiratory, cardiovascular, and central nervous systems. *J Fam Pract.* 1975;2:29.

when strong evidence of effectiveness is lacking. Primary care clinicians encounter a healthier population than do specialists, and they should not be reluctant to require evidence of benefit before adopting recommendations from expert specialty sources. Resources for obtaining evidence-based preventive recommendations are described in Table 21.3.

Integrating the delivery of preventative services into the flow of patient care can be facilitated through the design of specific templates utilized in the electronic medical record in the practice.

Ultimately, clinicians must agree with the interventions contained in their practice's health maintenance schedule. After all, they are the ones who must implement the schedule, and they are the ones who will experience both the rewards and the frustrations that result from their efforts.

TABLE 21.3 Evidence-Based Preventive Medicine Guideline Resources

- **Agency for Healthcare Research and Quality**
www.ahrq.gov
Home of the U.S. Preventive Services Task Force (USPSTF) and the Put Prevention into Practice (PPIP) programs (see page 532); maintains a ListServ which sends e-mail notification of new USPSTF and PPIP recommendations

  - **U.S. Preventive Services Task Force (USPSTF):**
http://www.ahrq.gov/clinic/uspstfix.htm

  - **Put Prevention into Practice** program materials:
http://www.ahrq.gov/clinic/ppipix.htm

  - **Electronic Preventive Services Selector:**
http://epss.ahrq.gov/PDA/index.jsp
An electronic resource allowing physicians to input a patient's characteristics to find applicable USPSTF preventive health care recommendations

- **National Guideline Clearinghouse**
www.guideline.gov
Single source for evidence-based guidelines on many topics including preventive services. Guidelines issued by specialty organizations can be accessed through this site
USPSTF Website
http://www.uspreventiveservicestaskforce.org
A Web-based resource of all active and inactive recommendations, as well as those referring to another organization, such as the CDC

- **Advisory Committee on Immunization Practices (ACIP)**
www.cdc.gov/vaccines/pubs/acip-list.htm
Authoritative source for immunization guidelines

- **American Cancer Society Guidelines for the Early Detection of Cancer**
http://Caonline.amcancersoc.org
Recommendations are in the January–February issue yearly

ESTABLISHING A GROUP PROCESS

Most clinicians practice in groups. Even clinicians in solo practice work closely with nurses and other health professionals. Therefore, a process is needed for the group to reach a consensus on the content of the health maintenance schedule. Although no single method for forging consensus is ideal for all groups, several common principles apply:

1. **Choose a leader.** In larger groups, there may be several clinicians with a particular interest in prevention. One of them is a logical choice to become the leader and should take charge of developing the health maintenance schedule. The leader should be respected by most of the group members. The leader should also be dedicated to the importance of disease prevention and be a good facilitator of group processes. It is helpful if the leader is knowledgeable about evidence-based preventive care recommendations. Such guidelines can be obtained from the resources listed in Table 21.3. Alternatively, an expert consultant can be retained to help the group understand the different prevention guidelines.

2. **Set a minimum standard.** The goal is not necessarily to develop full consensus but to develop a protocol that establishes a minimum acceptable standard for the practice. The schedule should not list every preventive service recommended by an expert group. The USPSTF assigns one of five letter grades (A, B, C, D, or I), providing definitions of and suggestions for practice services for low-risk adults, and many more for patients with one or more known risk factors can be found in Appendix A. It is difficult and unnecessary for all the clinicians in a practice to reach a consensus on an identical schedule. What is necessary, however, is that the group agrees upon a *minimum* standard. Most of the proven benefits of early detection accrue from screening for a few conditions, namely, risk factors for coronary artery disease and cancer of the breast, cervix, colon, and rectum. Clinicians who wish to add other procedures or adopt more frequent intervals may do so. In reality, most clinicians will find it challenging enough to comply with even the minimum standard for all patients. Screening is hard work.

3. **Group process.** The process should involve as many clinicians as possible. Ideally, unless the group is very large, all members should participate. Clinicians are unlikely to perform procedures on the health maintenance schedule that they do not believe are worthwhile. Clinicians' involvement in the development process is the best way to help them understand the rationale for each intervention. Depending on the size and dynamics of the group, it is desirable to involve nurses and nonmedical personnel when developing

the health maintenance schedule. Clinician buy-in is essential to creating a health maintenance schedule that reflects the views of the group and will be used by the practice. If specific clinicians disagree with the schedule, they should be given the opportunity to suggest an alternate schedule and to discuss the merits of each option. An acceptable compromise is most easily reached by emphasizing the concept that the group schedule is a minimum acceptable protocol, allowing clinicians the freedom to do more if they wish.

4. **Reevaluate.** The practice should not be reluctant to try an intervention for a specified time and to reevaluate its value at a later date. Developing a health maintenance schedule is a dynamic process that should result in changes to the document over time. If a major controversy over the schedule develops within the practice, the group should make a temporary decision about what to include and should also commit itself to reevaluate the issue at a later date. The experience of either undertaking or not undertaking the intervention will, over time, help inform the clinicians' opinions about whether the schedule needs to be revised.

CHOOSING SPECIFIC INTERVENTIONS

Most practices will use a set of published guidelines as the starting point for deciding which interventions to include when developing a health maintenance schedule. Table 21.3 lists some of the major groups that issue evidence-based guidelines relating to prevention. The USPSTF, sponsored by the Agency for Healthcare Research and Quality (AHRQ), is considered the most comprehensive, authoritative, and unbiased source of clinical preventive recommendations. Appendix A in this book lists interventions recommended by the USPSTF for low-risk adults. The Advisory Committee on Immunization Practices, sponsored by the Centers for Disease Control and Prevention, is the leading source of recommendations relating to immunizations for vaccine-preventable disease (see Chapter 17). The American Cancer Society recommendations regarding cancer prevention are widely known and followed by many clinicians and the lay public. The National Guideline Clearinghouse is a website maintained by AHRQ, which catalogs evidence-based guidelines on a wide range of medical topics, including preventive medicine. Most guidelines issued by specialty organizations can be accessed through this site. An AHRQ initiative has produced an Electronic Preventive Services Selector (ePSS) that can be used online or can be downloaded to a personal digital assistant or smartphone to provide ready access to the USPSTF recommendations. The tool is not meant to replace clinical judgment or individualized patient care.

Before a practice decides to include or exclude controversial interventions, the recommendations of several authoritative groups should be compared so that members understand the reasons that the experts disagree. The practice may find it useful to consider interventions for different age groups separately. Developing separate schedules for children (e.g., age 18 yr and younger), young adults (e.g., ages 19–39 yr), middle-aged adults (e.g., ages 40–64 yr), and older adults (e.g., age 65 yr and older) may be helpful.

The rationale for each potential recommendation should be understood. Clinicians should not hesitate to question or be critical of any recommendation, regardless of its acceptance in the medical community. Medicine has many examples of accepted screening interventions, such as pelvic examinations for the detection of ovarian cancer, for which there is little supporting scientific evidence. Although there is no recommendation against performing a routine pelvic examination, continued use of clinical judgment is encouraged and more research is called for. In addition to the scientific validity of the recommendation, the clinicians should consider the relevance of the recommendation to their patient population and the feasibility of implementing the recommendation under current practice conditions.

The definition of some preventive services in the health maintenance schedule may need special clarification. For example, the meaning of blood pressure measurement is obvious, whereas the exact operational meaning of "healthy diet and physical activity counseling" could have multiple interpretations, and examples of clinical considerations should be accessed where effective interventions are discussed such as in the Final Recommendation Statements available on the USPSTF website. The practice should spell out in detail what is expected of the clinician to comply with the recommendation. If the practice cannot decide exactly what a recommendation means or how it should be implemented, then it may be decided that one be excluded from the schedule.

Keep the schedule simple. When developing health maintenance schedules, there may be a tendency to become idealistic and include a variety of interventions with marginal evidence of benefit. As a general rule, if an adult or pediatric schedule cannot be clearly outlined in a flow sheet or table and limited to a single page, then it is too complex. A complex schedule will not be used routinely by clinicians because its implementation requires too much time and attention, and frustration can ensue. Clinicians will then likely ignore the schedule altogether, omitting worthwhile as well as marginal interventions.

The basic schedule should focus on interventions applicable to the general, low-risk population. The USPSTF outlines grade A recommendations, approximately 16, which are recommended as a service with high certainty that the net benefit is substantial. Grade B services, approximately 34, are recommendations with a high certainty that the net benefit is moderate or there is a moderate certainty that the net benefit is moderate to substantial. Suggestions for practice include both grade A and B services. Given the caveats reviewed in Chapter 20, discussing the benefits and harms of prostate cancer screening with men older than 50 years and helping them decide if they wish to have screening is an essential intervention.[5]

Interventions that do not fulfill the above-mentioned criteria should be considered optional. A practice can be more selective in deciding whether or not to include optional interventions in its health maintenance schedule. A few interventions relevant to large high-risk groups, such as influenza vaccination, might be included. Including services for all high-risk groups is unnecessary and should be avoided, however, or a service with a grade C, which depends on individual circumstances. Whatever the content of the practice's health maintenance schedule, most clinicians will individualize preventive care to the particular patient. This is partly because each patient has a unique set of risk factors and concurrent diagnoses, but it also reflects such factors as patient preferences. It is virtually impossible to account for all these factors in a preset schedule. Rather, the schedule can be seen as a basic guide to be modified, augmented, or pruned to reflect the needs of the individual patient.

FREQUENCY OF INTERVENTIONS

In addition to listing recommended interventions, the health maintenance schedule should specify the frequency for offering each intervention. For some recommendations, such as certain immunizations, the proper timing of the intervention is well established. For other preventive services, such as smoking cessation counseling, there are few scientific data to support a specific frequency. For most preventive interventions the evidence supports a range of frequencies (e.g., every 3–5 yr for Pap smears).

The two most important determinants of screening frequency are the sensitivity of the screening test and the rate of progression of the disease. The risk of acquiring the disease (e.g., incidence rate) should not play a factor in determining screening frequency. For example, consider a cancer with a slow rate of progression of 10 years from dysplasia to an incurable stage. If a screening test with a sensitivity of 80% is performed every 3 years, the first screening will detect 80% of cases, the second will detect 80% of the remainder (96% of cases), and the third will detect 80% of the remainder (99% of cases). Unless the rate of progression of the disease or the sensitivity of the test changes,[6] the same proportion of cases will be detected regardless of the patient's risk of acquiring the disease. Therefore, the health maintenance schedule should not recommend a shorter interval between screening tests for persons at high risk of disease simply because they are at higher risk. High-risk patients should receive more intensive outreach efforts to ensure their involvement in the health maintenance program of the practice, but they need not be screened more frequently. A patient's risk status does influence the cost-effectiveness of screening, however. Screening for tuberculosis, for example, will have a very low yield in an affluent suburban population but is very important in a correctional facility. Therefore, risk status influences the decision of whether or not to screen more than it affects the decision of how often to screen.

For many preventive interventions, a frequency cannot be specified based on scientific evidence and must be determined by the clinician. An excessively frequent interval will increase costs and take time away from other important tasks. In addition, more frequent testing increases the probability of generating false-positive results and unnecessary workups. Too long a screening interval will increase the risk of missing important disease. Because the practice will have to make an arbitrary decision about the recommended frequency that will appear in the schedule, the concept of a minimum schedule, with tolerance of individual variation, is again useful.

ANNUAL COMPLETE PHYSICAL EXAMINATIONS

The proper frequency of health maintenance *visits*, an issue separate from the frequency of performing specific *procedures*, is a subject of much controversy. The appropriateness of the "annual physical" has been debated since the 1940s, and the proper schedule for well child examinations has received greater attention in recent years. Several important questions underlie this controversy: What is the role of the annual complete physical examination (CPE)? How is the CPE different from the periodic health examination (PHE)? Should preventive interventions be delivered during acute-care visits or just during dedicated prevention visits?

The CPE was first popularized in the 1920s by the life insurance industry and became more entrenched after World War II. With increased acceptance of evidence-based preventive medicine in the 1970s and 1980s, however, major authoritative groups, including the Canadian Task Force on the Periodic Health Examination, the American Medical Association, and the USPSTF, recommended replacing the annual CPE with selective interventions tailored to the individual patient. Despite these recommendations, the annual CPE remains very popular with clinicians, patients, and the media. Most adults in the United States believe that annual comprehensive physical examinations are important and a 2002 study showed that more than 90% endorse the value of routine examination of the heart, lungs, abdomen, reflexes, and prostate.[3] Several factors may explain the enduring appeal of the CPE. It is a simple concept that most health consumers have embraced, whereas the argument for a complex health maintenance schedule is less intuitive. This chapter has stressed the need for a system to deliver preventive care. The annual CPE is a system, which may be better than no system, which may be the only alternative for practices that have not organized themselves to generate patient and clinician reminders. Finally, the CPE provides more time than an acute visit to focus on lifestyle issues and the delivery of preventive services.

There are disadvantages to the annual CPE, however. First, there is not enough time to perform a CPE on all patients. The average primary care clinician, with 2000 patients in the practice and 200 workdays per year, would have to perform 10 CPEs every day and would have little time to do anything else. Therefore, clinicians who profess that the annual CPE is their system for delivering preventive care are probably offering it to selected patients. Patients who elect to have annual CPEs and PHEs tend to be the affluent with relatively healthy lifestyles. Therefore, in what has been called *reverse targeting*, patients who are in less need of preventive services may receive more preventive services than they need, whereas high-risk patients most in need of preventive services may receive little or no organized preventive care.

The annual CPE is also expensive and inefficient. "Complete" implies doing many tests, many of which offer no benefit to the asymptomatic patient but do generate false-positive results that must be evaluated, often at substantial costs (see Chapter 20). The word complete may also imply (falsely) to patients that everything possible has been done and that their good health can be assured for the next year. A final disadvantage of the annual CPE is that they are not covered by many third-party payers (including Medicare and Medicaid). New Medicare beneficiaries (within 6 mo of enrollment) are eligible to receive a "Welcome to Medicare" visit in which some preventive services can be delivered, including a medical history, recommended immunizations, and screenings and perhaps further tests depending on current health and medical history.

The concept of the PHE is distinct from the annual CPE in that its periodicity and content can be specified by the practice and tailored to individual patients. The PHE is dedicated to prevention and is less about the physical examination and laboratory testing, which are done for specific indications, and more about risk assessment and risk reduction (see Chapter 2). Evidence of the effectiveness of the PHE was reviewed by AHRQ in 2006 (see http://www.ahrq.gov/clinic/tp/phetp.htm). Practices may choose to include the PHE in their health maintenance schedule at specified intervals depending on age and gender. The schedule should specify the minimum content of those visits.

Clinicians can and do deliver preventive services during both acute and chronic care visits. Flocke et al., in a direct observation study of family physicians, reported that preventive services were delivered during 32% of illness visits.[7] The limited time available to patients and clinicians during CPEs, PHEs, and illness visits can be put to best use by implementing reminder systems to help office staff quickly identify which preventive interventions are indicated when a patient checks in. Reminder systems enable the nurse to appropriately prepare the patient so that the clinician can more efficiently implement the scheduled preventive service. Chapter 2 discusses the role of previsit procedures, reminders, prompts, and flow sheets to help clinicians rapidly identify preventive services needing attention.

Delivering preventive care during either acute or chronic illness visits captures the patient population that does not schedule CPEs or PHEs.
Although lack of time is often considered the major disadvantage of implementing prevention during illness visits, most preventive interventions are
brief and can be easily worked into the pace of acute care. This does not apply
when patients are new to the practice, have multiple issues to address, or
require a comprehensive health risk appraisal. The most effective strategy
to maximize the delivery of preventive care to as many patients as possible
is for the clinician to try to address preventive health needs during all illness
visits and to recommend PHEs as needed for those patients who require
a more complete health risk appraisal and prevention plan. Components
of the physical examination recommended for the asymptomatic adult
include blood pressure screening every 1 to 2 years, periodic measurement
of body mass index, Pap smears beginning at age 21 years for sexually active
women with a cervix every 3 years up to the age of 65 years.[8]

As discussed in Chapter 2, continuity (longitudinal) relationships also
enable primary care clinicians to initiate preventive services at a given
visit and to return to the topic, or address other needed services, at future
appointments. Preventive services recommended by the USPSTF are listed
on their website.

SUMMARY AND CONCLUSION

Developing a health maintenance schedule requires an upfront effort to
create the health maintenance protocol, an ongoing practice commitment, and cooperation. The group should select a designated leader to
champion the effort. Participation and support should be sought from as
many clinicians as possible. The schedule should include essential preventive interventions and optional services of proven effectiveness. It should
provide a minimum standard for the group, based on the latest recommendations, with the understanding that it may be individually tailored
to the particular patient and clinician. The frequency of specific screening
interventions is not determined by the patient's risk but by the sensitivity
of the screening test and rate of progression of the disease. A structured
approach should be developed to ensure that the health maintenance
schedule is offered to all patients. A system for delivering preventive services, which is discussed in the following chapter, rests upon the foundation of a well-defined health maintenance schedule.

SUGGESTED RESOURCES AND MATERIALS

Agency for Healthcare Research and Quality
www.ahrq.gov
*Home of the U.S. Preventive Services Task Force (USPSTF) and the Put Prevention into
   Practice (PPIP) programs (see page 532); maintains a ListServ which sends e-mail
   notification of new USPSTF and PPIP recommendations*

U.S. Preventive Services Task Force (USPSTF):
http://www.ahrq.gov/clinic/uspstfix.htm

Put Prevention into Practice program materials:
http://www.ahrq.gov/clinic/ppipix.htm

Electronic Preventive Services Selector:
http://epss.ahrq.gov/PDA/index.jsp
An electronic resource allowing physicians to input a patient's characteristics to find applicable USPSTF preventive health care recommendations

National Guideline Clearinghouse
www.guideline.gov
Single source for evidence-based guidelines on many topics including preventive services. Guidelines issued by specialty organizations can be accessed through this site

USPSTF Website
http://www.uspreventiveservicestaskforce.org
A Web-based resource of all active and inactive recommendations, as well as those referring to another organization, such as the CDC

Advisory Committee on Immunization Practices (ACIP)
www.cdc.gov/vaccines/pubs/acip-list.htm
Authoritative source for immunization guidelines

American Cancer Society Guidelines for the Early Detection of Cancer
http://Caonline.amcancersoc.org
Recommendations are in the January–February issue yearly

REFERENCES

1. Frame PS. Health maintenance in clinical practice: strategies and barriers. *Am Fam Physician.* 1992;45:1192-1200.
2. Yarnall KS, Pollak KI, Ostbye T, et al. Primary care: is there enough time for prevention? *Am J Pub Health.* 2003;93:635-641.
3. Oboler SK, Prochazka AV, Gonzales R, et al. Public expectations and attitudes for annual physical examinations and testing. *Ann Intern Med.* 2002;136:652-659.
4. Mitka M. Studies continue to show no benefit from annual physicals in healthy adults. *JAMA.* 2012;308(22):2321-2322. doi:10.1001/jama.2012.36756.
5. Woolf SH. Screening for prostate cancer with prostate-specific antigen. *N Eng J Med.* 1995;333:1401-1405.
6. Frame PS, Frame JS. Determinants of cancer screening frequency: the example of screening for cervical cancer. *J Am Board Fam Pract.* 1998;11:87-95.
7. Flocke SA, Stange KC, Goodwin MA. Patient and visit characteristics associated with opportunistic preventive services delivery. *J Fam Pract.* 1998;47:202-208.
8. Bloomfield HE, Wilt TJ. *Evidence brief: role of the annual comprehensive physical examination in the asymptomatic adult.* In: *VA Evidence-based Synthesis Program Evidence Briefs [Internet].* Washington, DC: Department of Veterans Affairs (US); 2011. Available from: https://www.ncbi.nlm.nih.gov/books/NBK82767/.

Please see Online Appendix: Apps and Digital Resources for additional information.

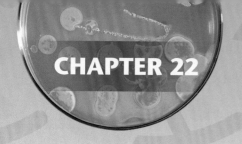

CHAPTER 22

Shared Decision Making: A Path to Patient-Centered Care

ERICA S. SPATZ

Shared decision making (SDM) is a model of care in which patients and clinicians work together to make a health care decision that is best for the patient. This process (Fig. 22.1) draws from the expertise of both the clinician and the patient.[1] In this bidirectional exchange, clinicians are charged with communicating scientific evidence from clinical trials and observational data about efficacy and safety, along with their knowledge and experience about the condition and the different options for diagnosis and/or treatment. In addition, patients are prompted to share their reaction to the information, along with their perspectives, values, and goals. Ultimately, when done well, clinicians and patients are better prepared to work together to determine what is feasible and likely to be beneficial and safe and to make decisions that are best aligned with the patients' preferences and goals.

Increasingly, SDM is being recognized not only for its potential to advance patient-centered care but also to improve patient safety and value in the health care system.[1-5] Patients who are engaged in a shared decision-making discussion have less decisional regret and are more likely to get the care they want and nothing more.[6,7] As such, when people are informed about their options, they are better able to flag concerns about side effects or safety, cost, convenience, and other burdens, the trade-offs of care that may ultimately compromise the effectiveness or benefits of the decided approach. In addition, there may be implications for spending, because "waste," or the care that patients would have otherwise declined had they had full knowledge of the available and reasonable treatment options, could be reduced. Second, some studies show that informed patients more often choose conservative and hence less expensive medical options, likely because they have more realistic expectations of the potential benefit and risks associated with a given therapy.[8,9] As an example, in a study by Arterburn et al. patients with hip or knee osteoarthritis who were exposed to a decision aid about treatment options were less likely to choose surgery than patients receiving usual care without the decision aid; the associated reduction in costs was estimated to be between 12% and 21%.[8]

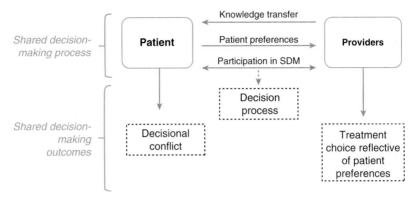

Figure 22.1   Shared decision making. Reprinted with permission from Spatz ES, Spertus JA. Shared decision making: a path toward improved patient-centered outcomes. *Circ Cardiovasc Qual Outcomes.* 2012;5(6):e75-e77.

SHARED DECISION MAKING IN ROUTINE CLINICAL CARE

SDM can occur in a multitude of practice settings and workflows. Commonly, SDM takes place during the clinical encounter, in which the patient and clinician sit down together to discuss a specific health care situation. However, SDM may also extend beyond the clinical encounter, either before or after a visit with the clinician; such workflows are designed to help better prepare patients for their visits with the clinician or to further process a discussion with their clinician, so that they may be more empowered to have meaningful discussions and develop informed preferences. For example, in a study of SDM in patients with hip or knee osteoarthritis, patients who received information about the treatment options before their visit with the orthopedist were better prepared to engage with their orthopedist, asked better questions, and were more likely to decide on a therapeutic approach at the initial consultation.[10]

SDM does not promote a singular model of decisional autonomy; in most cases, neither patients nor clinicians desire complete abdication of the clinician recommendation. Rather, clinician recommendations are informed by multiple considerations, including the patient's goals, such that the paradigm is not "What would you do if it were you, doctor?" but instead, "Knowing what you now know about me, what would you recommend?"

Patient decision aids, tools that provide evidence-based information about the reasonable options for management, can help facilitate patient understanding and enable patients to engage in a more confident and equal way with clinicians. Decision aids can also be useful for clinicians by consolidating known evidence about the intervention/s. Decision aids may take the form of a Web-based tool, video, or pamphlet and may be administered in the office or even independently by patients before their visit. Rigorous criteria, developed by the International Patient Decision Aid Standards Collaboration, have been used to assess the quality and effectiveness of decision aids.[11] More recently, the National Quality Forum drafted a list of criteria to certify decision aids as high-quality tools.[12] Decision aids to support SDM have been studied in a range of diseases, including prostate cancer, osteoporosis, osteoarthritis, hyperlipidemia, coronary artery disease, atrial fibrillation, and heart failure.[8–10,13–17] In a Cochrane review of 115 randomized controlled trials, decision aids, compared with usual care, were found to result in improved knowledge and confidence in decisions, including better decisional attributes (e.g., improved knowledge transfer, realistic perception of outcomes) and decisional processes (e.g., less decisional conflict, increased attention to personal values).[6]

WHEN TO USE SHARED DECISION MAKING: PREFERENCE-SENSITIVE CONDITIONS

The field of SDM has predominantly evolved to support "preference-sensitive conditions," a term used to describe conditions for which there is more than one reasonable option for management and in which the available options may involve significant trade-offs affecting the patient's quality and/or length of life.[18] Conditions considered to be of the highest priority for SDM include joint replacement for hip or knee osteoarthritis; treatment of herniated disk and spinal stenosis; treatment of clinically localized prostate cancer; maternal and fetal care, including birthing options; and percutaneous coronary intervention for stable ischemic heart disease. In an article by Oshima Lee and Emanuel, they call for the development of decision aids to support the 20 most frequently performed procedures, which would include procedures for the high-priority conditions noted earlier.[4]

Already, several clinical guidelines incorporate recommendations for SDM as a best practice, especially when the evidence is either unclear or supports two or more reasonable strategies. For example, in the American Heart Association/American College of Cardiology guidelines for cholesterol management, SDM is recommended as the preferred strategy when considering statin therapy in patients with low to moderate risk.[19] Other guidelines that incorporate recommendations for SDM in specific situations include the guidelines for the management of hypertension, advanced heart failure, and stable ischemic heart disease; the screening of lung cancer; and the treatment of localized prostate cancer.

Recently, SDM has been tied to several payment coverage determinations. The Centers for Medicare and Medicaid Services mandated that SDM with a certified (if available) decision aid be used before proceeding with a low-dose computed tomography to screen for lung cancer, left atrial appendage closure to prevent thromboembolic events in patients with atrial fibrillation, and insertion of an implantable cardioverter defibrillator to prevent sudden cardiac death in patients with advanced heart failure.[20–22] These decisions have prompted health care systems to figure out ways to incorporate SDM, to identify and access decision aids, and to educate and train clinicians on how best to meet this mandate.

BARRIERS TO IMPLEMENTATION

Despite decades of research, there is limited uptake of SDM into routine clinical practice, in part because of patient, physician, and system-level barriers.[23–25] One study identified pervasive physician and system-level barriers, summarized as "professional indifference," and "organizational inertia."[24] They found a lack of physician buy-in (e.g., lack of trust or agreement with content in decision aids, lack of comfort with the SDM tools); time constraints and competing priorities; lack of reimbursement; perceived burden; and cost. These concerns are legitimate and need to be considered when evaluating SDM adoption.

There is persistent concern among some clinicians that there can be unintentional harm in sharing evidence with patients. Some clinicians believe that the information will be too complicated for patients to comprehend, and that if offered the choice, patients will opt for more aggressive care than they need.[26] Others worry that patients would not go along with proven strategies because of a lack of perceived benefit. For example, many decision aids present information about the likelihood of benefits and risks in a graphic form showing the number needed to treat; yet, some worry that this translation of evidence will dampen enthusiasm for a given option, leading patients to opt for a less aggressive intervention or no intervention at all. Still, evidence suggests that patients value this information, and some studies show that the number needed to treat may not be the main factor on which patients make decsions.[27,28]

ADOPTION INTO CLINICAL PRACTICE

To guide the implementation of high-quality and achievable SDM, several steps are needed.[5] There is an urgent need for rapid certification of patient decision aids. This certification is necessary for clinicians, patients, and health systems to trust the quality of the data presented to patients and their source, ensuring that the information presented to patients is evidence based, balanced, and free of bias. Moreover, certification standards can ensure that developers employ a user-centered design, assuring that the information presented is of import to patients, is comprehendible, and is presented in a manner that helps patients develop informed preferences.

Second, there is a need to educate and train clinicians about SDM. The three elements of SDM are acknowledging with patients that a decision is required; knowing the treatment options and the associated risk, benefits, and trade-offs of each option, informed by the best available evidence; and incorporating the patient's values and preferences into the decision.[29] These concepts are further outlined in the "three-talk model" (Fig. 22.2), which breaks the discussion down into three components: Team Talk, Option Talk, and Decision Talk.[30] In addition, the Agency for Healthcare Research and Quality has developed the SHARE (seek, help, approach, reach, evaluate) approach, a five-step process for SDM.[31]

Third, shared decision-making tools need to be tied to the dissemination of clinical evidence.[32] Specifically, clinical guidelines that incorporate a recommendation for SDM should provide links to high-quality, certified, decision aids, which can consolidate the guideline evidence and support patient-clinician discussion.

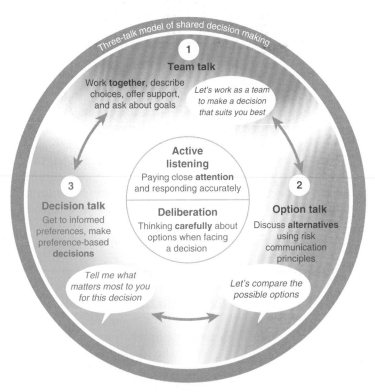

Figure 22.2 Three-talk model of shared decision making. Reprinted with permission from Elwyn G, Durand MA, Song J, et al. A three-talk model for shared decision making: multistage consultation process. *BMJ.* 2017;359:j4891.

SUMMARY

The concepts inherent to SDM can help to ensure that patients have the information they need to make decisions that are aligned with their preferences, values, and goals. When done well, SDM also helps to build strong relationships between clinicians and patients that are based on mutual respect, transparency, and trust. Clinicians need more training in SDM and specifically in eliciting patients' preferences, values, and goals, so that they can support patients in the decision-making process to the extent that the patient desires. Decision aids can help to facilitate these conversations, although are not a replacement for good communication. Ultimately, tying SDM and decision-making tools to clinical practice guidelines and to value-based programs can help to integrate SDM into the culture and practice of medicine.

REFERENCES

1. Spatz ES, Spertus JA. Shared decision making: a path toward improved patient-centered outcomes. *Circ Cardiovasc Qual Outcomes.* 2012;5(6):e75-e77.
2. Barry MJ, Edgman-Levitan S. Shared decision making – the pinnacle of patient-centered care. *N Engl J Med.* 2012;366(9):780-781.
3. Krumholz HM. Informed consent to promote patient-centered care. *JAMA.* 2010;303(12):1190-1191.
4. Oshima Lee E, Emanuel EJ. Shared decision making to improve care and reduce costs. *N Engl J Med.* 2013;368(1):6-8.
5. Spatz ES, Krumholz HM, Moulton BW. Prime time for shared decision making. *JAMA.* 2017;317(13):1309-1310.
6. Stacey D, Legare F, Col NF, et al. Decision aids for people facing health treatment or screening decisions. *Cochrane Database Syst Rev.* 2014;1:CD001431.
7. Mulley A, Trimble C, Elwyn G. *Patients' Preferences Matter: Stop the Silent Misdiagnosis.* The King's Fund; 2012.
8. Arterburn D, Wellman R, Westbrook E, et al. Introducing decision aids at group health was linked to sharply lower hip and knee surgery rates and costs. *Health Aff.* 2012;31(9):2094-2104.
9. Allen LA, McIlvennan CK, Thompson JS, et al. Effectiveness of an intervention supporting shared decision making for destination therapy left ventricular assist device: the DECIDE-LVAD randomized clinical trial. *JAMA Intern Med.* 2018;178(4):520-529.
10. Bozic KJ, Belkora J, Chan V, et al. Shared decision making in patients with osteoarthritis of the hip and knee: results of a randomized controlled trial. *J Bone Joint Surg Am.* 2013;95(18):1633-1639.
11. Volk RJ, Llewellyn-Thomas H, Stacey D, Elwyn G. Ten years of the international patient decision aid standards collaboration: evolution of the core dimensions for assessing the quality of patient decision aids. *BMC Med Inform Decis Mak.* 2013;13(suppl 2):S1.
12. Elwyn G, Burstin H, Barry MJ, et al. A proposal for the development of national certification standards for patient decision aids in the US. *Health Policy.* 2018;122(7):703-706.
13. Arnold SV, Decker C, Ahmad H, et al. Converting the informed consent from a perfunctory process to an evidence-based foundation for patient decision making. *Circ Cardiovasc Qual Outcomes.* 2008;1(1):21-28.

14. Spertus JA, Bach R, Bethea C, et al. Improving the process of informed consent for percutaneous coronary intervention: patient outcomes from the Patient Risk Information Services Manager (ePRISM) study. *Am Heart J.* 2015;169(2):234-241 e231.

15. Coylewright M, Dick S, Zmolek B, et al. PCI choice decision aid for stable coronary artery disease: a randomized trial. *Circ Cardiovasc Qual Outcomes.* 2016;9(6):767-776.

16. LeBlanc A, Wang AT, Wyatt K, et al. Encounter decision aid vs. Clinical decision support or usual care to support patient-centered treatment decisions in osteoporosis: the osteoporosis choice randomized trial II. *PLoS One.* 2015;10(5):e0128063.

17. Weymiller AJ, Montori VM, Jones LA, et al. Helping patients with type 2 diabetes mellitus make treatment decisions: statin choice randomized trial. *Arch Intern Med.* 2007;167(10):1076-1082.

18. *Preference-sensitive Care.* Lebanon, NH: Dartmouth Atlas Project; 2007.

19. Stone NJ, Robinson J, Lichtenstein AH, et al. 2013 ACC/AHA guideline on the treatment of blood cholesterol to reduce atherosclerotic cardiovascular risk in adults. A report of the American College of Cardiology/American heart association task force on practice guidelines. 2013;129:S1-S45.

20. Centers for Medicare & Medicaid Services (CMS). *Decision Memo for Screening for Lung Cancer With Low Dose Computed Tomography (LDCT) (CAG-00439N)*; 2015. Available at: https://www.cms.gov/medicare-coverage-database/details/nca-decision-memo.aspx?NCAId=274. Accessed 5 July 2016.

21. Centers for Medicare & Medicaid Services (CMS). *Decision Memo for Percutaneous Left Atrial Appendage (LAA) Closure Therapy (CAG-00445N)*; 2016. Available at: https://www.cms.gov/medicare-coverage-database/details/nca-decision-memo.aspx?NCAId=281. Accessed 5 March 2017.

22. Centers for Medicare & Medicaid Services (CMS). *Decision Memo for Implantable Cardioverter Defibrillators (CAG-00157R4)*; 2018. Available at: https://www.cms.gov/medicare-coverage-database/details/nca-decision-memo.aspx?NCAId=288. Accessed 15 June 2018.

23. Legare F, Stacey D, Forest PG, et al. Milestones, barriers and beacons: shared decision making in Canada inches ahead. *Z Evid Fortbild Qual Gesundhwes.* 2017;123-124:23-27.

24. Elwyn G, Scholl I, Tietbohl C, et al. "Many miles to go…": a systematic review of the implementation of patient decision support interventions into routine clinical practice. *BMC Med Inform Decis Mak.* 2013;13(suppl 2):S14.

25. Gravel K, Legare F, Graham ID. Barriers and facilitators to implementing shared decision-making in clinical practice: a systematic review of health professionals' perceptions. *Implement Sci.* 2006;1:16.

26. Probst MA, Kanzaria HK, Hoffman JR, et al. Emergency physicians' perceptions and decision-making processes regarding patients presenting with palpitations. *J Emerg Med.* 2015;49(2):236-243 e232.

27. Halvorsen PA, Selmer R, Kristiansen IS. Different ways to describe the benefits of risk-reducing treatments: a randomized trial. *Ann Intern Med.* 2007;146(12):848-856.

28. Halvorsen P, Kristiansen I. Decisions on drug therapies by numbers needed to treat: a randomized trial. *Arch Inter Med.* 2005;165(10):1140-1146.

29. Legare F, Witteman HO. Shared decision making: examining key elements and barriers to adoption into routine clinical practice. *Health Aff.* 2013;32(2):276-284.

30. Elwyn G, Durand MA, Song J, et al. A three-talk model for shared decision making: multistage consultation process. *BMJ.* 2017;359:j4891.

31. Agency for Healthcare Research and Quality. The Shared Approach. https://www. ahrq.gov/professionals/education/curriculum-tools/shareddecisionmaking/ index.html. Accessed 1 April 2018.
32. Montori VM, Brito JP, Murad MH. The optimal practice of evidence-based medicine: incorporating patient preferences in practice guidelines. *JAMA.* 2013;310(23):2503-2504.

Please see Online Appendix: Apps and Digital Resources for additional information.

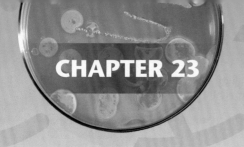

CHAPTER 23

The Future of Health Promotion and Disease Prevention in Clinical Practice

SUSANNE J. PHILLIPS

POLICY SHIFT IN ACCESS TO HEALTH PROMOTION AND DISEASE PREVENTION SERVICES

Arguably one of the most important policy changes in the delivery of health promotion and disease prevention (HPDP) services in the United States is the enactment of the Patient Protection and Affordable Care Act (PPACA) of 2010.[1] The PPACA removes barriers to the delivery of preventive services by mandating that nearly all private health plans with plan-years beginning on or after September 23, 2010, cover these services without cost to the patient.[2] Leading scientific and medical authorities, with federal support, have provided evidence documenting the cost-effectiveness of evidence-based preventive services,[3] ultimately resulting in the mandate for all private health plans to provide evidence-based screening and counseling, routine immunizations, preventive services for children and youth, and preventive services for women. In 2015, the Assistant Secretary for Planning and Evaluation estimated 137 million existing and newly insured Americans had access to no-cost coverage for preventive services, including 28.5 million children, 55.6 million women, and 53.5 million men.[4] Research over time will demonstrate whether access to no-cost clinical prevention services equates to improved health outcomes. One thing is clear, HPDP services stepped into the spotlight in 2010. So where are we now?

TEN YEARS LATER—WHERE ARE WE NOW?

In the second edition of this book, which predates the passage of the PPACA, a discussion of future trends by Dr. Kevin Patrick provides good context of this subject and a present-day jumping off point for our look

610

into the future.[5] Dr. Patrick's discussion of future trends in health care and preventive service delivery, including population growth, increasing diversity, and demographic trends; resource competition and allocation in an environment where medical care costs continue to rise; the rapid pace at which the growth in science and technology affects access to and the delivery of health care; and increasing economic globalization are astonishingly spot on. One of the scenarios Dr. Patrick provided was that HPDP would take center stage and be a focal point of future health care reform. His final words emphasized the impact and importance of local adoption, implementation, and evaluation of current evidence-based prevention services while seeking new science to improve our current knowledge and understanding. The current state of HPDP has improved since 2008. If change to policy and increased funding to improve access to preventive services as provided by the PPACA was the only measurable change, it would be a sufficiently monumental improvement, given the recent past and present political climate, to show huge movement in the needle measuring improvement to the state of HPDP delivery 10 years later. This shows the current climate of addressing HPDP as a central organizing principle as Dr. Patrick described.

AS I SEE IT: THE FUTURE OF HEALTH PROMOTION AND DISEASE PREVENTION IN PRIMARY CARE

A basic assumption in the discussion of HPDP services is that these services encompass screening, counseling, and appropriate immunizations to promote physical, emotional, dental, and visual health. Let us take a theoretical leap forward into the future where changes in HPDP have created optimal health care provisioning. Here are several key areas that have created this possible future.

Community-Based Centers of Health Promotion and Disease Prevention

Team-based delivery of health care has evolved as *community-based centers of HPDP* were adopted into the team-based primary care model. Funding for community-based HPDP services have grown as local, state, and federal legislators and public and private agencies demanded increased access to and provisioning of screening, education, and vaccination based on the latest science and evidence. Growth and national recognition of what we now call nurse-managed *"community-based centers of excellence in HPDP"* have flourished in workplace settings, primary and secondary schools, senior wellness centers, and community centers fully reimbursed by health plans and government health programs. These leverage the services of health care professionals traditionally relegated to staff positions of large health systems: registered nurses, mental health professionals, dieticians, dental hygienists, and public health professionals. These professionals now independently deliver screening, counseling, and immunization services at the top of their license, greatly expanding direct access in the community where people live, work, and play. The federally reimbursed prevention services[6] have evolved and improved as the United States Prevention Services Task Force evidence-based recommendations for adults, children, and women (including pregnant women) have increased.

Both federally funded and privately funded grant opportunities have burgeoned as pilot projects in the community setting not only demonstrate improved access and delivery but also have improved the health of citizens in the community. Positive research results have fostered policy change in how and where primary prevention services are rendered. Capitalizing on the expanding use of electronic health records, community-based programs seamlessly communicate screening findings to existing or new primary care teams. The pool of primary care teams is now greatly expanded by the removal of state and federal regulatory scope of practice restrictions. The current community health clinic and primary care provider systems remain undisrupted as clients move seamlessly between community centers for HPDP and community health and dental clinics, academic medical and dental centers, private health care offices, optometry centers, and dental offices for primary care follow-up, diagnostic testing, and treatment. The overarching goal to foster a team-based primary care provider system, free up physicians, advanced practice registered nurses, physician assistants, dentists and optometrists to practice at the top of their licenses, and allow them to focus on management of acute and chronic illness has been achieved.

Expansion, Recognition, and Reimbursement of Health Promotion and Disease Prevention Professionals

The current system of delivering health promotion services, buckling under the weight of reliance on access to sparse health care professionals authorized and reimbursed to deliver screening, counseling, and immunization services, undergoes a critical policy shift. Full expansion in access to and delivery of services has now been attained because all professionals educated and prepared to provide these services are recognized by health care payers and health systems and their scope and roles are delineated by statute and regulation. By allowing direct reimbursement for care delivered at the top of their license, registered nurses, dieticians, physician assistants, dental hygienists, pharmacists, and other licensed independent practitioners greatly impact access where clients live, work, and play. New policy is designed and implemented, authorizing public health professionals to deliver and be reimbursed for appropriate screening and counseling services.

Currently licensed health care providers, such as registered nurses, physician assistants, dieticians, dental hygienists, and pharmacists, have education, training, and scope of practice authority to deliver many of the covered screening, counseling, and vaccination services. But the current system allows limited or no direct access, often requiring referral from physicians, oversight by a physician or dentist, disallowing direct reimbursement, or some combination of these. In this possible future, these licensed providers have both statutory and regulatory authority to deliver and be reimbursed for preventive services.

The creation of a paradigm shift in health care delivery required a growing supply of professionals who were prepared and available to impact access and overall health outcomes. Scope of practice turf battles have dissolved since professional stakeholders and state legislatures embraced the value of team-based care where services are accessible, timely, and in a space where consumers have a choice of where health promotion services are delivered. Now that physicians, nurses, allied health professionals, and public health professionals place the patient at the center of the health care team as the leader, which allowed patients to determine where they receive their care and by whom, the debate over who will lead the team disappeared.

The addition of prepared, recognized, and reimbursed HPDP professionals does not fragment the system, it instead adds value to the primary care health team by increasing access to diagnostic and therapeutic services within the scope of practice of primary care providers, such as physicians, advanced practice registered nurses, and physician assistants. Now, because patients are presenting to their primary care providers with their updated screening results, vaccinations, and already-completed HPDP counseling, the efficiency of care delivery has improved time to diagnosis and treatment of identified health concerns and has improved health outcomes. In addition, primary care providers report less burn-out because student health care professionals (physicians, APRNs, physician assistants, dentists, etc.) select primary care over specialty care as a viable, efficient, and appropriately reimbursed specialty.

Scope of Practice Expands and Turf Battles Are Eliminated

How very little can be done under the spirit of fear.
Florence Nightingale

Scope of practice limitations and professional health care provider turf battles, grounded in fear, are now a mere footnote in health care policy history after decades of discussion, debate, research, and published policy recommendations by state legislatures, regulatory bodies, patient advocacy groups, and federal government agencies. Political funding to undermine advancement of scope of practice measures was eliminated, which freed professional associations to focus on professional issues unique to the care provider they represent. Stakeholders recognize, because providers are now utilized to the fullest extent of their scope of practice authorization, there is an ample supply of health care providers today and in the future to deliver high-quality, safe care uniquely suited to their specialty in a team-based setting. Federal policy, which eliminated restraint of trade practices, empowered existing and new types of health care providers to create bold and unique delivery systems. For example, pharmacists, with their extensive scientific background in clinical pharmacology, lead chronic disease management programs in partnership with other providers and provide unique direct-patient access to services. Nurses lead delivery of timely HPDP services in community and home-based settings, as well traditional health care settings, with authority to assess, order, and deliver health screening, counseling, and vaccination services. Patients found at risk for health conditions as a result of screening and counseling services are provided immediate intervention; timely referral to physicians, APRNs, physician assistants, optometrists, mental health professionals, dentists, dental hygienists, and pharmacists for further intervention and diagnostic services as appropriate; or a combination of these.

Success and evaluation of the new prevention-focused system is facilitated by a standardized electronic health system (EHS). Creation of a single, centralized EHS was impractical given the competitive, creative, and adaptable capabilities, as well as the economic interest, of multiple system vendors. However, EHSs are now designed with standardized communication protocols that provided seamless communication among EHSs. Health care providers are free to choose a system that best suits their needs but have the ability, upon patient approval, to share or transfer all or part of a patient record to another provider to give each health care giver a comprehensive picture of the patient.

Wellness Technology and Genomics Drive Health Promotion and Disease Prevention Services

Inherent in the shift to a patient-centered approach to care, breakthroughs in technology and mass adoption of wearable fitness devices, high utilization of fitness technology, and expanded genetic testing have significantly improved primary care data collection and identification of health risk. Randomly controlled trials demonstrate that the positive impact on overall health and improvement in health outcomes has grown, and continues to grow, as the result of research initiatives in this area that continue to be highly funded by public and private stakeholders. The U.S. Precision Medicine Initiative[7] and other public and private organizations successfully tackled challenges in genetic testing, including documenting scientific evidence to support valid genetic tests and the development and dissemination of evidence-based practice recommendations for genetic testing. What is more, genetic information and decision support tools have been incorporated into the standardized EHS for use by clinicians.

Consumers engage using individualized wellness technology both as an intervention and a measurement tool for HPDP initiatives. Patient privacy, confidentiality, and the integrity of the health data captured are secured through technological advances and through public policy adoption. Coverage for genetic counseling and screening for some of the leading causes of death and disability, including heart disease, cancer, stroke, diabetes, and Alzheimer disease risk,[8] have been adopted similar to the way the PPACA provisions covering genetic counseling as a preventive service for women with increased risk of BRCA 1/2 mutations and genetic testing for all people newly diagnosed with colorectal cancer[9] was adopted years ago. Harnessing reliable and secure screening data from wearable devices and genetic testing, health care providers interpreting risk are freed to pursue recommended diagnostic testing, pharmaceutical and procedural intervention, and treatment without delay.

Integration of Behavioral Health Into Primary Care Prevention

Behavioral health is center stage in the future of HPDP in primary care. Utilization of appropriately trained providers in the community setting in addition to the primary care setting improved access to behavioral health services traditionally underfunded and underutilized.[10] Expanding on PPACA-mandated cost-free screening and counseling for alcohol and drug misuse, depression, tobacco use, domestic and interpersonal violence, autism, and developmental delay, programs such as the Centers for Medicare and Medicaid Services Psychiatric Collaborative Care Model add behavioral health care managers (such as social workers, nurses, and psychologists) to the primary care team providing treatment of mental health disorders to patients and interspecialty consultation.[11]

Access to behavioral screening and counseling services provided in the community is supported through recognition of and reimbursement to clinical social workers, mental health counselors, certified alcohol and drug abuse counselors, nurse psychotherapists, and marriage and family therapists providing services at the workplace, school, and community centers. Using evidence-based prevention and early-intervention strategies, the incidence of mental health and substance use conditions have diminished over time. Reimbursement and operational barriers, such as reimbursement and implementation, to integration of behavioral health treatment and management into primary care, and provision of screening and counseling services external but connected to primary care teams were identified and eliminated through policy reform at institutional, state, and federal levels.

CONCLUSION

The previous discussion represents one vision, a few potential scenarios, defining the future of HPDP in primary care. Incorporation of community-based HPDP centers of excellence, expansion of health care professionals recognized and reimbursed for delivery of HPDP services, technological advancement and standardization of EHRs along with utilization and safeguarding of patient-initiated health monitoring and genetic testing, and incorporation of behavioral health into the primary care team improves access to and timely delivery of HPDP services. Ultimately, patients are now recognized as the health care team leader.

The importance placed on this futuristic vision are in no way exhaustive, as the complexity of HPDP funding, policy, and delivery is purposefully omitted in the discussion to allow possibility for an unencumbered vision. There is no room for quick dismissal of these ideas; they are in fact worthy ideals for a bright future. Providing opportunity for readers to discuss and debate how this vision for HPDP in primary care can be realized, future and current health care providers are challenged to consider the vision presented, assess the current state of HPDP policy, discuss possible goals and measurable outcomes, and develop strategies for potential change. Consider in detail the complex issues of policy development and change, funding, and implementation and evaluation. Persist.

"First they ignore you, then they laugh at you, then they fight you, then you win."—Mahatma Gandhi.

REFERENCES

1. Patient Protection and Affordable Care Act of 2010, Pub. L. No. 111–148. Retrieved from: https://www.gpo.gov/fdsys/pkg/PLAW-111publ148/content-detail.html.
2. Preventive Services Covered by Private Health Plans under the Affordable Care Act, The Henry J. Kaiser Family Foundation, last modified August 2015, https://www.kff.org/health-reform/fact-sheet/preventive-services-covered-by-private-health-plans/.
3. Maciosek MV. Greater use of preventive services in U.S. health care could save lives at little or no cost. *Health Aff.* 2010;29(9):1656-1660.
4. The Affordable Care Act is Improving Access to Preventive Services for Millions of Americans, Assistant Secretary for Planning and Evaluation, last modified May 14, 2015. https://aspe.hhs.gov/pdf-report/affordable-care-act-improving-access-preventive-services-millions-americans.
5. Patrick K. The future of health promotion and disease prevention in clinical practice. In: Woolf SH, Jonas S, Kaplan-Liss E, eds. *Health Promotion & Disease Prevention in Clinical Practice.* 2nd ed. Pennsylvania: Lippincott Williams & Wilkins; 2008.
6. Preventive Services Covered Under the Affordable Care Act, *National Conference of State Legislatures,* last modified June 30, 2014, http://www.ncsl.org/research/health/american-health-benefit-exchanges-b.aspx.

7. Handelsman J. Precision Medicine: Improving Health and Treating Disease. Last modified January 21, 2015, https://obamawhitehouse.archives.gov/blog/2015/01/21/precision-medicine-improving-health-and-treating-disease.
8. Centers for Disease Control and Prevention. Leading Causes of Death. https://www.cdc.gov/nchs/fastats/leading-causes-of-death.htm. Accessed 14 April 2018.
9. Genomics, HealthyPeople.gov. https://www.healthypeople.gov/2020/topics-objectives/topic/genomics#11. Accessed 14 April 2018.
10. Vogel ME, Kanzler KE, Aikens JE, Goodie JL. Integration of behavioral health and primary care: current knowledge and future directions. *J Behav Med.* 2017;40:69-84.
11. Press MJ, Howe R, Schoenbaum M, et al. Medicare payment for behavioral health integration. *N Engl J Med.* 2017;376:405-407. http://www.nejm.org/doi/full/10.1056/NEJMp1614134. Accessed 14 April 2018.

Please see Online Appendix: Apps and Digital Resources for additional information.

Index

Note: Page numbers followed by "f" indicate figures, "t" indicate tables, and "b" indicate boxes.

ProQuad, 437, 438, 461, 477t
Prostate cancer, 130–132, 536–537
　abnormal screening tests, 536
　diagnostic strategy, 536
　follow-up, 537
　prostate-specific antigen, screening with
　　abnormal result definition, 131–132
　　accuracy and reliability, 132
　　potential adverse effects, 132
　　standard counseling, 131
　screening, 562
　treatment options, 537
Prostate-specific antigen, 130–132
Protein, 216
Protein-sparing modified fast, 243–245
Pseudoaddiction, 307
Put Prevention into Practice Initiative
　(PPI), 593t
Pyrazinamide, 550

Q

Quadracel, 432, 476t
Question period, 54
Quick Start, 322
Quit lines, 276

R

RabAvert, 474t
Rabies vaccination, 478
Raloxifene, 48, 391–393
　in breast cancer, 391
Reality. *See* Female condoms
Reciprocal determinism model, 160
Recombivax, 442
Recombivax HB, 449, 472t
Rectal examination. *See* Digital rectal
　examination
Reflective listening, motivational inter-
　viewing, 169–172
Regular exercise, 178–196
　basic concepts, 180–182
　　aerobic and nonaerobic, 181
　　epidemiology, 180
　　objectives, 181–182
　　risks, 182
　counseling, 185–195
　　activity or sport, choosing, 189–191
　　duration and frequency, 187–189
　　equipment, 194–195
　　generic training program, 192–193
　　getting started, 185–187
　　making exercise fun, 191–192
　　technique, 193–194
　　and vital signs, 179
　first thoughts, 178–179
　office and clinic organization, 195–196

patient education materials, 196–198
recommendation vs. prescription,
　182–183
risk assessment, 183–185
wearable devices and smart phone
　technology, 183
Reminder systems, 481
Resistance, 73
Resting metabolic rate (RMR), 240
Reverse targeting, 599
Reversible hormonal contraceptive meth-
　ods, 312
Rifampin, 550
Risedronate, 547
Risk assessment principles, 32–50
　exercise recommendation, 183–185
　illness-based *vs.* risk factor–based
　　thinking processes, 36–38
　importance of, 35–36
　individualize, tools to, 45–48
　limits and priorities, 38–40
　　potential interventions, 39
　　risk factor detection, 39–40
　　target condition seriousness, 39
　in practice, 48–50
　priorities, setting, 44–45
Rivastigmine, 373t
Rosuvastatin, 528t
Rotarix, 467, 475t
RotaTeq, 467, 475t
Rotavirus (Rota)
　administration, 467
　indications, 467
　precautions and contraindications,
　　468
　RotaTeq (Merck), 467
　vaccine, 466–468
5 R's framework
　relevance, 173
　repetition, 174
　rewards, 173
　risks, 173
　roadblocks, 174
Rubella, vaccines for, 436–439

S

SDM. *See* Shared decision making (SDM)
Safer sexual practices, 343–350
Safety guidance for children. *See* Anticipa-
　tory guidance in pediatrics
Scoliosis examination, children, 496
Screening and prevention, benefits of,
　563–569
　individuals could benefit, low disease
　　prevalence, 565
　intensity of screening, 568–569